Drugs Used in Ps

This guide contains color reproductions of some [...]
apeutic drugs. This guide mainly illustrates pro[...]
preceding the name of a drug indicates that other doses are available. Check directly
with the manufacturer. (*Although the photos are intended as accurate reproductions
of the drug, this guide should be used only as a quick identification aid.*)

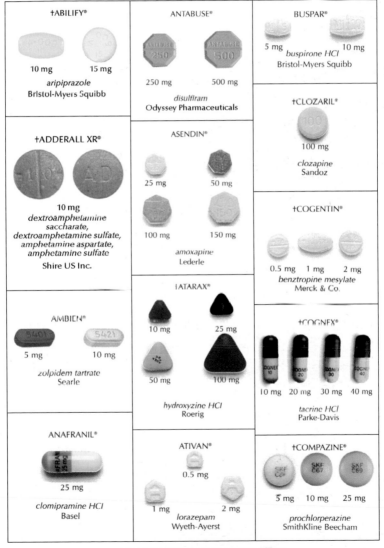

†ABILIFY®

10 mg   15 mg

aripiprazole
Bristol-Myers Squibb

ANTABUSE®

250 mg   500 mg

disulfiram
Odyssey Pharmaceuticals

BUSPAR®

5 mg   10 mg
buspirone HCl
Bristol-Myers Squibb

†CLOZARIL®

100 mg

clozapine
Sandoz

†ADDERALL XR®

10 mg
*dextroamphetamine
saccharate,
dextroamphetamine sulfate,
amphetamine aspartate,
amphetamine sulfate*
Shire US Inc.

ASENDIN®

25 mg   50 mg

100 mg   150 mg

amoxapine
Lederle

†COGENTIN®

0.5 mg   1 mg   2 mg
benztropine mesylate
Merck & Co.

AMBIEN®

5 mg   10 mg

zolpidem tartrate
Searle

ATARAX®

10 mg   25 mg

50 mg   100 mg

hydroxyzine HCl
Roerig

†COGNEX®

10 mg   20 mg   30 mg   40 mg

tacrine HCl
Parke-Davis

ANAFRANIL®

25 mg

clomipramine HCl
Basel

ATIVAN®

0.5 mg

1 mg   2 mg
lorazepam
Wyeth-Ayerst

†COMPAZINE®

5 mg   10 mg   25 mg

prochlorperazine
SmithKline Beecham

LIPPINCOTT WILLIAMS & WILKINS©

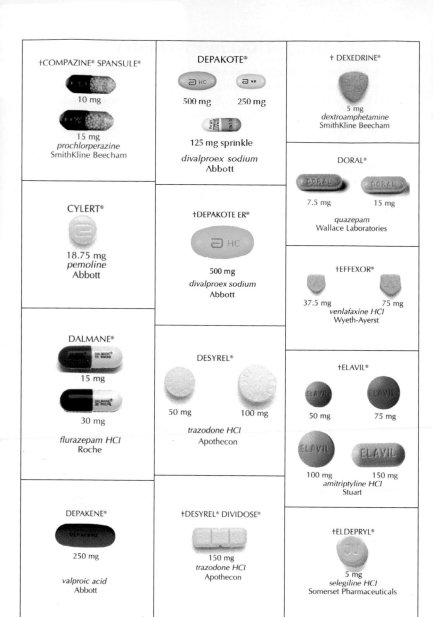

†COMPAZINE® SPANSULE®

10 mg

15 mg
prochlorperazine
SmithKline Beecham

DEPAKOTE®

500 mg   250 mg

125 mg sprinkle

divalproex sodium
Abbott

† DEXEDRINE®

5 mg
dextroamphetamine
SmithKline Beecham

DORAL®

7.5 mg   15 mg

quazepam
Wallace Laboratories

CYLERT®

18.75 mg
pemoline
Abbott

†DEPAKOTE ER®

500 mg
divalproex sodium
Abbott

†EFFEXOR®

37.5 mg   75 mg
venlafaxine HCl
Wyeth-Ayerst

DALMANE®

15 mg

30 mg

flurazepam HCl
Roche

DESYREL®

50 mg   100 mg

trazodone HCl
Apothecon

†ELAVIL®

50 mg   75 mg

100 mg   150 mg
amitriptyline HCl
Stuart

DEPAKENE®

250 mg

valproic acid
Abbott

†DESYREL® DIVIDOSE®

150 mg
trazodone HCl
Apothecon

†ELDEPRYL®

5 mg
selegiline HCl
Somerset Pharmaceuticals

LIPPINCOTT WILLIAMS & WILKINS©

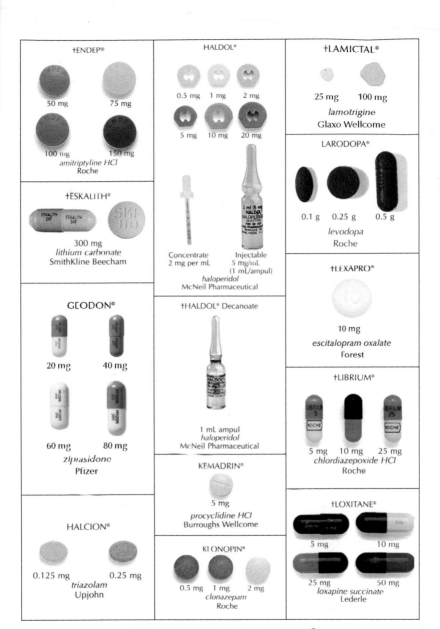

†ENDEP®

50 mg 75 mg

100 mg 150 mg

amitriptyline HCl
Roche

†ESKALITH®

300 mg
lithium carbonate
SmithKline Beecham

GEODON®

20 mg 40 mg

60 mg 80 mg

ziprasidone
Pfizer

HALCION®

0.125 mg 0.25 mg
triazolam
Upjohn

HALDOL®

0.5 mg 1 mg 2 mg

5 mg 10 mg 20 mg

Concentrate   Injectable
2 mg per mL   5 mg/mL
                   (1 mL/ampul)
haloperidol
McNeil Pharmaceutical

†HALDOL® Decanoate

1 mL ampul
haloperidol
McNeil Pharmaceutical

KEMADRIN®

5 mg
procyclidine HCl
Burroughs Wellcome

KLONOPIN®

0.5 mg 1 mg 2 mg
clonazepam
Roche

†LAMICTAL®

25 mg 100 mg
lamotrigine
Glaxo Wellcome

LARODOPA®

0.1 g 0.25 g 0.5 g

levodopa
Roche

†LEXAPRO®

10 mg
escitalopram oxalate
Forest

†LIBRIUM®

5 mg 10 mg 25 mg
chlordiazepoxide HCl
Roche

†LOXITANE®

5 mg 10 mg

25 mg 50 mg
loxapine succinate
Lederle

LIPPINCOTT WILLIAMS & WILKINS©

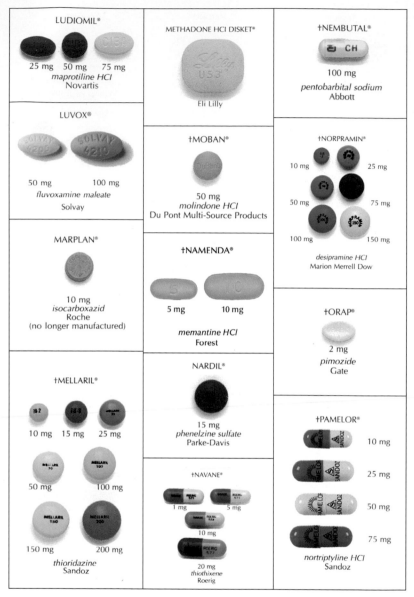

LUDIOMIL®

25 mg 50 mg 75 mg
maprotiline HCl
Novartis

LUVOX®

50 mg 100 mg
fluvoxamine maleate
Solvay

MARPLAN®

10 mg
isocarboxazid
Roche
(no longer manufactured)

†MELLARIL®

10 mg 15 mg 25 mg

50 mg 100 mg

150 mg 200 mg

thioridazine
Sandoz

METHADONE HCl DISKET®

Eli Lilly

†MOBAN®

50 mg
molindone HCl
Du Pont Multi-Source Products

†NAMENDA®

5 mg 10 mg

memantine HCl
Forest

NARDIL®

15 mg
phenelzine sulfate
Parke-Davis

†NAVANE®

1 mg 5 mg

10 mg

20 mg
thiothixene
Roerig

†NEMBUTAL®

100 mg
pentobarbital sodium
Abbott

†NORPRAMIN®

10 mg 25 mg

50 mg 75 mg

100 mg 150 mg

desipramine HCl
Marion Merrell Dow

†ORAP®

2 mg
pimozide
Gate

†PAMELOR®

10 mg

25 mg

50 mg

75 mg

nortriptyline HCl
Sandoz

LIPPINCOTT WILLIAMS & WILKINS©

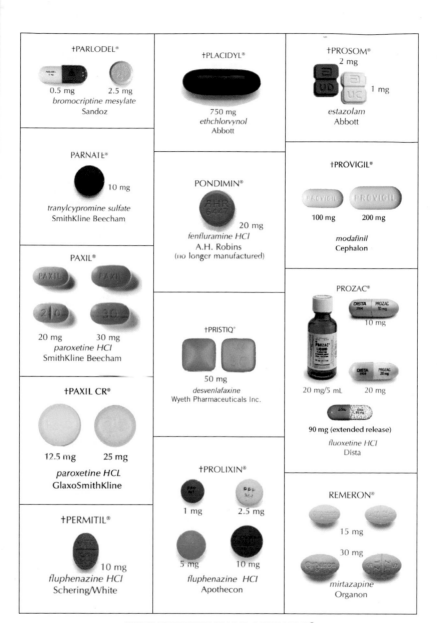

†PARLODEL®

0.5 mg   2.5 mg
bromocriptine mesylate
Sandoz

†PLACIDYL®

750 mg
ethchlorvynol
Abbott

†PROSOM®
2 mg

1 mg
estazolam
Abbott

PARNATE®

10 mg
tranylcypromine sulfate
SmithKline Beecham

PONDIMIN®

20 mg
fenfluramine HCl
A.H. Robins
(no longer manufactured)

†PROVIGIL®

100 mg   200 mg
modafinil
Cephalon

PAXIL®

20 mg   30 mg
paroxetine HCl
SmithKline Beecham

†PRISTIQ®

50 mg
desvenlafaxine
Wyeth Pharmaceuticals Inc.

PROZAC®

10 mg

20 mg/5 mL   20 mg

90 mg (extended release)
fluoxetine HCl
Dista

†PAXIL CR®

12.5 mg   25 mg
paroxetine HCL
GlaxoSmithKline

†PROLIXIN®

1 mg   2.5 mg

5 mg   10 mg
fluphenazine HCl
Apothecon

REMERON®

15 mg

30 mg
mirtazapine
Organon

†PERMITIL®

10 mg
fluphenazine HCl
Schering/White

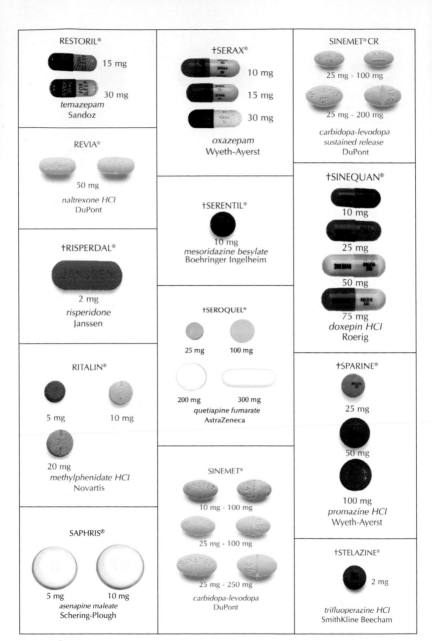

RESTORIL®

15 mg
30 mg

temazepam
Sandoz

REVIA®

50 mg

naltrexone HCl
DuPont

†RISPERDAL®

2 mg

risperidone
Janssen

RITALIN®

5 mg   10 mg

20 mg

methylphenidate HCl
Novartis

SAPHRIS®

5 mg   10 mg

asenapine maleate
Schering-Plough

†SERAX®

10 mg
15 mg
30 mg

oxazepam
Wyeth-Ayerst

†SERENTIL®

10 mg
mesoridazine besylate
Boehringer Ingelheim

†SEROQUEL®

25 mg   100 mg

200 mg   300 mg
quetiapine fumarate
AstraZeneca

SINEMET®

10 mg - 100 mg

25 mg - 100 mg

25 mg - 250 mg

carbidopa-levodopa
DuPont

SINEMET® CR

25 mg - 100 mg

25 mg - 200 mg

carbidopa-levodopa
sustained release
DuPont

†SINEQUAN®

10 mg

25 mg

50 mg

75 mg
doxepin HCl
Roerig

†SPARINE®

25 mg

50 mg

100 mg
promazine HCl
Wyeth-Ayerst

†STELAZINE®

2 mg

trifluoperazine HCl
SmithKline Beecham

LIPPINCOTT WILLIAMS & WILKINS©

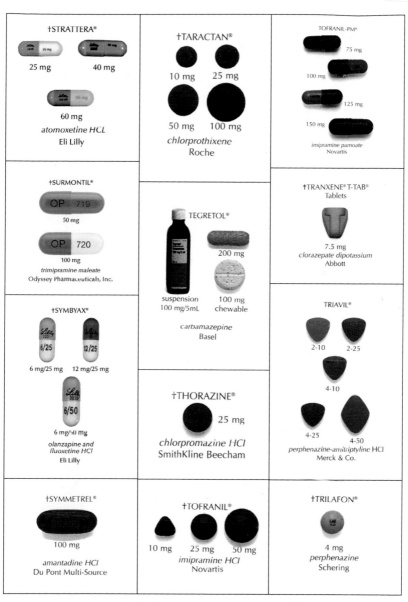

†STRATTERA®
25 mg　40 mg
60 mg
atomoxetine HCL
Eli Lilly

†TARACTAN®
10 mg　25 mg
50 mg　100 mg
chlorprothixene
Roche

TOFRANIL-PM®
75 mg
100 mg
125 mg
150 mg
imipramine pamoate
Novartis

†SURMONTIL®
OP 719
50 mg
OP 720
100 mg
trimipramine maleate
Odyssey Pharmaceuticals, Inc.

TEGRETOL®
200 mg
100 mg
chewable
suspension
100 mg/5mL
carbamazepine
Basel

†TRANXENE® T-TAB®
Tablets
7.5 mg
clorazepate dipotassium
Abbott

†SYMBYAX®
6/25　12/25
6 mg/25 mg　12 mg/25 mg
6/50
6 mg/50 mg
olanzapine and
fluoxetine HCl
Eli Lilly

†THORAZINE®
25 mg
chlorpromazine HCl
SmithKline Beecham

TRIAVIL®
2-10　2-25
4-10
4-25　4-50
perphenazine-amitriptyline HCl
Merck & Co.

†SYMMETREL®
100 mg
amantadine HCl
Du Pont Multi-Source

†TOFRANIL®
10 mg　25 mg　50 mg
imipramine HCl
Novartis

†TRILAFON®
4 mg
perphenazine
Schering

LIPPINCOTT WILLIAMS & WILKINS©

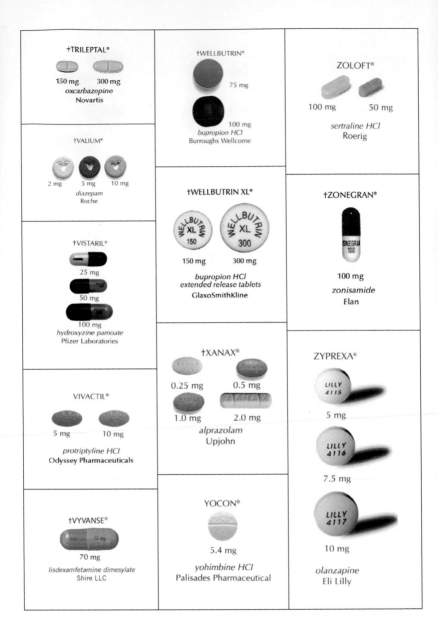

†TRILEPTAL®
150 mg 300 mg
oxcarbazepine
Novartis

†VALIUM®
2 mg 5 mg 10 mg
diazepam
Roche

†VISTARIL®
25 mg
50 mg
100 mg
hydroxyzine pamoate
Pfizer Laboratories

VIVACTIL®
5 mg 10 mg
protriptyline HCl
Odyssey Pharmaceuticals

†VYVANSE®
70 mg
lisdexamfetamine dimesylate
Shire LLC

†WELLBUTRIN®
75 mg
100 mg
bupropion HCl
Burroughs Wellcome

†WELLBUTRIN XL®
150 mg 300 mg
bupropion HCl
extended release tablets
GlaxoSmithKline

†XANAX®
0.25 mg 0.5 mg
1.0 mg 2.0 mg
alprazolam
Upjohn

YOCON®
5.4 mg
yohimbine HCl
Palisades Pharmaceutical

ZOLOFT®
100 mg 50 mg
sertraline HCl
Roerig

†ZONEGRAN®
100 mg
zonisamide
Elan

ZYPREXA®
LILLY 4115
5 mg
LILLY 4116
7.5 mg
LILLY 4117
10 mg
olanzapine
Eli Lilly

LIPPINCOTT WILLIAMS & WILKINS©

KAPLAN & SADOCK'S
POCKET HANDBOOK
OF CLINICAL
PSYCHIATRY

Fifth Edition

SENIOR CONTRIBUTING EDITOR

Gary S. Belkin, M.D., PhD, MPH

Associate Professor of Psychiatry and Director, Program in Global Mental Health, New York University School of Medicine, Senior Director for Psychiatric Services, New York City Health and Behavioral Health

CONTRIBUTING EDITORS

Norman Sussman, M.D.

Professor of Psychiatry, New York University School of Medicine, Director of Psychopharmacology Research and Consultation Service, Bellevue Hospital Center, New York, New York

Richard Perry, M.D.

Clinical Professor of Child and Adolescent Psychiatry, NYU School of Medicine and Attending Psychiatrist, Pediatric Psychiatry Consultation-Liaison Unit, Bellevue Hospital Center, New York

Samoon Ahmad, M.D.

Clinical Assistant Professor, Co-Director of Continuing Medical Education, Attending Physician, Department of Psychiatry, NYU School of Medicine, Attending Physician, Department of Psychiatry, Bellevue Hospital Center, New York, New York

KAPLAN & SADOCK'S POCKET HANDBOOK OF CLINICAL PSYCHIATRY

Fifth Edition

BENJAMIN J. SADOCK, M.D.

Menas S. Gregory Professor of Psychiatry
New York University School of Medicine
Attending Psychiatrist, Tisch Hospital
Attending Psychiatrist, Bellevue Hospital Center
Honorary Medical Staff, Lenox Hill Hospital
New York, New York

VIRGINIA A. SADOCK, M.D.

Professor of Psychiatry
Department of Psychiatry
New York University School of Medicine
Attending Psychiatrist, Tisch Hospital
Attending Psychiatrist, Bellevue Hospital Center
New York, New York

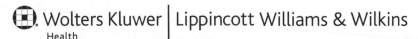

Wolters Kluwer | Lippincott Williams & Wilkins
Health

Philadelphia · Baltimore · New York · London
Buenos Aires · Hong Kong · Sydney · Tokyo

Acquisitions Editor: Lisa McAllister
Product Manager: Tom Gibbons
Manufacturing Manager: Benjamin Rivera
Vendor Manager: Bridgett Dougherty
Marketing Manager: Brian Freiland
Design Coordinator: Steven Druding
Production Service: Aptara® Inc.

Library of Congress Cataloging-in-Publication Data

Sadock, Benjamin J.
  Kaplan & Sadock's pocket handbook of clinical psychiatry / Benjamin J. Sadock, Virginia A. Sadock.—5th ed. / contributing editors, Gary S. Belkin ... [et al.]
    p. ; cm.
  Companion v. to: Kaplan & Sadock's comprehensive textbook of psychiatry / editors, Benjamin J. Sadock, Virginia A. Sadock. 9th ed. c2009.
  Includes bibliographical references and index.
  ISBN-13: 978-1-60547-264-5 (alk. paper)
  ISBN-10: 1-60547-264-6 (alk. paper)
  1. Psychiatry—Textbooks.   I. Sadock, Virginia A.   II. Belkin, Gary S.   III. Kaplan & Sadock's comprehensive textbook of psychiatry.   IV. Title.   V. Title: Pocket handbook of clinical psychiatry.
VI. Title: Kaplan and Sadock's pocket handbook of clinical psychiatry.
  [DNLM: 1. Mental Disorders—Handbooks.   WM 34 S126k 2010]
  RC454.C637 2010
  616.89—dc22

                                                                          2009047238

CCS0310

To Celia and Emily

Preface

This is the fifth edition of *Kaplan & Sadock's Pocket Handbook of Clinical Psychiatry*, which is used as a ready reference to diagnose the full range of psychiatric disorders in adults and children. Both psychiatrists and nonpsychiatric physicians have found it to be a useful guide, as have medical students, especially during their rotations through psychiatry. It is also used by psychologists, social workers, nurses, and others who work with the mentally ill.

Every section has been updated and revised, and all diagnoses conform to the criteria listed in the latest edition of the *American Psychiatric Association's Diagnostic and Statistical Manual of Mental Disorders* (DSM-IV-TR; the TR standing for "text revision").

All aspects of both psychological and pharmacologic management are discussed, and as in other Kaplan & Sadock books, completely up-to-date colored plates of all the major drugs used in psychiatry are included.

The *Pocket Handbook* is the minicompanion to the much larger and more encyclopedic ninth edition of *Kaplan & Sadock's Comprehensive Textbook of Psychiatry* (IX). The *Pocket Handbook* provides brief summaries of psychiatric disorders, which include key aspects of etiology, epidemiology, clinical features, and treatment. Psychopharmacologic principles and prescribing methods are briefly but thoroughly discussed. Each chapter ends with references to the more detailed, relevant sections in CTP/IX.

ACKNOWLEDGMENTS

We thank our contributing editors, Gary Belkin, M.D., Samoon Ahmad, M.D., Norman Sussman, M.D., and Richard Perry, M.D., for their enormous help, particularly in the area of psychopharmacology, in which major advances have occurred since the publication of the last edition.

Other persons who helped in previous editions of this text whom we wish to acknowledge are Barry Reisberg, M.D.; Matthew Smith, M.D.; Henry Weinstein, M.D.; and Myrl Manley, M.D. Particular thanks are extended to Victoria Sadock Gregg, M.D., and James Sadock, M.D., experts in child and adult emergency medicine, respectively, for their assistance.

Our staff at NYU, Nitza Jones, who served as project editor, and her associate Sara Brown, deserve our deepest thanks. They worked with skill and enthusiasm. As always, our publishers continued to maintain their high standards for which we are indebted.

We hope this book fulfills the expectations of all those for whom it is intended—the busy doctor-in-training and the clinical practitioner.

Benjamin J. Sadock, M.D.
Virginia A. Sadock, M.D.

New York University Langone Medical Center
New York, New York

Contents

1

Classification and Diagnosis
in Psychiatry

I. Introduction

The *Diagnostic and Statistical Manual of Mental Disorders, Text Revision*, fourth edition (*DSM-IV-TR*), published in 2000 by the American Psychiatric Association, is the official classification system used by all mental health professionals to diagnosis psychiatric disorders. *DSM-IV-TR* contains diagnostic criteria for 17 major categories of mental disorders (Table 1–1), comprising 375 discrete illnesses. All of those disorders are covered in this book, in separate chapters.

A similar system is used in Europe called the *International Statistical Classification of Diseases and Related Health Problems* (ICD). Both *ICD* and *DSM-IV-TR* use the same numerical codes (which are used in medical reports and insurance forms) for each disorder. All terminology in this book conforms to the official *DSM-IV-TR* nomenclature, and the diagnostic *DSM-IV-TR* criteria are contained in the discussion of each disorder.

The *DSM-IV-TR* classification and code numbers are listed on page 555 of this handbook.

II. Basic Features *DSM-IV-TR*

A. Diagnostic criteria

1. The *DSM-IV-TR* diagnostic system lists diagnostic criteria for each disorder.
2. If a sufficient number of signs and symptoms are elicited from the patient in the history and mental status (see Chapter 2), the diagnosis can be made.
3. Specific diagnostic criteria increase reliability (e.g., different observers get the same results).

B. Descriptive approach

1. *DSM-IV-TR* only describes mental disorders. It is atheoretical with regard to cause. Etiology and treatment are not covered in *DSM*.
2. The descriptive approach increases validity. It measures what it is supposed to measure (e.g., a patient diagnosed with schizophrenia really is schizophrenic).

III. Definition of Mental Disorder

A mental disorder is an illness with psychological or behavioral manifestations associated with significant distress and impaired functioning caused by a biologic, social, psychological, genetic, physical, or chemical disturbance. It is measured in terms of deviation from some normative concept. Each illness has characteristic signs and symptoms.

Table 1–1
Groups of Conditions in *DSM-IV-TR* *

Disorders usually first diagnosed in infancy, childhood, or adolescence
Delirium, dementia, amnestic, and other cognitive disorders
Mental disorders due to a general medical condition
Substance-related disorders
Schizophrenia and other psychotic disorders
Mood disorders
Anxiety disorders
Somatoform disorders
Factitious disorders
Dissociative disorders
Sexual and gender identity disorders
Eating disorders
Sleep disorders
Impulse-control disorders not elsewhere classified
Adjustment disorders
Personality disorders
Other conditions that may be a focus of clinical attention

*Each of the disorders is discussed in a separate chapter in this book.

In addition to the *DSM-IV-TR* classifications, other terms that are used in psychiatry to describe mental illness are as follows:

A. Psychotic. Loss of reality testing with delusions and hallucinations (e.g., schizophrenia).

B. Neurotic. No loss of reality testing; based on mainly intrapsychic conflicts or life events that cause anxiety; symptoms include obsession, phobia, and compulsion.

C. Functional. No known structural damage or clear-cut biological cause to account for impairment.

D. Organic. Illness caused by a specific agent producing structural change in the brain; usually associated with cognitive impairment, delirium, or dementia (e.g., Pick's disease). The term *organic* is not used in *DSM-IV-TR* because it implies that some mental disorders do not have a biological or chemical component; however, it still remains in common use.

E. Primary. No known cause; also called *idiopathic* (similar to *functional*).

F. Secondary. Known to be a symptomatic manifestation of a systemic, medical, or cerebral disorder (e.g., delirium resulting from infectious brain disease).

IV. Classification of Disorders in *DSM-IV-TR*

A. Disorders usually first diagnosed in infancy, childhood, or adolescence

1. **Mental retardation.** Below-average intellectual functioning; onset before age 10. Associated with impaired maturation and learning and social maladjustment; classified according to intelligence quotient (IQ) as **mild** (50–55 to 70), **moderate** (35–40 to 50–55), **severe** (20–25 to 35–40), or **profound** (below 20–25).

2. **Learning disorders.** Maturational deficits in development associated with difficulty in acquiring specific skills in **mathematics, writing,** and **reading.**

3. **Motor skills disorder.** Impairments in the development of motor coordination (**developmental coordination disorder**). Children with the disorder are often clumsy and uncoordinated.

4. **Communication disorders.** Developmental impairment resulting in difficulty in producing age-appropriate sentences (**expressive language disorder**), difficulty in using and understanding words (**mixed receptive–expressive language disorder**), difficulty in articulation (**phonological disorder**), and disturbances in fluency, rate, and rhythm of speech (**stuttering**).

5. **Pervasive developmental disorders.** Characterized by autistic, atypical, and withdrawn behavior; gross immaturity; inadequate development; divided into **autistic disorder** (stereotyped behavior usually without speech), **Rett's disorder** (loss of speech and motor skills with decreased head growth), **childhood disintegrative disorder** (loss of acquired speech and motor skills before age 10), **Asperger's disorder** (stereotyped behavior with some ability to communicate), and a **not otherwise specified** (NOS) type.

6. **Attention-deficit and disruptive behavior disorders.** Characterized by inattention, overaggressiveness, delinquency, destructiveness, hostility, and feelings of rejection, negativism, or impulsiveness. Divided into **attention-deficit/hyperactivity disorder** (poor attention span, impulsiveness), **conduct disorder** (delinquency), and **oppositional defiant disorder** (negativism).

7. **Feeding and eating disorders of infancy or early childhood.** Characterized by disturbed or bizarre feeding and eating habits that usually begin in childhood or adolescence and continue into adulthood. Divided into **pica** (eating nonnutritional substances) and **rumination disorder** (regurgitation or rechewing).

8. **Tic disorders.** Characterized by sudden, involuntary, recurrent, stereotyped movement or vocal sounds. Divided into **Tourette's disorder** (vocal tic and coprolalia), **chronic motor** or **vocal tic disorder,** and **transient tic disorder.**

9. **Elimination disorders.** Inability to maintain bowel control (**encopresis**) or bladder control (**enuresis**) because of physiologic or psychological immaturity.

10. **Other disorders of infancy, childhood, or adolescence. Selective mutism** (voluntary refusal to speak), **reactive attachment disorder of infancy or early childhood** (severe impairment of ability to relate, beginning before age 5), **stereotypic movement disorder** (thumb sucking, head banging, nail biting, skin picking), and **separation anxiety disorder** (cannot separate from home, e.g., school refusal, because of anxiety).

B. **Delirium, dementia, and amnestic and other cognitive disorders.** Disorders characterized by change in brain structure and function that result in impaired learning, orientation, judgment, memory, and intellectual functions.

1. **Delirium.** Marked by short-term confusion and changes in cognition caused by a **general medical condition** (e.g., infection), **substances** (e.g., cocaine, opioids, phencyclidine), or **multiple etiologies** (e.g., head trauma and kidney disease). **Delirium NOS** may have other causes (e.g., sleep deprivation).

2. **Dementia.** Marked by severe impairment in memory, judgment, orientation, and cognition; **dementia of the Alzheimer's type**—usually occurs in persons over 65 years of age and manifested by progressive intellectual disorientation and dementia, delusions, or depression; **vascular dementia**—caused by vessel thrombosis or hemorrhage; dementia caused by **other medical conditions**—HIV disease or head trauma; miscellaneous group—Pick's disease, Jakob–Creutzfeldt disease (caused by a mutated protein called a prion); also may be **substance-induced** caused by toxin or medication—gasoline fumes, atropine, or **multiple etiologies** and **NOS.**

3. **Amnestic disorder.** Marked by memory impairment and forgetfulness. Caused by **medical condition** (e.g., hypoxia, toxin), or **substance** (e.g., marijuana, diazepam [Valium]).

C. **Mental disorders caused by a general medical condition.** Signs and symptoms of psychiatric disorders that occur as a direct result of medical disease. Includes disorders associated with syphilis, encephalitis, abscess, cardiovascular disease or trauma, epilepsy, intracranial neoplasm, endocrine disorders, pellagra, avitaminosis, systemic infection (e.g., typhoid, malaria), and degenerative central nervous system (CNS) diseases (e.g., multiple sclerosis). May produce **catatonic disorder** (e.g., immobility resulting from stroke) or **personality change** (e.g., resulting from brain tumor). Also may produce **delirium, dementia, amnestic disorder, psychotic disorder, mood disorder, anxiety disorder, sexual dysfunction,** and **sleep disorder.**

D. **Substance-related disorders**

1. **Substance use disorders. Dependence** on or **abuse** of any psychoactive drug (previously called *drug addiction*). Covers patients addicted to or dependent on such drugs as **alcohol, nicotine** (tobacco), and **caffeine.** Patients may be dependent on **opioids** (e.g., opium, opium alkaloids and their derivatives, and synthetic analgesics with morphine-like effects); **hallucinogens** (e.g., lysergic acid diethylamide [LSD]); **phencyclidine; hypnotics, sedatives, or anxiolytics; cocaine; cannabis** (hashish, marijuana); **amphetamines;** and **inhalants.**

2. **Substance-induced disorders.** Psychoactive drugs and other substances may cause **intoxication** and **withdrawal** syndromes in addition to **delirium, persisting dementia, persisting amnestic disorder, psychotic disorder, mood disorder, anxiety disorder, sexual dysfunction,** and **sleep disorder.**

3. **Alcohol-related disorders.** Subclass of substance-related disorders that includes **alcohol intoxication** (simple drunkenness); **intoxication delirium** (from being drunk for several days); **alcohol withdrawal delirium** (also called *delirium tremens* [DTs]); **alcohol-induced**

psychotic disorder (includes alcohol hallucinosis—differentiated from DTs by clear sensorium); **alcohol-induced persisting amnestic disorder** ([Korsakoff's syndrome]—often preceded by Wernicke's encephalopathy, a neurologic condition of ataxia, ophthalmoplegia, and confusion, or the two may coexist [Wernicke–Korsakoff syndrome]); and **alcohol-induced persisting dementia** (differentiated from Korsakoff's syndrome by multiple cognitive deficits). **Mood disorder, anxiety disorder,** and **sleep disorder** induced by alcohol may also occur.

E. **Schizophrenia and other psychotic disorders.** Covers disorders manifested by disturbances of thinking and misinterpretation of reality, often with delusions and hallucinations.

1. **Schizophrenia.** Characterized by changes in affect (ambivalent, constricted, and inappropriate responsiveness; loss of empathy with others), behavior (withdrawn, aggressive, bizarre), thinking (distortion of reality, sometimes with delusions and hallucinations), and cognition. Schizophrenia includes five types: (1) **disorganized** (hebephrenic) **type**—disorganized thinking, giggling, shallow and inappropriate affect, silly and regressive behavior and mannerisms, frequent somatic complaints, and occasional transient and unorganized delusions and hallucinations; (2) **catatonic type**—the *excited subtype* is characterized by excessive and sometimes violent motor activity, and the *withdrawn subtype* is characterized by generalized inhibition, stupor, mutism, negativism, waxy flexibility, and in some cases a vegetative state; (3) **paranoid type**—schizophrenia characterized by persecutory or grandiose delusions and sometimes by hallucinations or excessive religiosity, and the patient is often hostile and aggressive; (4) **undifferentiated type**—disorganized behavior with prominent delusions and hallucinations; and (5) **residual type**— signs of schizophrenia, after a psychotic schizophrenic episode, in patients who are no longer psychotic. (**Postpsychotic depressive disorder of schizophrenia** can occur during the residual phase.)

2. **Delusional (paranoid) disorder.** Psychotic disorder associated with persistent delusions (e.g., erotomanic, grandiose, jealous, persecutory, somatic, unspecified). *Paranoia* is a rare condition characterized by the gradual development of an elaborate delusional system with grandiose ideas; it has a chronic course; the rest of the personality remains intact.

3. **Brief psychotic disorder.** Psychotic disorder of less than 4 weeks' duration brought on by an external stressor.

4. **Schizophreniform disorder.** Similar to schizophrenia, with delusions, hallucinations, and incoherence, but lasts less than 6 months.

5. **Schizoaffective disorder.** Characterized by a mixture of schizophrenic symptoms and pronounced elation (bipolar type) or depression (depressive type).

6. **Shared psychotic disorder.** Same delusion occurs in two persons, one of whom is less intelligent than or more dependent on the other (also known as *shared delusional disorder, folie à deux*).

7. **Psychotic disorder resulting from a general medical condition.** Hallucinations or delusions that result from medical illness (e.g., temporal lobe epilepsy, avitaminosis, meningitis).
8. **Substance-induced psychotic disorder.** Symptoms of psychosis caused by psychoactive or other substances (e.g., hallucinogens, cocaine).
9. **Psychotic disorder NOS** (also known as *atypical psychosis*). Psychotic features that are related to (1) a specific culture (koro—found in South and East Asia, fear of shrinking penis); (2) a certain time or event (postpartum psychosis—48 to 72 hours after childbirth); or (3) a unique set of symptoms (Capgras' syndrome—patients think they have a double).

F. **Mood disorders** (previously called *affective disorders*). Characterized by a change in mood (e.g., depression) that dominates the patient's mental life and is responsible for diminished functioning. Mood disorders may be caused by a **medical condition** or by a **substance** (e.g., psychoactive drugs [cocaine] or medication [antineoplastic agents, reserpine]).

1. **Bipolar disorders.** Marked by severe mood swings between depression and elation and by remission and recurrence. **Bipolar I**—full manic or mixed episode, usually with major depressive episode; **bipolar II**—major depressive episode and hypomanic episode (less intense than mania); **cyclothymic disorder**—less severe type of bipolar disorder.
2. **Depressive disorders. Major depressive disorder**—severely depressed mood, mental and motor retardation, apprehension, uneasiness, perplexity, agitation, feelings of guilt, suicidal ideation, usually recurrent. **Dysthymic disorder**—less severe form of depression, usually caused by identifiable event or loss (previously called *depressive neurosis*). **Postpartum depression** occurs within 1 month after childbirth. **Seasonal pattern depression** (also called *seasonal affective disorder* [SAD]) occurs most often during the winter months.

G. **Anxiety disorders.** Characterized by massive and persistent anxiety (**generalized anxiety disorder**), often to the point of panic (**panic disorder**) and fears of going outside the home (**agoraphobia**); fear of specific situations or objects (**specific phobia**) or of performance and public speaking (**social phobia**); involuntary and persistent intrusions of thoughts, desires, urges, or actions (**obsessive–compulsive disorder**). Includes **posttraumatic stress disorder**—follows extraordinary life stress (war, catastrophe) and is characterized by anxiety, nightmares, agitation, and sometimes depression; **acute stress disorder**—similar to posttraumatic stress disorder but lasts for 4 weeks or less. May also be caused by a (1) **medical condition** (e.g., hyperthyroidism) or (2) **substance** (e.g., cocaine).

H. **Somatoform disorders.** Marked by preoccupation with the body and fears of disease. Classified into **somatization disorder**—multiple somatic complaints without organic pathology; **conversion disorder** (previously called *hysteria, Briquet's syndrome*)—the special senses or voluntary nervous system is affected, with resultant blindness, deafness, anosmia, anesthesias, paresthesias, paralysis, ataxia, akinesia, or dyskinesia; patients may show inappropriate lack of concern (*la belle indifference*) and may derive some benefits from their actions (secondary gain); **hypochondriasis** (hypochondriacal neurosis)—marked by preoccupation with the body and persistent fears of presumed disease; **pain disorder**—preoccupation with pain in which psychological factors play a part; **body dysmorphic disorder**—unrealistic concern that part of the body is deformed.

I. **Factitious disorders.** Characterized by the intentional production or feigning of psychological symptoms, physical symptoms, or both to assume sick role (also called *Munchausen syndrome*).

J. **Dissociative disorders.** Characterized by sudden, temporary change in consciousness or identity. **Dissociative** (psychogenic) **amnesia**—loss of memory without organic cause; **dissociative** (psychogenic) **fugue**—unexplained wandering from home; **dissociative identity disorder** (multiple personality disorder)—person has two or more separate identities; **depersonalization disorder**—feelings that things are unreal.

K. **Sexual and gender identity disorders.** Divided into paraphilias, gender identity disorders, and sexual dysfunctions. In **paraphilia,** a person's sexual interests are primarily directed toward objects rather than other people, toward sexual acts not usually associated with coitus, or toward coitus performed under bizarre circumstances. Included are **exhibitionism, fetishism, frotteurism, pedophilia, sexual masochism, sexual sadism, transvestite fetishism** (cross-dressing), and **voyeurism.** Sexual dysfunctions include disorders of **desire (hypoactive sexual desire disorder, sexual aversion disorder), arousal (female sexual arousal disorder, male erectile disorder** [i.e., impotence]), **orgasm (female orgasmic disorder** [i.e., anorgasmia]), **male orgasmic disorder** (i.e., delayed or retarded ejaculation, premature ejaculation), and **sexual pain (dyspareunia, vaginismus).** Sexual dysfunction may be caused by a **medical condition** (e.g., multiple sclerosis) or **substance abuse** (e.g., amphetamine). **Gender identity disorders** (including transsexualism) are characterized by persistent discomfort with one's biologic sex and the desire to lose one's sex characteristics (e.g., castration).

L. **Eating disorders.** Characterized by marked disturbance in eating behavior. Includes **anorexia nervosa** (loss of body weight, refusal to eat) and **bulimia nervosa** (binge eating with or without vomiting).

M. **Sleep disorders.** Covers (1) **dyssomnias,** in which the person cannot fall asleep or stay asleep (**insomnia**) or sleeps too much (**hypersomnia**); (2) **parasomnias,** such as **nightmares, sleepwalking,** or **sleep terror disorder** (person wakes up in an immobilized state of terror); (3) **narcolepsy** (sleep attacks with loss of muscle tone [cataplexy]); (4) **breathing-related sleep disorders** (snoring, apnea); and (5) **circadian rhythm sleep disorder** (daytime sleepiness, jet lag). Sleep disorders can also be caused by **medical disease** (e.g., Parkinson's disease) and **substance abuse** (e.g., alcoholism).

N. **Impulse-control disorders not elsewhere classified.** Covers disorders in which persons cannot control impulses and act out. Includes **intermittent explosive disorder** (aggression), **kleptomania** (stealing), **pyromania** (setting fires), **trichotillomania** (pulling hair), and **pathological gambling**.

O. **Adjustment disorder.** Maladaptive reaction to a clearly defined life stress. Divided into six subtypes depending on symptoms—with **anxiety, depressed mood, mixed anxiety and depressed mood, disturbance of conduct,** and **mixed disturbance of emotions and conduct**.

P. **Personality disorder.** Disorders characterized by deeply ingrained, generally lifelong maladaptive patterns of behavior that are usually recognizable at adolescence or earlier.

1. **Paranoid personality disorder.** Characterized by unwarranted suspicion, hypersensitivity, jealousy, envy, rigidity, excessive self-importance, and a tendency to blame and ascribe evil motives to others.

2. **Schizoid personality disorder.** Characterized by shyness, oversensitivity, seclusiveness, avoidance of close or competitive relationships, eccentricity, daydreaming, an ability to express hostility and aggression; no loss of capacity to recognize reality.

3. **Schizotypal personality disorder.** Similar to schizoid, but the person exhibits slight loss of reality testing, has odd beliefs, and is aloof and withdrawn.

4. **Obsessive–compulsive personality disorder.** Characterized by excessive concern with conformity and standards of conscience; patient may be rigid, overconscientious, overdutiful, overinhibited, and unable to relax (three *P*s—punctual, parsimonious, precise).

5. **Histrionic personality disorder.** Characterized by emotional instability, excitability, overreactivity, vanity, immaturity, dependency, and self-dramatization that is attention seeking and seductive.

6. **Avoidant personality disorder.** Characterized by low levels of energy, easy fatigability, lack of enthusiasm, inability to enjoy life, and oversensitivity to stress.

7. **Antisocial personality disorder.** Covers persons in conflict with society. They are incapable of loyalty and are selfish, callous, irresponsible, impulsive, and unable to feel guilt or learn from experience; they have a low level of frustration tolerance and a tendency to blame others.

8. **Narcissistic personality disorder.** Characterized by grandiose feelings, sense of entitlement, envy, manipulativeness, lack of empathy, and need for attention and admiration.

9. **Borderline personality disorder.** Characterized by instability, impulsiveness, chaotic sexuality, suicidal acts, self-mutilating behavior, identity problems, ambivalence, and feeling of emptiness and boredom.

10. **Dependent personality disorder.** Characterized by passive and submissive behavior; person is unsure of himself or herself and becomes entirely dependent on others.

Q. **Other conditions that may be a focus of clinical attention.** Include conditions in which no mental disorder is present, but the problem is the focus of diagnosis or treatment.

1. **Psychological factors affecting physical condition.** Disorders characterized by physical symptoms caused or affected by emotional factors; usually involve a single organ system with autonomic nervous system

control or input. Examples are atopic dermatitis, backache, bronchial asthma, hypertension, migraine, ulcer, irritable colon, and colitis (also called *psychosomatic disorders*).

2. **Medication-induced movement disorders. Disorders caused by medications,** especially dopamine receptor antagonists (e.g., chlorpromazine [Thorazine]). Includes **parkinsonism, neuroleptic malignant syndrome** (muscle rigidity, hypothermia), **acute dystonia** (muscle spasm), **acute akathisia** (restlessness), **tardive dyskinesia** (choreiform movements), and **postural tremor.**

3. **Relational problems.** Impaired social interaction within a relational unit. Includes **parent–child problem, spouse** or **partner problem,** and **sibling problem.** May also result when one member is mentally or physically ill and the other is stressed as a result.

4. **Problems related to abuse or neglect.** Includes **physical abuse** and **sexual abuse** of children and adults.

R. **Additional conditions that may be a focus of clinical attention.** Conditions in which persons have problems not severe enough to warrant a psychiatric diagnosis but that interfere with functioning. Classified into **adult** and **child or adolescent antisocial behavior** (repeated criminal acts), **borderline intellectual functioning** (IQ, 71–84), **malingering** (voluntary production of symptoms), **noncompliance with treatment, occupational** or **academic problem, phase of life problem** (parenthood, unemployment), **bereavement, age-related cognitive decline** (normal forgetfulness of old age), **identity problem** (career choice), **religious or spiritual problem,** and **acculturation problem** (immigration).

S. **Other categories.** In addition to the diagnostic categories listed above, other categories of illness are listed in *DSM-IV-TR* that require further study before they become an official part of *DSM-IV-TR* or that are controversial. These include the following:

1. **Postconcussional disorder.** Cognitive impairment, headache, sleep problems, irritability, dizziness, change in personality occurring after head injury.

2. **Mild neurocognitive disorder.** Disturbances in memory, comprehension, and attention as a result of medical disease (e.g., electrolyte imbalance, hypothyroidism, early stages of multiple sclerosis).

3. **Caffeine withdrawal.** Fatigue, depression, headaches, and anxiety after cessation of coffee intake.

4. **Postpsychotic depressive disorder of schizophrenia.** A depressive episode, which may be prolonged, arising in the aftermath of a schizophrenic illness.

5. **Simple deteriorative disorder (simple schizophrenia).** Characterized by oddities of conduct, inability to meet demands of society, blunting of affect, loss of volition, and social impoverishment. Delusions and hallucinations are evident.

6. **Minor depressive disorder, recurrent brief depressive disorder, and premenstrual dysphoric disorder. Minor depressive disorder**

is associated with mild symptoms, such as worry and overconcern with minor autonomic symptoms (tremor and palpitations). **Recurrent brief depressive disorder** is characterized by recurrent episodes of depression, each of which lasts less than 2 weeks (typically 2 to 3 days) and each of which ends with complete recovery. **Premenstrual dysphoric disorder** occurs 1 week before menses (luteal phase) and is characterized by depressed mood, anxiety, irritability, lethargy, and sleep disturbances.

 7. **Mixed anxiety–depressive disorder.** Characterized by symptoms of both anxiety and depression, neither of which predominates (called *neurasthenia* in ICD).

 8. **Factitious disorder by proxy.** Also known as *Munchausen syndrome by proxy*; parents feign illness in their children.

 9. **Dissociative trance disorder.** Marked by temporary loss of sense of personal identity and awareness of the surroundings; patient acts as if taken over by another personality, spirit, or force.

10. **Binge-eating disorder.** Variant of bulimia nervosa, characterized by recurrent episodes of binge eating without self-induced vomiting and laxative abuse.

11. **Depressive personality disorder.** Marked by pessimism, anhedonia, chronic unhappiness, and loneliness.

12. **Passive–aggressive personality disorder.** Marked by stubbornness, procrastination, and intentional inefficiency multiplied by underlying aggression (also called *negativistic personality disorder*).

For a more detailed discussion of this topic, see Classification in Psychiatry, Chapter 9, p. 1108, CTP/IX.

2

Psychiatric History and Mental Status

I. Introduction

A. Psychiatric history. The psychiatric history is the record of the patient's life; it allows the psychiatrist to understand who the patient is, where the patient has come from, and where the patient is likely to go in the future. The history is the patient's life story told in the patient's own words from his or her own point of view. It may include information about the patient from other sources, such as parents or spouse. A thorough psychiatric history is essential to making a correct diagnosis and formulating a specific and effective treatment plan.

B. Mental status. The mental status examination (MSE) is a description of the patient's appearance, speech, actions, and thoughts during the interview. It is a systematic format for recording findings about thinking, feeling, and behavior. A patient's history remains stable, whereas the mental status can change daily or hourly. Only phenomena observed at the time of the interview are recorded in the mental status. Other data are recorded in the history. A comprehensive psychiatric history and mental status are described below.

The reader is referred to the glossary of signs and symptoms at the end of the book for a definition of terms.

II. Psychiatric History

A. Identification
1. Name, age, marital status, sex, occupation, language if other than English, race, nationality, religion.
2. Previous admissions to a hospital for the same or a different condition.
3. Persons with whom the patient lives.

B. Chief Complaint (CC)
1. Describe exactly why the patient came to the psychiatrist, preferably in the patient's own words.
2. If that information does not come from the patient, note who supplied it.

C. History of Present Illness (HPI)
1. Chronological background and development of the symptoms or behavioral changes that culminated in the patient seeking assistance.
2. Patient's life circumstances at the time of onset.
3. Personality when well; how illness has affected life activities and personal relations—changes in personality, interests, mood, attitudes toward others, dress, habits, level of tenseness, irritability, activity, attention, concentration, memory, speech.
4. Psychophysiological symptoms—nature and details of dysfunction; pain—location, intensity, fluctuation.
5. Level of anxiety—generalized and nonspecific (free floating) or specifically related to particular situations, activities, or objects.

6. How anxieties are handled—avoidance, repetition of feared situation.

7. Use of drugs or other activities for alleviation.

D. Past psychiatric and medical history

1. Emotional or mental disturbances—extent of incapacity, type of treatment, names of hospitals, length of illness, effect of treatment.

2. Psychosomatic disorders: hay fever, arthritis, colitis, chronic fatigue, recurrent colds, skin conditions.

3. Medical conditions—customary review of systems, sexually transmitted diseases, alcohol or other substance abuse, at risk for acquired immune deficiency syndrome (AIDS).

4. Neurological disorders—headache, craniocerebral trauma, loss of consciousness, seizures, or tumors.

E. Family history

1. Elicited from patient and from someone else, because quite different descriptions may be given of the same people and events.

2. Ethnic, national, and religious traditions.

3. List other people in the home and descriptions of them—personality and intelligence—and their relationship to the patient.

4. Role of illness in the family and family history of mental illness.

5. Where the patient lives—neighborhood and particular residence of the patient; is the home crowded; privacy of family members from each other and from other families.

6. Sources of family income, public assistance (if any) and attitudes about it; will the patient lose his or her job or apartment by remaining in the hospital.

7. Child care arrangements.

F. Personal history (anamnesis)

 CLINICAL HINT:

It is seldom necessary to describe all of the following categories below for all patients. For example, early developmental history may not be as relevant for adults as for children and adolescents.

---

1. *Early childhood (through 3 years of age)*

   a. Prenatal history and mother's pregnancy and delivery: length of pregnancy, spontaneity and normality of delivery, birth trauma, whether the patient was planned and wanted, birth defects.

   b. Feeding habits: breast-fed or bottle-fed, eating problems.

   c. Early development: maternal deprivation, language development, motor development, signs of unmet needs, sleep pattern, object constancy, stranger anxiety, separation anxiety.

   d. Toilet training: age, attitude of parents, feelings about it.

   e. Symptoms of behavior problems: thumb sucking, temper tantrums, tics, head bumping, rocking, night terrors, fears, bed-wetting or bed soiling, nail biting, masturbation.

    f. Personality and temperament as a child: shy, restless, overactive, withdrawn, studious, outgoing, timid, athletic, friendly patterns of play, reactions to siblings.

    g. Early or recurrent dreams or fantasies.

2. *Middle childhood (3 to 11 years of age)*

    a. Early school history—feelings about going to school.

    b. Early adjustment, gender identification.

    c. Conscience development, punishment.

    d. Social relationships.

    e. Attitudes toward siblings and playmates.

3. *Later childhood (prepuberty through adolescence)*

    a. Peer relationships: number and closeness of friends, leader or follower, social popularity, participation in group or gang activities, idealized figures, patterns of aggression, passivity, anxiety, antisocial behavior.

    b. School history: how far the patient went in school, adjustment to school, relationships with teachers—teacher's pet or rebellious — favorite studies or interests, particular abilities or assets, extracurricular activities, sports, hobbies, relationships of problems or symptoms to any school period.

    c. Cognitive and motor development: learning to read and other intellectual and motor skills, minimal cerebral dysfunction, learning disabilities—their management and effects on the child.

    d. Particular adolescent emotional or physical problems: nightmares, phobias, bed-wetting, running away, delinquency, smoking, drug or alcohol use, weight problems, feeling of inferiority.

    e. Psychosexual history.

        (1) Early curiosity, infantile masturbation, sex play.

        (2) Acquiring of sexual knowledge, attitude of parents toward sex, sexual abuse.

        (3) Onset of puberty, feelings about it, kind of preparation, feelings about menstruation, development of secondary sexual characteristics.

        (4) Adolescent sexual activity: crushes, parties, dating, petting, masturbation, wet dreams (nocturnal emissions) and attitudes toward them.

        (5) Attitudes toward same and opposite sex: timid, shy, aggressive, need to impress, seductive, sexual conquests, anxiety.

        (6) Sexual practices: sexual problems, homosexual and heterosexual experiences, paraphilias, promiscuity.

    f. Religious background: strict, liberal, mixed (possible conflicts), relationship of background to current religious practices.

4. *Adulthood*

    a. Occupational history: choice of occupation, training, ambitions, and conflicts; relations with authority, peers, and subordinates; number of jobs and duration; changes in job status; current job and feelings about it.

    b. Social activity: whether patient has friends; whether he or she is withdrawn or socializing well; social, intellectual, and physical interests; relationships with same sex and opposite sex; depth, duration, and quality of human relations.

    c. Adult sexuality.

      (1) Premarital sexual relationships, age of first coitus, sexual orientation.

      (2) Marital history: common-law marriages; legal marriages; description of courtship and role played by each partner; age at marriage; family planning and contraception; names and ages of children; attitudes toward raising children; problems of any family members; housing difficulties, if important to the marriage; sexual adjustment; extramarital affairs; areas of agreement and disagreement; management of money; role of in-laws.

      (3) Sexual symptoms: anorgasmia, impotence (erectile disorder), premature ejaculation, lack of desire.

      (4) Attitudes toward pregnancy and having children; contraceptive practices and feelings about them.

      (5) Sexual practices: paraphilias, such as sadism, fetishes, voyeurism; attitude toward fellatio, cunnilingus; coital techniques, frequency.

    d. Military history: general adjustment, combat, injuries, referral to psychiatrists, type of discharge, veteran status.

    e. Value systems: whether children are seen as a burden or a joy; whether work is seen as a necessary evil, an avoidable chore, or an opportunity; current attitude about religion; belief in after life.

III. Mental Status

A. Appearance

    1. Personal identification: may include a brief nontechnical description of the patient's appearance and behavior, as a novelist might write it. Attitude toward examiner can be described here: cooperative, attentive, interested, frank, seductive, defensive, hostile, playful, ingratiating, evasive, or guarded.

    2. Behavior and psychomotor activity: gait, mannerisms, tics, gestures, twitches, stereotypes, picking, touching examiner, echopraxia, clumsy, agile, limp, rigid, retarded, hyperactive, agitated, combative, or waxy.

    3. General description: posture, bearing, clothes, grooming, hair, nails; healthy, sickly, angry, frightened, apathetic, perplexed, contemptuous, ill at ease, poised, old looking, young looking, effeminate, masculine; signs of anxiety—moist hands, perspiring forehead, restlessness, tense posture, strained voice, wide eyes; shifts in level of anxiety during interview or with particular topic; eye contact (50% is normal).

B. Speech: rapid, slow, pressured, hesitant, emotional, monotonous, loud, whispered, slurred, mumbled, stuttering, echolalia, intensity, pitch, ease, spontaneity, productivity, manner, reaction time, vocabulary, prosody.

C. **Mood and affect**
  1. Mood (a pervasive and sustained emotion that colors the person's perception of the world): how does patient say he or she feels; depth, intensity, duration, and fluctuations of mood—depressed, despairing, irritable, anxious, terrified, angry, expansive, euphoric, empty, guilty, awed, futile, self-contemptuous, anhedonic, alexithymic.
  2. Affect (the outward expression of the patient's inner experiences): how the examiner evaluates the patient's affects—broad, restricted, blunted or flat, shallow, amount and range of expression; difficulty in initiating, sustaining, or terminating an emotional response; whether the emotional expression is appropriate to the thought content, culture, and setting of the examination; examples should be given if emotional expression is not appropriate.

D. **Thinking and perception**
  1. **Form of thinking**
     a. Productivity: overabundance of ideas, paucity of ideas, flight of ideas, rapid thinking, slow thinking, hesitant thinking; whether the patient speaks spontaneously or only when questions are asked; stream of thought, quotations from patient.
     b. Continuity of thought: whether the patient's replies really answer questions and are goal directed, relevant, or irrelevant; loose associations; lack of cause-and-effect relationships in the patient's explanations; illogical, tangential, circumstantial, rambling, evasive, persevering statements; blocking or distractibility.
     c. Language impairments: impairments that reflect disordered mentation, such as incoherent or incomprehensible speech (word salad), clang associations, neologisms.
  2. **Content of thinking**
     a. Preoccupations about the illness, environmental problems.
     b. Obsessions, compulsions, phobias.
     c. Obsessions or plans about suicide and/or homicide.
     d. Hypochondriacal symptoms, specific antisocial urges or impulses.
  3. **Thought disturbances**
     a. Delusions: content of any delusional system, its organization, the patient's convictions as to its validity, how it affects his or her life; persecutory delusions—isolated or associated with pervasive suspiciousness; mood-congruent or mood-incongruent.
     b. Ideas of reference and ideas of influence: how ideas began, their content, and the meaning that the patient attributes to them.
     c. Thought broadcasting—thoughts being heard by others.
     d. Thought insertion—thoughts being inserted into a person's mind by others.
  4. **Perceptual disturbances**
     a. Hallucinations and illusions: whether the patient hears voices or sees visions; content, sensory system involvement, circumstances of

the occurrence; hypnagogic or hypnopompic hallucinations; thought broadcasting.

b. Depersonalization and derealization: extreme feelings of detachment from self or from the environment.

5. Dreams and fantasies

a. Dreams: prominent ones, if the patient recalls them; nightmares.

b. Fantasies: recurrent, favorite, or unshakable daydreams.

E. Sensorium

 CLINICAL HINT:
This section includes an assessment of several cognitive functions. Collectively, they help describe the overall intactness of the central nervous system, as different functions are served by different brain regions. Abnormalities of the sensorium are seen in delirium and dementia, and they raise the suspicion of an underlying medical or drug-related cause of symptoms. See Table 2–1 for a scored general intelligence test that can be used to increase the reliability and validity of the diagnosis of cognitive disorder.

1. Alertness: awareness of environment, attention span, clouding of consciousness, fluctuations in levels of awareness, somnolence, stupor, lethargy, fugue state, coma.

2. Orientation

a. Time: whether the patient identifies the day or the approximate date and the time of day correctly; if in a hospital, whether the patient knows how long he or she has been there; whether the patient behaves as though oriented to the present.

b. Place: whether the patient knows where he or she is.

c. Person: whether the patient knows who the examiner is and the roles or names of the persons with whom the patient is in contact.

3. Concentration and calculation: whether the patient can subtract 7 from 100 and keep subtracting 7s; if the patient cannot subtract 7s, whether easier tasks can be accomplished—4×9 and 5×4; whether the patient can calculate how many nickels are in $1.35; whether anxiety or some disturbance of mood or concentration seems to be responsible for difficulty.

4. Memory: impairment, efforts made to cope with impairment—denial, confabulation, catastrophic reaction, circumstantiality used to conceal deficit; whether the process of registration, retention, or recollection of material is involved.

a. Remote memory: childhood data, important events known to have occurred when the patient was younger or free of illness, personal matters, neutral material.

b. Recent past memory: past few months.

c. Recent memory: past few days, what did the patient do yesterday and the day before, what did the patient have for breakfast, lunch, and dinner.

Table 2–1
Scored General Intelligence Test*

Indications: When a cognitive disorder is suspected because of apparent intellectual, defects, impairment in the ability to make generalizations, the ability to maintain a trend of thought, or to show good judgment, a scored test can be of value. It can confirm the diagnosis of impairment with greater reliability and validity.

Directions: Ask the following questions as part of the mental status examination. A conversational manner should be used and the questions may be adapted to cultural differences.

Scoring: If the patient obtains a score of 25 or under (out of a maximum of 40), it is indicative of a cognitive problem and further examination should follow.

Questions: There are 13 questions that follow.

1. What are houses made of? (Any material you can think of).............................1–4
   One point for each item, up to four.
2. What is sand used for?..1, 2, or 4
   Four points for manufacture of glass. Two points for mixing with concrete, road building, or other constructive use. One point for play or sandboxes. Credit not cumulative.
3. If the flag floats to the south, from what direction is the wind?..........................3
   Three points for north, no partial credits. It is permissible to say: 'Which way is the wind coming from?'
4. Tell me the names of some fish..1–4
   One point for each, up to four. If the subject stops with one, encourage him or her to go on.
5. At what time of day is your shadow shortest?...3
   Noon, three points. If correct response is suspected of being a guess, inquire why.
6. Give the names of some large cities..1–4
   One point for each, up to four. When any state is named as a city, no credit, that is, New York unless specified as New York City. No credit for hometown, except when it is an outstanding city.
7. Why does the moon look larger than the stars?.....................................2, 3, or 4
   Make it clear that the question refers to any particular star, and give assurance that the moon is actually smaller than any star. Encourage the subject to guess. Two points for "Moon is lower down." Three points for nearer or closer. Four points for generalized statement that nearer objects look larger than more distant objects.
8. What metal is attracted by a magnet?...2 or 4
   Four points for iron, two for steel.
9. If your shadow points to the northeast, where is the sun?...............................4
   Four points for southwest, no partial credits.
10. How many stripes are in the American flag?..2
    Thirteen, two points. A subject who responds 50 may be permitted to correct the mistake. Explain, if necessary, that the white stripes are included as well as the red ones.
11. What does ice become when it melts?...1
    Water, one point.
12. How many minutes in an hour?..1
    60, one point.
13. Why is it colder at night than in the daytime?......................................1–2
    Two points for "sun goes down," or any recognition of direct rays of sun as source of heat. Question may be reversed: "What makes it warmer in the daytime than at night?" Only one point for answer to reverse question.

*This test was developed and validated by N. D. C. Lewis, MD. Adapted by B. J. Sadock, MD.

    d. Immediate retention and recall: ability to repeat six figures after the examiner dictates them—first forward, then backward, then after a few minutes' interruption; other test questions; whether the same questions, if repeated, called forth different answers at different times.

    e. Effect of defect on patient: mechanisms the patient has developed to cope with the defect.

  5. Fund of knowledge

    a. Estimate of the patient's intellectual capability and whether the patient is capable of functioning at the level of his or her basic endowment.

  b. General knowledge; questions should have relevance to the patient's educational and cultural background.
6. Abstract thinking: disturbances in concept formation; manner in which the patient conceptualizes or handles his or her ideas; similarities (e.g., between apples and pears), differences, absurdities; meanings of simple proverbs, such as "a rolling stone gathers no moss"; answers may be concrete (giving specific examples to illustrate the meaning) or overly abstract (giving generalized explanation); appropriateness of answers.
7. Insight: the recognition of having a mental disorder and degree of personal awareness and understanding of illness.
  a. Complete denial of illness.
  b. Slight awareness of being sick and needing help but denying it at the same time.
  c. Awareness of being sick but blaming it on others, external factors, or medical or unknown organic factors.
  d. Intellectual insight: admission of illness and recognition that symptoms or failures in social adjustment are due to irrational feelings or disturbances, without applying that knowledge to future experiences.
  e. True emotional insight: emotional awareness of the motives and feelings within and of the underlying meaning of symptoms, whether the awareness leads to changes in personality and future behavior, openness to new ideas and concepts about self and the important people in the patient's life.

 CLINICAL HINT:
Test for insight by asking: "Do you think you have a problem?" "Do you need treatment?" "What are your plans for the future?" Insight is severely impaired in cognitive disorders, psychosis, and borderline IQ.

---

8. Judgment
  a. Social judgment: subtle manifestations of behavior that are harmful to the patient and contrary to acceptable behavior in the culture, whether the patient understands the likely outcome of personal behavior and is influenced by that understanding, examples of impairment.
  b. Test judgment: the patient's prediction of what he or she would do in imaginary situations; for instance, what the patient would do with a stamped, addressed letter found in the street or if medication was lost.

 CLINICAL HINT:
Judgment is severely impaired in manic episodes of bipolar disorders and in cognitive disorders (e.g., delirium and dementia).

  A summary of questions and clinical hints to elicit psychiatric history and mental status data is provided in Table 2–2.

Table 2–2
Common Questions for the Psychiatric History and Mental Status

Topic	Questions	Comments and Clinical Hints
Identifying data	Be direct in obtaining identifying data. Request specific answers.	If patient cannot cooperate, get information from family member or friend; if referred by a physician, obtain medical record.
Chief complaint (CC)	Why are you going to see a psychiatrist? What brought you to the hospital? What seems to be the problem?	Record answers verbatim; a bizarre complaint points to psychotic process.
History of present illness (HPI)	When did you first notice something happening to you? Were you upset about anything when symptoms began? Did they begin suddenly or gradually?	Record in patient's own words as much as possible. Get history of previous hospitalizations and treatment. Sudden onset of symptoms may indicate drug-induced disorder.
Previous psychiatric and medical disorders	Did you ever lose consciousness? Have a seizure?	Ascertain extent of illness, treatment, medications, outcomes, hospitals, doctors. Determine whether illness serves some additional purpose (secondary gain).
Personal history	Do you know anything about your birth? If so, from whom? How old was your mother when you were born? Your father?	Older mothers (>35) have high risk for Down syndrome baby; older father (>45) may contribute damaged sperm producing deficits including schizophrenia.
Childhood	Toilet training? Bed-wetting? Sex play with peers? What is your first childhood memory?	Separation anxiety and school phobia are associated with adult depression; enuresis associated with fire setting. Childhood memories before the age of 3 are usually imagined, not real.
Adolescence	Adolescents may refuse to answer questions, but they should be asked. Adults may distort memories of emotionally charged adolescent experiences. Sexual molestation?	Poor school performance is a sensitive indicator of emotional disorder. Schizophrenia begins in late adolescence.
Adulthood	Open-ended questions are preferable. Tell me about your marriage. Be nonjudgmental: What role does religion play in your life, if any? What is your sexual preference in a partner?	Depending on chief complaint, some areas require more detailed inquiry. Manic patients frequently go into debt or are promiscuous. Overvalued religious ideas associated with paranoid personality disorder.
Sexual history	Are there or have there been any problems or concerns about your sex life? How did you learn about sex? Has there been any change in your sex drive?	Be nonjudgmental. Asking *when* masturbation began is a better approach than asking *do you* or *did you ever* masturbate.

(continued)

Table 2–2—*continued*
Common Questions for the Psychiatric History and Mental Status

Topic	Questions	Comments and Clinical Hints
Family history	Have any members in your family been depressed? Alcoholic? In a mental hospital? In jail? Describe your living conditions. Did you have your own room?	Genetic loading in anxiety, depression, schizophrenia. Get medication history of family (medications effective in family members for similar disorders may be effective in patient).
Mental status		
General appearance	Introduce yourself and direct patient to take a seat. In the hospital, bring your chair to bedside; do not sit on the bed.	Unkempt and disheveled in cognitive disorder, pinpoint pupils in narcotic addiction, withdrawal and stooped posture in depression.
Motoric behavior	Have you been more active than usual? Less active? You may ask about obvious mannerisms, e.g., "I notice that your hand still shakes, can you tell me about that?" Stay aware of smells, e.g., alcoholism/ ketoacidosis.	Fixed posturing, odd behavior in schizophrenia. Hyperactive with stimulant (cocaine) abuse and in mania. Psychomotor retardation in depression; tremors with anxiety or medication side effect (lithium). Eye contact is normally made approximately half the time during the interview. Minimal eye contact in schizophrenia. Scanning of environment in paranoid states.
Attitude during interview	You may comment about attitude: You seem irritated about something; is that an accurate observation?	Suspiciousness in paranoia; seductive in hysteria; apathetic in conversion disorder (*la belle indifference*); punning (*witzlesucht*) in frontal lobe syndromes.
Mood	How do you feel? How are your spirits? Do you have thoughts that life is not worth living or that you want to harm yourself? Do you have plans to take your own life? Do you want to die? Has there been a change in your sleep habits?	Suicidal ideas in 25% of depressives; elation in mania. Early morning awakening in depression; decreased need for sleep in mania.
Affect	Observe nonverbal signs of emotion, body movements, facies, rhythm of voice (prosody). Laughing when talking about sad subjects, e.g., death, is inappropriate.	Changes in affect usual with schizophrenia: loss of prosody in cognitive disorder, catatonia. Do not confuse medication adverse effect with flat affect.
Speech	Ask patient to say "Methodist Episcopalian" to test for dysarthria.	Manic patients show pressured speech; paucity of speech in depression; uneven or slurred speech in cognitive disorders.
Perceptual disorders	Do you ever see things or hear voices? Do you have strange experiences as you fall asleep or upon awakening? Has the world changed in any way? Do you have strange smells?	Visual hallucinations suggest schizophrenia. Tactile hallucinations suggest cocainism, delirium tremens (DTs). Olfactory hallucinations common in temporal lobe epilepsy.

(continued)

Table 2–2—*continued*
Common Questions for the Psychiatric History and Mental Status

Topic	Questions	Comments and Clinical Hints
Thought content	Do you feel people want to harm you? Do you have special powers? Is anyone trying to influence you? Do you have strange body sensations? Are there thoughts that you can't get out of your mind? Do you think about the end of the world? Can people read your mind? Do you ever feel the TV is talking to you? Ask about fantasies and dreams.	Are delusions congruent with mood (grandiose delusions with elated mood) or incongruent? Mood-incongruent delusions point to schizophrenia. Illusions are common in delirium. Thought insertion is characteristic of schizophrenia.
Thought process	Ask meaning of proverbs to test abstraction, e.g., "People in glass houses should not throw stones." Concrete answer is, "Glass breaks." Abstract answers deal with universal themes or moral issues. Ask similarity between bird and butterfly (both alive), bread and cake (both food).	Loose associations point to schizophrenia; flight of ideas, to mania; inability to abstract, to schizophrenia, brain damage.
Sensorium	What place is this? What is today's date? Do you know who I am? Do you know who you are?	Delirium or dementia shows clouded or wandering sensorium. Orientation to person remains intact longer than orientation to time or place.
Remote memory (long-term memory)	Where were you born? Where did you go to school? Date of marriage? Birthdays of children? What were last week's newspaper headlines?	Patients with dementia of the Alzheimer's type retain remote memory longer than recent memory. Gaps in memory may be localized or filled in with confabulatory details. Hypermnesia is seen in paranoid personality.
Recent memory (short-term memory)	Where were you yesterday? What did you eat at your last meal?	In brain disease, recent memory loss (amnesia) usually occurs before remote memory loss.
Immediate memory (very short-term memory)	Ask patient to repeat six digits forward, then backward (normal responses). Ask patient to try to remember three nonrelated items; test patient after 5 minutes.	Loss of memory occurs with cognitive, dissociative, or conversion disorder. Anxiety can impair immediate retention and recent memory. Anterograde memory loss (amnesia) occurs after taking certain drugs, e.g., benzodiazepines. Retrograde memory loss occurs after head trauma.
Concentration and calculation	Ask patient to count from 1 to 20 rapidly; do simple calculations (2×3, 4×9); do serial 7 test, i.e., subtract 7 from 100 and keep subtracting 7. How many nickels in $1.35?	Rule out medical cause for any defects versus anxiety or depression (pseudodementia). Make tests congruent with educational level of patient.

(continued)

Table 2–2—*continued*
Common Questions for the Psychiatric History and Mental Status

Topic	Questions	Comments and Clinical Hints
Information and intelligence	Distance from New York City to Los Angeles. Name some vegetables. What is the largest river in the United States?	Check educational level to judge results. Rule out mental retardation, borderline intellectual functioning.
Judgment	What is the thing to do if you find an envelope in the street that is sealed, stamped, and addressed?	Impaired in brain disease, schizophrenia, borderline intellectual functioning, intoxication.
Insight level	Do you think you have a problem? Do you need treatment? What are your plans for the future?	Impaired in delirium, dementia, frontal lobe syndrome, psychosis, borderline intellectual functioning.

For further reading on this topic, see Psychiatric Interview, History, and Mental Status Examination, Section 7.1, p. 886, CTP/IX.

3
Psychiatric Report and Medical Record

The psychiatric report consists of the findings from the psychiatric history and the mental status written up in summary form. In addition, the report includes a diagnosis, prognosis, psychodynamic formulation, and comprehensive treatment plan.

A. How to record the psychiatric history and mental status

 CLINICAL HINT:
By the end of the examination, you must be able to judge: (1) presence or absence of psychosis, (2) cognitive defect, and (3) if patient is suicidal or homicidal.

1. The summary of the history and mental status is written up with each of the categories described including identification of the patient, chief complaint, history of present illness, past psychiatric history and medical history, family history, and so on. It includes a final summary of both positive and negative findings. Use specific examples of what questions are asked and how they are answered. Try to summarize the case not only from a descriptive approach, but also from an interpretive standpoint.

2. Clarity of thinking is reflected in clarity or writing and psychiatric terms should be used with precision. When summarizing the mental status, for example, the phrase "patient denies hallucinations and delusions" is not as precise as "patient denies hearing voices or thinking that he is being followed." The latter indicates the specific questions asked and the specific response given. Similarly, in the conclusion of the report, one would write, "Hallucinations and delusions were not elicited."

3. The examiner addresses critical questions in the report: Are future diagnostic studies needed, and if so, which ones? Is a consultant needed? Is a comprehensive neurological workup needed including an electroencephalogram (EEG) or computerized tomography (CT) scan? Are psychological tests indicated by a clinical psychologist? Are social work services needed?

B. How to record the diagnosis

1. Diagnostic classification is made according to the *Diagnostic and Statistical Manual of Mental Disorders, Text Revision*, fourth edition (*DSM-IV-TR*) (see Chapter 1).

2. The diagnosis is made using a multiaxial classification, which consists of five axes, each of which should be covered in the diagnosis. They are as follows:

    a. *Axis I*: includes all clinical syndromes (e.g., mood disorders, schizophrenia, generalized anxiety disorder) and other conditions that may be the focus of clinical attention.

    b. *Axis II*: includes personality disorders and mental retardation.

Table 3–1
DSM-IV-TR Severity of Psychosocial Stressors Scale in Adults

		Examples of Stressors	
Code	Term	Acute Events	Enduring Circumstances
1	None	No acute events that may be relevant to the disorder	No enduring circumstances that may be relevant to the disorder
2	Mild	Broke up with boyfriend or girlfriend; started or graduated from school; child left home	Family arguments; job dissatisfaction; residence in high-crime neighborhood
3	Moderate	Marriage: marital separation; loss of job; retirement; miscarriage	Marital discord; serious financial problems; trouble with boss; being a single parent
4	Severe	Divorce: birth of first child	Unemployment: poverty
5	Extreme	Death of spouse; serious physical illness diagnosed; victim of rape	Serious chronic illness in self or child; ongoing physical or sexual abuse
6	Catastrophic	Death of child; suicide of spouse; devastating natural disaster	Captivity as hostage; concentration camp experience
0	Inadequate information, or no change in condition		

 CLINICAL HINT:
Diagnosis on Axis I and Axis II can coexist. The Axis I or II condition that is responsible for bringing the patient to the psychiatrist or hospital is called the principle or main diagnosis.

    c. *Axis III*: includes any general medical conditions (e.g., epilepsy, cardiovascular disease, endocrine disorders). Please note: If a medical disorder is considered the cause of the psychiatric disorder, it is listed on Axis I.

    d. *Axis IV*: used to describe psychosocial and environmental problems (e.g., divorce, injury, death of a loved one) relevant to the illness (Table 3–1).

    e. *Axis V*: assesses global assessment of functioning exhibited by the patient during the interview (e.g., social, occupational, and psychological functioning); a rating scale with the continuum from 100 (superior functioning) to 1 (grossly impaired functioning) is used (see Table 4–3 in Chapter 4, Psychiatric Rating Scales).

3. How to record multiple diagnoses

    a. It is possible for a patient to have more than one diagnosis.

    b. The *principle* or *main diagnosis* is usually the one that was responsible for admission to a hospital or a visit to the psychiatrist.

    c. In some cases, it may not be possible to determine which diagnosis is the main one because each may have contributed equally to the need for treatment. In such cases, the term *dual diagnosis* is used (e.g., amphetamine dependence accompanied by schizophrenia).

    d. A *provisional diagnosis* is used when there is insufficient data to fulfill the criteria for a definitive diagnosis.

C. How to record severity of disorder. Depending on the clinical picture and the presence or absence of signs and symptoms and their intensity, the severity of a disorder may be classified as follows:

    1. Mild. Few if any symptoms are present and no more than minor impairment in social or occupational functioning.

    2. Moderate. Symptoms or functional impairment between *mild* and *severe* are present.

    3. Severe. Many symptoms or particularly severe symptoms are present that result in marked impairment in social or occupational functioning.

    4. In partial remission. The full criteria for the disorder were previously met, but currently only some of the symptoms or signs of the disorder remain.

    5. In full remission. There are no longer any symptoms or signs of the disorder.

D. How to record psychodynamic formulation. Note the causes of the patient's psychodynamic breakdown—influences in the patient's life that contributed to present disorder (environmental, genetic)—and personality factors relevant to determining patient's symptoms; primary and secondary gains; outline the major defense mechanism used by the patient. Table 3–2 presents a glossary of defense mechanisms and coping styles.

Table 3–2
Glossary of Specific Defense Mechanisms

acting out The individual deals with emotional conflict or internal or external stressors by actions rather than reflections or feelings. This definition is broader than the original concept of the acting out of transference feelings or wishes during psychotherapy and is intended to include behavior arising both within and outside the transference relationship. Defensive acting out is not synonymous with "bad behavior" because it requires evidence that the behavior is related to emotional conflicts.

altruism The individual deals with emotional conflict or internal or external stressors by dedication to meeting the needs of others. Altruism differs from the self-sacrifice sometimes characteristic of reaction formation in that the individual receives gratification either vicariously or from the response of others.

anticipation The individual deals with emotional conflict or internal or external stressors by experiencing emotional reactions in advance of, or anticipating consequences of, possible future events and considering realistic, alternative responses or solutions.

denial The individual deals with emotional conflict or internal or external stressors by refusing to acknowledge some painful aspect of external reality or subjective experience that would be apparent to others. The term *psychotic denial* is used when gross impairment in reality testing is present.

displacement The individual deals with emotional conflict or internal or external stressors by transferring a feeling about, or a response to, one object onto another (usually less threatening) substitute object.

dissociation The individual deals with emotional conflict or internal or external stressors with a breakdown in the usually integrated functions of consciousness, memory, perception of self or the environment, or sensory/motor behavior.

humor The individual deals with emotional conflict or external stressors by emphasizing the amusing or ironic aspects of the conflict or stressor.

idealization The individual deals with emotional conflict or internal or external stressors by attributing exaggerated positive qualities to others.

(continued)

Table 3–2—*continued*
Glossary of Specific Defense Mechanisms

intellectualization   The individual deals with emotional conflict or internal or external stressors by the excessive use of abstract thinking or the making of generalizations to control or minimize disturbing feelings.

isolation of affect   The individual deals with emotional conflict or internal or external stressors by the separation of ideas from the feelings originally associated with them. The individual loses touch with the feelings associated with a given idea (e.g., a traumatic event) while remaining aware of the cognitive elements of it (e.g., descriptive details).

omnipotence   The individual deals with emotional conflict or internal or external stressors by feeling or acting as if he or she possesses special powers or abilities and is superior to others.

projection   The individual deals with emotional conflict or internal or external stressors by falsely attributing to another his or her own unacceptable feelings, impulses, or thoughts.

projective identification   As in projection, the individual deals with emotional conflict or internal or external stressors by falsely attributing to another his or her own unacceptable feelings, impulses, or thoughts. However, the individual does not fully disavow what is projected, as in simple projection. Instead, the individual remains aware of his or her own affects or impulses but misattributes them as justifiable reactions to the other person. Not infrequently, the individual induces the very feelings in others that were first mistakenly believed to be there, making it difficult to clarify who did what to whom first.

rationalization   The individual deals with emotional conflict or internal or external stressors by concealing the true motivations for his or her own thoughts, actions, or feelings through the elaboration of reassuring or self-serving but incorrect explanations.

reaction formation   The individual deals with emotional conflict or internal or external stressors by substituting behavior, thoughts, or feelings that are diametrically opposed to his or her own unacceptable thoughts or feelings (this usually occurs in conjunction with their repression).

repression   The individual deals with emotional conflict or internal or external stressors expelling disturbing wishes, thoughts, or experiences from conscious awareness. The feeling component may remain conscious, detached from its associated ideas.

splitting   The individual deals with emotional conflict or internal or external stressors by compartmentalizing opposite affect states and failing to integrate the positive and negative qualities of the self or others into cohesive images. Because ambivalent affects cannot be experienced simultaneously, more balanced views and expectations of self or others are excluded from emotional awareness. Self and object images tend to alternate between polar opposites: exclusively loving, powerful, worthy, nurturant, and king—or exclusively bad, hateful, angry, destructive, rejecting, or worthless.

sublimation   The individual deals with emotional conflict or internal or external stressors by channeling potentially maladaptive feelings or impulses into socially acceptable behavior (e.g., contact sports to channel angry impulses).

suppression   The individual deals with emotional conflict or internal or external stressors by intentionally avoiding thinking about disturbing problems, wishes, feelings, or experiences.

undoing   The individual deals with emotional conflict or internal or external stressors by words or behavior designed to negate or to make amends symbolically for unacceptable thoughts, feelings, or actions.

From American Psychiatric Association. *Diagnostic and Statistical Manual of Mental Disorders,* text revision, 4th ed. Washington, DC: American Psychiatric Association; 2000, with permission.

E. How to formulate a treatment plan

   1. Modalities of treatment recommended; role of medication; inpatient or outpatient treatment; frequency of sessions; probable duration of therapy; type of psychotherapy; individual, group, or family therapy; symptoms or problems to be treated.

   2. Initially, treatment must be directed toward any life-threatening situations, such as suicidal risk or risk of danger to others, which require psychiatric hospitalization. Danger to self or others is an acceptable reason (both legally and medically) for involuntary hospitalization.

3. In the absence of the need for confinement, a variety of outpatient treatment alternatives are available: day hospitals, supervised residences, outpatient psychotherapy, or pharmacotherapy, among others.

4. Treatment plan must attend to vocational and psychosocial skills training and sometimes legal or forensic issues.

5. A therapeutic team approach using the skills of psychologists, social workers, nurses, and activity and occupational therapists may be needed.

6. Referral to self-help groups (e.g., Alcoholics Anonymous [AA]), if needed. If either the patient or family members are unwilling to accept the recommendations of treatment and the clinician thinks that the refusal of the recommendations may have serious consequences, the patient, parent, or guardian should sign a statement to the effect that the recommended treatment was refused.

F. **How to use the medical record.** The medical record is more than the psychiatric report. It is a narrative that documents all events that occur during the course of treatment, most often referring to the patient's stay in the hospital. Progress notes record every interaction between doctor and patient, reports of all special studies including laboratory tests, and prescriptions and orders for all medications. The patient's course should be described with particular attention to the following questions:

1. Is the patient beginning to respond to treatment?

2. Are there times during the day or night when symptoms get worse or remit?

3. Are there adverse effects or complaints by the patient about prescribed medication?

4. Are there signs of agitation or violence or mention of suicide?

5. If the patient requires restraints or seclusion, are the proper supervisory procedures being followed?

Table 3–3
Medical Record

There shall be an individual record for each person admitted to the psychiatric inpatient unit. Patient records shall be safeguarded for confidentiality and be accessible only to authorized persons. Each case record shall include:

1. Legal admission documents
2. Identifying information on the individual and family
3. Source of referral, date of commencing service, and name of staff member carrying overall responsibility for treatment and care
4. Initial, intercurrent, and final diagnoses, including psychiatric or mental retardation diagnoses in official terminology
5. Reports of all diagnostic examinations and evaluations, including findings and conclusions
6. Reports of all special studies performed, including X-rays, clinical laboratory tests, clinical psychological testing, electroencephalograms, and psychometric tests
7. The individual written plan of care, treatment, and rehabilitation
8. Progress notes written and signed by all staff members having significant participation in the program of treatment and care
9. Summaries of case conferences and special consultations
10. Dated and signed prescriptions or orders for all medications, with notation of termination dates
11. A closing summary of the course of treatment and care
12. Documentation of any referrals to another agency

Adapted from guidelines of the New York State Office of Mental Health.

Taken as a whole, the medical record tells what happened to the patient since first making contact with the health care system. It concludes with a discharge summary that provides a concise overview of the patient's course with recommendations for future treatment, if necessary. Evidence of contact with a referral agency should be documented in the medical record to establish continuity of care if further intervention is necessary (Table 3–3).

For further reading on this topic, see Psychiatric Report, Medical Record, and Medical Error, Section 7.2, p. 907 in CTP/IX.

4

Psychiatric Rating Scales

I. Introduction

Psychiatric rating scales or rating instruments are used in treatment planning to help establish a diagnosis, identify comorbid conditions, and assess levels of functioning. They also provide a baseline for follow-up of the progress of an illness over time or in response to specific interventions. This is particularly useful in the conduct of psychiatric research.

II. Rating Scales Used in *DSM-IV-TR*

Rating scales form an integral part of the text revision of the fourth edition of the *Diagnostic and Statistical Manual of Mental Disorders* (*DSM-IV-TR*). The rating scales used are broad and measure the overall severity of a patient's illness.

A. Global Assessment of Functioning Scale (GAF)
1. Used in Axis V of *DSM-IV-TR*.
2. Used to report a clinician's judgment of a patient's overall level of functioning.
3. Information is used to decide on a treatment plan and later to measure the plan's effect (Table 4–1).

B. Social and Occupational Functioning Assessment Scale (SOFAS)
1. Can be used to track a patient's progress in social and occupational areas.
2. Is independent of the psychiatric diagnosis and the severity of the patient's psychological symptoms (Table 4–2).

C. Global Assessment of Relational Functioning (GARF)
1. Measures the overall functioning of a family or other ongoing relationship (Table 4–3).
2. The development of mental illness is higher in dysfunctional families.
3. Slow recovery in the absence of a supportive social network.

D. Defensive Functioning Scale (DFS)
1. Covers the defense mechanisms used by the patient to cope with stressors (Table 4–4).
2. Humor, suppression, anticipation, and sublimation are among the healthiest defense mechanisms.
3. Denial, acting-out, projection, and projective identification are some of the most pathological defense mechanisms.

III. Other Scales

A. Brief Psychiatric Rating Scale (BPRS)
1. Measures the severity of psychiatric symptomatology.
2. Used as an outcome measure in treatment studies of schizophrenia.
3. Most useful for patients with fairly significant impairment.

Table 4–1
Global Assessment of Functioning (GAF) Scale

Consider psychological, social, and occupational functioning on a hypothetical continuum of mental health–illness. Do not include impairment in functioning due to physical (or environmental) limitations.

Code	**Note:** Use intermediate codes when appropriate, e.g., 45, 68, 72.
100–91	Superior functioning in a wide range of activities, life's problems never seem to get out of hand, is sought out by others because of his or her many positive qualities. No symptoms.
90–81	Absent or minimal symptoms (e.g., mild anxiety before an exam), good functioning in all areas, interested and involved in a wide range of activities, socially effective, generally satisfied with life, no more than everyday problems or concerns (e.g., an occasional argument with family members).
80–71	If symptoms are present, they are transient and expectable reactions to psychosocial stressors (e.g., difficulty concentrating after family argument); no more than slight impairment in social, occupational, or school functioning (e.g., temporarily falling behind in schoolwork).
70–61	Some mild symptoms (e.g., depressed mood and mild insomnia) OR some difficulty in social, occupational, or school functioning (e.g., occasional truancy, or theft within the household), but generally functioning pretty well, has some meaningful interpersonal relationships.
60–51	Moderate symptoms (e.g., flat affect and circumstantial speech, occasional panic attacks) OR moderate difficulty in social, occupational, or school functioning (e.g., few friends, conflicts with peers or coworkers).
50–41	Serious symptoms (e.g., suicidal ideation, severe obsessional rituals, frequent shoplifting) OR any serious impairment in social, occupational, or school functioning (e.g., no friends, unable to keep a job).
40–31	Some impairment in reality testing or communication (e.g., speech is at times illogical, obscure, or irrelevant) OR major impairment in several areas, such as work or school, family relations, judgment, thinking, or mood (e.g., depressed man avoids friends, neglects family, and is unable to work; child frequently beats up younger children, is defiant at home, and is failing at school).
30–21	Behavior is considerably influenced by delusions or hallucinations OR serious impairment in communication or judgment (e.g., sometimes incoherent, acts grossly inappropriately, suicidal preoccupation) OR inability to function in almost all areas (e.g., stays in bed all day; no job, home, or friends).
20–11	Some danger of hurting self or others (e.g., suicide attempts without clear expectation of death, frequently violent, manic excitement) OR occasionally fails to maintain minimal personal hygiene (e.g., smears feces) OR gross impairment in communication (e.g., largely incoherent or mute).
10–1	Persistent danger of severely hurting self or others (e.g., recurrent violence) OR persistent inability to maintain minimal personal hygiene OR serious suicidal act with clear expectation of death.
0	Inadequate information.

The GAF Scale is a revision of the GAS (Endicott J, Spitzer RL, Fleiss JL, Cohen I. The Global Assessment Scale: a procedure for measuring overall severity of psychiatric disturbance. *Arch Gen Psychiatry.* 1976;33:766) and CGAS (Shaffer D, Gould MS, Brasio J, Ambrosini PJ, Fisher PW, Bird HR, Aluwahlia S. Children's Global Assessment Scale (CGAS). *Arch Gen Psychiatry.* 1983;40:1228). They are revisions of the Global Scale of the Health-Sickness Rating Scale (Luborsky I. Clinicians' judgments of mental health. *Arch Gen Psychiatry.* 1962;7:407).
From American Psychiatric Association. *Diagnostic and Statistical Manual of Mental Disorders*, 4th ed. Text rev. Washington, DC: American Psychiatric Association; 2000, with permission.

B. Hamilton Rating Scales for Depression and Anxiety (HAM-D and HAM-A, respectively)

1. Used to monitor the severity of depression and anxiety.

Text continues on page 34.

Table 4–2
Social and Occupational Functioning Assessment Scale (SOFAS)

Consider social and occupational functioning on a continuum from excellent functioning to grossly impaired functioning. Include impairments in functioning due to physical limitations, as well as those due to mental impairments. To be counted, impairment must be a direct consequence of mental and physical health problems; the effects of lack of opportunity and other environmental limitations are not to be considered.

Code	(**Note:** Use intermediate codes when appropriate, e.g., 45, 68, 72.)
100–91	Superior functioning in a wide range of activities.
90–81	Good functioning in all areas, occupationally and socially effective.
80–71	No more than a slight impairment in social, occupational, or school functioning (e.g., infrequent interpersonal conflict, temporarily falling behind in schoolwork).
70–61	Some difficulty in social, occupational, or school functioning, but generally functioning well, has some meaningful interpersonal relationships.
60–51	Moderate difficulty in social, occupational, or school functioning (e.g., few friends, conflicts with peers or coworkers).
50–41	Serious impairment in social, occupational, or school functioning (e.g., no friends, unable to keep a job).
40–31	Major impairment in several areas, such as work or school, family relations (e.g., depressed man avoids friends, neglects family, and is unable to work; child frequently beats up younger children, is defiant at home, and is failing at school).
30–21	Inability to function in almost all areas (e.g., stays in bed all day; no job, home, or friends).
20–11	Occasionally fails to maintain minimal personal hygiene; unable to function independently.
10–1	Persistent inability to maintain minimal personal hygiene. Unable to function without harming self or others or without considerable external support (e.g., nursing care and supervision).
0	Inadequate information.

Note: The rating of overall psychological functioning on a scale of 0–100 was operationalized by Luborsky in the Health-Sickness Rating Scale. (Luborsky L. Clinicians' judgments of mental health. *Arch Gen Psychiatry.* 1962;7:407). Spitzer and colleagues developed a revision of the Health-Sickness Rating Scale called the Global Assessment Scale (GAS) (Endicott J, Spitzer RL, Fleiss JL, Cohen J. The Global Assessment Scale: a procedure for measuring overall severity of psychiatric disturbance. *Arch Gen Psychiatry.* 1976;33:766). The SOFAS is derived from the GAS and its development is described in Goldman HH, Skodol AE, Lave TR. Revising Axis V for *DSM-IV*: a review of measures of social functioning. *Am J Psychiatry.* 1992;149.1148.
From American Psychiatric Association. *Diagnostic and Statistical Manual of Mental Disorders.* 4th ed. Text rev. Washington, DC: American Psychiatric Association; 2000, with permission.

Table 4–3
Global Assessment of Relational Functioning (GARF)

INSTRUCTIONS: The GARF Scale can be used to indicate an overall judgment of the functioning of a family or other ongoing relationship on a hypothetical continuum ranging from competent, optimal relational functioning to a disrupted, dysfunctional relationship. It is analogous to Axis V (Global Assessment of Functioning Scale) provided for individuals in *DSM-IV-TR.* The GARF Scale permits the clinician to rate the degree to which a family or other ongoing relational unit meets the affective and/or instrumental needs of its members in the following areas:

A. *Problem solving*—skills in negotiating goals, rules, and routines: adaptability to stress; communication skills; ability to resolve conflict.

B. *Organization*—maintenance of interpersonal roles and subsystem boundaries; hierarchical functioning, coalitions and distribution of power, control and responsibility.

C. *Emotional climate*—tone and range of feelings; quality of caring, empathy, involvement and attachment/commitment; sharing of values; mutual affective responsiveness, respect, and regard; quality of sexual functioning.

In most instances, the GARF Scale should be used to rate functioning during the current period (i.e., the level of relational functioning at the time of the evaluation). In some settings, the GARF Scale may also be used to rate functioning for other time periods (i.e., the highest level of relational

(continued)

Table 4–3—*continued*
Global Assessment of Relational Functioning (GARF)

functioning for at least a few months during the past year). **Note:** Use specific, intermediate codes when possible, for example, 45, 68, 72. If detailed information is not adequate to make specific ratings, use midpoints of the five ranges, that is, 90, 70, 50, 30, or 10.

(81–100) Overall: Relational unit is functioning satisfactorily from self-report of participants and from perspectives of observers.

Agreed-on patterns or routines exist that help meet the usual needs of each family/couple member; there is flexibility for change in response to unusual demands or events; occasional conflicts and stressful transitions are resolved through problem-solving communication and negotiation.

There is a shared understanding and agreement about roles and appropriate tasks; decision making is established for each functional area, and there is recognition of the unique characteristics and merit of each subsystem (e.g., parents/spouses, siblings, and individuals).

There is a situationally appropriate, optimistic atmosphere in the family; there is a wide range of feelings is freely expressed and managed within the family; there is a general atmosphere of warmth, caring, and sharing of values among all family members. Sexual relations of adult members are satisfactory.

(61–80) Overall: Functioning of relational unit is somewhat unsatisfactory. Over a period of time, many but not all difficulties are resolved without complaints.

Daily routines are present but there is some pain and difficulty in responding to the unusual. Some conflicts remain unresolved, but do not disrupt family functioning.

Decision making is usually competent, but efforts at control of one another quite often are greater than necessary or are ineffective. Individuals and relationships are clearly demarcated but sometimes a specific subsystem is depreciated or scapegoated.

A range of feeling is expressed, but instances of emotional blocking or tension are evident. Warmth and caring are present but are marred by a family member's irritability and frustrations. Sexual activity of adult members may be reduced or problematic.

(41–60) Overall: Relational unit has occasional times of satisfying and competent functioning together, but clearly dysfunctional, unsatisfying relationships tend to predominate.

Communication is frequently inhibited by unresolved conflicts that often interfere with daily routines; there is significant difficulty in adapting to family stress and transitional change.

Decision making is only intermittently competent and effective; either excessive rigidity or significant lack of structure is evident at these times. Individual needs are quite often submerged by a partner or coalition.

Pain or ineffective anger or emotional deadness interferes with family enjoyment. Although there is some warmth and support for members, it is usually unequally distributed. Troublesome sexual difficulties between adults are often present.

(21–40) Overall: Relational unit is obviously and seriously dysfunctional; forms and time periods of satisfactory relating are rare.

Family/couple routines do not meet the needs of members; they are grimly adhered to or blithely ignored. Life cycle changes, such as departures or entries into the relational unit, generate painful conflict and obviously frustrating failures of problem solving.

Decision making is tyrannical or quite ineffective. The unique characteristics of individuals are unappreciated or ignored by either rigid or confusingly fluid coalitions.

There are infrequent periods of enjoyment of life together; frequent distancing or open hostility reflects significant conflicts that remain unresolved and quite painful. Sexual dysfunction among adult members is commonplace.

(1–20) Overall: Relational unit has become too dysfunctional to retain continuity of contact and attachment.

Family/couple routines are negligible (e.g., no mealtime, sleeping, or waking schedule); family members often do not know where others are or when they will be in or out; there is little effective communication among family members.

Family/couple members are not organized in such a way that personal or generational responsibilities are recognized. Boundaries of relational unit as a whole and subsystems cannot be identified or agreed upon. Family members are physically endangered or injured or sexually attacked.

Despair and cynicism are pervasive; there is little attention to the emotional needs of others; there is almost no sense of attachment, commitment, or concern about one another's welfare.

0 Inadequate information.

From American Psychiatric Association. *Diagnostic and Statistical Manual of Mental Disorders.* 4th ed. Text rev. Washington, DC: American Psychiatric Association; 2000, with permission.

Table 4–4
Defensive Functioning Scale

High adaptive level. This level of defensive functioning results in optimal adaptation in the handling of stressors. These defenses usually maximize gratification and allow the conscious awareness of feelings, ideas, and their consequences. They also promote an optimum balance among conflicting motives. Examples of defenses characteristically at this level are

- anticipation
- affiliation
- altruism
- humor
- self-assertion
- self-observation
- sublimation
- suppression

Mental inhibitions (compromise formation) level. Defensive functioning at this level keeps potentially threatening ideas, feelings, memories, wishes, or fears out of awareness. Examples are

- displacement
- dissociation
- intellectualization
- isolation of affect
- reaction formation
- repression
- undoing

Minor image-distorting level. This level is characterized by distortions in the image of the self, body, or others that may be employed to regulate self-esteem. Examples are

- devaluation
- idealization
- omnipotence

Disavowal level. This level is characterized by keeping unpleasant or unacceptable stressors, impulses, ideas, affect, or responsibility out of awareness with or without a misattribution of these to external causes. Examples are

- denial
- projection
- rationalization

Major image-distorting level. This level is characterized by gross distortion or misattribution of the image of self or others. Examples are

- autistic fantasy
- projective identification
- splitting of self-image or image of others

Action level. This level is characterized by defensive functioning that deals with internal or external stressors by action or withdrawal. Examples are

- acting out
- apathetic withdrawal
- help-rejecting complaining
- passive aggression

Level of defensive dysregulation. This level is characterized by failure of defensive regulation to contain the individual's reaction to stressors, leading to a pronounced break with objective reality. Examples are

- delusional projection
- psychotic denial
- psychotic distortion

From American Psychiatric Association. *Diagnostic and Statistical Manual of Mental Disorders.* 4th ed. Text rev. Washington, DC: American Psychiatric Association; 2000, with permission.

2. Are scored from 0 to 4; score totals greater than 9 are considered the borderline of pathology.

3. Useful in measuring the effects of treatment, particularly with pharmacological agents.

C. Scales for the Assessment of Positive Symptoms (SAPS) and Assessment of Negative Symptoms (SANS)

1. Measure negative and positive symptoms of schizophrenia.

2. Used primarily in research to measure change induced by psychopharmacological agents over the course of treatment. (For this scale, see *Kaplan and Sadock: Synopsis of Psychiatry,* 10th ed., pp. 316–317.)

D. Positive and Negative Syndrome Scale (PANSS)

1. Measures negative and positive symptoms of schizophrenia and other psychotic disorders.

2. Has become the standard tool for assessing clinical outcome in treatment studies in schizophrenia.

For further reading on this topic, see Psychiatric Rating Scales, Section 7.10, p. 1032 in CTP/IX.

Laboratory Tests in Psychiatry

Laboratory testing is an integral part of psychiatric assessment and treatment. Compared to other medical specialists, however, psychiatrists depend more on the clinical examination and observation of signs and symptoms to make the diagnosis than they do on laboratory tests. For example, no test can establish or rule out a diagnosis of schizophrenia or mood disorder. Nevertheless, advances in neuropsychiatry and biological psychiatry have made laboratory tests more and more useful to psychiatrists in the management of emotional illness.

I. Neuroendocrine Tests

A. Thyroid function tests

1. Include tests for thyroxine (T_4) by competitive protein binding (T_4D), radioimmunoassay (T_4RIA) involving a specific antigen–antibody reaction, free T_4 index (FT_4I), triiodothyronine uptake, and total serum triiodothyronine measured by radioimmunoassay (T_3RIA).
2. Tests are used to rule out hypothyroidism, which can appear with symptoms of depression.
3. Up to 10% of patients complaining of depression and associated fatigue have incipient hypothyroid disease. Neonatal hypothyroidism results in mental retardation and is preventable if the diagnosis is made at birth.
4. Thyrotropin-releasing hormone (TRH) stimulation test indicated in patients whose marginally abnormal thyroid test results suggest subclinical hypothyroidism, which may account for clinical depression.
5. **Procedure**
   a. At 8 AM, after an overnight fast, have the patient lie down and warn of a possible urge to urinate after the injection.
   b. Measure baseline levels of thyroid-stimulating hormone, triiodothyronine (T_3), thyroxine (T_4), and T_3 resin uptake.
   c. Inject 500 μg of thyroid-releasing hormone intravenously.
   d. Measure thyroid-stimulating hormone levels at 15, 30, 60, and 90 minutes.

B. Dexamethasone suppression test (DST)

1. **Procedure**
   a. Give 1 mg of dexamethasone orally at 11 PM.
   b. Measure plasma cortisol at 4 PM and 11 PM the next day (may also take 8 PM sample).
   c. Any plasma cortisol level above 5 μg/dL is abnormal (although the normal range should be adjusted according to the local assay so that 95% of normals are within the normal range).
   d. Baseline plasma cortisol level may be helpful.

2. Indications

a. To help confirm a diagnostic impression of major depressive disorder. Not routinely used because it is unreliable. Abnormal results may confirm need for somatic treatment.

b. To follow a depressed nonsuppressor through treatment of depression.

c. To differentiate major depression from minor dysphoria.

d. Some evidence indicates that depressed nonsuppressors are more likely to respond positively to treatment with electroconvulsive therapy or tricyclic antidepressants.

e. Proposed utility in predicting outcome of treatment, but DST results may normalize before depression resolves.

f. Proposed utility in predicting relapse in patients who are persistent nonsuppressors or whose DST results revert to abnormal.

g. Possible utility in differentiating delusional from nondelusional depression.

h. Highly abnormal plasma cortisol levels (>10 $\mu g/dL$) are more significant than mildly elevated levels.

3. Reliability.

The problems associated with the DST include varying reports of sensitivity or specificity. False-positive and false-negative results are common. The sensitivity of the DST is considered to be 45% in major depressive disorders and 70% in major depressive episodes with psychotic features. The specificity is 90% compared with controls and 77% compared with other psychiatric diagnoses. Some evidence indicates that patients with a positive DST result (especially 10 $\mu g/dL$) will have a good response to somatic treatment, such as electroconvulsive therapy or cyclic antidepressant therapy.

C. Catecholamines

1. Level of serotonin metabolite 5-hydroxyindoleacetic acid (5-HIAA) is elevated in the urine of patients with carcinoid tumors.

2. Elevated levels are noted at times in patients who take phenothiazine medication and in those who eat foods high in serotonin (i.e., walnuts, bananas, and avocados).

3. The amount of 5-HIAA in cerebrospinal fluid (CSF) is low in some people who are in a suicidal depression and in postmortem studies of those who have committed suicide in particularly violent ways.

4. Low CSF 5-HIAA levels are associated with violence in general.

5. Norepinephrine and its metabolic products—metanephrine, normetanephrine, and vanillylmandelic acid—can be measured in urine, blood, and plasma.

6. Plasma catecholamine levels are markedly elevated in pheochromocytoma, which is associated with anxiety, agitation, and hypertension.

7. High levels of urinary norepinephrine and epinephrine have been found in some patients with posttraumatic stress disorder (PTSD).

8. The norepinephrine metabolic 3-methoxy-4-hydroxyphenylglycol level is decreased in patients with severe depressive disorders, especially in those patients who attempt suicide.

Table 5–1
Other Laboratory Testing for Patients Taking Lithium

Test	Frequency
1. Complete blood count	Before treatment and yearly
2. Serum electrolytes	Before treatment and yearly
3. Fasting blood glucose	Before treatment and yearly
4. Electrocardiogram	Before treatment and yearly
5. Pregnancy testing for women of childbearing age[a]	Before treatment

[a]Test more frequently when compliance with treatment plan is uncertain. Reprinted with permission from MacKinnon RA, Yudofsky SC. *Principles of the Psychiatric Evaluation.* Philadelphia: JB Lippincott; 1991:106.

D. Other endocrine tests. In addition to thyroid hormones, these hormones include the anterior pituitary hormone prolactin, growth hormone, somatostatin, gonadotropin-releasing hormone, and the sex steroids—luteinizing hormone, follicle-stimulating hormone, testosterone, and estrogen. Melatonin from the pineal gland has been implicated in seasonal affective disorder (called *mood disorder with seasonal pattern* in the text revision of the fourth edition of the *Diagnostic and Statistical Manual of Mental Disorders* [*DSM-IV-TR*]).

II. Renal and Hepatic Tests

A. Renal function tests. Serum blood urea nitrogen (BUN) and creatinine are monitored in patients taking lithium (Eskalith). If the serum BUN or creatinine is abnormal, the patient's 2-hour creatinine clearance and, ultimately, the 24-hour creatinine clearance are tested. Table 5–1 summarizes other laboratory testing for patients taking lithium.

B. Liver function tests

1. Total bilirubin and direct bilirubin values are elevated in hepatocellular injury and intrahepatic bile stasis, which can occur with phenothiazine or tricyclic medication and with alcohol and other substance abuse.

2. Liver damage or disease, which is reflected by abnormal findings in liver function tests (LFTs), may manifest with signs and symptoms of a cognitive disorder, including disorientation and delirium.

3. LFTs must be monitored routinely when using certain drugs, such as carbamazepine (Tegretol) and valproate (Depakene).

III. Blood Test for Sexually Transmitted Diseases (STDs)

A. Venereal Disease Research Laboratory (VDRL) test is used as a screening test for syphilis. If positive, the result is confirmed by using the specific fluorescent treponemal antibody-absorption test (FTA-ABS test), in which the spirochete *Treponema pallidum* is used as the antigen.

B. A positive HIV test result indicates that a person has been exposed to infection with the virus that causes AIDS.

IV. Tests Related to Psychotropic Drugs

A. Benzodiazepines

1. No special tests are needed. Among the benzodiazepines metabolized in the liver by oxidation, impaired hepatic function increases the half-life.

2. Baseline LFTs are indicated in patients with suspected liver damage. Urine testing for benzodiazepines is used routinely in cases of substance abuse.

B. Antipsychotics

1. No specific tests are needed, although it is good to obtain baseline values for liver function and a complete blood cell count. Antipsychotics are metabolized primarily in the liver, with metabolites excreted primarily in urine. Many metabolites are active. Peak plasma concentration usually is reached 2 to 3 hours after an oral dose. Elimination half-life is 12 to 30 hours but may be much longer. Steady state requires at least 1 week at a constant dose (months at a constant dose of depot antipsychotics).

2. With the exception of clozapine (Clozaril), all antipsychotics acutely cause an elevation in serum prolactin (secondary to tuberoinfundibular activity). A normal prolactin level often indicates either noncompliance or nonabsorption. Side effects include leukocytosis, leucopenia, impaired platelet function, mild anemia (both aplastic and hemolytic), and agranulocytosis. Bone marrow and blood element side effects can occur abruptly, even when the dosage has remained constant. Low-potency antipsychotics are most likely to cause agranulocytosis, which is most common bone marrow side effect. These agents may cause hepatocellular injury and intrahepatic biliary stasis (indicated by elevated total and direct bilirubin and elevated transaminases). They also can cause electrocardiographic changes (not as frequently as with tricyclic antidepressants), including a prolonged QT interval; flattened, inverted, or bifid T waves; and U waves. Dose-plasma concentration relations differ widely among patients.

3. **Clozapine.** Because of the risk of agranulocytosis (1% to 2%), patients who are being treated with clozapine must have a baseline white blood cell (WBC) and differential count before the initiation of treatment, a WBC count every week throughout treatment, and a WBC count for 4 weeks after the discontinuation of clozapine. Physicians and pharmacists who provide clozapine are required to be registered through Clozaril National Registry (1-800-448-5938).

C. Tricyclic and tetracyclic drugs. An electrocardiogram (ECG) should be given before starting a regimen of cyclic drugs to assess for conduction delays, which may lead to heart blocks at therapeutic levels. Some clinicians believe that all patients receiving prolonged cyclic drug therapy should have an annual ECG. At therapeutic levels, the drugs suppress arrhythmias through a quinidinelike effect.

Blood levels should be tested routinely when using imipramine (Tofranil), desipramine (Norpramin), or nortriptyline (Pamelor) in the treatment of depressive disorders. Taking blood levels may also be of use in patients for whom there is an urgent need to know whether a therapeutic or toxic plasma level of the drug has been reached. Blood level tests should also include the measurement of active metabolites (e.g., imipramine is converted to desipramine, amitriptyline [Elavil] to nortriptyline). Some characteristics of tricyclic drug plasma levels are described as follows.

1. **Imipramine (Tofranil).** The percentage of favorable responses to imipramine correlates with plasma levels in a linear manner between 200 and 250 ng/mL, but some patients may respond at a lower level. At levels that exceed 250 ng/mL, there is no improved favorable response, and side effects increase.

2. **Nortriptyline (Pamelor).** The therapeutic window (the range within which a drug is most effective) of nortriptyline is between 50 and 150 ng/mL. There is a decreased response rate at levels greater than 150 ng/mL.

3. **Desipramine (Norpramin).** Levels of desipramine greater than 125 ng/mL correlate with a higher percentage of favorable responses.

4. **Amitriptyline (Elavil).** Different studies have produced conflicting results with regard to blood levels of amitriptyline, but they range from 75 to 175 ng/mL.

5. **Procedure for determining blood concentrations.** The blood specimen should be drawn 10 to 14 hours after the last dose, usually in the morning after a bedtime dose. Patients must be receiving stable daily dosage for at least 5 days for the test to be valid. Some patients are unusually poor metabolizers of cyclic drugs and may have levels as high as 2,000 ng/mL while taking normal dosages and before showing a favorable clinical response. Such patients must be monitored closely for cardiac side effects. Patients with levels greater than 1,000 ng/mL are generally at risk for cardiotoxicity.

D. **Monamine oxidase inhibitors (MAOIs).** Patients taking MAOIs are instructed to avoid tyramine-containing foods because of the danger of a potential hypertensive crisis. A baseline normal blood pressure (BP) must be recorded, and the BP must be monitored during treatment. MAOIs may also cause orthostatic hypotension as a direct drug side effect unrelated to diet. Other than their potential for causing elevated BP when taken with certain foods, MAOIs are relatively free of other side effects. A test used both in a research setting and in current clinical practice involves correlating the therapeutic response with the degree of platelet MAO inhibition.

E. **Lithium.** Patients receiving lithium should have baseline thyroid function tests, electrolyte monitoring, a WBC count, renal function tests (specific gravity, BUN, and creatinine), and a baseline ECG. The rationale for these tests is that lithium can cause renal concentrating defects, hypothyroidism, and leukocytosis; sodium depletion can cause toxic lithium levels; and approximately 95% of lithium is excreted in the urine. Lithium has also been shown to cause ECG changes, including various conduction defects.

Lithium is most clearly indicated in the prophylactic treatment of manic episodes (its direct antimanic effect may take up to 2 weeks) and is commonly coupled with antipsychotics for the treatment of acute manic episodes. Lithium itself may also have antipsychotic activity. The maintenance level is 0.6 to 1.2 mEq/L, although acutely manic patients can tolerate up to 1.5 to 1.8 mEq/L. Some patients may respond at lower levels, whereas others may require higher levels. A response below 0.4 mEq/L is probably a placebo. Toxic reactions may occur with levels over 2.0 mEq/L. Regular lithium monitoring is essential; there is a narrow therapeutic range beyond which cardiac problems and central nervous system effects can occur.

Lithium levels are drawn 8 to 12 hours after the last dose, usually in the morning after the bedtime dose. The level should be measured at least twice a week while stabilizing the patient and may be drawn monthly thereafter.

F. **Carbamazepine.** A pretreatment complete blood count, including platelet count, should be done. Reticulocyte count and serum iron tests are also desirable. These tests should be repeated weekly during the first 3 months of treatment and monthly thereafter. Carbamazepine can cause aplastic anemia, agranulocytosis, thrombocytopenia, and leucopenia. Because of the minor risk of hepatoxicity, LFTs should be done every 3 to 6 months. The medication should be discontinued if the patient shows any signs of bone marrow suppression as measured with periodic complete blood counts. The therapeutic level of carbamazepine is 8 to 12 ng/mL, with toxicity most often reached at levels of 15 ng/mL. Most clinicians report that levels as high as 12 ng/mL are hard to achieve.

G. **Valproate.** Serum levels of valproic acid (Depakene) and divalproex (Depakote) are therapeutic in the range of 45 to 50 ng/mL. When levels exceed 125 ng/mL, side effects occur, including thrombocytopenia. Serum levels should be obtained periodically, and LFTs should be obtained every 6 to 12 months.

H. **Tacrine (Cognex).** Tacrine may cause liver damage. A baseline of liver function should be established, and follow-up serum transaminase levels should be obtained every other week for approximately 5 months. Patients who develop jaundice or who have bilirubin levels higher than 3 mg/dL must be withdrawn from the drug. It is rarely prescribed because of hepatotoxicity.

V. **Provocation of Panic Attacks with Sodium Lactate**

Up to 72% of patients with panic disorder have a panic attack when administered an intravenous (IV) injection of sodium lactate. Therefore, lactate provocation is used to confirm a diagnosis of panic disorder. Lactate provocation has also been used to trigger flashbacks in patients with PTSD. Hyperventilation, another known trigger of panic attacks in predisposed persons, is not as sensitive as lactate provocation in inducing panic attacks. Carbon dioxide inhalation also precipitates panic attacks in those so predisposed. Panic attacks triggered by sodium lactate are not inhibited by peripherally acting β-blockers but are inhibited by alprazolam (Xanax) and tricyclic drugs.

VI. **Lumbar Puncture**

Lumbar puncture is of use in patients who have a sudden manifestation of new psychiatric symptoms, especially changes in cognition. The clinician should be especially vigilant if there is fever or neurological symptoms, such as seizure. Lumbar puncture is of use in diagnosing central nervous system (CNS) infection (i.e., meningitis).

Table 5–2
Substances of Abuse That Can Be Tested in Urine

Substance	Length of Time Detected in Urine
Alcohol	7–12 hr
Amphetamine	48 hr
Barbiturate	24 hr (short-acting)
	3 weeks (long-acting)
Benzodiazepine	3 days
Cannabis	3 days to 4 weeks (depending on use)
Cocaine	6–8 hr (metabolites 2–4 days)
Codeine	48 hr
Heroin	36–72 hr
Methadone	3 days
Methaqualone	7 days
Morphine	48–72 hr
Phencyclidine (PCP)	8 days
Propoxyphene	6–48 hr

VII. Urine Testing for Substance Abuse

A number of substances may be detected in a patient's urine if the urine is tested within a specific (and variable) period after ingestion. Knowledge of urine substance testing is becoming crucial for practicing physicians in view of mandatory or random substance testing. Table 5–2 provides a summary of substances of abuse that can be tested in the urine.

Laboratory tests are also used in the detection of substances that may be contributing to cognitive disorders.

VIII. Screening Tests for Medical Illnesses

Rule out organic causes for the psychiatric disorder. A thorough screening battery of laboratory tests administered on admission may detect a significant degree of morbidity. See Table 5–3. The routine admission workup includes the following:

A. Complete blood cell count with differential.

B. Complete blood chemistries (including measurements of electrolytes, glucose, calcium, and magnesium and tests of hepatic and renal function).

C. Thyroid function tests.

D. Rapid plasma reagent (RPR) or VDRL test.

E. Urinalysis.

F. Urine toxicology screen.

G. ECG.

IX. Biochemical Markers

Many potential biochemical markers, including neurotransmitters and their metabolites, may help in the diagnosis and treatment of psychiatric disorders. Research in this area is still evolving.

A. **Monoamines**

1. Plasma homovanillic as (pHVA), a major dopamine metabolite, may have value in identifying schizophrenic patients who respond to antipsychotics.

Text continues on page 49.

Table 5–3
Psychiatric Indications for Diagnostic Tests

Test	Indications	Comments
Acid phosphatase	Cognitive/medical workup	Increased in prostate cancer, benign prostatic hypertrophy, excessive platelet destruction, bone disease
Adrenocorticotropic hormone (ACTH)	Cognitive/medical workup	Changed in steroid abuse; may be increased in seizures, psychoses, and Cushing's disease, and in response to stress Decreased in Addison's disease
Alanine aminotransferase (ALT)	Cognitive/medical workup	Increased in hepatitis, cirrhosis, liver metastases Decreased in pyridoxine (vitamin B_6) deficiency
Albumin	Cognitive/medical workup	Increased in dehydration Decreased in malnutrition, hepatic failure, burns, multiple myeloma, carcinomas
Aldolase	Eating disorders Schizophrenia	Increased in patients who abuse ipecac (e.g., bulimic patients), some patients with schizophrenia
Alkaline phosphatase	Cognitive/medical workup Use of psychiatric medications	Increased in Paget's disease, hyperparathyroidism, hepatic disease, liver metastases, heart failure, phenothiazine use Decreased in pernicious anemia (vitamin B_{12} deficiency)
Ammonia, serum	Cognitive/medical workup	Increased in hepatic encephalopathy, liver failure, Reye's syndrome; increases with gastrointestinal hemorrhage and severe congestive heart failure
Amylase, serum	Eating disorders	May be increased in bulimia nervosa
Antinuclear antibodies	Cognitive/medical workup	Found in systemic lupus erythematosus (SLE) and drug-induced lupus (e.g., secondary to phenothiazines, anticonvulsants); SLE can be associated with delirium, psychosis, mood disorder
Aspartate aminotransferase (AST)	Cognitive/medical workup	Increased in heart failure, hepatic disease, pancreatitis, eclampsia, cerebral damage, alcoholism Decreased in pyridoxine (vitamin B_6) deficiency and terminal stages of liver disease
Bicarbonate, serum	Panic disorder	Decreased in hyperventilation syndrome, panic disorder, anabolic steroid abuse
	Eating disorders	May be elevated in patients with bulimia nervosa, in laxative abuse, psychogenic vomiting
Bilirubin	Cognitive/medical workup	Increased in hepatic disease
Blood urea nitrogen (BUN)	Delirium Use of psychiatric medications	Elevated in renal disease, dehydration Elevations associated with lethargy, delirium If elevated, can increase toxic potential of psychiatric medications, especially lithium and amantadine (Symmetrel)

(continued)

Table 5–3—*continued*
Psychiatric Indications for Diagnostic Tests

Test	Indications	Comments
Bromide, serum	Dementia	Bromide intoxication can cause psychosis, hallucinations, delirium
	Psychosis	Part of dementia workup, especially when serum chloride is elevated
Caffeine level, serum	Anxiety/panic disorder	Evaluation of patients with suspected caffeinism
Calcium (Ca), serum	Cognitive/medical workup	Increased in hyperparathyroidism, bone metastases
	Mood disorders	Increase associated with delirium, depression, psychosis
	Psychosis	Decreased in hypoparathyroidism, renal failure
	Eating disorders	Decrease associated with depression, irritability, delirium, chronic laxative abuse
Carotid ultrasonography	Dementia	Occasionally included in dementia workup, especially to rule out multiinfarct dementia
		Primary value is in search for possible infarct causes
Catecholamines, urinary and plasma	Panic attacks Anxiety	Elevated in pheochromocytoma
Cerebrospinal fluid (CSF)	Cognitive/medical workup	Increased protein and cells in infection, positive VDRL in neurosyphilis, bloody CSF in hemorrhagic conditions
Ceruloplasmin, serum; copper, serum	Cognitive/medical workup	Low in Wilson's disease (hepatolenticular disease)
Chloride (Cl), serum	Eating disorders	Decreased in patients with bulimia and psychogenic vomiting
	Panic disorder	Mild elevation in hyperventilation syndrome, panic disorder
Cholecystokinin (CCK)	Eating disorders	Compared with controls, blunted in bulimic patients after eating meal (may normalize after treatment with antidepressants)
CO_2 inhalation; sodium bicarbonate infusion	Anxiety/panic attacks	Panic attacks produced in subgroup of patients
Coombs' test, direct and indirect	Hemolytic anemias secondary to psychiatric medications	Evaluation of drug induced hemolytic anemias, such as those secondary to chlorpromazine, phenytoin, levodopa, and methyldopa
Copper, urine	Cognitive/medical workup	Elevated in Wilson's disease
Cortisol (hydrocortisone)	Cognitive/medical workup Mood disorders	Excessive level may indicate Cushing's disease associated with anxiety, depression, and a variety of other conditions
Creatine phosphokinase (CPK)	Use of antipsychotic agents Use of restraints Substance abuse	Increased in neuroleptic malignant syndrome, intramuscular injection rhabdomyolysis (secondary to substance abuse), patients in restraints, patients experiencing dystonic reactions; asymptomatic elevation with use of antipsychotic drugs

(continued)

Table 5–3—*continued*
Psychiatric Indications for Diagnostic Tests

Test	Indications	Comments
Creatinine, serum	Cognitive/medical workup	Elevated in renal disease (see BUN)
Dopamine (DA) (levodopa stimulation of dopamine)	Depression	Inhibits prolactin Test used to assess functional integrity of dopaminergic system, which is impaired in Parkinson's disease, depression
Doppler ultrasonography	Erectile disorder (ED) Cognitive/medical workup	Carotid occlusion, transient ischemic attack (TIA), reduced penile blood flow in ED
Electrocardiogram (ECG)	Panic disorder	Among patients with panic disorder, 10% to 40% show mitral valve prolapse
Electroencephalogram (EEG)	Cognitive/medical workup	Seizures, brain death, lesions; shortened rapid eye movement (REM) latency in depression High-voltage activity in stupor, low-voltage fast activity in excitement, functional nonorganic cases (e.g., dissociative states); alpha activity present in the background, which responds to auditory and visual stimuli Biphasic or triphasic slow bursts seen in dementia of Creutzfeldt–Jacob disease
Epstein-Barr virus (EBV); cytomegalovirus (CMV)	Cognitive/medical workup	Part of herpesvirus group EBV is causative agent for infectious mononucleosis, which can present with depression, fatigue, and personality change
	Anxiety	CMV can produce anxiety, confusion, mood disorders
	Mood disorders	EBV may be associated with chronic mononucleosislike syndrome associated with chronic depression and fatigue
Erythrocyte sedimentation rate (ESR)	Cognitive/medical workup	An increase in ESR represents a nonspecific test of infectious, inflammatory, autoimmune, or malignant disease; sometimes recommended in the evaluation of anorexia nervosa
Estrogen	Mood disorder	Decreased in menopausal depression and premenstrual syndrome; variable changes in anxiety
Ferritin, serum	Cognitive/medical workup	Most sensitive test for iron deficiency
Folate (folic acid), serum	Alcohol abuse	Usually measured with vitamin B_{12} deficiencies associated with psychosis, paranoia, fatigue, agitation, dementia, delirium
	Use of specific medications	Associated with alcoholism, use of phenytoin, oral contraceptives, estrogen

(continued)

Table 5–3—*continued*
Psychiatric Indications for Diagnostic Tests

Test	Indications	Comments
Follicle-stimulating hormone (FSH)	Depression	High normal in anorexia nervosa, higher values in postmenopausal women; low levels in patients with panhypopituitarism
Glucose, fasting blood (FBS)	Panic attacks Anxiety Delirium	Very high FBS associated with delirium
	Depression	Very low FBS associated with delirium, agitation, panic attacks, anxiety, depression
Glutamyl transaminase, serum	Alcohol abuse	Increased in alcohol abuse, cirrhosis, liver disease
Gonadotropin-releasing hormone (GnRH)	Cognitive/medical workup	Decreased in schizophrenia; increased in anorexia; variable in depression, anxiety
Growth hormone (GH)	Depression Anxiety Schizophrenia	Blunted GH responses to insulin-induced hypoglycemia in depressed patients; increased GH responses to dopamine agonist challenge in schizophrenic patients; increased in some cases of anorexia
Hematocrit (Hct); hemoglobin (Hb)	Cognitive/medical workup	Assessment of anemia (anemia may be associated with depression and psychosis)
Hepatitis A viral antigen (HAAg)	Mood disorders Cognitive/medical workup	Less severe, better prognosis than hepatitis B; may present with anorexia, depression
Hepatitis B surface antigen (HBsAg); hepatitis B core antigen (HBcAg)	Mood disorders Cognitive/medical workup	Active hepatitis B infection indicates greater degree of infectivity and progression to chronic liver disease May present with depression
Holter monitor	Panic disorder	Evaluation of panic-disordered patients with palpitations and other cardiac symptoms
HIV	Cognitive/medical workup	CNS involvement; AIDS dementia organic personality disorder, organic mood disorder, acute psychosis
17-Hydroxycorticosteroid	Depression	Deviations detect hyperadrenocorticalism, which can be associated with major depression Increased in steroid abuse
5-Hydroxyindoleacetic acid (5-HIAA)	Depression Suicide Violence	Decreased in CSF in aggressive or violent patients with suicidal or homicidal impulses May be indicator of decreased impulse control and predictor of suicide
Iron, serum	Cognitive/medical workup	Iron-deficiency anemia
Lactate dehydrogenase (LDH)	Cognitive/medical workup	Increased in myocardial infarction, pulmonary infarction, hepatic disease, renal infarction, seizures, cerebral damage, megaloblastic (pernicious) anemia, factitious elevations secondary to rough handling of blood specimen tube

(continued)

Table 5–3—*continued*
Psychiatric Indications for Diagnostic Tests

Test	Indications	Comments
Lupus anticoagulant (LA)	Use of phenothiazines	An antiphospholipid antibody, which has been described in some patients using phenothiazines, especially chlorpromazine; often associated with elevated PTT; associated with anticardiolipin antibodies
Lupus erythematosus (LE) test	Depression Psychosis Delirium Dementia	Positive test associated with systemic LE, which may present with various psychiatric disturbances, such as psychosis, depression, delirium, dementia; also tested with antinuclear antibody (ANA) and anti-DNA antibody tests
Luteinizing hormone (LH)	Depression	Low in patients with panhypopituitarism; decrease associated with depression
Magnesium, serum	Alcohol abuse Cognitive/medical workup	Decreased in alcoholism; low levels associated with agitation, delirium, seizures
Monoamine oxidase (MAO), platelet	Depression	Low in depression; has been used to monitor MAO inhibitor therapy
MCV (mean corpuscular volume) (average volume of a red blood cell)	Alcohol abuse	Elevated in alcoholism and vitamin B_{12} and folate deficiency
Melatonin	Seasonal affective disorder	Produced by light and pineal gland and decreased in seasonal affective disorder
Metal (heavy) intoxication (serum or urinary)	Cognitive/medical workup	Lead—apathy, irritability, anorexia, confusion Mercury—psychosis, fatigue, apathy, decreased memory, emotional lability, "mad hatter" Manganese—manganese madness, Parkinson-like syndrome Aluminum—dementia Arsenic—fatigue, blackouts, hair loss
3-Methoxy-4-hydroxyphenylglycol (MHPG)	Depression Anxiety	Most useful in research; decreases in urine may indicate decreases centrally; may predict response to certain antidepressants
Myoglobin, urine	Phenothiazine use Substance abuse Use of restraints	Increased in neuroleptic malignant syndrome; in phencyclidine (PCP), cocaine, or lysergic acid diethylamide (LSD) intoxication; and in patients in restraints
Nicotine	Anxiety Nicotine addiction	Anxiety, smoking
Nocturnal penile tumescence	Erectile disorder (ED)	Quantification of penile circumference changes, penile rigidity, frequency of penile tumescence Evaluation of erectile function during sleep Erections associated with REM sleep Helpful in differentiation between organic and functional causes of ED

(continued)

Table 5–3—*continued*
Psychiatric Indications for Diagnostic Tests

Test	Indications	Comments
Parathyroid hormone (parathormone)	Anxiety	Low level causes hypocalcemia and anxiety
	Cognitive/medical workup	Dysregulation associated with wide variety of organic mental disorders
Partial thromboplastin time (PTT)	Treatment with antipsychotics, heparin	Monitor anticoagulant therapy; increased in presence of lupus anticoagulant and anticardiolipin antibodies
Phosphorus, serum	Cognitive/medical workup Panic disorder	Increased in renal failure, diabetic acidosis hypoparathyroidism, hypervitaminosis D; decreased in cirrhosis, hypokalemia, hyperparathyroidism, panic attacks, hyperventilation syndrome
Platelet count	Use of psychotropic medications	Decreased by certain psychotropic medications (carbamazepine, clozapine, phenothiazines)
Porphobilinogen (PBG)	Cognitive/medical workup	Increased in acute porphyria
Porphyria-synthesizing enzyme	Psychosis Cognitive/medical workup	Acute neuropsychiatric disorder can occur in acute porphyria attack, which may be precipitated by barbiturates, imipramine
Potassium (K), serum	Cognitive/medical workup Eating disorders	Increased in hyperkalemic acidosis; increase associated with anxiety in cardiac arrhythmia
		Decreased in cirrhosis, metabolic alkalosis, laxative abuse, diuretic abuse; decrease is common in bulimic patients and in psychogenic vomiting, anabolic steroid abuse
Prolactin, serum	Use of antipsychotic medications	Antipsychotics, by decreasing dopamine, increased prolactin synthesis and release, especially in women
	Cocaine use	Elevated prolactin levels may be seen secondary to cocaine withdrawal
	Pseudoseizures	Lack of prolactin rise after seizure suggests pseudoseizure
Protein, total serum	Cognitive/medical workup	Increased in multiple myeloma, myxedema, lupus
		Decreased in cirrhosis, malnutrition, overhydration
	Use of psychotropic medications	Low serum protein can result in greater sensitivity to conventional doses of protein-bound medications (lithium is not protein bound)
Prothrombin time (PT)	Cognitive/medical workup	Elevated in significant liver damage (cirrhosis)
Reticulocyte count (estimate of red blood cell production in bone marrow)	Cognitive/medical workup	Low in megaloblastic or iron-deficiency anemia and anemia of chronic disease
	Use of carbamazepine	Must be monitored in patient taking carbamazepine
Salicylate, serum	Organic hallucinosis Suicide attempts	Toxic levels may be seen in suicide attempts; may also cause organic hallucinosis with high levels

(continued)

Table 5–3—*continued*
Psychiatric Indications for Diagnostic Tests

Test	Indications	Comments
Sodium (Na), serum	Cognitive/medical workup	Decreased with water intoxication, syndrome of inappropriate secretion of antidiuretic hormone (SIADH) Decreased in hypoadrenalism, myxedema, congestive heart failure, diarrhea, polydipsia, use of carbamazepine, anabolic steroids
	Use of lithium	Low levels associated with greater sensitivity to conventional dose of lithium
Testosterone, serum	Erectile disorder (ED)	Increased in anabolic steroid abuse May be decreased in organic workup of ED
	Inhibited sexual desire	Decrease may be seen with inhibited sexual desire Follow-up of sex offenders treated with medroxyprogesterone Decreased with medroxyprogesterone treatment
Thyroid function tests	Cognitive/medical workup Depression	Detection of hypothyroidism or hyperthyroidism Abnormalities can be associated with depression, anxiety, psychosis, dementia, delirium, lithium treatment
Urinalysis	Cognitive/medical workup Pretreatment workup of lithium Drug screening	Provides clues to cause of various cognitive disorders (assessing general appearance, pH, specific gravity, bilirubin, glucose, blood, ketones, protein); specific gravity may be affected by lithium
Urinary creatinine	Cognitive/medical workup Substance abuse Lithium use	Increased in renal failure, dehydration Part of pretreatment workup for lithium; sometimes used in follow-up evaluations of patients treated with lithium
Venereal Disease Research Laboratory (VDRL)	Syphilis	Positive (high titers) in secondary syphilis (may be positive or negative in primary syphilis); rapid plasma reagent (RPR) test also used Low titers (or negative) in tertiary syphilis
Vitamin A, serum	Depression Delirium	Hypervitaminosis A is associated with a variety of mental status changes, headache
Vitamin B_{12}, serum	Cognitive/medical workup	Part of workup of megaloblastic anemia and dementia
	Dementia	B_{12} deficiency associated with psychosis, paranoia, fatigue, agitation, dementia, delirium
	Mood disorder	Often associated with chronic alcohol abuse
White blood cell (WBC) count	Use of psychiatric medications	Leukopenia and agranulocytosis associated with certain psychotropic medications, such as phenothiazines, carbamazepine, clozapine Leukocytosis associated with lithium and neuroleptic malignant syndrome

Table by Richard B. Rosse, M.D., Lynn H. Deutsch, D.O., and Stephen J. Deutsch, M.D., Ph.D.

2. 3-Methoxy-4-hydroxyphenylglycol (MHPG) is a norepinephrine metabolite.
3. 5-Hydroxyindoleacetic acid is associated with suicidal behavior, aggression, poor impulse control, and depression. Elevated levels may be associated with anxious, obsessional, and inhibited behaviors.

B. Alzheimer's disease

1. Apolipoprotein E allele—associated with increased risk for Alzheimer's disease. Reduced glucose metabolism noted on PET in some asymptomatic middle-aged persons, similar to findings in Alzheimer's patients.
2. Neural thread protein—reported to be increased in patients with Alzheimer's disease. CSF neural thread protein is marketed as a diagnostic test.
3. Other potential CSF tests include CSF tau (increased), CSF amyloid (decreased), ratio of CSF albumin to serum albumin (normal in Alzheimer's disease, elevated in vascular dementia), and inflammatory markers (e.g., CSF acute-phase reactive proteins). The gene for the amyloid precursor protein is considered to be of possible etiological significance, but further research is needed.

For further reading on this topic, see Medical Assessment and Laboratory Testing in Psychiatry, Section 7.8, p. 995 in CTP/IX.

6
Brain Imaging in Psychiatry

I. Introduction

Neuroimaging methodologies allow measurement of the structure, function, and chemistry of the living human brain. Computer tomography (CT) scanners, the first widely used neuroimaging devices, allowed assessment of structural brain lesions, such as tumors or strokes. Magnetic resonance imaging (MRI) scans, developed next, distinguish gray and white matter better than CT scans do and allow visualizations of smaller brain lesions as well as white matter abnormalities. In addition to structural neuroimaging with CT and MRI, a revolution in functional neuroimaging has enabled clinical scientists to obtain unprecedented insights into brain function using positron emission tomography (PET) and single photon emission computer tomography (SPECT).

II. Uses of Neuroimaging

A. Indications for ordering neuroimaging in clinical practice

1. **Neurological deficits.** In a neurological examination, any change that can be localized to the brain or spinal cord requires neuroimaging. Consider neuroimaging for patients with new-onset psychosis and acute changes in mental status.

 CLINICAL HINT:

The clinical examination always assumes priority, and neuroimaging is ordered on the basis of clinical suspicion of a central nervous system (CNS) disorder.

---

2. **Dementia.** The most common cause of dementia is Alzheimer's disease, which does not have a characteristic appearance on routine neuroimaging but, rather, is associated with diffuse loss of brain volume. One treatable cause of dementia that requires neuroimaging for diagnosis is *normal pressure hydrocephalus*, a disorder of the drainage of cerebrospinal fluid (CSF).

3. **Strokes.** Strokes are easily seen on MRI scans. In addition to major strokes, extensive atherosclerosis in brain capillaries can cause countless tiny infarctions of brain tissue; patients with this phenomenon may develop dementia as fewer and fewer neural pathways participate in cognition. This state, called *vascular dementia*, is characterized on MRI scans by patches of increased signal in the white matter.

4. **Degenerative disorders.** Certain degenerative disorders of basal ganglia structures, associated with dementia, may have a characteristic appearance on MRI scans. Huntington's disease typically produces atrophy on the caudate nucleus; thalamic degeneration can interrupt the neural links to the cortex.

Space-occupying lesions can cause dementia and are apparent with neuroimaging techniques (e.g., chronic subdural hematomas, cerebral contusions, brain tumors).

5. **Chronic infections.** Chronic infections, including neurosyphilis, cryptococcosis, tuberculosis, and Lyme disease, may produce a characteristic enhancement of the meninges, especially at the base of the brain. Serological studies are needed to complete the diagnosis. Human immunodeficiency virus (HIV) infection can cause dementia directly, in which case is seen a diffuse loss of brain volume, or it can allow proliferation to the Creutzfeldt–Jakob virus to yield progressive multifocal leukoencephalopathy, which affects white matter tracts and appears as increased white matter signal on MRI scans. Multiple sclerosis plaques are easily seen on MRI scans as periventricular patches of increased signal intensity.

III. Brain Imaging Methods
A. Computed tomography (CT)
1. Clinical indications—dementia or depression, general cognitive and medical workup, and routine workup for any first-break psychosis.
2. Research
   a. Differentiating subtypes of Alzheimer's disease.
   b. Cerebral atrophy in alcohol abusers.
   c. Cerebral atrophy in benzodiazepine abusers.
   d. Cortical and cerebellar atrophy in schizophrenia.
   e. Increased ventricle size in schizophrenia.
B. Magnetic resonance imaging (MRI). Formally called *nuclear magnetic resonance*.
1. Measures radio frequencies emitted by different elements in the brain following application of an external magnetic field and produces slice images.
2. Measures structure, not function.
3. Provides much higher resolution than CT, particularly in gray matter.
4. No radiation involved; minimal or no risk to patients from strong magnetic fields.
5. Can image deep midline structures well.
6. Does not actually measure tissue density; measures density of particular nucleus being studied.
7. A major problem is the time needed to make a scan ($\pm$ 40 minutes).
8. May offer information about cell function in the future, but stronger magnetic fields are needed.
9. The ideal technique for evaluating multiple sclerosis (MS) and other demyelinating diseases.
C. Positron emission tomography (PET)
1. Positron emitters (e.g., carbon 11 or fluorine 18) are used to label glucose, amino acids, neurotransmitter precursors, and many other molecules (particularly high-affinity ligands), which are used to measure receptor densities.

2. Can follow the distribution and fate of these molecules.
3. Produces slice images, as CT does.
4. Labeled antipsychotics can map out location and density of dopamine receptors.
5. Dopamine receptors have been shown to decrease with age (through PET).
6. Can assess regional brain function and blood flow.
7. 2-Deoxyglucose (a glucose analogue) is absorbed into cells as easily as glucose but is not metabolized. Can be used to measure regional glucose uptake.
8. Measure brain function and physiology.
9. Potential for increasing our understanding of brain function and sites of action of drugs.
10. Research.
   a. Usually compares laterality, anteroposterior gradients, and cortical-to-subcortical gradients.
   b. Findings reported in schizophrenia.
      (1) Cortical hypofrontality (also found in depressed patients).
      (2) Steeper subcortical-to-cortical gradient.
      (3) Uptake decreased in left compared with right cortex.
      (4) Higher rate of activity in left temporal lobe.
      (5) Lower rate of metabolism in left basal ganglia.
      (6) Higher density of dopamine receptors (replicated studies needed).
      (7) Greater increase in metabolism in anterior brain regions in response to unpleasant stimuli, but this finding is not specific to patients with schizophrenia.

D. Brain electrical activity mapping (BEAM)
1. Topographic imaging of EEG and evoked potentials.
2. Shows areas of varying electrical activity in the brain through scalp electrodes.
3. New data-processing techniques produce new ways of visualizing massive quantities of data produced by EEG and evoked potentials.
4. Each point on the map is given a numeric value representing its electrical activity.
5. Each value is computed by linear interpolation among the three nearest electrodes.
6. Some preliminary results show differences in schizophrenic patients. Evoked potentials differ spatially and temporally; asymmetric beta-wave activity is increased in certain regions; delta-wave activity is increased, most prominently in the frontal lobes.

E. Regional cerebral blood flow (rCBF)
1. Yields a two-dimensional cortical image representing blood flow to different brain areas.
2. Blood flow is believed to correlate directly with neuronal activity.

3. Xenon 133 (radioisotope that emits low-energy gamma rays) is inhaled. Crosses blood–brain barrier freely but is inert.

4. Detectors measure rate at which xenon 133 is cleared from specific brain areas and compare with calculated control to obtain a mean transit time for the tracer.
   a. Gray matter—clears quickly.
   b. White matter—clears slowly.

5. rCBF may have great potential in studying diseases that involve a decrease in the amount of brain tissue (e.g., dementia, ischemia, atrophy).

6. Highly susceptible to transient artifacts (e.g., anxiety, hyperventilation, low carbon dioxide pressure, high rate of CBF).

7. Test is fast, equipment relatively inexpensive.

8. Low levels of radiation.

9. Compared with PET, spatial resolution less, but temporal resolution is better.

10. Preliminary data show that in schizophrenia patients, CBF in the dorsolateral frontal lobe may be decreased and CBF in the left hemisphere may be increased during activation (e.g., when subjected to the Wisconsin Card Sorting Test).

11. No differences have been found in resting schizophrenic patients.

F. **Single photon emission computed tomography (SPECT)**

1. Adaptation of rCBF techniques to obtain slice tomograms rather than two-dimensional surface images.

2. Presently can obtain tomograms 2, 6, and 10 cm above and parallel to the canthomeatal line.

3. Aids in diagnosis of Alzheimer's disease. Typically shows decrease in bilateral temporoparietal perfusion in Alzheimer's disease and single perfusion defects or multiple areas of hypoperfusion in vascular dementia.

G. **Functional MRI (fMRI)**

1. May provide functional brain images with clarity of MRI.

2. fMRI can be correlated with high-resolution three-dimensional MRI.

3. Schizophrenic patients show less frontal activation and more left temporal activation during a word fluency task in comparison with controls.

4. Used in research clinical settings in other disorders (e.g., panic disorder, phobias, and substance-related disorders).

H. **Magnetic resonance spectroscopy (MRS)**

1. Uses powerful magnetic fields to evaluate brain function and metabolism.

2. Provides information regarding brain intracellular pH and phospholipids, carbohydrate, protein, and high-energy phosphate metabolism.

3. Can provide information about lithium and fluorinated psychopharmacological agents.

4. Has detected decreased adenosine triphosphate and inorganic orthophosphate levels, suggestive of dorsal prefrontal hypoactivity, in schizophrenic patients in comparison with controls.

5. Further use in research is expected with refinements in technique.

I. Magnetoencephalography

1. Research tool.

2. Uses conventional and computerized EEG data.

3. Detects magnetic fields associated with neuronal electrical activity in cortical and deep brain structures.

4. Noninvasive with no radiation exposure.

For further reading on this topic, see Nuclear Magnetic Resonance Imaging and Spectroscopy, Section 1.16, p. 248, and Radiotracer Imaging with Position Emission Tomography and Single Photon Emission Computed Tomography, Section 1.17, p. 273, in CTP/IX.

Delirium and Dementia

I. Delirium

Delirium is defined by the acute onset of fluctuating cognitive impairment and a disturbance of consciousness. Delirium is a syndrome, not a disease, and it has many causes, all of which result in a similar pattern of signs and symptoms relating to the patient's level of consciousness and cognitive impairment.

A. **Epidemiology.** Delirium is a common disorder. According to text revision of the fourth edition of the *Diagnostic Statistical Manual of Mental Disorders* (*DSM-IV-TR*), the point prevalence of delirium in the general population is 0.4% for people 18 years of age and older and 1.1% for people 55 and older. Approximately 10% to 30% of medically ill patients who are hospitalized exhibit delirium. Approximately 30% of patients in surgical intensive care units and cardiac intensive care units and 40% to 50% of patients who are recovering from surgery for hip fractures have an episode of delirium. The highest rate of delirium is found in postcardiotomy patients—more than 90% in some studies. An estimated 20% of patients with severe burns and 30% to 40% of patients with acquired immunodeficiency syndrome (AIDS) have episodes of delirium while they are hospitalized.

B. **Risk factors**
   1. **Advanced age.** A major risk factor for the development of delirium is advanced age. Approximately 30% to 40% of hospitalized patients older than age 65 years have an episode of delirium, and another 10% to 15% of elderly persons exhibit delirium on admission to the hospital.
   2. **Nursing home residents.** Of residents older than age 75 years, 60% have repeated episodes of delirium.
   3. **Pre-existing brain damage.** Such as dementia, cerebrovascular disease, and tumor.
   4. **Other risk factors.** A history of delirium, alcohol dependence, and malnutrition.
   5. **Male gender.** An independent risk factor for delirium.

C. **Etiology.** The major causes of delirium are central nervous system disease (e.g., epilepsy), systemic disease (e.g., cardiac failure), and either intoxication or withdrawal from pharmacological or toxic agents. When evaluating patients with delirium, clinicians should assume that any drug that a patient has taken may be etiologically relevant to the delirium.

D. **Diagnosis and clinical features.** The *DSM-IV-TR* gives separate diagnostic criteria for each type of delirium: (1) delirium due to a general medical condition (Table 7–1), (2) substance intoxication delirium (Table 7–2),

Table 7–1
***DSM-IV-TR* Diagnostic Criteria for Delirium Due to a General Medical Condition**

A. Disturbance of consciousness (i.e., reduced clarity of awareness of the environment) with reduced ability to focus, sustain, or shift attention.
B. A change in cognition (such as memory deficit, disorientation, language disturbance) or the development of a perceptual disturbance that is not better accounted for by a pre-existing, established, or evolving dementia.
C. The disturbance develops over a short period of time (usually hours to days) and tends to fluctuate during the course of the day.
D. There is evidence from the history, physical examination, or laboratory findings that the disturbance is caused by the direct physiologic consequences of a general medical condition.

From American Psychiatric Association. *Diagnostic and Statistical Manual of Mental Disorders.* 4th ed. Text rev. Washington, DC: American Psychiatric Association; 2000, with permission.

(3) substance withdrawal delirium (Table 7–3), (4) delirium due to multiple etiologies (Table 7–4), and (5) delirium not otherwise specified (Table 7–5) for a delirium of unknown cause or of causes not listed, such as sensory deprivation. The syndrome, however, is the same, regardless of cause.

The core features of delirium include

1. **Altered consciousness.** Such as decreased level of consciousness.
2. **Altered attention.** Can include diminished ability to focus, sustain, or shift attention.
3. **Disorientation.** Especially to time and space.
4. **Decreased memory.**
5. **Rapid onset.** Usually hours to days.
6. **Brief duration.** Usually days to weeks.
7. **Fluctuations.**
8. **Sometimes worse at night (sundowning).** May range from periods of lucidity to quite severe cognitive impairment and disorganization.
9. **Disorganization of thought.** Ranging from mild tangentiality to frank incoherence.
10. **Perceptual disturbances.** Such as illusions and hallucinations.
11. **Disruption of the sleep–wake cycle.** Often manifested as fragmented sleep at night, with or without daytime drowsiness.

Table 7–2
***DSM-IV-TR* Diagnostic Criteria for Substance Intoxication Delirium**

A. Disturbance of consciousness (i.e., reduced clarity of awareness of the environment) with reduced ability to focus, sustain, or shift attention.
B. A change in cognition (such as memory deficit, disorientation, language disturbance) or the development of a perceptual disturbance that is not better accounted for by a pre-existing, established, or evolving dementia.
C. The disturbance develops over a short period of time (usually hours to days) and tends to fluctuate during the course of the day.
D. There is evidence from the history, physical examination, or laboratory findings of either (1) or (2):
    1. The symptoms in Criteria A and B developed during substance intoxication.
    2. Medication use is etiologically related to the disturbance.

From American Psychiatric Association. *Diagnostic and Statistical Manual of Mental Disorders.* 4th ed. Text rev. Washington, DC: American Psychiatric Association; 2000, with permission.

Table 7–3
DSM-IV-TR Diagnostic Criteria for Substance Withdrawal Delirium

A. Disturbance of consciousness (i.e., reduced clarity of awareness of the environment) with reduced ability to focus, sustain, or shift attention.

B. A change in cognition (such as memory deficit, disorientation, language disturbance) or the development of a perceptual disturbance that is not better accounted for by a pre-existing, established, or evolving dementia.

C. The disturbance develops over a short period of time (usually hours to days) and tends to fluctuate during the course of the day.

D. There is evidence from the history, physical examination, or laboratory findings that the symptoms in Criteria A and B developed during, or shortly after, a withdrawal syndrome.

Note: This diagnosis should be made instead of a diagnosis of substance withdrawal only when the cognitive symptoms are in excess of those usually associated with the withdrawal syndrome and when the symptoms are sufficiently severe to warrant independent clinical attention.

Code (Specific substance) withdrawal delirium:

(Alcohol; Sedative, hypnotic, or anxiolytic; Other (or unknown) substance)

From American Psychiatric Association. *Diagnostic and Statistical Manual of Mental Disorders.* 4th ed. Text rev. Washington, DC: American Psychiatric Association; 2000, with permission.

Table 7–4
DSM-IV-TR Diagnostic Criteria for Delirium Due to Multiple Etiologies

A. Disturbance of consciousness (i.e., reduced clarity of awareness of the environment) with reduced ability to focus, sustain, or shift attention.

B. A change in cognition (such as memory deficit, disorientation, language disturbance) or the development of a perceptual disturbance that is not better accounted for by a pre-existing, established, or evolving dementia.

C. The disturbance develops over a short period of time (usually hours to days) and tends to fluctuate during the course of the day.

D. There is evidence from the history, physical examination, or laboratory findings that the delirium has more than one etiology (e.g., more than one etiological general medical condition, a general medical condition plus substance intoxication or medication side effect).

Coding note: Use multiple codes reflecting specific delirium and specific etiologies, e.g., Delirium due to viral encephalitis; Alcohol withdrawal delirium.

From American Psychiatric Association. *Diagnostic and Statistical Manual of Mental Disorders.* 4th ed. Text rev. Washington, DC: American Psychiatric Association; 2000, with permission.

Table 7–5
DSM-IV-TR Diagnostic Criteria for Delirium Not Otherwise Specified

This category should be used to diagnose a delirium that does not meet criteria for any of the specific types of delirium described in this section.

Examples include

1. A clinical presentation of delirium that is suspected to be due to a general medical condition or substance use but for which there is insufficient evidence to establish a specific etiology.

2. Delirium due to causes not listed in this section (e.g., sensory deprivation).

From American Psychiatric Association. *Diagnostic and Statistical Manual of Mental Disorders.* 4th ed. Text rev. Washington, DC: American Psychiatric Association; 2000, with permission.

12. **Mood alterations.** From subtle irritability to obvious dysphoria, anxiety, or even euphoria.

13. **Altered neurological function.** For example, autonomic hyperactivity or instability, myoclonic jerking, and dysarthria.

E. **Physical and laboratory examinations.** Delirium is usually diagnosed at the bedside and is characterized by the sudden onset of symptoms. The physical examination often reveals clues to the cause of the delirium. The presence of a known physical illness or a history of head trauma or alcohol or other substance dependence increases the likelihood of the diagnosis.

The laboratory workup of a patient with delirium should include standard tests and additional studies indicated by the clinical situation. In delirium, the EEG characteristically shows a generalized slowing of activity and may be useful in differentiating delirium from depression or psychosis. The EEG of a delirious patient sometimes shows focal areas of hyperactivity.

F. **Differential diagnosis**

1. **Delirium versus dementia.** The developmental time of delirium symptoms is usually short, and, except for vascular dementia caused by stroke, it is usually gradual and insidious in dementia. A patient with dementia is usually alert; a patient with delirium has episodes of decreased consciousness. Occasionally, delirium occurs in a patient with dementia, a condition known as *beclouded dementia*. A dual diagnosis of delirium can be made when there is a definite history of pre-existing dementia. See Table 7–6.

2. **Delirium versus schizophrenia or depression.** The hallucinations and delusions of patients with schizophrenia are more constant and better

Table 7–6
Clinical Differentiation of Delirium and Dementia[a]

	Delirium	Dementia
History	Acute disease	Chronic disease
Onset	Rapid	Insidious (usually)
Duration	Days to weeks	Months to years
Course	Fluctuating	Chronically progressive
Level of consciousness	Fluctuating	Normal
Orientation	Impaired, at least periodically	Intact initially
Affect	Anxious, irritable	Labile but not usually anxious
Thinking	Often disordered	Decreased amount
Memory	Recent memory markedly impaired	Both recent and remote impaired
Perception	Hallucinations common (especially visual)	Hallucinations less common (except sundowning)
Psychomotor function	Retarded, agitated, or mixed	Normal
Sleep	Disrupted sleep–wake cycle	Less disruption of sleep–wake cycle
Attention and awareness	Prominently impaired	Less impaired
Reversibility	Often reversible	Majority not reversible

[a]Demented patients are more susceptible to delirium, and delirium superimposed on dementia is common.

organized than those of patients with delirium. Patients with hypoactive symptoms of delirium may appear somewhat similar to severely depressed patients, but they can be distinguished on the basis of an EEG.

3. **Dissociative disorders.** May show spotty amnesia but lack the global cognitive impairment and abnormal psychomotor and sleep patterns of delirium.

G. **Course and prognosis.** The symptoms of delirium usually persist as long as the causally relevant factors are present, although delirium generally lasts less than a week. After identification and removal of the causative factors, the symptoms of delirium usually recede over a 3- to 7-day period, although some symptoms may take up to 2 weeks to resolve completely. Recall of what occurred during a delirium, once it is over, is characteristically spotty. The occurrence of delirium is associated with a high mortality rate in the ensuing year, primarily because of the serious nature of the associated medical conditions that lead to delirium. Periods of delirium are sometimes followed by depression or posttraumatic stress disorder (PTSD).

H. **Treatment.** The primary goal is to treat the underlying cause. When the underlying condition is anticholinergic toxicity, the use of physostigmine salicylate (Antilirium), 1 to 2 mg intravenously or intramuscularly, with repeated doses in 15 to 30 minutes may be indicated. Physical support is necessary so that delirious patients do not get into situations in which they may have accidents. Patients with delirium should be neither sensory deprived nor overly stimulated by the environment. Delirium can sometimes occur in older patients wearing eye patches after cataract surgery ("black-patch delirium"). Such patients can be helped by placing pinholes in the patches to let in some stimuli or by occasionally removing one patch at a time during recovery.

1. **Pharmacotherapy.** The two major symptoms of delirium that may require pharmacological treatment are psychosis and insomnia. A commonly used drug for psychosis is haloperidol (Haldol), a butyrophenone antipsychotic drug. The initial dose may range from 2 to 6 mg intramuscularly, repeated in an hour if the patient remains agitated. The effective total daily dose of haloperidol may range from 5 to 40 mg for most patients with delirium. Phenothiazines should be avoided in delirious patients because these drugs are associated with significant anticholinergic activity.

   Use of second-generation antipsychotics, such as risperidone (Risperdal), clozapine (Clozaril), olanzapine (Zyprexa), quetiapine (Seroquel), ziprasidone (Geodon), and aripiprazole (Abilify), may be considered for delirium management, but clinical trial experience with these agents for delirium is limited. Insomnia is best treated with benzodiazepines with short or intermediate half-lives (e.g., lorazepam [Ativan] 1 to 2 mg at bedtime). Benzodiazepines with long half-lives and barbiturates should be avoided unless they are being used as part of the treatment for the underlying disorder (e.g., alcohol withdrawal).

II. Dementia

Dementia is defined as a progressive impairment of cognitive functions occurring in clear consciousness (e.g., in the absence of delirium). Global impairment of intellect is the essential feature, manifested as difficulty with memory, attention, thinking, and comprehension. Other mental functions can often be affected, including mood, personality, judgment, and social behavior.

A. **Epidemiology.** The prevalence of dementia is rising. The prevalence of moderate to severe dementia in different population groups is approximately 5% in the general population older than 65 years of age, 20% to 40% in the general population older than 85 years of age, 15% to 20% in outpatient general medical practices, and 50% in chronic care facilities. Of all patients with dementia, 50% to 60% have the most common type of dementia, dementia of the Alzheimer's type (Alzheimer's disease). The second most common type of dementia is vascular dementia, which is causally related to cerebrovascular diseases. Other common causes of dementia, each representing 1% to 5% of all cases, include head trauma, alcohol-related dementias, and various movement disorder–related dementias, such as Huntington's disease and Parkinson's disease.

B. **Etiology.** The most common causes of dementia in individuals older than 65 years of age are (1) Alzheimer's disease, (2) vascular dementia, and (3) mixed vascular and Alzheimer's dementia. Other illnesses that account for approximately 10% include Lewy body dementia; Pick's disease; frontotemporal dementias; normal pressure hydrocephalus (NPH); alcoholic dementia; infectious dementia, such as that due to infection with human immunodeficiency virus (HIV) or syphilis; and Parkinson's disease (Table 7–7).

C. **Diagnosis, signs, and symptoms.** The major defects in dementia involve orientation, memory, perception, intellectual functioning, and reasoning. Marked changes in personality, affect, and behavior can occur. Dementias are commonly accompanied by hallucinations (20% to 30% of patients) and delusions (30% to 40%). Symptoms of depression and anxiety are present in 40% to 50% of patients with dementia. Dementia is diagnosed according to etiology (Table 7–8).

D. **Laboratory tests.** First, identify a potentially reversible cause for the dementia, and then identify other treatable medical conditions that may otherwise worsen the dementia (cognitive decline is often precipitated by other medical illness). The workup should include vital signs, complete blood cell count with differential sedimentation rate (ESR), complete blood chemistries, serum B_{12} and folate levels, liver and renal function tests, thyroid function tests, urinalysis, urine toxicology, ECG, chest roentgenography, computed tomography (CT) or magnetic resonance imaging (MRI) of the head, and lumbar puncture. Single photon emission computed tomography (SPECT) can be used to detect patterns of brain metabolism in certain types of dementia. See Table 7–9.

Table 7–7
Causes of Dementia

Tumor	**Physiologic**
Primary cerebral[a]	Epilepsy[a]
Trauma	Normal-pressure hydrocephalus[a]
Hematomas[a]	**Metabolic**
Posttraumatic dementia[a]	Vitamin deficiencies[a]
Infection (chronic)	Chronic metabolic disturbances[a]
Metastatic[a]	Chronic anoxic states[a]
Syphilis	Chronic endocrinopathies[a]
Creutzfeldt–Jakob disease[b]	**Degenerative dementias**
AIDS dementia complex[c]	Alzheimer's disease[b]
Cardiac/vascular	Pick's disease (dementias of frontal lobe type)[b]
Single infarction[a]	Parkinson's disease[a]
Multiple infarctions[b]	Progressive supranuclear palsy[c]
Large infarction	Idiopathic cerebral ferrocalcinosis (Fahr's
Locunar infarction	disease)[c]
Binswanger's disease	Wilson's disease[a]
(subcortical arteriosclerotic	**Demyelinating disease**
encephalopathies)	Multiple sclerosis[c]
Hemodynamic type[a]	**Drugs and toxins**
Congenital/hereditary	Alcohol[a]
Huntington's disease[c]	Heavy metals[a]
Metachromatic leukodystrophy[c]	Carbon monoxide poisoning[a]
Primary psychiatric	Medications[a]
Pseudodementia[a]	Irradiation[a]

[a] Variable or mixed pattern.
[b] Predominantly cortical pattern.
[c] Predominantly subcortical pattern.
Table by Eric D. Caine, M.D., Hillel Grossman, M.D., and Jeffrey M. Lyness, M.D.

Table 7–8
DSM-IV-TR Diagnostic Criteria for Dementia Due to Other General Medical Conditions

A. The development of multiple cognitive deficits manifested by both
1. memory impairment (impaired ability to learn new information or to recall previously learned information)
2. one (or more) of the following cognitive disturbances:
    a. aphasia (language disturbance)
    b. apraxia (impaired ability to carry out motor activities despite intact motor function)
    c. agnosia (failure to recognize or identify objects despite intact sensory function)
    d. disturbance in executive functioning (i.e., planning, organizing, sequencing, abstracting)
B. The cognitive deficits in Criteria A1 and A2 each cause significant impairment in social or occupational functioning and represent a significant decline from a previous level of functioning.
C. There is evidence from the history, physical examination, or laboratory findings that the disturbance is the direct physiologic consequence of a general medical condition other than Alzheimer's disease or cerebrovascular disease (e.g., HIV infection, traumatic brain injury, Parkinson's disease, Huntington's disease, Pick's disease, Creutzfeldt-Jakob disease, normal-pressure hydrocephalus, hypothyroidism, brain tumor, or vitamin B_{12} deficiency).
D. The deficits do not occur exclusively during the course of delirium.
Code based on presence or absence of a clinically significant behavioral disturbance:
    Without behavioral disturbance: if the cognitive disturbance is not accompanied by any clinically significant behavioral disturbance.
    With behavioral disturbance: if the cognitive disturbance is accompanied by a clinically significant behavioral disturbance (e.g., wandering, agitation).
Coding note: Also, code the general medical condition on Axis III (e.g., HIV infection, head injury, Parkinson's disease, Huntington's disease, Pick's disease, Creutzfeldt-Jakob disease).

From American Psychiatric Association. *Diagnostic and Statistical Manual of Mental Disorders*, text revision, 4th ed. Washington, DC: American Psychiatric Association; 2000, with permission.

Table 7–9
Comprehensive Workup of Dementia

Physical examination, including thorough neurological examination
Vital signs
Mental status examination
Review of medications and drug levels
Blood and urine screens for alcohol, drugs, and heavy metals[a]
Physiological workup
    Serum electrolytes/glucose/Ca^{++}, Mg^{++}
    Liver, renal function tests
    SMA-12 or equivalent serum chemistry profile
    Urinalysis
    Complete blood cell count with differential cell type count
    Thyroid function tests (including TSH level)
    RPR (serum screen)
    FTA-ABS (if CNS disease suspected)
    Serum B_{12}
    Folate levels
    Urine corticosteroids[a]
    Erythrocyte sedimentation rate (Westergren)
    Antinuclear antibody[a](ANA), C_3C_4, Anti-DS DNA[a]
    Arterial blood gases[a]
    HIV screen[a,b]
    Urine porphobilinogens[a]
Chest radiograph
Electrocardiogram
Neurological workup
    CT or MRI of head[a]
    SPECT[b]
    Lumbar puncture[a]
    EEG[a]
    Neuropsychological testing[c]

[a] All indicated by history and physical examination.
[b] Requires special consent and counseling.
[c] May be useful in differentiating dementia from other neuropsychiatric syndromes if it cannot be done clinically.
Adapted from Stoudemire A, Thompson TL. Recognizing and treating dementia. *Geriatrics.* 1981;36:112, with permission.

E. Differential diagnosis

1. **Age-associated memory impairment (normal aging).** There is a decreased ability to learn new material and a slowing of thought processes as a consequence of normal aging. In addition, there is a syndrome of benign senescent forgetfulness, which does not show a progressively deteriorating course.

2. **Depression.** Depression in the elderly may present as symptoms of cognitive impairment, which has led to the term *pseudodementia*. The apparently demented patient is really depressed and responds well to antidepressant drugs or electroconvulsive therapy (ECT). Many demented patients also become depressed as they begin to comprehend their progressive cognitive impairment. In patients with both dementia and depression, a treatment trial with antidepressants is often warranted. ECT may be of help in refractory cases. Table 7–10 differentiates dementia from depression.

Table 7–10
Dementia Versus Depression

Feature	Dementia	Pseudodementia
Age	Usually elderly	Nonspecific
Onset	Vague	Days to weeks
Course	Slow, worse at night	Rapid, even through day
History	Systemic illness or drugs	Mood disorder
Awareness	Unaware, unconcerned	Aware, distressed
Organic signs	Often present	Absent
Cognition[a]	Prominent impairment	Personality changes
Mental status examination	Consistent, spotty deficits	Variable deficits in different modalities
	Approximates, confabulates, perseverates	Apathetic, "I don't know"
	Emphasizes trivial accomplishments	Emphasizes failures
	Shallow or stable mood	Depressed
Behavior	Appropriate to degree of cognitive impairment	Incongruent with degree of cognitive impairment
Cooperation	Cooperative but frustrated	Uncooperative with little effort
CT and EEG	Abnormal	Normal

[a] Benzodiazepines and barbiturates worsen cognitive impairments in the demented patient, whereas they help the depressed patient to relax.

3. **Delirium.** Also characterized by global cognitive impairment. Demented patients often have a superimposed delirium. Dementia tends to be chronic and lacks the prominent features of rapid fluctuations, sudden onset, impaired attention, changing level of consciousness, psychomotor disturbance, acutely disturbed sleep–wake cycle, and prominent hallucinations or delusions that characterize delirium.

F. **Course and prognosis.** Dementia may be progressive, remitting, or stable. Because about 15% of dementias are reversible (e.g., hypothyroidism, central nervous system [CNS] syphilis, subdural hematoma, vitamin B_{12} deficiency, uremia, hypoxia), the course in these cases depends on how quickly the cause is reversed. If the cause is reversed too late, the patient may have residual deficits with a subsequently stable course if extensive brain damage has not occurred. For dementia with no identifiable cause (e.g., dementia of the Alzheimer's type), the course is likely to be one of slow deterioration. The patient may become lost in familiar places, lose the ability to handle money, later fail to recognize family members, and eventually become incontinent of stool and urine.

G. **Treatment.** Treatment is generally supportive. Ensure proper treatment of any concurrent medical problems. Maintain proper nutrition, exercise, and activities. Provide an environment with frequent cues for orientation to day, date, place, and time. As functioning decreases, nursing home placement may be necessary. Often, cognitive impairment may become worse at night (sundowning). Some nursing homes have successfully developed a schedule of nighttime activities to help manage this problem.

1. **Psychological.** Supportive therapy, group therapy, and referral to organizations for families of demented patients can help them to cope and feel less frustrated and helpless.
2. **Pharmacologic.** In general, barbiturates and benzodiazepines should be avoided because they can worsen cognition. For agitation, low doses of an antipsychotic may be effective (e.g., 2 mg of haloperidol orally or intramuscularly or 0.25 to 1.0 mg of risperidone per day orally). However, black box warnings have been issued for conventional and atypical antipsychotics alerting clinicians to reports of elevated mortality in demented, agitated elderly patients treated with these agents. Some studies also question their efficacy. Practice is evolving in this area, as few alternatives are available. When using antipsychotics, use the lowest effective dose and review progress frequently. Some clinicians suggest a short-acting benzodiazepine for sleep (e.g., 0.25 mg of triazolam [Halcion] orally), but this may cause further memory deficits the next day.

III. Dementia of the Alzheimer's Type (DAT)

A. **Definition.** A progressive dementia in which all known reversible causes have been ruled out. Two types—with late onset (onset after age 65) and with early onset (onset before or at age 65).

B. **Diagnosis, signs, and symptoms.** Multiple cognitive deficits with behavioral disturbances. See Table 7–11.

C. **Epidemiology.** Most common cause of dementia. DAT accounts for 50% to 60% of all dementias. May affect as many as 5% of persons over age 65 and 15% to 20% of persons age 85 or older. Risk factors include female sex, history of head injury, and having a first-degree relative with the disorder. Incidence increases with age. Patients with DAT occupy more than 50% of nursing home beds.

 CLINICAL HINT:
DAT patients can be impulsively violent. If agitation is present, be prepared for such events.

D. **Etiology.** Genetic factors play a role; up to 40% of patients have a family history of DAT. Concordance rate for monozygotic twins is 43%, versus 8% for dizygotic twins. Several cases have documented autosomal dominant transmission. Down syndrome is associated with DAT. The gene for amyloid precursor protein on chromosome 21 may be involved. The neurotransmitters most often implicated are acetylcholine and norepinephrine. Both are believed to be hypoactive. Degeneration of cholinergic neurons in the nucleus basalis of Meynert in addition to decreased brain concentrations of acetylcholine and its key synthetic enzyme choline acetyltransferase have been noted. Further evidence for a cholinergic hypothesis includes the beneficial effects of cholinesterase inhibitors and the further impairment

Table 7–11
DSM-IV-TR Diagnostic Criteria for Dementia of the Alzheimer's Type

A. The development of multiple cognitive deficits manifested by both
   1. memory impairment (impaired ability to learn new information or to recall previously learned information)
   2. one (or more) of the following cognitive disturbances:
      a. aphasia (language disturbance)
      b. apraxia (impaired ability to carry out motor activities despite intact motor function)
      c. agnosia (failure to recognize or identify objects despite intact sensory function)
      d. disturbance in executive functioning (i.e., planning, organizing, sequencing, abstracting)
B. The cognitive deficits in Criteria A1 and A2 each cause significant impairment in social or occupational functioning and represent a significant decline from a previous level of functioning.
C. The course is characterized by gradual onset and continuing cognitive decline.
D. The cognitive deficits in Criteria A1 and A2 are not due to any of the following:
   1. other central nervous system conditions that cause progressive deficits in memory and cognition (e.g., cerebrovascular disease, Parkinson's disease, Huntington's disease, subdural hematoma, normal-pressure hydrocephalus, brain tumor)
   2. systemic conditions that are known to cause dementia (e.g., hypothyroidism, vitamin B_{12} or folic acid deficiency, niacin deficiency, hypercalcemia, neurosyphilis, HIV infection)
   3. substance-induced conditions
E. The deficits do not occur exclusively during the course of a delirium.
F. The disturbance is not better accounted for by another Axis I disorder (e.g., major depressive disorder, schizophrenia).
Code based on presence or absence of a clinically significant behavioral disturbance:
   Without behavioral disturbance: if the cognitive disturbance is not accompanied by any clinically significant behavioral disturbance.
   With behavioral disturbance: if the cognitive disturbance is accompanied by a clinically significant behavioral disturbance (e.g., wandering, agitation).
Specify subtype:
   With early onset: if onset is at age 65 years or below
   With late onset: if onset is after age 65 years
Coding note: Also code Alzheimer's disease on Axis III. Indicate other prominent clinical features related to the Alzheimer's disease on Axis I (e.g., mood disorder due to Alzheimer's disease, with depressive features, and personality change due to Alzheimer's disease, aggressive type).

From American Psychiatric Association. *Diagnostic and Statistical Manual of Mental Disorders*, text revision, 4th ed. Washington, DC: American Psychiatric Association; 2000, with permission.

of cognition associated with anticholinergics. Some evidence has been found of a decrease in norepinephrine-containing neurons in the locus ceruleus. Decreased levels of corticotropin and somatostatin may also be involved. Other proposed causes include abnormal regulation of cell membrane phospholipid metabolism, aluminum toxicity, and abnormal brain glutamate metabolism.

E. **Neuropathology.** The characteristic neuropathological changes, first described by Alois Alzheimer, are neurofibrillary tangles, senile plaques, and granulovacuolar degenerations. These changes can also appear with normal aging, but they are always present in the brains of DAT patients. They are most prominent in the amygdala, hippocampus, cortex, and basal forebrain. A definitive diagnosis of Alzheimer's disease can be made only by histopathology. The aluminum toxicity etiological theory is based on the fact that these pathological structures in the brain contain high amounts of aluminum. The clinical diagnosis of DAT should be considered only either possible or probable in Alzheimer's disease. Other abnormalities that have

Table 7–12
Approved Medications for Alzheimer's Disease

Medication	Preparations	Initial Dosage	Maintenance Dosage	Comment
Tacrine (Cognex)	10-, 20-, 30-, and 40-mg capsules	10 mg 4×/day	30 or 40 mg 4×/day	Reversible direct hepatotoxicity in approximately one third of patients, requiring initial biweekly transaminase monitoring. Not commonly used.
Donepezil (Aricept)	5- and 10-mg tablets	5 mg/day	5–10 mg/day	10 mg may be somewhat more efficacious, but with more adverse effects.
Rivastigmine (Exelon)	1.5-, 3.0-, 4.5-, and 6.0-mg capsules	1.5 mg 2×/day	3.0, 4.5, or 6.0 mg 2×/day	Doses of 4.5 mg 2×/day may be most optimal. May be taken with food.
Galantamine (Reminyl)	4-, 8-, and 12-mg capsules; solution, 4 mg/mL	4 mg 2×/day	8 or 12 mg 2×/day	8 mg 2×/day has fewer adverse events.
Memantine (Namenda)	5- and 10-mg tablets	5 mg/day	10 mg 2×/day	10 mg/day was effective in a trial in nursing home patients.
Rivastigmine (Exelon)	1.5-, 3.0-, 4.5-, and 6.0-mg capsules	3–5 mg/day	3–6 mg/day	Transdermal patch preparation (9.5 mg/day) available

been found in DAT patients include diffuse cortical atrophy on CT or MRI, enlarged ventricles, and decreased brain acetylcholine metabolism. The finding of low levels of acetylcholine explains why these patients are highly susceptible to the effects of anticholinergic medication and has led to development of choline-replacement strategies for treatment.

F. Course and prognosis
1. Onset usually insidious in person in their 50s or 60s; slowly progressive.
2. Aphasia, apraxia, and agnosia often present after several years.
3. Motor and gait disturbances may develop later; patient may become bedridden.
4. Mean survival is 8 years; ranges from 1 to 20 years.

G. Treatment. Donepezil (Aricept), rivastigmine (Exelon), galantamine (Reminyl), and tacrine (Cognex) are cholinesterase inhibitors. These drugs can enhance cognition and slow the cognitive decline in some patients with mild to moderate Alzheimer's disease. The last drug introduced, memantine (Namenda), acts on glutamate receptors. None of these alters the underlying disease process. Tacrine is rarely used because of liver toxicity. See Table 7–12.

IV. Vascular Dementia
    A. Definition. The second most common type of dementia is dementia resulting from cerebrovascular disease. Vascular dementia usually progresses

Table 7–13
DSM-IV-TR Diagnostic Criteria for Vascular Dementia

A. The development of multiple cognitive deficits manifested by both
  1. memory impairment (impaired ability to learn new information or to recall previously learned information)
  2. one (or more) of the following cognitive disturbances:
    a. aphasia (language disturbance)
    b. apraxia (impaired ability to carry out motor activities despite intact motor function)
    c. agnosia (failure to recognize or identify despite intact sensory function)
    d. disturbance in executive functioning (i.e., planning, organizing, sequencing, abstracting)
B. The cognitive deficits in Criteria A1 and A2 each cause significant impairment in social or occupational functioning and represent a significant decline from a previous level of functioning.
C. Focal neurologic signs and symptoms (e.g., exaggeration of deep tendon reflexes, extensor plantar response, pseudobulbar palsy, gait abnormalities, weakness of an extremity) or laboratory evidence indicative of cerebrovascular disease (e.g., multiple infarctions involving cortex and underlying white matter) that are judged to be etiologically related to the disturbance.
D. The deficits do not occur exclusively during the course of a delirium.
Code based on predominant features:
  With delirium: if delirium is superimposed on the dementia
  With delusions: if delusions are the predominant feature
  With depressed mood: If depressed mood (including presentations that meet full symptom criteria for a major depressive episode) is the predominant feature. A separate diagnosis of mood disorder due to a general medical condition is not given.
  Uncomplicated: if none of the above predominates in the current clinical presentation
Specify if:
With behavioral disturbance
Coding note: Also code cerebrovascular condition on Axis III.

From American Psychiatric Association. *Diagnostic and Statistical Manual of Mental Disorders,* 4th ed. Text rev. Washington, DC: American Psychiatric Association; 2000, with permission.

in a stepwise fashion with each recurrent infarct. Some patients notice one specific moment when their functioning became worse and improved slightly over subsequent days until their next infarct. Other patients have a progressively downhill course.

B. **Diagnosis, signs, and symptoms.** Multiple cognitive impairments and behavioral changes. Neurological signs are common; small and medium-sized cerebral vessels are usually affected. Infarcts may be caused by occlusive plaque or thromboembolism. Physical findings may include carotid bruit, funduscopic abnormalities, and enlarged cerebral chambers. Cognitive impairment may be patchy, with some areas intact. See Table 7–13.

C. **Epidemiology.** Accounts for 15% to 30% of all dementia; most common in persons 60 to 70 years of age. Less common than DAT. More common in men than in women. Onset is at an earlier age than onset of DAT. Risk factors include hypertension, heart disease, and other risk factors for stroke.

D. **Laboratory tests.** CT or MRI will show infarcts.

E. **Differential diagnosis**
  1. **DAT.** Vascular dementia may be difficult to differentiate from DAT. Obtain a good history of the course of the disease, noting whether the onset was abrupt, whether the course was insidious or stepwise,

and whether neurological impairment was present. Identify vascular disease risk factors and obtain brain image. If a patient has features of both vascular dementia and DAT, then the diagnosis should be dementia with multiple causes.

2. **Depression.** Patients with vascular dementia may become depressed, like patients with pseudodementia, as previously described. Depression is unlikely to produce focal neurological findings. If present, depression should be diagnosed and treated.

3. **Strokes and transient ischemic attacks (TIAs).** Generally do not lead to a progressively demented patient. TIAs are brief episodes of focal neurological dysfunction lasting less than 24 hours (usually 5 to 15 minutes). A patient with a completed stroke may have some cognitive deficits, but unless the loss of brain tissue is massive, a single stroke generally will not cause dementia.

F. **Treatment.** The treatment is to identify and reverse the cause of the strokes. Hypertension, diabetes, and cardiac disease must be treated. Nursing home placement may be necessary if impairment is severe. Treatment is supportive and symptomatic. Antidepressants, psychostimulants, antipsychotic medication, and benzodiazepines can be used, but any psychoactive drug may cause adverse effects in a brain-damaged patient.

V. Pick's disease

This relatively rare primary degenerative dementia is clinically similar to DAT. Pick's disease accounts for approximately 5% of all irreversible dementias. The frontal lobe is prominently involved, and frontal signs of disinhibited behavior may present early. With a relative preservation of cognitive functions, Klüver–Bucy syndrome (hypersexuality, hyperorality, and placidity) is more common in Pick's disease than in DAT. The frontal and temporal lobes show atrophy, neuronal loss, gliosis, and intraneural deposits called *Pick's bodies*. The diagnosis often is made at autopsy, although CT or MRI can reveal prominent frontal lobe involvement.

VI. Prion Disorders

Prion diseases are rapidly progressive degenerative dementing diseases caused by a prion infection. A prion is a replicative protein that, when it mutates, causes a variety of spongiform diseases. Prions can mutate spontaneously, and abnormal prions can be transmitted by the use of contaminated dura mater or corneal grafts, or by ingesting meat from cattle infected with bovine spongiform encephalopathy. Prion disorders are discussed more fully in Chapter 9, Mental Disorders Due to a Medical Condition.

VII. Huntington's Disease

A. **Definition.** A genetic autosomal dominant disease with complete penetrance (chromosome 4) characterized by choreoathetoid movement and dementia. The chance for the development of the disease in a person who has one parent with Huntington's disease is 50%.

B. **Diagnosis.** Onset usually is in a patient's 30s to 40s (the patient frequently already has children). Choreiform movements usually present first and become progressively more severe. Dementia presents later, often with psychotic features. Dementia may first be described by the patient's family as a personality change. Look for a family history.

C. **Associated psychiatric symptoms and complications**
1. Personality changes (25%).
2. Schizophreniform (25%).
3. Mood disorder (50%).
4. Presentation with sudden-onset dementia (25%).
5. Development of dementia in patients (90%).

D. **Epidemiology.** Incidence is two to six cases a year per 100,000 persons. More than 1,000 cases have been traced to two brothers who immigrated to Long Island from England. Incidence is equal in men and women.

E. **Pathophysiology.** Atrophy of brain with extensive involvement of the basal ganglia and the caudate nucleus in particular.

F. **Differential diagnosis.** When choreiform movements are first noted, they are often misinterpreted as inconsequential habit spasms or tics. Up to 75% of patients with Huntington's disease are initially misdiagnosed with a primary psychiatric disorder. Features distinguishing it from DAT are the high incidence of depression and psychosis and the classic choreoathetoid movement disorder.

G. **Course and prognosis.** The course is progressive and usually leads to death 15 to 20 years after diagnosis. Suicide is common.

II. **Treatment.** Institutionalization may be needed as chorea progresses. Symptoms of insomnia, anxiety, and depression can be relieved with benzodiazepines and antidepressants. Psychotic symptoms can be treated with antipsychotic medication, usually of the atypical or second-generation group. Genetic counseling is the most important intervention.

VIII. **Parkinson's Disease**
A. **Definition.** An idiopathic movement disorder with onset usually late in life, characterized by bradykinesia, resting tremor, pill-rolling tremor, masklike face, cogwheel rigidity, and shuffling gait. Intellectual impairment is common, and 40% to 80% of patients become demented. Depression is extremely common.

B. **Epidemiology.** Annual prevalence in the Western Hemisphere is 200 cases per 100,000 persons.

C. **Etiology.** Unknown for most patients. Characteristic findings are decreased cells in the substantia nigra, decreased dopamine, and degeneration of dopaminergic tracts. Parkinsonism can be caused by repeated head trauma and a contaminant of an illicitly made synthetic heroin, N-methyl-4-phenyl-1,2,3,6-tetrahydropyridine (MPTP).

D. **Treatment.** Levodopa (Larodopa) is a dopamine precursor and is often prepared with carbidopa (Sinemet), a dopa decarboxylase inhibitor, to increase brain dopamine levels. Amantadine (Symadine) has also been used synergistically with levodopa. Some surgeons have tried implanting adrenal medulla tissue into the brain to produce dopamine, with equivocal results. Depression is treatable with antidepressants or ECT.

IX. Other Dementias

Other dementias include those associated with Wilson's disease, supranuclear palsy, normal-pressure hydrocephalus (dementia, ataxia, incontinence), and brain tumors.

Systemic causes of dementia include thyroid disease, pituitary diseases (Addison's disease and Cushing's disease), liver failure, dialysis, nicotinic acid deficiency (pellagra causes the three *D*s: dementia, dermatitis, diarrhea), vitamin B_{12} deficiency, folate deficiency, infections, heavy-metal intoxication, and chronic alcohol abuse. See Chapter 9, Mental Disorders Associated with a Medical Condition, for other causes of delirium and dementia.

For a more detailed discussion of this topic, see Delirium, Section 10.2, p. 1153 and Dementia, Section 10.3, p. 1167, in CTP/IX.

8

Amnestic Disorders

I. Introduction
The amnestic disorders are a broad category that includes a variety of diseases and conditions that present with amnesia or loss of memory. Three types exist: (1) amnestic disorder due to a general medical condition (such as head trauma), (2) substance-induced persisting amnestic disorder (such as due to carbon monoxide poisoning or chronic alcohol consumption), and (3) amnestic disorder not otherwise specified (NOS) for cases in which the etiology is unclear. There are two modifiers for this condition: (1) *transient*, for conditions lasting less than 1 month, and (2) *chronic*, for conditions lasting more than 1 month.

II. Epidemiology
A. No adequate studies have reported on incidence or prevalence.
B. Most commonly found in alcohol use disorders and in head injury.
C. Frequency of amnesia related to chronic alcohol abuse has decreased, and the frequency of amnesia related to head trauma has increased.

III. Etiology
Most common form is caused by thiamine deficiency associated with alcohol dependence. May also result from head trauma, surgery, hypoxia, infarction, and herpes simplex encephalitis. Typically, any process that damages certain diencephalic and medial temporal structures (e.g., mammillary bodies, fornix, and hippocampus) can cause the disorder. See Table 8–1.

IV. Diagnosis, Signs, and Symptoms
The essential feature is the acquired impaired ability to learn and recall new information coupled with the inability to recall past events. Impaired recent, short-term memory and long-term memory is caused by systemic medical or primary cerebral disease. Patient is normal in other areas of cognition.

Amnestic disorders are diagnosed according to their etiology: amnestic disorder resulting from a general medical condition, substance-induced persisting amnestic disorder, and amnestic disorder NOS.

V. Clinical Features and Subtypes
A. Impairment in the ability to learn new information (anterograde amnesia).
B. The inability to recall previously remembered knowledge (retrograde amnesia).
C. Short-term and recent memory are usually impaired and patients cannot remember what they had for breakfast or lunch or the name of the doctors.
D. Memory for learned information or events from the remote past, such as childhood experiences, is preserved, but memory for events from the less remote past (the past decade) is impaired.

Table 8–1
Major Causes of Amnestic Disorders

Systemic medical conditions
  Thiamine deficiency (Korsakoff's syndrome)
  Hypoglycemia
Primary brain conditions
  Seizures
  Head trauma (closed and penetrating)
  Cerebral tumors (especially thalamic and temporal lobe)
  Cerebrovascular diseases (especially thalamic and temporal lobe)
  Surgical procedures on the brain
  Encephalitis due to herpes simplex
  Hypoxia (including nonfatal hanging attempts and carbon monoxide poisoning)
  Transient global amnesia
  Electroconvulsive therapy
  Multiple sclerosis
  Prion disorders
Substances
  Alcohol
  Neurotoxins
  Benzodiazepines (and other sedative–hypnotics)
  Many over-the-counter preparations

    E. The onset of symptoms can be sudden, as in trauma, cerebrovascular events, and neurotoxic chemical assaults, or gradual, as in nutritional deficiency and cerebral tumors. The amnesia can be of short duration specified by the *Diagnostic and Statistical Manual of Mental Disorders, Text Revision*, fourth edition (*DSM-IV-TR*) as transient if less than 1 month or chronic if lasting more than 1 month.

    F. Subtle and gross changes in personality can occur and patients may be apathetic, lack initiative, have unprovoked episodes of agitation, or appear to be overly friendly or agreeable. Patients with amnestic disorders can also appear bewildered and confused, and may attempt to cover their confusion with confabulatory answers to questions.

    G. Patients with amnestic disorders do not have good insight into their neuropsychiatric conditions.

VI. Pathophysiology

    A. Structures involved in memory loss include diencephalic structures, such as dorsomedial and midline nuclei of the thalamus and midtemporal lobe structures such as the hippocampus, the mammillary bodies, and the amygdala.

    B. Amnesia is usually the result of bilateral damage to these structures; and left hemisphere may be more critical than the right hemisphere in the development of memory disorders. Many studies of memory and amnesia in animals have suggested that other brain areas may also be involved in the symptoms accompanying amnesia.

    C. Frontal lobe involvement can result in such symptoms as confabulation and apathy, which can be seen in patients with amnestic disorders.

VII. Pathology and Laboratory Examination

A. Laboratory findings diagnostic of amnestic disorder may be obtained using quantitative neuropsychological testing. Standardized tests also are available to assess recall of well-known historical events or public figures to characterize an individual's inability to remember previously learned information.

B. Subtle deficits in other cognitive functions may be noted in individuals with amnestic disorder. Memory deficits, however, constitute the predominant feature of the mental status examination and account largely for any functional deficits. No specific or diagnostic features are detectable on imaging studies, such as magnetic resonance imaging (MRI) or computed tomography (CT). Damage of midtemporal lobe structures is common, however, and may be reflected in enlargement of third ventricle or temporal horns or in structural atrophy detected by MRI.

VIII. Differential Diagnosis

A. Delirium and dementia, involve impairments in many other areas of cognition (e.g., confusion, disorientation).

B. Factitious disorders may simulate amnesia, but the amnestic deficits will be inconsistent. There is often secondary gain to forgetting.

C. Patients with dissociative disorders are more likely to have lost their orientation to self and may have more selective memory deficits than do patients with amnestic disorders. They can also lay down new memories. Dissociative disorders are also often associated with emotionally stressful life events involving money, the legal system, or troubled relationships.

D. The deficits in Alzheimer's disease extend beyond memory to general knowledge (semantic memory), language, praxis, and general function. These are spared in amnestic disorders.

E. The dementias associated with Parkinson's disease, acquired immunodeficiency syndrome (AIDS), and other subcortical disorders demonstrate disproportionate impairment of retrieval but relatively intact encoding and consolidation and, thus, can be distinguished from amnestic disorders.

F. Subcortical pattern dementias are also likely to display motor symptoms, such as bradykinesia, chorea, or tremor, that are not components of the amnestic disorders.

IX. Course and Prognosis

A. Generally, the amnestic disorder has a static course. Little improvement is seen over time, but also no progression of the disorder occurs.

B. Acute amnesias, such as transient global amnesia, resolve entirely over hours to days.

C. Amnestic disorder associated with head trauma improves steadily in the months subsequent to the trauma.

D. Amnesia secondary to processes that destroy brain tissue, such as stroke, tumor, and infection, are irreversible, although, again, static, once the acute infection or ischemia has been staunched.

X. Treatment
   A. Treat the underlying cause of the disorder (e.g., infection, trauma).
   B. Supportive prompts about the date, the time, and the patient's location can be helpful and can reduce the patient's anxiety.
   C. After resolution of the amnestic episode, psychotherapy of some type (cognitive, psychodynamic, or supportive) may help patients incorporate the amnestic experience into their lives.

For a more detailed discussion of this topic, see Amnestic Disorders and Mild Cognitive Impairment, Section 10.4, p. 1198, in CTP IX.

Mental Disorders Due to a Medical Condition

I. Introduction
General medical conditions may cause and be associated with a variety of mental disorders. The psychiatrist should always be aware of (1) any general medical condition that a patient may have and (2) any prescription, nonprescription, or illegal substances that a patient may be taking.

II. Mood Disorder Due to a General Medical Condition
A. Epidemiology
1. Appears to affect men and women equally.
2. As many as 50% of all poststroke patients experience depressive illness. A similar prevalence pertains to individuals with pancreatic cancer.
3. Forty percent of patients with Parkinson's disease are depressed.
4. Major and minor depressive episodes are common after certain illnesses such as Huntington's disease, human immunodeficiency virus (HIV) infection, and multiple sclerosis (MS).

 CLINICAL HINT:
Depressive disorders associated with terminal or painful conditions carry the greatest risk of suicide.

B. Diagnosis and clinical features
1. Patients with depression may experience psychological symptoms (e.g., sad mood, lack of pleasure or interest in usual activities, tearfulness, concentration disturbance, and suicidal ideation) or somatic symptoms (e.g., fatigue, sleep disturbance, and appetite disturbance), or both psychological and somatic symptoms.
2. Diagnosis in the medically ill can be confounded by the presence of somatic symptoms related purely to medical illness, not to depression. In an effort to overcome the underdiagnosis of depression in the medically ill, most practitioners favor including somatic symptoms in identifying mood syndromes (Table 9–1).
C. Differential diagnosis
1. **Substance-induced mood disorder.** Mood disorder due to a general medical condition can be distinguished from substance-induced mood disorder by examination of time course of symptoms, response to correction of suspect medical conditions or discontinuation of substances, and, occasionally, urine or blood toxicology results.

Table 9–1
DSM-IV-TR Criteria for Mood Disorder Due to a General Medical Condition

A. A prominent and persistent disturbance in mood predominates in the clinical picture and is characterized by either (or both) of the following:
 1. Depressed mood or markedly diminished pleasure in all, or almost all, activities
 2. Elevated, expansive, or irritable mood.
B. There is evidence from the history, physical examination, or laboratory findings that the disturbance is the direct physiological consequence of a general medical condition.
C. The disturbance is not better accounted for by another mental disorder (e.g., adjustment disorder with depressed mood in response to the stress of having a general medical condition).
D. The disturbance does not occur exclusively during the course of a delirium.
E. The symptoms cause clinically significant distress or impairment in social, occupational, or other important areas of functioning.
Specify:
With depressive features: if the predominant mood is depressed, but the full criteria are not met for a major depressive disorder
With major depressive-like episode: if all criteria for major depressive episode are met, except, clearly, for the criterion that the symptoms are not due to the physiological effects of a substance or a general medical condition
With manic features: if the predominant mood is elevated, euphoric, or irritable
With mixed features: if the symptoms of mania and depression are present, but neither predominates

From American Psychiatric Association. *Diagnostic and Statistical Manual of Mental Disorders.* 4th ed. Text rev. Washington, DC: American Psychiatric Association; 2000, with permission.

2. **Delirium.** Mood changes occurring during the course of delirium are acute and fluctuating and should be attributed to that disorder.
3. **Pain syndromes.** Pain syndromes can depress mood through psychological, not physiological means, and may appropriately lead to a diagnosis of primary mood disorder.
4. **Sleep disorders, anorexia, and fatigue.** In the medically ill, somatic complaints, such as sleep disturbance, anorexia, and fatigue, may be counted toward a diagnosis of major depressive episode or mood disorder due to a general medical condition, unless those complaints are purely attributable to the medical illness.
D. **Course and prognosis.** Prognosis for mood symptoms is best when etiological medical illnesses or medications are most susceptible to correction (e.g., treatment of hypothyroidism and cessation of alcohol use).
E. **Treatment**
 1. **Pharmacotherapy.** The underlying medical cause should be treated as effectively as possible. Standard treatment approaches for the corresponding primary mood disorder should be used, although the risk of toxic effects from psychotropic drugs may require more gradual dose increases. Standard antidepressant medications, including tricyclic drugs, monoamine oxidase inhibitors (MAOIs), selective serotonin reuptake inhibitors (SSRIs), and psychostimulants, are effective in many patients.
 2. **Psychotherapy.** At a minimum, psychotherapy should focus on psychoeducational issues. The concept of a behavioral disturbance secondary to medical illness may be new or difficult for many patients and

families to understand. Specific intrapsychic, interpersonal, and family issues are addressed as indicated in psychotherapy.

III. Psychotic Disorder Due to a General Medical Condition

To establish the diagnosis of psychotic disorder due to a general medical condition, the clinician first must exclude syndromes in which psychotic symptoms may be present in association with cognitive impairment (e.g., delirium and dementia of the Alzheimer's type). Disorders in this category are not associated usually with changes in the sensorium.

A. Epidemiology

1. The incidence and prevalence in the general population are unknown.
2. As many as 40% of individuals with temporal lobe epilepsy experience psychosis.
3. The prevalence of psychotic symptoms is increased in selected clinical populations, such as nursing home residents, but it is unclear how to extrapolate these findings to other patient groups.

B. Etiology.

Virtually any cerebral or systemic disease that affects brain function can produce psychotic symptoms. Degenerative disorders, such as Alzheimer's disease or Huntington's disease, can present initially with new-onset psychosis, with minimal evidence of cognitive impairment at the earliest stages.

C. Diagnosis and clinical features.

Two subtypes exist for psychotic disorder due to a general medical condition: *with delusions*, to be used if the predominant psychotic symptoms are delusional, and *with hallucinations*, to be used if hallucinations of any form comprise the primary psychotic symptoms (Table 9–2). To establish the diagnosis of a secondary psychotic syndrome, determine that the patient is not delirious, as evidenced by a stable level of consciousness. Conduct a careful mental status assessment to exclude significant cognitive impairments, such as those encountered in dementia or amnestic disorder.

D. Differential diagnosis

1. **Psychotic disorders and mood disorders.** Features may present with symptoms identical or similar to psychotic disorder due to a general medical condition; however, in primary disorders, no medical or substance cause is identifiable, despite laboratory workup.

Table 9–2
DSM-IV-TR Criteria for Psychotic Disorder Due to a General Medical Condition

A. Prominent hallucinations or delusions.
B. There is evidence from the history, physical examination, or laboratory findings that the disturbance is the direct physiological consequence of a general medical condition.
C. The disturbance is not better accounted for by another mental disorder.
D. The disturbance does not occur exclusively during the course of a delirium.
Specify:
With delusions: if delusions are the predominant symptom
With hallucinations: if hallucinations are the predominant symptom

From American Psychiatric Association. *Diagnostic and Statistical Manual of Mental Disorders*. 4th ed. Text rev. Washington, DC: American Psychiatric Association; 2000, with permission.

2. **Delirium.** May be present with psychotic symptoms; however, delirium-related psychosis is acute and fluctuating, commonly associated with disturbance in consciousness and cognitive defects.

3. **Dementia.** Psychosis resulting from dementia may be diagnosed as psychotic disorder due to a general medical condition, except in the case of vascular dementia, which should be diagnosed as vascular dementia with delusions.

4. **Substance-induced psychosis.** Most cases of nonauditory hallucinosis are due to medical conditions, substances, or both. Auditory hallucinations can occur in primary and induced psychoses. Stimulant (e.g., amphetamine and cocaine) intoxication psychosis may involve a perception of bugs crawling under the skin (formication). Diagnosis may be assisted by chronology of symptoms, response to removal of suspect substances or alleviation of medical illnesses, and toxicology results.

E. **Course and prognosis.** Psychosis caused by certain medications (e.g., immunosuppressants) may gradually subside even when use of those medications is continued. Minimizing doses of such medications consistent with therapeutic efficacy often facilitates resolution of psychosis. Certain degenerative brain disorders (e.g., Parkinson's disease) can be characterized by episodic lapses into psychosis, even as the underlying medical condition advances. If abuse of substances persists over a lengthy period, psychosis (e.g., hallucinations from alcohol) may fail to remit even during extended intervals of abstinence.

F. **Treatment.** The principles of treatment for a secondary psychotic disorder are similar to those for any secondary neuropsychiatric disorder, namely, rapid identification of the etiological agent and treatment of the underlying cause. Antipsychotic medication can provide symptomatic relief.

IV. **Anxiety Disorder Due to a General Medical Condition**
The individual experiences anxiety that represents a direct physiological, not emotional, consequence of a general medical condition. In *substance-induced anxiety disorder*, the anxiety symptoms are the product of a prescribed medication or stem from intoxication or withdrawal from a nonprescribed substance, typically a drug of abuse.

A. **Epidemiology**

1. Medically ill individuals in general have higher rates of anxiety disorder than do the general population.

2. Rates of panic and generalized anxiety are especially high in neurological, endocrine, and cardiology patients.

3. Approximately one third of patients with hypothyroidism and two thirds of patients with hyperthyroidism may experience anxiety symptoms.

4. As many as 40% of patients with Parkinson's disease have anxiety disorders. Prevalence of most anxiety disorders is higher in women than in men.

B. **Etiology.** Causes most commonly described in anxiety syndromes include substance-related states (intoxication with caffeine, cocaine,

Table 9–3
DSM-IV-TR Criteria for Anxiety Disorder Due to a General Medical Condition

A. Prominent anxiety, panic attacks, or obsessions or compulsions predominate in the clinical picture.
B. There is evidence from the history, physical examination, or laboratory findings that the disturbance is the direct physiological consequence of a general medical condition.
C. The disturbance is not better accounted for by another mental disorder (e.g., adjustment disorder with anxiety in which the stressor is a serious general medical condition).
D. The disturbance does not occur exclusively during the course of a delirium.
E. The disturbance causes clinical significant distress or impairment in social, occupational, or other important areas of functioning.
Specify:
With generalized anxiety: if excessive anxiety or worry about a number of events or activities predominates in the clinical presentation
With panic attacks: if panic attacks predominate in the clinical presentation
With obsessive-compulsive symptoms: if obsessions or compulsions predominate in the clinical presentation

From American Psychiatric Association. *Diagnostic and Statistical Manual of Mental Disorders*. 4th ed. Text rev. Washington, DC: American Psychiatric Association; 2000, with permission.

amphetamines, and other sympathomimetic agents; withdrawal from nicotine, sedative–hypnotics, and alcohol), endocrinopathies (especially pheochromocytoma, hyperthyroidism, hypercortisolemic states, and hyperparathyroidism), metabolic derangements (e.g., hypoxemia, hypercalcemia, and hypoglycemia), and neurological disorders (including vascular, trauma, and degenerative types). Many of these conditions are either inherently transient or easily remediable.

C. **Diagnosis and clinical features.** Anxiety stemming from a general medical condition or substance may present with physical complaints (e.g., chest pain, palpitation, abdominal distress, diaphoresis, dizziness, tremulousness, and urinary frequency), generalized symptoms of fear and excessive worry, outright panic attacks associated with fear of dying or losing control, recurrent obsessive thoughts or ritualistic compulsive behaviors, or phobia with associated avoidant behavior (Table 9–3).

D. **Differential diagnosis**

1. **Primary anxiety disorders.** Anxiety disorder due to a general medical condition symptomatically can resemble corresponding primary anxiety disorders. Acute onset, lack of family history, and occurrence within the context of acute medical illness or introduction of new medications or substances suggest a nonprimary cause.

2. **Delirium.** Individuals with delirium commonly experience anxiety and panic symptoms, but these fluctuate and are accompanied by other delirium symptoms such as cognitive loss and inattentiveness; furthermore, anxiety symptoms diminish as delirium subsides.

3. **Dementia.** Dementia often is associated with agitation or anxiety, especially at night (called *sundowning*), but an independent anxiety diagnosis is warranted only if it becomes a source of prominent clinical attention.

4. **Psychosis.** Patients with psychosis of any origin can experience anxiety commonly related to delusions or hallucinations.

5. **Mood disorders.** Depressive disorders often present with anxiety symptoms, mandating that the clinician inquire broadly about depressive symptoms in any patient whose primary complaint is anxiety.
6. **Adjustment disorders.** Adjustment disorders with anxiety arising within the context of a psychological reaction to medical or other life stressors should not be diagnosed as anxiety disorder due to a general medical condition.

E. **Course and prognosis**
   1. Medical conditions responsive to treatment or cure (e.g., correction of hypothyroidism and reduction in caffeine consumption) often provide concomitant relief of anxiety symptoms, although such relief may lag behind the rate or extent of improvement in the underlying medical condition.
   2. Chronic, incurable medical conditions associated with persistent physiological insult (e.g., chronic obstructive pulmonary disease) or recurrent relapse to substance use can contribute to seeming refractoriness of associated anxiety symptoms.
   3. In medication-induced anxiety, if complete cessation of the offending factor (e.g., immunosuppressant therapy) is not possible, dose reduction, when clinically feasible, often brings substantial relief.

F. **Treatment.** Aside from treating the underlying causes, benzodiazepines are helpful in decreasing anxiety symptoms; supportive psychotherapy (including psychoeducational issues focusing on the diagnosis and prognosis) may also be useful. More specific therapies in secondary syndromes (e.g., antidepressant medications for panic attacks, SSRIs for obsessive–compulsive symptoms, behavior therapy for simple phobias) may be of use.

V. **Sleep Disorder Due to a General Medical Condition**
   A. **Diagnosis.** Sleep disorders can manifest in four ways: by an excess of sleep (hypersomnia), by a deficiency of sleep (insomnia), by abnormal behavior or activity during sleep (parasomnia), and by a disturbance in the timing of sleep (circadian rhythm sleep disorders). Primary sleep disorders occur unrelated to any other medical or psychiatric illness (Table 9–4).
   B. **Treatment.** The diagnosis of a secondary sleep disorder hinges on the identification of an active disease process known to exert the observed effect on sleep. Treatment first addresses the underlying neurological or medical disease. Symptomatic treatments focus on behavior modification, such as improvement of sleep hygiene. Pharmacological options can also be used, such as benzodiazepines for restless legs syndrome or nocturnal myoclonus, stimulants for hypersomnia, and tricyclic antidepressant medications for manipulation of rapid eye movement (REM) sleep.

VI. **Sexual Dysfunction Due to a General Medical Condition**
   Sexual dysfunction often has psychological and physical underpinnings. *Sexual dysfunction due to a general medical condition* subsumes multiple forms

Table 9–4
DSM-IV-TR Criteria for Sleep Disorder Due to a General Medical Condition

A. A prominent disturbance in sleep that is sufficiently severe to warrant independent clinical attention.
B. There is evidence from the history, physical examination, or laboratory findings that the sleep disturbance is the direct physiological consequence of a general medical condition.
C. The disturbance is not better accounted for by another mental disorder (e.g., an adjustment disorder in which the stressor is a serious medical illness).
D. The disturbance does not occur exclusively during the course of a delirium.
E. The disturbance does not meet the criteria for breathing-related sleep disorder or narcolepsy.
F. The sleep disturbance causes clinically significant distress or impairment in social, occupational, or other important areas of functioning.
Specify type:
Insomnia type: if the predominant sleep disturbance is insomnia
Hypersomnia type: if the predominant sleep disturbance is hypersomnia
Parasomnia type: if the predominant sleep disturbance is a parasomnia
Mixed type: if more than one sleep disturbance is present and none predominate of comparable sexual dysfunction that was not substance induced

From American Psychiatric Association. *Diagnostic and Statistical Manual of Mental Disorders.* 4th ed. Text rev. Washington, DC: American Psychiatric Association; 2000, with permission.

of medically-induced sexual disturbance, including erectile dysfunction, pain during sexual intercourse, low sexual desire, and orgasmic disorders (Table 9–5).

A. Epidemiology

1. Little is known regarding the prevalence of sexual dysfunction due to general medical illness.

Table 9–5
DSM-IV-TR Criteria for Sexual Dysfunction Due to a General Medical Condition

A. Clinically significant sexual dysfunction that results in marked distress or interpersonal difficulty predominates in the clinical picture.
B. There is evidence from the history, physical examination, or laboratory findings that the sexual dysfunction is fully explained by the direct physiological effects of a general medical condition.
C. The disturbance is not better accounted for by another mental disorder (e.g., major depressive disorder).
Select code and term based on the predominant sexual dysfunction:
Female hypoactive sexual desire disorder due to . . . (insert general medical condition here): if deficient or absent sexual desire is the predominant feature.
Male hypoactive sexual desire disorder due to . . . (insert general medical condition here): if deficient or absent sexual desire is the predominant feature.
Male erectile disorder due to . . . (insert general medical condition here): if male erectile dysfunction is the predominant feature.
Female dyspareunia due to . . . (insert general medical condition here): if pain associated with intercourse is the predominant feature.
Male dyspareunia due to . . . (insert general medical condition here): if pain associated with intercourse is the predominant feature.
Other female sexual dysfunction due to . . . (insert general medical condition here): if some other feature is predominant (e.g., orgasmic disorder) or if no feature predominates.
Other male sexual dysfunction due to . . . (insert general medical condition here): if some other feature is predominant (e.g., orgasmic disorder) or if no feature predominates.

From American Psychiatric Association. *Diagnostic and Statistical Manual of Mental Disorders.* 4th ed. Text rev. Washington, DC: American Psychiatric Association; 2000, with permission.

   2. Prevalence rates for sexual complaints are highest for female hypoactive sexual desire and orgasm problems and for premature ejaculation in men.
   3. High rates of sexual dysfunction are described in patients with cardiac conditions, cancer, diabetes, and HIV.
   4. Forty percent to 50% of individuals with MS describe sexual dysfunction.
   5. Cerebrovascular accident impairs sexual functioning, with the possibility that, in men, greater impairment follows right-hemispheric cerebrovascular injury than left-hemispheric injury.
   6. Delayed orgasm can affect as many as 90% of individuals taking SSRIs.
B. Etiology. The type of sexual dysfunction is affected by the cause, but specificity is rare; that is, a given cause can manifest as one (or more than one) of several syndromes. General categories include medications and drugs of abuse, local disease processes that affect the primary or secondary sexual organs, and systemic illnesses that affect sexual organs via neurological, vascular, or endocrinological routes.
C. Course and prognosis. Varies widely, depending on the cause. Drug-induced syndromes generally remit with discontinuation (or dose reduction) of the offending agent. Endocrine-based dysfunctions also generally improve with restoration of normal physiology. By contrast, dysfunctions caused by neurological disease can run protracted, even progressive, courses.
D. Treatment. When reversal of the underlying cause is not possible, supportive and behaviorally oriented psychotherapy with the patient (and perhaps the partner) may minimize distress and increase sexual satisfaction (e.g., by developing sexual interactions that are not limited by the specific dysfunction). Support groups for people with specific types of dysfunctions are available. Other symptom-based treatments can be used in certain conditions; for example, sildenafil (Viagra) administration or surgical implantation of a penile prosthesis may be used in the treatment of male erectile dysfunction. (See Chapter for 18, Sexual Dysfunctions for a further discussion of sexual disorders).

VII. Mental Disorders Due to a General Medical Condition Not Elsewhere Classified
   The *Diagnostic and Statistical Manual of Mental Disorders*, fourth edition, Text Revision (*DSM-IV-TR*) has three additional diagnostic categories for clinical presentations of mental disorders due to a general medical condition that does not meet the diagnostic criteria for specific diagnoses. The first of the diagnoses is catatonic disorder due to a general medical condition (Table 9–6). The second is personality change due to a general medical condition. The third diagnosis is mental disorder not otherwise specified due to a general medical condition (Table 9–7).
   A. Catatonia due to a medical condition. Catatonia can be caused by a variety of medical or surgical conditions. It is characterized usually by

Table 9–6
***DSM-IV-TR* Diagnostic Criteria for Catatonic Disorder Due to a General Medical Condition**

A. The presence of catatonia as manifested by motoric immobility, excessive motor activity (that is apparently purposeless and not influenced by external stimuli), extreme negativism or mutism, peculiarities of voluntary movement, or echolalia or echopraxia.
B. There is evidence from the history, physical examination, or laboratory findings that the disturbance is the direct physiological consequence of a general medical condition.
C. The disturbance is not better accounted for by another mental disorder (e.g., a manic episode).
D. The disturbance does not occur exclusively during the course of a delirium.
Coding note: Include the name of the general medical condition on Axis I, for example, Catatonic disorder due to hepatic encephalopathy; also code the general medical condition on Axis III.

From American Psychiatric Association. *Diagnostic and Statistical Manual of Mental Disorders.* 4th ed. Text rev. Washington, DC: American Psychiatric Association; 2000, with permission.

fixed posture and waxy flexibility. Mutism, negativism, and echolalia may be associated features.

1. **Epidemiology.** Catatonia is an uncommon condition. Among inpatients with catatonia, 25% to 50% are related to mood disorders (e.g., major depressive episode, recurrent, with catatonic features), and approximately 10% are associated with schizophrenia. Data are scant on catatonia's rate of occurrence due to medical conditions or substances.
2. **Diagnosis and clinical features.** Peculiarities of movement are the most characteristic feature, usually rigidity. Hyperactivity and psychomotor agitation can also occur (Table 9–6). A thorough medical workup is necessary to confirm the diagnosis.
3. **Course and prognosis.** The course and prognosis are intimately related to the cause. Neoplasms, encephalitis, head trauma, diabetes, and other metabolic disorders can manifest with catatonic features. If the underlying disorder is treatable, the catatonic syndrome will resolve.
4. **Treatment.** Treatment must be directed to the underlying cause. Antipsychotic medications may improve postural abnormalities even though they have no effect on the underlying disorder. Schizophrenia must always be ruled out in patients who present with catatonic symptoms. ECT has been shown to be a useful method of treatment.

B. **Personality Change Due to a General Medical Condition.** Personality change means that the person's fundamental means of interacting

Table 9–7
***DSM-IV-TR* Diagnostic Criteria for Mental Disorder Not Otherwise Specified Due to a General Medical Condition**

This residual category should be used for situations in which it has been established that the disturbance is caused by the direct physiological effects of a general medical condition, but the criteria are not met for a specific mental disorder due to a general medical condition (e.g., dissociative symptoms due to complex partial seizures).
Coding note: Include the name of the general medical condition on Axis I, for example, mental disorder not otherwise specified due to HIV disease; also code the general medical condition on Axis III.

HIV, human immunodeficiency virus.
From American Psychiatric Association. *Diagnostic and Statistical Manual of Mental Disorders.* 4th ed. Text rev. Washington, DC: American Psychiatric Association; 2000, with permission.

and behaving have been altered. When a true personality change occurs in adulthood, the clinician should always suspect brain injury. However, almost every medical disorder can be accompanied by personality change.

1. **Epidemiology.** No reliable epidemiological data exist on personality trait changes in medical conditions. Specific personality trait changes for particular brain diseases—for example, passive and self-centered behaviors in patients with dementia of the Alzheimer's type—have been reported. Similarly, apathy has been described in patients with frontal lobe lesions.

2. **Etiology**
   a. Diseases that preferentially affect the frontal lobes or subcortical structures are more likely to manifest with prominent personality change.
   b. Head trauma is a common cause. Frontal lobe tumors, such as meningiomas and gliomas, can grow to considerable size before coming to medical attention because they can be neurologically silent (i.e., without focal signs).
   c. Progressive dementia syndromes, especially those with a subcortical pattern of degeneration, such as acquired immunodeficiency syndrome (AIDS) dementia complex, Huntington's disease, or progressive supranuclear palsy, often cause significant personality disturbance.
   d. MS can impinge on the personality, reflecting subcortical white matter degeneration.
   e. Exposure to toxins with a predilection for white matter, such as irradiation, can also produce significant personality change disproportionate to the cognitive or motor impairment.

3. **Diagnosis and clinical features.** The *DSM-IV-TR* diagnostic criteria for personality change due to a general medical condition are listed in Table 9–8.

4. **Course and prognosis.** Course depends on the nature of the medical or neurological insult. Personality changes resulting from medical conditions likely to yield to intervention (e.g., correction of hypothyroidism) are more amenable to improvement than are personality changes due to medical conditions that are static (e.g., brain injury after head trauma) or progressive in nature (e.g., Huntington's disease).

5. **Treatment**
   a. **Pharmacotherapy.** Lithium carbonate (Eskalith), carbamazepine (Tegretol), and valproic acid (Depakote) have been used for the control of affective lability and impulsivity. Aggression or explosiveness can be treated with lithium, anticonvulsant medications, or a combination of lithium and an anticonvulsant agent. Centrally active β-adrenergic receptor antagonists, such as propranolol (Inderal), have some efficacy as well. Apathy and inertia have occasionally improved with psychostimulant agents.

Table 9–8
DSM-IV-TR Diagnostic Criteria for Personality Change Due to a General Medical Condition

A. A persistent personality disturbance that represents a change from the individual's previous characteristic personality pattern. (In children, the disturbance involves a marked deviation from normal development or a significant change in the child's usual behavior patterns lasting at least 1 year.)
B. There is evidence from the history, physical examination, or laboratory findings that the disturbance is the direct physiological consequence of a general medical condition.
C. The disturbance is not better accounted for by another mental disorder (including other mental disorders due to a general medical condition).
D. The disturbance does not occur exclusively during the course of a delirium.
E. The disturbance causes clinically significant distress or impairment in social, occupational, or other important areas of functioning.
Specify type:
Labile type: if the predominant feature is affective lability
Disinhibited type: if the predominant feature is poor impulse control as evidenced by sexual indiscretions, etc.
Aggressive type: if the predominant feature is aggressive behavior
Apathetic type: if the predominant feature is marked apathy and indifference
Paranoid type: if the predominant feature is suspiciousness or paranoid ideation
Other type: if the presentation is not characterized by any of the above subtypes
Combined type: if more than one feature predominates in the clinical picture
Unspecified type
Coding note: Include the name of the general medical condition on Axis I, for example, personality change due to temporal lobe epilepsy; also code the general medical condition on Axis III.

From American Psychiatric Association. *Diagnostic and Statistical Manual of Mental Disorders.* 4th ed. Text rev. Washington, DC: American Psychiatric Association; 2000, with permission.

b. Psychotherapy. Families should be involved in the therapy process, with a focus on education and understanding the origins of the patient's inappropriate behaviors. Issues such as competency, disability, and advocacy are frequently of clinical concern with these patients in light of the unpredictable and pervasive behavior change.

VIII. Specific Disorders

A. Epilepsy

1. Ictal and postictal confusional syndromes.
2. Prevalence of psychosis in epilepsy is 7%.
3. Epilepsy is three to seven times more common in psychotic patients.
4. Lifetime prevalence of psychosis in patients with epilepsy is 10%.
5. Seizures versus pseudoseizures (Table 9–9).
6. Temporal lobe epilepsy (TLE)
   a. TLE is the most likely type to produce psychiatric symptoms.
   b. Often involves schizophrenialike psychosis.
   c. Often difficult to distinguish from schizophrenia with aggressiveness.
   d. Varied and complex auras that may masquerade as functional illness (e.g., hallucinations, depersonalization, derealization).
   e. Automatisms, autonomic effects, and visceral sensations (e.g., epigastric aura, stomach churning, salivation, flushing, tachycardia, dizziness).

Table 9–9
Clinical Features Distinguishing Seizures and Pseudoseizures*ᵃ*

Features	Seizure	Pseudoseizure
Aura	Common stereotyped	Rare
Timing	Nocturnal common	Only when awake
Incontinence	Common	Rare
Cyanosis	Common	Rare
Postictal confusion	Yes	No
Body movement	Tonic or clonic	Nonstereotyped and asynchronous
Self-injury	Common	Rare
EEG	May be abnormal	Normal
Affected by suggestion	No	Yes
Secondary gain	No	Yes

*ᵃ*Some patients with organic seizure disorders may also have pseudoseizures.

    f. Altered perceptual experiences (e.g., distortions, hallucinations, depersonalization, feeling remote, feeling something has a peculiar significance [*déjà vu, jamais vu*]).
    g. Hallucinations of taste and smell are common and may be accompanied by lip smacking or pursing, chewing, or tasting and swallowing movements.
    h. Subjective disorders of thinking and memory.
    i. Strong affective experiences, most commonly fear and anxiety.

 CLINICAL HINT:
If patient complains of only smelling bad odors (burning hair, feces), then TLE is the most likely diagnosis.

B. Brain tumors
    1. Neurological signs, headache, nausea, vomiting, seizures, visual loss, papilledema, virtually any psychiatric symptoms are possible.
    2. Symptoms often are caused by raised intracranial pressure or mass effects rather than by direct effects of tumor.
    3. Suicidal ideation is present in 10% of patients, usually during headache paroxysms.
    4. Slow tumors produce personality change. Rapid tumors produce cognitive change.
    5. Frontal lobe tumors—depression, inappropriate affect, disinhibition, dementia, impaired coordination, psychotic symptoms. Often misdiagnosed as primary degenerative dementia; neurological signs often are absent. May have bowel or bladder incontinence.
    6. Temporal lobe tumors—anxiety, depression, hallucinations (especially gustatory and olfactory), TLE symptoms, schizophrenialike psychosis. May have impaired memory and speech.
    7. Parietal lobe tumors—fewer psychiatric symptoms (anosognosia, apraxia, aphasia); may be mistaken for hysteria.

Table 9–10
***DSM-IV-TR* Research Criteria for Postconcussional Disorder**

A. A history of head trauma that has caused significant cerebral concussion.
   Note: The manifestations of concussion include loss of consciousness, posttraumatic amnesia, and, less commonly, posttraumatic onset of seizures. The specific method of defining this criterion needs to be established by further research.
B. Evidence from neuropsychological testing or quantified cognitive assessment of difficulty in attention (concentrating, shifting focus of attention, performing simultaneous cognitive tasks) or memory (learning or recalling information).
C. Three (or more) of the following occur shortly after the trauma and last at least 3 months:
   1. becoming fatigued easily
   2. disordered sleep
   3. headache
   4. vertigo or dizziness
   5. irritability or aggression on little or no provocation
   6. anxiety, depression, or affective lability
   7. changes in personality (e.g., social or sexual inappropriateness)
   8. apathy or lack of spontaneity
D. The symptoms in Criteria B and C have their onset following head trauma or else represent a substantial worsening of pre-existing symptoms.
E. The disturbance causes significant impairment in social or occupational functioning and represents a significant decline from a previous level of functioning. In school-aged children, the impairment may be manifested by a significant worsening in school or academic performance dating from the trauma.
F. The symptoms do not meet criteria for dementia due to head trauma and are not better accounted for by another mental disorder (e.g., amnestic disorder due to head trauma, personality change due to head trauma).

From American Psychiatric Association. *Diagnostic and Statistical Manual of Mental Disorders.* 4th ed. Text rev. Washington, DC: American Psychiatric Association; 2000, with permission.

8. Colloid cysts—not a tumor. Located in third ventricle and can place pressure on diencephalon. Can produce depression, psychosis, mood lability, and personality change. Classically produces position-dependent intermittent headaches.

C. Head trauma. Head trauma can result in an array of mental symptoms (Table 9–10).

  1. Pathophysiology

    a. An estimated 2 million incidents involve head trauma each year.

    b. Most commonly occurs in people 15 to 25 years of age and has a male-to-female predominance of approximately 3 to 1.

    c. Virtually all patients with serious head trauma, more than half of patients with moderate head trauma, and about 10% of patients with mild head trauma have ongoing neuropsychiatric sequelae resulting from the head trauma.

  2. Symptoms. The most common cognitive problems are decreased speed in information processing, decreased attention, increased distractibility, deficits in problem solving and in the ability to sustain effort, and problems with memory and learning new information. A variety of language disabilities can also occur. Behaviorally, the major symptoms involve depression, increased impulsivity, increased aggression, and changes in personality.

3. **Treatment.** Standard antidepressants can be used to treat depression, and either anticonvulsants or antipsychotics can be used to treat aggression and impulsivity. Other approaches to the symptoms include lithium, calcium channel blockers, and β-adrenergic receptor antagonists. Clinicians must support patients through individual or group psychotherapy and should support the major caretakers through couples and family therapy. All involved parties need help to adjust to any changes in the patient's personality and mental abilities.

D. **Demyelinating disorders**
   1. **Multiple sclerosis**
      a. More common in Northern Hemisphere.
      b. Psychiatric changes are common (75%).
      c. Depression is seen early in course.
      d. With frontal lobe involvement, disinhibition and maniclike symptoms occur, including euphoria.
      e. Intellectual deterioration is common (60%), ranging from mild memory loss to dementia.
      f. Psychosis is reported, but rates are unclear.
      g. Hysteria is common, especially late in disease.
      h. Symptoms are exacerbated by physical or emotional trauma.
      i. MRI is needed for workup.
   2. **Amyotrophic lateral sclerosis (ALS)**
      a. Rare progressive noninherited disease causing asymmetric muscle atrophy.
      b. Atrophy of all muscle except cardiac and ocular.
      c. Deterioration of anterior horn cells.
      d. Rapidly progressive, usually fatal within 4 years.
      e. Concomitant dementia rare. Patients with pseudobulbar palsy may show emotional lability.

E. **Infectious diseases**
   1. **Herpes simplex encephalitis**
      a. Most commonly affects the frontal and temporal lobes.
      b. Symptoms often include anosmia, olfactory and gustatory hallucinations, and personality changes and can also involve bizarre or psychotic behaviors.
      c. Complex partial epilepsy may also develop in patients with herpes simplex encephalitis.
      d. Although the mortality rate for the infection has decreased, many patients exhibit personality changes, symptoms of memory loss, and psychotic symptoms.
   2. **Rabies encephalitis**
      a. The incubation period ranges from 10 days to 1 year, after which symptoms of restlessness, overactivity, and agitation can develop.
      b. Hydrophobia, present in up to 50% of patients.
      c. Is fatal within days or weeks.

3. **Neurosyphilis (general paresis)**
   a. Appears 10 to 15 years after the primary *Treponema* infection.
   b. Penicillin has made it a rare disorder, although AIDS is associated with reintroducing neurosyphilis into medical practice in some urban settings.
   c. Generally affects the frontal lobes and results in personality changes, development of poor judgment, irritability, and decreased care for self.
   d. Delusions of grandeur develop in 10% to 20% of affected patients.
   e. Progresses with the development of dementia and tremor, until patients are paretic.
4. **Chronic meningitis.** Now seen more often than in the recent past because of the immunocompromised condition of people with AIDS. The usual causative agents are *Mycobacterium tuberculosis*, *Cryptococcus*, and *Coccidioides*. The usual symptoms are headache, memory impairment, confusion, and fever.
5. **Lyme disease**
   a. Caused by infection with the spirochete *Borrelia burgdorferi* transmitted through the bite of the deer tick (*Ixodes scapularis*).
   b. About 16,000 cases are reported annually in the United States.
   c. Associated with impaired cognitive functioning and mood changes (i.e., memory lapses, difficulty concentrating, irritability, depression).
   d. No clear-cut diagnostic test is available.
   e. About 50% of patients become seropositive to *B. burgdorferi*.
   f. Treatment consists of a 14- to 21-day course of doxycycline (Vibramycin).
   g. Specific psychotropic drugs can be targeted to treat the psychiatric sign or symptom (e.g., diazepam [Valium] for anxiety).
   h. Approximately 60% of persons develop a chronic condition if left untreated.
   i. Support groups provide emotional support that help improve quality of life.
6. **Prion disease.** Prion disease is a group of related disorders caused by a transmissible infectious protein known as a *prion*. Included in this group are Creutzfeldt–Jakob disease (CJD), Gerstmann–Straussler syndrome (GSS), fatal familial insomnia (FFI), and kuru. Collectively, these disorders are also known as *subacute spongiform encephalopathy* because of shared neuropathological changes that consist of (1) spongiform vacuolization, (2) neuronal loss, and (3) astrocyte proliferation in the cerebral cortex. Amyloid plaques may or may not be present.
   a. **Etiology.** Prions are mutated proteins generated from the human prion protein gene (PrP), which is located on the short arm of chromosome 20. The PrP mutates into a disease-related isoform PrP-Super-C (PrP^{Sc}) that can replicate and is infectious. The

neuropathological changes that occur in prion disease are presumed to be caused by direct neurotoxic effects of PrP^{Sc}.

    b. Creutzfeldt–Jakob disease. Psychiatric manifestations are protean and include emotional lability, anxiety, euphoria, depression, delusions, hallucinations, or marked personality changes. The disease progresses over months, leading to dementia, akinetic mutism, coma, and death. The rates of CJD range from 1 to 2 cases per 1 million persons a year, worldwide.

    c. Variant CJD. The psychiatric presentation of vCJD is not specific. Most patients reported depression, withdrawal, anxiety, and sleep disturbance. Paranoid delusions have occurred. No cure exists, and death usually occurs within 2 to 3 years after diagnosis. Prevention is dependent on careful monitoring of cattle for disease and feeding them grain instead of meat by-products.

    d. Kuru. Found in New Guinea and is caused by cannibalistic funeral rituals in which the brains of the deceased are eaten. The cerebellum is most affected. Since the cessation of cannibalism in New Guinea, the incidence of the disease has decreased drastically.

    e. Gerstmann–Straussler–Scheinker disease. Is characterized by ataxia, chorea, and cognitive decline leading to dementia. The disease is inherited and genetic testing can confirm the presence of the abnormal genes before onset. Onset of the disease occurs between 30 and 40 years of age and is fatal within 5 years of onset.

    f. Fatal familial insomnia. A syndrome of insomnia and autonomic nervous system dysfunction consisting of fever, sweating, labile blood pressure, and tachycardia occurs that results in death.

F. Immune disorders

    1. Systemic lupus erythematosus. An autoimmune disease that involves inflammation of multiple organ systems. Between 5% and 50% of patients have mental symptoms at the initial presentation, and approximately 50% eventually show neuropsychiatric manifestations. The major symptoms are depression, insomnia, emotional lability, nervousness, and confusion. Treatment with steroids commonly induces further psychiatric complications, including mania and psychosis.

G. Endocrine disorders

    1. Thyroid disorders. Hyperthyroidism is characterized by confusion, anxiety, and an agitated, depressive syndrome. Patients may also complain of being easily fatigued and of feeling generally weak. Insomnia, weight loss despite increased appetite, tremulousness, palpitations, and increased perspiration are also common symptoms. Serious psychiatric symptoms include impairments in memory, orientation, and judgment; manic excitement; delusions; and hallucinations.

    2. Parathyroid disorders

        a. Dysfunction of the parathyroid gland results in the abnormal regulation of calcium metabolism.

  b. Excessive secretion of parathyroid hormone causes hypercalcemia, which can result in delirium, personality changes, and apathy in 50% to 60% of patients and cognitive impairments in approximately 25% of patients.

  c. Neuromuscular excitability, which depends on proper calcium ion concentration, is reduced, and muscle weakness may appear.

  d. Hypocalcemia can occur with hypoparathyroid disorders and can result in neuropsychiatric symptoms of delirium and personality changes.

  e. Other symptoms of hypocalcemia are cataract formation, seizures, extrapyramidal symptoms, and increased intracranial pressure.

3. Adrenal disorders

  a. Addison's disease: adrenal insufficiency.

  (1) Most common causes are adrenocortical atrophy or tubercular or fungal infection of adrenals.

  (2) Patients may have apathy, irritability, fatigue, and depression.

  (3) Rarely have confusion or psychosis.

  (4) Treatment with cortisone or the equivalent is usually effective.

  b. Cushing's syndrome

  (1) Excessive cortisol produced by an adrenocortical tumor or hyperplasia.

  (2) Causes secondary mood disorder of agitated depression and often suicide.

  (3) Patient may have memory deficits, decreased concentration, and psychosis.

  (4) Physical findings include truncal obesity, moon facies, buffalo hump, purple striae, hirsutism, and excessive bruising.

  (5) Severe depression can follow the termination of steroid therapy.

4. Pituitary disorders. Patients with total pituitary failure can exhibit psychiatric symptoms, particularly postpartum women who have hemorrhaged into the pituitary, a condition known as *Sheehan's syndrome*. Patients have a combination of symptoms, especially of thyroid and adrenal disorders, and can show virtually any psychiatric symptom.

H. Metabolic disorders

1. Hepatic encephalopathy

  a. Can result in hepatic encephalopathy, characterized by asterixis, hyperventilation, EEG abnormalities, and alterations in consciousness.

  b. The alterations in consciousness can range from apathy to drowsiness to coma.

  c. Associated psychiatric symptoms are changes in memory, general intellectual skills, and personality.

2. Uremic encephalopathy

  a. Renal failure is associated with alterations in memory, orientation, and consciousness. Restlessness, crawling sensations on the limbs, muscle twitching, and persistent hiccups are associated symptoms.

   b. In young people with brief episodes of uremia, the neuropsychiatric symptoms tend to be reversible; in elderly people with long episodes of uremia, the neuropsychiatric symptoms can be irreversible.
3. **Hypoglycemic encephalopathy**
   a. Can be caused either by excessive endogenous production of insulin or by excessive exogenous insulin administration.
   b. Premonitory symptoms include nausea, sweating, tachycardia, and feelings of hunger, apprehension, and restlessness.
   c. As the disorder progresses, disorientation, confusion, and hallucinations, as well as other neurological and medical symptoms can develop. Stupor and coma can occur, and a residual and persistent dementia can sometimes be a serious neuropsychiatric sequela of the disorder.
4. **Diabetic ketoacidosis**
   a. Begins with feelings of weakness, easy fatigability, and listlessness and increasing polyuria and polydipsia.
   b. Headache and sometimes nausea and vomiting appear.
   c. Patients with diabetes mellitus have an increased likelihood of chronic dementia with general arteriosclerosis.
5. **Acute intermittent porphyria**
   a. An autosomal dominant disorder that affects more women than men and has its onset between ages 20 and 50.
   b. Psychiatric symptoms include anxiety, insomnia, lability of mood, depression, and psychosis.
   c. Some studies have found that between 0.2% and 0.5% of chronic psychiatric patients may have undiagnosed porphyrias.

 CLINICAL HINT:
Barbiturates can precipitate and aggravate the disorder and thus are contraindicated in patients with porphyria.

I. Nutritional disorders
1. **Niacin deficiency**
   a. Seen in association with alcohol abuse, vegetarian diets, and extreme poverty and starvation.
   b. Neuropsychiatric symptoms include apathy, irritability, insomnia, depression, and delirium; the medical symptoms include dermatitis, peripheral neuropathies, and diarrhea.
   c. Course has traditionally been described as "five Ds": dermatitis, diarrhea, delirium, dementia, and death.
   d. The response to treatment with nicotinic acid is rapid, but dementia from prolonged illness may improve only slowly and incompletely.
2. **Thiamine (vitamin B_1) deficiency**
   a. Leads to beriberi, characterized chiefly by cardiovascular and neurological changes, and to Wernicke–Korsakoff's syndrome, which is most often associated with chronic alcohol abuse.

      b. Psychiatric symptoms include apathy, depression, irritability, nervousness, and poor concentration; severe memory disorders can develop with prolonged deficiencies.

  3. Cobalamin (vitamin B$_{12}$) deficiency

      a. Mental changes such as apathy, depression, irritability, and moodiness are common. In a few patients, encephalopathy and its associated delirium, delusions, hallucinations, dementia, and, sometimes, paranoid features are prominent and are sometimes called megaloblastic madness.

      b. The neurological manifestations of vitamin B$_{12}$ deficiency can be rapidly and completely arrested by early and continued administration of parenteral vitamin therapy.

J. Toxins

  1. Mercury. Mercury poisoning can be caused by either inorganic or organic mercury. Inorganic mercury poisoning results in the "mad hatter" syndrome with depression, irritability, and psychosis. Associated neurological symptoms are headache, tremor, and weakness. Organic mercury poisoning can be caused by contaminated fish or grain and can result in depression, irritability, and cognitive impairment. Associated symptoms are sensory neuropathies, cerebellar ataxia, dysarthria, paresthesias, and visual field defects. Mercury poisoning in pregnant women causes abnormal fetal development. No specific therapy is available, although chelation therapy with dimercaprol has been used in acute poisoning.

  2. Lead. It takes several months for toxic symptoms to appear. When lead reaches levels above 200 mg/mL, symptoms of severe lead encephalopathy occur, with dizziness, clumsiness, ataxia, irritability, restlessness, headache, and insomnia. Later, an excited delirium occurs, with associated vomiting and visual disturbances, and progresses to convulsions, lethargy, and coma. The treatment of choice to facilitate lead excretion is intravenous administration of calcium disodium edetate (calcium disodium versenate) daily for 5 days.

  3. Manganese. Sometimes called *manganese madness* and causes symptoms of headache, irritability, joint pains, and somnolence. An eventual picture appears of emotional lability, pathological laughter, nightmares, hallucinations, and compulsive and impulsive acts associated with periods of confusion and aggressiveness. Lesions involving the basal ganglia and pyramidal system result in gait impairment, rigidity, monotonous or whispering speech, tremors of the extremities and tongue, masked facies (manganese mask), micrographia, dystonia, dysarthria, and loss of equilibrium. The psychological effects tend to clear 3 or 4 months after the patient's removal from the site of exposure, but neurological symptoms tend to remain stationary or to progress. No specific treatment exists for manganese poisoning, other than removal from the source of poisoning.

  4. Arsenic. Most commonly results from prolonged exposure to herbicides containing arsenic or from drinking water contaminated with arsenic. Early signs of toxicity are skin pigmentation, gastrointestinal complaints, renal and hepatic dysfunction, hair loss, and a characteristic garlic odor to the breath. Encephalopathy eventually occurs, with generalized sensory and motor loss. Chelation therapy with dimercaprol has been used successfully to treat arsenic poisoning.

For more detailed discussion of this topic, see Other Cognitive and Mental Disorders Due to a General Medical Condition, Section 10.5, p. 1207, in CTP/IX.

Neuropsychiatric Aspects of HIV and AIDS

I. Introduction

The human immunodeficiency virus (HIV) epidemic was identified in the 1980s, and neurologists described several HIV-related central nervous system (CNS) syndromes within the first several years of the epidemic. These include acquired immunodeficiency syndrome (AIDS) dementia, the associated AIDS mania, increased rates of major depression, and psychiatric consequences of CNS injuries. More than 50% of infected persons have neuropsychiatric manifestations, which is often the first presenting complaint. Neuropathological changes have been found in up to 90% of AIDS patients at autopsy.

II. HIV Transmission

HIV is a retrovirus related to the human T-cell leukemia virus (HTLV) and to retroviruses that infect animals, including nonhuman primates. HIV-1 is the primary causative agent for most HIV-related disorders. HIV is present in blood, semen, cervical and vaginal secretions, and, to a lesser extent, saliva, tears, breast milk, and the cerebrospinal fluid of those who are infected. The modes of transmission include heterosexual and homosexual intercourse, needles, blood products, and medical accidents. Children can be infected in utero. Oral sex has been rarely implicated. Transmission also occurs through exposure to contaminated needles, thus accounting for the high incidence of HIV infection among drug users. HIV is also transmitted by infusions of whole blood, plasma, and clotting factors, but not immune serum globulin or hepatitis B vaccine. The risk for transmission is higher with higher viral loads and with the coexistence of sexually transmitted diseases that compromise skin or mucosal integrity.

AIDS develops 8 to 11 years after infection. This time has been increased by early intervention with antiretroviral drugs. The virus binds to the CD4 receptor on T4 (also called CD4) lymphocytes. The virus injects ribonucleic acid (RNA) into the lymphocyte. HIV pathophysiological mechanisms gradually disable all T4 lymphocytes and destroy cell-mediated immunity, and opportunistic infections develop.

III. Epidemiology

It is estimated that 33 million people have been infected with HIV worldwide, with more than 12 million deaths as a result. In the United States, an estimated 1.1 million persons are infected with the virus, and another 320,000 have full-blown AIDS. According to the Centers for Disease Control and Prevention (CDC), over 800,000 people in the United States are living with HIV infection or AIDS. The chance of becoming infected after a single exposure to an HIV-infected person is relatively low: 0.8% to 3.2% for unprotected receptive anal intercourse, 0.05% to 0.15% with unprotected vaginal sex, 0.32% after puncture with an HIV-contaminated needle, and 0.67% after using a contaminated needle to inject drugs. The risk of infection of health care workers after a needlestick is rare, about 1 in 300 incidents. The proportion of African Americans and Hispanics with AIDS has increased. Worldwide, the vast majority (>95%) of AIDS cases and deaths occur in developing countries, mostly in young adults, with an increasing proportion of cases in women.

IV. **Diagnosis and Clinical Picture**
   A. **Serum testing.** Techniques are widely available to detect the presence of anti-HIV antibodies in human serum. The conventional test uses blood (time to result, 3 to 10 days), and the rapid test uses an oral swab (time to result, 20 minutes). Two available techniques for detection of antibodies to HIV are the enzyme-linked immunosorbent assay (ELISA) and the Western blot. The ELISA is the initial screen. The Western blot is more specific and is used to confirm positive ELISA results. Seroconversion is the change after HIV infection from a negative HIV antibody test result to a positive HIV antibody test result. Seroconversion usually occurs 6 to 12 weeks after infection but may take 6 to 12 months. Possible indications for HIV testing are outlined in Tables 10–1.

   Some of the issues involved in pretest and posttest counseling are described in Tables 10–2 and 10–3.
   B. **Nonneurological clinical manifestations.** About 30% of persons infected with HIV experience a flulike syndrome 3 to 6 weeks after becoming infected; most never notice any symptoms immediately or shortly after their infection. When symptoms do appear, the flulike syndrome includes fever, myalgia, headaches, fatigue, gastrointestinal symptoms, and sometimes a rash. The syndrome may be accompanied by splenomegaly and lymphadenopathy. Rare neurological manifestations include Guillain-Barré syndrome, encephalopathy, and meningitis. An asymptomatic stage follows that lasts a median of 10 years. During this time, the number of CD4+ cells declines from a normal of more than $1,000/mm^3$ to fewer than $200/mm^3$.

Table 10–1
Possible Indications for HIV Testing

1. Patients who belong to a high-risk group: (1) men who have had sex with another man since 1977, (2) intravenous drug abusers since 1977, (3) hemophiliacs or other patients who have received blood or blood product transfusions not screened for HIV since 1977, (4) sexual partners of people from any of these groups, (5) sexual partners of people with known HIV exposure—people with cuts, wounds, sores, or needlesticks whose lesions have had direct contact with HIV-infected blood.
2. Patients who request testing; not all patients will admit to the presence of risk factors (e.g., because of shame, fear).
3. Patients with symptoms of AIDS or HIV infection.
4. Women belonging to a high-risk group who are planning pregnancy or who are pregnant.
5. Blood, semen, or organ donors.
6. Patients with dementia in a high-risk group.

Adapted from Rosse RB, Giese AA, Deutsch SI, Morihisa JM. *Laboratory & Diagnostic Testing in Psychiatry.* Washington, DC: American Psychiatric Press; 1989:54, with permission.

Table 10–2
Pretest HIV Counseling

1. Discuss meaning of a positive result and clarify distortions (e.g., the test detects exposure to the AIDS virus; it is not a test for AIDS).
2. Discuss the meaning of a negative result (e.g., seroconversion requires time; recent high-risk behavior might require follow-up testing).
3. Be available to discuss the patient's fears and concerns (unrealistic fears might require appropriate psychological intervention).
4. Discuss why the test is necessary (not all patients will admit to high-risk behaviors).
5. Explore the patient's potential reactions to a positive result (e.g., "I'll kill myself if I'm positive"). Take appropriate necessary steps to intervene in a potentially catastrophic reaction.
6. Explore past reactions to severe stresses.
7. Discuss the confidentiality issues relevant to the testing situation (e.g., whether it is an anonymous or a nonanonymous setting). Inform the patient of other possible testing options wherein the counseling and testing can be done completely anonymously (e.g., where the result would not be made a permanent part of a hospital chart). Discuss who might have access to the test results.
8. Discuss with the patient how being seropositive can potentially affect social status (e.g., health and the insurance coverage, employment, housing).
9. Explore high-risk behaviors and recommend risk-reducing interventions.
10. Document discussions in chart.
11. Allow the patient time to ask questions.

From Rosse RB, Giese AA, Deutsch SI, Morihisa JM. *Laboratory & Diagnostic Testing in Psychiatry.* Washington, DC: American Psychiatry Press; 1989:55, with permission.

Patients are at high risk for AIDS-defining complications when CD4+ cells drop to below 200. The two most common coinfections in persons infected with HIV who have AIDS are *Pneumocystis carinii* pneumonia and Kaposi's sarcoma.

C. **Classification.** The CDC classifies AIDS based on CD4+ counts and the presence or absence of HIV-associated clinical conditions. Category A represents primarily asymptomatic patients; category B includes patients with AIDS-defining conditions, such a *Pneumocystis* pneumonia.

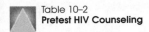

Table 10–3
Posttest HIV Counseling

1. Interpretation of test result: clarify distortion (e.g., "A negative test still means you could contract the virus in the future—it does not mean you are immune to AIDS"). Ask the patient about his or her understanding and emotional reaction to the test result.
2. Recommendations for prevention of transmission (careful discussion of high-risk behaviors and guidelines for prevention of transmission).
3. Recommendations on the follow-up of sexual partners and needle contacts.
4. If test result is positive, recommendations against donating blood, sperm, or organs and against sharing razors, toothbrushes, and anything else that might have blood on it.
5. Referral for appropriate psychological support: HIV-positive persons often need to have available a mental health team (assess need for inpatient versus outpatient care; consider individual or group supportive therapy). Common themes include shock of diagnosis, fear of death and social consequences, grief over potential losses, and dashed hope for good news. Also, look for depression, hopelessness, anger, frustration, guilt, and obsessional themes. Activate supports available to patient (e.g., family, friends, community services).

From Rosse RB, Giese AA, Deutsch SI, Morihisa JM. *Laboratory & Diagnostic Testing in Psychiatry.* Washington, DC: American Psychiatric Press; 1989:58, with permission.

Table 10–4
Neurobiological Complications of HIV-1 Infection

I. Primary neurobiological complications
  A. HIV-1 neurocognitive disorders
    1. Asymptomatic neurocognitive impairment
    2. HIV-1 mild neurocognitive disorder
    3. HIV-1–associated dementia
  B. Other HIV-1 neurobiological complications
    1. HIV-1 meningitis
    2. HIV-1 vacuolar myelopathy
    3. HIV-1 neuropathies
      a. Acute demyelinating (Guillain-Barré) syndrome
      b. Relapsing or progressive demyelinating disease (e.g., mononeuritis multiplex)
      c. Predominantly sensory polyneuropathy
    4. HIV-1 myopathy
II. Secondary neurobiological complications (generally causing delirium)
  A. Infections
    1. *Toxoplasma* encephalitis/abscess
    2. *Cryptococcus* meningitis
    3. Cytomegalovirus (CMV) encephalitis
    4. Progressive multifocal leukoencephalopathy
    5. Other infections of the central nervous system (CNS)
  B. Neoplasia
    1. Primary or secondary CNS lymphoma
    2. Kaposi's sarcoma of the CNS
    3. Other neoplasia
  C. Cerebrovascular disease related to HIV infection
  D. Other delirium
    1. Adverse effects of drugs
    2. Hypoxemia, hypercapnia (e.g., with *Pneumocystis carinii* pneumonia)
    3. Other metabolic and nutritional disorders

Table by Igor Grant, M.D., F.R.C.P.(C), and J. Hampton Atkinson, Jr., M.D.

V. Neurobiological Aspects of HIV Infection

A. Introduction. An extensive array of disease processes can affect the brain of HIV-infected patients, even in the absence of other signs or symptoms of AIDS. Primary neurobiological complications are those attributed directly to the virus itself. Secondary complications are those that arise from HIV-associated illnesses and treatments. Mental disorders associated with HIV infection include dementia, acute psychosis, mood disorder, and personality change resulting from a general medical condition. Diseases that occasionally cause dementia in patients with AIDS include cerebral toxoplasmosis, cryptococcal meningitis, and primary brain lymphoma. The neurobiological complications of HIV-1 infection are listed in Table 10–4.

B. Neurocognitive disorders. In HIV infection of brain macrophage microglia, neurotoxins are produced that ultimately cause neuronal injury. Cardinal features include impaired cognition, motor slowing, incoordination, and mood disturbances. Table 10–5 summarizes HIV-1 cognitive disorders.

C. Psychiatric syndromes

  1. Delirium. Can result from the same variety of causes that lead to dementia in HIV-infected patients. Clinicians have classified delirious states characterized by both increased and decreased activity. Delirium in patients

Table 10–5
HIV-1–Associated Cognitive Disorders

As Defined by Grant and Atkinson	As Proposed by American Academy of Neurology (AAN) Working Group
HIV-1–associated neurocognitive disorders	HIV-1–associated cognitive/motor complex
A. HIV-1–associated dementia	A. Probable[b] HIV-1–associated dementia complex
1. *Marked acquired impairment in cognitive functioning*, involving at least two ability domains (e.g., memory, attention); typically the impairment is in multiple domains, especially in learning of new information, slowed information processing, and defective attention or concentration. The cognitive impairment can be ascertained by history, mental status examination, or neuropsychological testing.	1. *Acquired abnormality in at least two of the following cognitive abilities* (present for at least 1 month): attention/concentration, speed of information processing, abstraction/reasoning, visuospatial skills, memory/learning, speech/language. Cognitive dysfunction causes impairment in work or activities of daily living.
2. The cognitive impairment produces marked interference with day-to-day functioning (work, home life, social activities).	2. *At least one of the following*: a. Acquired abnormality in motor functioning. b. Decline in motivation or emotional control or change in social behavior.
3. The marked cognitive impairment has been present for at least 1 month.	3. Absence of clouding of consciousness during a period long enough to establish presence of No. 1.
4. The pattern of cognitive impairment does not meet criteria for delirium (e.g., clouding of consciousness is not a prominent feature); or, if delirium is present, criteria for dementia need to have been met on a prior examination when delirium was not present.	4. Absence of another cause of the above cognitive, motor, or behavioral symptoms or signs (e.g., active CNS opportunistic infection or malignancy, psychiatric disorders, substance abuse).
5. There is no evidence of another, preexisting cause that could explain the dementia (e.g., other CNS infection, CNS neoplasm, cerebrovascular disease, preexisting neurological disease, or severe substance abuse compatible with CNS disorder).	
B. HIV-1–associated mild neurocognitive disorder (MND)	B. Probable[b] HIV-1–associated minor cognitive/motor disorder
1. Acquired impairment in cognitive functioning, involving at least two ability domains, documented by performance of at least 1.0 standard deviation below the mean for age- or education-appropriate norms on standardized neuropsychological tests. The neuropsychological assessment must survey at least the following abilities: verbal/language, attention/speeded processing, abstraction/executive, memory (learning, recall), complex perceptual-motor performance, motor skills.	1. Acquired cognitive/motor/behavior abnormalities (must have both a and b) a. At least two of the following symptoms present for at least 1 month verified by a reliable history: 1. Impaired attention or concentration. 2. Mental slowing. 3. Impaired memory. 4. Slowed movements. 5. Incoordination. b. Acquired cognitive/motor abnormality verified by clinical neurological examination or neuropsychological testing.

(continued)

Table 10–5—*continued*
HIV-1–Associated Cognitive Disorders

2. The cognitive impairment produces at least mild interference in daily functioning (at least one of the following):
  a. Self-report of reduced mental acuity, inefficiency in work, homemaking, or social functioning.
  b. Observation by knowledgeable others that the individual has undergone at least mild decline in mental acuity with resultant inefficiency in work, homemaking, or social functioning.
	2. Cognitive/motor/behavioral abnormality causes mild impairment of work or activities of daily living (objectively verifiable or by report of key informant).

3. The cognitive impairment has been present for at least 1 month.	3. Absence of another cause of the above cognitive/motor/behavioral abnormality (e.g., active CNS opportunistic infection or malignancy, psychiatric disorders, substance abuse).
4. Does not meet criteria for delirium or dementia.	
5. There is no evidence of another preexisting cause for the MND.	

a If the individual with suspected MND also satisfies criteria for a major depressive episode or substance dependence, the diagnosis of MND should be deferred to a subsequent examination conducted at a time when the major depression has remitted or at least 1 month has elapsed following termination of dependent substance use.
b The designation probable is used when criteria are met, there is no other likely cause, and data are complete. The designation possible is used if another potential cause is present whose contribution is unclear, when a dual diagnosis is possible, or if the evaluation is not complete.
Table by Igor Grant, M.D., F.R.C.P.(C), and J. Hampton Atkinson, Jr., M.D.

infected with HIV is probably underdiagnosed, but it should always precipitate a medical workup of a patient infected with HIV to determine whether a new CNS-related process has begun.

2. **Anxiety disorders.** Patients with HIV infection may have any of the anxiety disorders, but generalized anxiety disorder, posttraumatic stress disorder (PTSD), and obsessive–compulsive disorder (OCD) are particularly common.

3. **Adjustment disorder.** Adjustment disorder with anxiety or depressed mood reportedly occurs in 5% to 20% of HIV-infected patients. The incidence of adjustment disorder in persons infected with HIV is higher than usual in some special populations, such as military recruits and prison inmates.

4. **Depressive disorders.** The range of HIV-infected patients reported to meet the diagnostic criteria for depressive disorders is 4% to 40%. Some of the criteria for depressive disorders (poor sleep and weight loss) can also be caused by the HIV infection itself. Depression is higher in women than in men.

5. **Mania.** Mood disorder with manic features, with or without hallucinations, delusions, or a disorder of thought process, can complicate any stage of HIV infection, but most commonly occurs in late-stage disease complicated by neurocognitive impairment.

6. **Psychotic disorder.** Psychotic symptoms are usually later-stage complications of HIV infection. They require immediate medical and neurological evaluation and often require management with antipsychotic medications.

7. **Substance abuse.** Patients may be tempted to use drugs regularly in an attempt to deal with depression or anxiety.

8. **Suicide.** Suicidal ideation and suicide attempts may be increased in patients with HIV infection and AIDS. The risk factors for suicide are having friends who died of AIDS-related causes, recent notification of HIV seropositivity, relapse, difficult social issues relating to homosexuality, inadequate social and financial support, dementia or delirium, and substance abuse.

9. **Worried well.** Persons in high-risk groups who, although they are seronegative and disease-free, are anxious or have an obsession about contracting the virus. Symptoms can include generalized anxiety, panic attacks, OCD, and hypochondriasis. Repeated negative serum test results can reassure some patients. For those who cannot be reassured, psychotherapy or pharmacotherapy may be indicated.

VI. Treatment

A. **Prevention.** All persons at any risk for HIV infection should be informed about safe sex practices and the need to avoid sharing hypodermic needles. Preventive strategies are complicated by the complex societal values surrounding sexual acts, sexual orientation, birth control, and substance abuse.

1. **Safe sex.** A common question that physicians should be prepared to answer is, "What is safe and unsafe sex?" Patients should be advised to follow the guidelines listed in Table 10–6.

2. **Postexposure prophylaxis.** Prompt administration of antiretroviral therapy following exposure to HIV can reduce the likelihood of infection developing by 80%. Combination treatment with zidovudine (Retrovir) and lamivudine (Epivir) for 4 weeks is usually recommended.

B. **Pharmacotherapy**

1. **Antiretroviral therapy** (Table 10–7). The goal of antiretroviral therapy is full viral suppression, as the viral load governs the rate of CD4-cell decline. Combination therapy with agents that act at different points in viral transcription has become standard.

2. **Antiretroviral therapy of neurocognitive disorders.** Pharmacotherapy with antiretroviral therapy appears to prevent or reverse the progression of HIV-related neurocognitive disorders. A significant percentage of patients show improvement on neuropsychological testing and improvement in pattern and severity of white matter signal abnormalities on MRI within 2 to 3 months of beginning therapy.

3. **Drug therapy of HIV-associated psychiatric syndromes.** Psychiatric syndromes associated with HIV should be treated as they would be in non–HIV-infected persons. In patients with more advanced HIV-related disease, lower drug doses should be used (initial doses of one half to one

Table 10–6
AIDS Safe Sex Guidelines

Remember: Any activity that allows for exchange of body fluids of one person and the mouth, anus, vagina, bloodstream, cuts, or sores of another person is considered unsafe at this time.

Safe sex practices
Massage, hugging, body-to-body rubbing
Dry social kissing
Masturbation
Acting out sexual fantasies (that do not include any unsafe sex practices)
Using vibrators or other instruments (provided they are not shared)

Low-risk sex practices (these activities are not considered completely safe)
French (wet) kissing (without mouth sores)
Mutual masturbation
Vaginal and anal intercourse with a condom
Oral sex, male (fellatio), with a condom
Oral sex, female (cunnilingus), with barrier
External contact with semen or urine provided there are no breaks in the skin

Unsafe sex practices
Vaginal or anal intercourse without a condom
Semen, urine, or feces in the mouth or vagina
Unprotected oral sex (fellatio or cunnilingus)
Blood contact of any kind
Sharing sex instruments or needles

From Moffatt B, Spiegel J, Parrish S, Helquist M. *AIDS: A Self-Care Manual.* Santa Monica, CA: IBS Press; 1987:125, with permission.

fourth of the usual starting doses) because of their heightened sensitivity to side effects.

Agitation associated with delirium and dementia or psychosis can be treated with low doses of high-potency antipsychotics (e.g., 0.5 mg of haloperidol [Haldol] initially) or serotonin–dopamine antagonists (e.g., 0.25 mg of risperidone [Risperdal] initially, 2.5 mg of olanzapine

Table 10–7
Antiretroviral Agents

Generic Name	Trade Name
Nucleoside reverse transcriptase inhibitors	
Zidovudine	Retrovir
Didanosine	Videx
Zalcitabine	Hivid
Stavudine	Zerit
Lamivudine	Epivir
Abacavir	Ziagen
Nonnucleoside reverse transcriptase inhibitors	
Nevirapine	Viramune
Delavirdine	Rescriptor
Efavirenz	Sustiva
Protease inhibitors	
Saquinavir	Invirase, Fortovase
Ritonavir	Norvir
Indinavir	Crixivan
Nelfinavir	Viracept
Amprenavir	Agenerase

Adapted from Igor Grant, M.D., F.R.C.P.(C), and J. Hampton Atkinson, Jr., M.D.

[Zyprexa] initially). One must be aware of the increased risk for anticholinergic delirium, seizures, and extrapyramidal side effects in this population.

Patients with neurocognitive syndromes may benefit from psychostimulants (e.g., 2.5 mg of methylphenidate twice a day with slow increases up to 20 mg/day).

Depression may also be treated with stimulants if a rapid response is required or typical antidepressants are not effective. For depression, selective serotonin reuptake inhibitors (SSRIs) or tricyclics with the lowest possible anticholinergic burden, such as desipramine (Norpramin, Pertofrane), are typically used. Injections of up to 400 mg of testosterone (DEPO–Testosterone) biweekly for 8 weeks may be effective for major depression and fatigue–anergia syndromes. Electroconvulsive therapy has also been effective.

Anxiety states are generally treated with benzodiazepines of short or medium half-life or buspirone (BuSpar). Manic states can be treated with lithium or anticonvulsant mood stabilizers. It appears that the anticonvulsants are better tolerated than lithium in this population. Mania secondary to zidovudine has been successfully treated with lithium to allow continuation of zidovudine. Medical, environmental, and social support are needed in addition to pharmacotherapy.

4. **Interactions of psychotropic drugs and antiretroviral drugs.** The antiretroviral agents have many adverse effects. Of importance to psychiatrists is that protease inhibitors are metabolized by the hepatic cytochrome P450 oxidase system and, therefore, can increase levels of certain psychotropic drugs that are similarly metabolized. Protease inhibitors may inhibit the metabolism of antidepressants, antipsychotics, and benzodiazepines resulting in increased blood levels. It is good practice to anticipate drug interactions and monitor patients for treatment-related emergent adverse events and, when possible, check plasma drug concentrations.

C. **Psychotherapy.** Major psychodynamic themes for patients infected with HIV involve self-blame, self-esteem, and issues regarding death. Major practical themes involve employment, medical benefits, life insurance, career plans, dating and sex, and relationships with families and friends. The entire range of psychotherapeutic approaches may be appropriate for patients with HIV-related disorders. Specific treatments for particular substance-related disorders should be initiated if necessary for the total well-being of the patient.

For more detailed discussion of this topic, see Neuropsychiatric Aspects of HIV Infection and AIDS, Sec 2.8, p. 506, in CTP/IX.

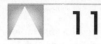

11

Alcohol, Opioids, and Other Substance-Related Disorders

I. Introduction

Despite the high prevalence and comorbid presence of substance disorders, clinicians variably include additional treatment in general practice. These disorders, however, have a growing array of psychopharmacological and psychotherapeutic treatments and reflect a complex set of biological, genetic, and social/environmental factors that impact and utilize the range of psychiatric clinical skills.

Substance abuse problems cause significant disabilities for a relatively high percentage of the population. Illicit substance abuse affects multiple areas of functioning, and comorbid diagnosis occurs in about 60% to 75% of patients with substance-related disorders. About 40% of the U.S. population have used an illicit substance at one time, and about 15% of persons over the age of 18 are estimated to have one of these disorders in their lifetime. Substance-induced syndromes can mimic the full range of psychiatric illnesses, including mood, psychotic, and anxiety disorders.

II. Classification

Brain-altering compounds are referred to as *substances* in the *Diagnostic and Statistical Manual of Mental Disorders,* fourth edition, text revision (*DSM-IV-TR*) and the related disorders as *substance-related disorders*. Diagnostic criteria for these generally capture patterns of toxicity, that is changes in mood, behavior, and cognition, as well as impairment in social or occupational functioning, tolerance, or dependence that results from continued and prolonged use of the offending drug or toxin. There are many classes of substances that are associated with these disorders.

A. Alcohol (ethanol): wood alcohol (methanol) may be used as an adulterant with ethanol and is toxic, also producing blindness.

B. Amphetamine: amphetaminelike substances are included here, such as 3, 4-methylenedioxyamphetamine (MDMA).

C. Caffeine.

D. Cannabis (marijuana).

E. Cocaine: *crack* is a rock base form of cocaine.

F. Hallucinogens: these include mescaline (present in the peyote cactus), psilocybin (present in mushrooms), and lysergic acid derivatives (LSD). These drugs are also known as *psychedelics.*

G. Inhalants: these include solvents such as toluene and gasoline and gases such as nitrous oxide.

H. Nicotine.

I. Opioids.

J. Phencyclidine (PCP).

K. **Sedatives, hypnotics, and anxiolytics:** depending on dose, these drugs are often interchangeable and can produce sedation (a calming effect), hypnosis (referring to promoting sleep), or act as anxiolytics (reducing anxiety).

L. **Prescribed drugs and over-the-counter (OTC) medications:** These include pain-killers, such as OxyContin (an opioid), and over-the-counter preparations, such as ephedra (a stimulant now banned from sale in the United States).

M. **Anabolic–androgenic steroids:** testosterone and human growth hormone (HGH). Each of these classes of drugs is discussed separately below.

III. Terminology

A. **Dependence.** The repeated use of a drug or chemical substance, with or without physical dependence. Physical dependence indicates an altered physiologic state due to repeated administration of a drug, the cessation of which results in a specific syndrome. (See Withdrawal Syndrome below.) See Table 11–1.

B. **Abuse.** Use of any drug, usually by self-administration, in a manner that deviates from approved social or medical patterns. See Table 11–2.

C. **Misuse.** Similar to abuse but usually applies to drugs prescribed by physicians that are not used properly.

D. **Addiction.** The repeated and increased use of a substance, the deprivation of which gives rise to symptoms of distress and an irresistible urge to use the agent again and which leads also to physical and mental deterioration. The term is no longer included in the official nomenclature, as it has been replaced by the term dependence, but it is a useful term in common usage.

E. **Intoxication.** A reversible syndrome caused by a specific substance (e.g., alcohol) that affects one or more of the following mental functions: memory, orientation, mood, judgment, and behavioral, social, or occupational functioning. See Table 11–3.

F. **Withdrawal.** A substance-specific syndrome that occurs after stopping or reducing the amount of the drug or substance that has been used regularly over a prolonged period of time. The syndrome is characterized by physiological signs and symptoms in addition to psychological changes such as disturbances in thinking, feeling, and behavior. Also called *abstinence syndrome* or *discontinuation syndrome.* See Table 11–4.

G. **Tolerance.** Phenomenon in which, after repeated administration, a given dose of a drug produces a decreased effect or increasingly larger doses must be administered to obtain the effect observed with the original dose. *Behavioral tolerance* reflects the ability of the person to perform tasks despite the effects of the drug.

H. **Cross-tolerance.** Refers to the ability of one drug to be substituted for another, each usually producing the same physiologic and psychological effect (e.g., diazepam and barbiturates). Also know as *cross-dependence.*

Table 11–1
DSM-IV-TR Diagnostic Criteria for Substance Dependence

A maladaptive pattern of substance use, leading to clinically significant impairment or distress, as manifested by three (or more) of the following, occurring at any time in the same 12-month period:
1. tolerance, as defined by either of the following:
   a. a need for markedly increased amounts of the substance to achieve intoxication or desired effect
   b. markedly diminished effect with continued use of the same amount of the substance
2. withdrawal, as manifested by either of the following:
   a. the characteristic withdrawal syndrome for the substance (refer to Criteria A and B of the criteria sets for Withdrawal from the specific substances)
   b. the same (or a closely related) substance is taken to relieve or avoid withdrawal symptoms
3. the substance is often taken in larger amounts or over a longer period than was intended
4. there is a persistent desire or unsuccessful efforts to cut down or control substance use
5. a great deal of time is spent in activities necessary to obtain the substance (e.g., visiting multiple doctors or driving long distances), use the substance (e.g., chain-smoking), or recover from its effects
6. important social, occupational, or recreational activities are given up or reduced because of substance use
7. the substance use is continued despite knowledge of having a persistent or recurrent physical or psychological problem that is likely to have been caused or exacerbated by the substance (e.g., current cocaine use despite recognition of cocaine-induced depression, or continued drinking despite recognition that an ulcer was made worse by alcohol consumption)

Specify if:
   With Physiologic Dependence: evidence of tolerance or withdrawal (i.e., either item 1 or 2 is present)
   Without Physiologic Dependence: no evidence of tolerance or withdrawal (i.e., neither item 1 nor 2 is present)
Course specifiers:
   Early Full Remission
   Early Partial Remission
   Sustained Full Remission
   Sustained Partial Remission
   On Agonist Therapy
   In a Controlled Environment

From American Psychiatric Association. *Diagnostic and Statistical Manual of Mental Disorders.* 4th ed. Text rev. Washington, DC: American Psychiatric Association; 2000, with permission.

Table 11–2
DSM-IV-TR Criteria for Substance Abuse

A. A maladaptive pattern of substance use leading to clinically significant impairment or distress, as manifested by one (or more) of the following, occurring within a 12-month period:
   1. recurrent substance use resulting in a failure to fulfill major role obligations at work, school, or home (e.g., repeated absences or poor work performance related to substance use; substance-related absences, suspensions, or expulsions from school; neglect of children or household)
   2. recurrent substance use in situations in which it is physically hazardous (e.g., driving an automobile or operating a machine when impaired by substance use)
   3. recurrent substance-related legal problems (e.g., arrests for substance-related disorderly conduct)
   4. continued substance use despite having persistent or recurrent social or interpersonal problems caused or exacerbated by the effects of the substance (e.g., arguments with spouse about consequences of intoxication, physical fights)
B. The symptoms have never met the criteria for Substance Dependence for this class of substance.

From American Psychiatric Association. *Diagnostic and Statistical Manual of Mental Disorders.* 4th ed. Text rev. Washington, DC: American Psychiatric Association; 2000, with permission.

Table 11-3
DSM-IV-TR Criteria for Substance Intoxication

A. The development of a reversible substance-specific syndrome due to recent ingestion of (or exposure to) a substance. **Note:** Different substances may produce similar or identical syndromes.
B. Clinically significant maladaptive behavioral or psychological changes that are due to the effect of the substance on the central nervous system (e.g., belligerence, mood lability, cognitive impairment, impaired judgment, impaired social or occupational functioning) and develop during or shortly after use of the substance.
C. The symptoms are not due to a general medical condition and are not better accounted for by another mental disorder.

From American Psychiatric Association. *Diagnostic and Statistical Manual of Mental Disorders.* 4th ed. Text rev. Washington, DC: American Psychiatric Association; 2000, with permission.

   I. Co-dependence. Term used to refer to family members affected by or influencing the behavior of the substance abuser. Related to the term *enabler,* which is a person who facilitates the abuser's addictive behavior (e.g., providing drugs directly or money to buy drugs). Enabling also includes the unwillingness of a family member to accept addiction as a medical–psychiatric disorder or to deny that the person is abusing a substance.

IV. Evaluation
Substance-abusing patients are often difficult to detect and evaluate. Not easily categorized, they almost always underestimate the amount of substance used, are prone to use denial, are often manipulative, and often fear the consequences of acknowledging the problem. Because these patients may be unreliable, it is necessary to obtain information from other sources, such as family members. Perhaps more than other disorders, understanding the interpersonal, social, and genetic contexts of those behaviors is central to evaluation and treatment.
   When dealing with these patients, clinicians must present clear, firm, and consistent limits, which will be tested frequently. Such patients usually require a confrontational approach. Although clinicians may feel angered by being manipulated, they should not act on these feelings.
   Psychiatric conditions are difficult to evaluate properly in the presence of ongoing substance abuse, which itself causes or complicates symptoms seen in other disorders. Substance abuse is frequently associated with personality disorders (e.g., antisocial, borderline, and narcissistic). Depressed, anxious, or

Table 11-4
DSM-IV-TR Criteria for Substance Withdrawal

A. The development of a substance-specific syndrome due to the cessation of (or reduction in) substance use that has been heavy and prolonged.
B. The substance-specific syndrome causes clinically significant distress or impairment in social, occupational, or other important areas of functioning.
C. The symptoms are not due to a general medical condition and are not better accounted for by another mental disorder.

From American Psychiatric Association. *Diagnostic and Statistical Manual of Mental Disorders.* 4th ed. Text rev. Washington, DC: American Psychiatric Association; 2000, with permission.

psychotic patients may self-medicate with either prescribed or nonprescribed substances.

 CLINICAL HINT:
Substance-induced disorders should always be considered in the evaluation of depression, anxiety, or psychosis. Underlying substance use is often present when psychiatric disorders do not respond to usual treatments.

A. **Toxicology.** Urine or blood tests are useful in confirming suspected substance use. The two types of tests are screening and confirmatory. Screening tests tend to be sensitive but not specific (many false-positive results). Confirm positive screening results with a specific confirmatory test for an identified drug. Although most drugs are well detected in urine, some are best detected in blood (e.g., barbiturates and alcohol). Absolute blood concentrations can sometimes be useful (e.g., a high concentration in the absence of clinical signs of intoxication would imply tolerance). Urine toxicology is usually positive for up to 2 days after the ingestion of most drugs. See Table 11–5.

B. **Physical examination**
   1. Carefully consider whether concomitant medical conditions are substance related. Look specifically for the following:
      a. **Subcutaneous or intravenous abusers:** AIDS, scars from intravenous or subcutaneous injections, abscesses, infections from contaminated injections, bacterial endocarditis, drug-induced or infectious hepatitis, thrombophlebitis, and tetanus.
      b. **Snorters of cocaine, heroin, or other drugs:** deviated or perforated nasal septum, nasal bleeding, and rhinitis.
      c. **Cocaine freebasers; smokers of crack, marijuana, or other drugs; inhalant abusers:** bronchitis, asthma, chronic respiratory conditions.

C. **History.** Determine the pattern of abuse. Is it continuous or episodic? When, where, and with whom is the substance taken? Is the abuse recreational or

 Table 11–5
Drugs of Abuse That Can Be Tested in Urine

Drug	Length of Time Detected in Urine
Alcohol	7–12 hr
Amphetamine	48 hr
Barbiturate	24 hr (short-acting)
	3 wk (long-acting)
Benzodiazepine	3 days
Cocaine	6–8 hr (metabolites 2–4 days)
Codeine	48 hr
Heroin	36–72 hr
Marijuana (tetrahydrocannabinol)	3 days–4 wk (depending on use)
Methadone	3 days
Methaqualone	7 days
Morphine	48–72 hr
Phencyclidine	8 days
Propoxyphene	6–48 hr

confined to certain social contexts? Find out how much of the patient's life is associated with obtaining, taking, withdrawing from, and recovering from substances. How much do the substances affect the patient's social and work functioning? How does he or she get and pay for the substances? Always specifically describe the substance and route of administration rather than the category (i.e., use "intravenous heroin withdrawal" rather than "opioid withdrawal"). If describing polysubstance abuse, list all substances. Substance abusers typically abuse multiple substances.

D. Diagnoses. Abuse is the chronic use of a substance that leads to impairment or distress and eventually produces dependence on the drug with tolerance and withdrawal symptoms.

E. Treatment. The management of dependence involves observation for possible overdose, evaluation for polysubstance intoxication and concomitant medical conditions, and supportive treatment, such as protecting the patient from injury. The management of abuse or dependence involves abstinence and long-term treatment often relies on creating adaptive social supports and problem solving, with psychopharmacologic strategies generally managing withdrawal, substituting for dependence antagonizing substance effects or mediating craving and reward mechanisms.

V. Specific Substance-Related Disorders

A. Alcohol-related disorders. Almost any presenting clinical problem can be related to the effects of alcohol abuse. Although alcoholism does not describe a specific mental disorder, the disorders associated with alcoholism generally can be divided into three groups: (1) disorders related to the direct effects of alcohol on the brain (including alcohol intoxication, withdrawal, withdrawal delirium, and hallucinosis), (2) disorders related to behavior associated with alcohol (alcohol abuse and dependence), and (3) disorders with persisting effects (including alcohol-induced persisting amnestic disorder, dementia, Wernicke's encephalopathy, and Korsakoff's syndrome). Table 11–6 lists all the *DSM-IV-TR* alcohol-related disorders.

B. Alcohol dependence and abuse

   1. Definitions. Alcohol dependence is a pattern of compulsive alcohol use, defined in *DSM-IV-TR* by the presence of three or more major areas of impairment related to alcohol occurring within the same 12 months. These areas may include tolerance or withdrawal, spending a great deal of time using the substance, returning to use despite adverse physical or psychological consequences, and repeated unsuccessful attempts to control alcohol intake. Alcohol abuse is diagnosed when alcohol is used in physically hazardous situations (e.g., driving). Alcohol abuse differs from alcohol dependence in that it does not include tolerance and withdrawal or a compulsive use pattern; rather, it is defined by negative consequences of repeated use. Alcohol abuse can develop into alcohol dependence, and maladaptive patterns of alcohol consumption may include continuous heavy use, weekend intoxication, or binges interspersed with periods of sobriety.

Table 11–6
***DSM-IV-TR* Alcohol-Related Disorders**

Alcohol use disorders
Alcohol dependence
Alcohol abuse
Alcohol-induced disorders
Alcohol intoxication
Alcohol withdrawal
Specify if:
With perceptual disturbances
Alcohol intoxication delirium
Alcohol withdrawal delirium
Alcohol-induced persisting dementia
Alcohol-induced persisting amnestic disorder
Alcohol-induced psychotic disorder, with delusions
Specify if:
With onset during intoxication
With onset during withdrawal
Alcohol-induced psychotic disorder, with hallucinations
Specify if:
With onset during intoxication
With onset during withdrawal
Alcohol-induced mood disorder
Specify if:
With onset during intoxication
With onset during withdrawal
Alcohol-induced anxiety disorder
Specify if:
With onset during intoxication
With onset during withdrawal
Alcohol-induced sexual dysfunction
Specify if:
With onset during intoxication
Alcohol-induced sleep disorder
Specify if:
With onset during intoxication
With onset during withdrawal
Alcohol-related disorder not otherwise specified

From American Psychiatric Association. *Diagnostic and Statistical Manual of Mental Disorders.* 4th ed. Text rev. Washington, DC: American Psychiatric Association; 2000, with permission.

2. **Pharmacology**
   a. **Pharmacokinetics.** About 90% of alcohol is absorbed through the stomach, the remainder from the small intestine. It is rapidly absorbed, highly water-soluble, and distributed throughout the body. Peak blood concentration is reached in 30 to 90 minutes. Rapid consumption of alcohol and consumption of alcohol on an empty stomach enhance absorption and decrease the time to peak blood concentration. Rapidly rising blood alcohol concentrations correlate with degree of intoxication. Intoxication is more pronounced when blood concentrations are rising rather than falling. Ninety percent of alcohol is metabolized by hepatic oxidation; the rest is excreted unchanged by the kidneys and lungs. Alcohol is converted by alcohol dehydrogenase into acetaldehyde, which is converted to acetic acid by aldehyde dehydrogenase.

The body metabolizes about 15 dL of alcohol per hour, which is equivalent to one moderately sized drink (12 g of ethanol—the content of 12 oz of beer, 4 oz of wine, or 1 to 1.5 oz of an 80-proof liquor). Patients who use alcohol excessively have up-regulated enzymes that metabolize alcohol quickly.

   b. **Neuropharmacology.** Alcohol is a depressant that produces somnolence and decreased neuronal activity. It can be categorized with the other sedative–anxiolytics, such as benzodiazepines, barbiturates, and carbamates. These agents are cross-tolerant with alcohol, produce similar profiles of intoxication and withdrawal, and are potentially lethal in overdose, especially when taken with other depressant drugs. According to the various theories regarding the mechanism of action of alcohol on the brain, alcohol may affect cell membrane fluidity, dopamine-mediated pleasure centers, benzodiazepine receptor complexes, glutamate-gated ionophore receptors that bind N-methyl-D-aspartate (NMDA), and the production of opioidlike alkaloids.

3. **Epidemiology.** Approximately 10% of women and 20% of men have met the diagnostic criteria for alcohol abuse during their lifetimes, and 3% to 5% of women and 10% of men have met the diagnostic criteria for the more serious diagnosis of alcohol dependence. See Table 11–7. The lifetime risk for alcohol dependence is about 10% to 15% for men and 3% to 5% for women. Whites have the highest rate of alcohol use—56%—and 60% of alcohol abusers are men. The higher the educational level, the more likely is the current use of alcohol, in contrast to the pattern for illicit drugs. Among religious groups, alcohol dependence is highest among liberal Protestants and Catholics. The orthodox religions appear to be protective against alcohol dependence in all religious groups. About 200,000 deaths each year are directly related to alcohol abuse, and about 50% of all automotive fatalities involve drunken drivers.

4. **Etiology.** Data supporting genetic influences in alcoholism include the following: (1) close family members have a fourfold increased risk, (2) the identical twin of an alcoholic person is at higher risk than a fraternal twin, and (3) adopted-away children of alcoholic persons have a fourfold increased risk. The familial association is strongest for the son of an

Table 11–7
Alcohol Epidemiology

Condition	Population (%)
Ever had a drink	90
Current drinker	60–70
Temporary problems	40+
Abuse[a]	Male: 10+
	Female: 5+
Dependence[a]	Male: 10
	Female: 3–5

[a]20%–30% of psychiatric patients.

alcohol-dependent father. Ethnic and cultural differences are found in susceptibility to alcohol and its effects. For example, many Asians show acute toxic effects (e.g., intoxication, flushing, dizziness, headache) after consuming only minimal amounts of alcohol. Some ethnic groups, such as Jews and Asians, have lower rates of alcohol dependence, whereas others, such as Native Americans, Inuits, and some groups of Hispanic men, show high rates. These findings have led to a genetic theory about the cause of alcoholism, but a definitive cause remains unknown.

5. **Comorbidity.** The sedative effect and its ready availability make alcohol the most commonly used substance for the relief of anxiety, depression, and insomnia. However, long-term use may cause depression, and withdrawal in a dependent person may cause anxiety. Proper evaluation of depressed or anxious patients who drink heavily may require observation and reevaluation after a period of sobriety lasting up to several weeks.

Many psychotic patients medicate themselves with alcohol when prescribed medications do not sufficiently reduce psychotic symptoms or when prescription medications are not available. In bipolar patients, heavy alcohol use often leads to a manic episode. Among patients with personality disorders, those with antisocial personalities are particularly likely to exhibit long-standing patterns of alcohol dependence. Alcohol abuse is prevalent in persons with other substance use disorders, and the correlation between alcohol dependence and nicotine dependence is particularly high.

6. **Diagnosis, signs, and symptoms**
   a. **Alcohol dependence.** See Table 11–8. Tolerance is a phenomenon in the drinker, who with time requires greater amounts of alcohol to obtain the same effect. The development of tolerance, especially marked tolerance, usually indicates dependence. Mild tolerance for alcohol is common, but severe tolerance, such as that possible with opioids and barbiturates, is uncommon. Tolerance varies widely among persons. Dependence may become apparent in the tolerant patient only when he or she is forced to stop drinking and withdrawal symptoms develop. The clinical course of alcohol dependence is given in Table 11–9.
   b. **Alcohol abuse.** Chronic use of alcohol that leads to dependence, tolerance, or withdrawal. See Table 11–10.
7. **Evaluation.** The proper evaluation of the alcohol user requires some suspicion on the part of the evaluator. In general, most people, when questioned, minimize the amount of alcohol they say that they consume.

 CLINICAL HINT:
When obtaining a history of the degree of alcohol use, it can be helpful to phrase questions in a manner likely to elicit positive responses. For example, ask "How much alcohol do you drink?" rather than "Do you drink alcohol?"

Table 11–8
DSM-IV-TR Diagnostic Criteria for Alcohol or Other Substance Dependence

A maladaptive pattern of substance use, leading to clinically significant impairment or distress, as manifested by three (or more) of the following, occurring at any time in the same 12-month period:

1. tolerance, as defined by either of the following:
   a. a need for markedly increased amounts of the substance to achieve intoxication or desired effect
   b. markedly diminished effect with continued use of the same amount of the substance
2. withdrawal, as manifested by either of the following:
   a. the characteristic withdrawal syndrome for the substance (refer to Criteria A and B of the criteria sets for Withdrawal from the specific substances)
   b. the same (or a closely related) substance is taken to relieve or avoid withdrawal symptoms
3. the substance is often taken in larger amounts or over a longer period than was intended
4. there is a persistent desire or unsuccessful efforts to cut down or control substance use
5. a great deal of time is spent in activities necessary to obtain the substance (e.g., visiting multiple doctors or driving long distances), use the substance (e.g., chain-smoking), or recover from its effects
6. important social, occupational, or recreational activities are given up or reduced because of substance use
7. the substance use is continued despite knowledge of having a persistent or recurrent physical or psychological problem that is likely to have been caused or exacerbated by the substance (e.g., current cocaine use despite recognition of cocaine-induced depression, or continued drinking despite recognition that an ulcer was made worse by alcohol consumption)

Specify if:
With physiologic dependence: evidence of tolerance or withdrawal (i.e., either item 1 or 2 is present)
Without physiologic dependence: no evidence of tolerance or withdrawal (i.e., neither item 1 nor 2 is present)

From American Psychiatric Association. *Diagnostic and Statistical Manual of Mental Disorders.* 4th ed. Text rev. Washington, DC: American Psychiatric Association; 2000, with permission.

Other questions that may provide important clues include how often and when the patient drinks, how often he or she has blackouts (amnesia while intoxicated), and how often friends or relatives have told the patient to cut down on drinking. Always look for subtle signs of alcohol abuse, and always inquire about the use of other substances. Physical findings may include palmar erythema, Dupuytren's contractures, and telangiectasia. Does the patient seem to be accident-prone (head injury, rib fracture, motor vehicle accidents)? Is he or she often in fights? Often absent from work? Are there social or family problems? Laboratory assessment can

Table 11–9
Clinical Course of Alcohol Dependence

Age at first drink[a]	13–15 years
Age at first intoxication[a]	15–17 years
Age at first problem[a]	16–22 years
Age at onset of dependence	25–40 years
Age at death	60 years
Fluctuating course of abstention, temporary control, alcohol problems	
Spontaneous remission in 20%	

[a]Same as general population.
Table by Marc A. Schuckitt, M.D.

Table 11–10
DSM-IV-TR Diagnostic Criteria for Alcohol or Substance Abuse

A. A maladaptive pattern of substance use leading to clinically significant impairment or distress, as manifested by one (or more) of the following, occurring within a 12-month period:
  1. recurrent substance use resulting in a failure to fulfill major role obligations at work, school, or home (e.g., repeated absences or poor work performance related to substance use; substance-related absences, suspensions, or expulsions from school; neglect of children or household)
  2. recurrent substance use in situations in which it is physically hazardous (e.g., driving an automobile or operating a machine when impaired by substance use)
  3. recurrent substance-related legal problems (e.g., arrests for substance-related disorderly conduct)
  4. continued substance use despite having persistent or recurrent social or interpersonal problems caused or exacerbated by the effects of the substance (e.g., arguments with spouse about consequences of intoxication, physical fights)
B. The symptoms have never met the criteria for substance dependence for this class of substance.

From American Psychiatric Association. *Diagnostic and Statistical Manual of Mental Disorders.* 4th ed. Text rev. Washington, DC: American Psychiatric Association; 2000, with permission.

be helpful. Patients may have macrocytic anemia secondary to nutritional deficiencies. Serum liver enzymes and γ-glutamyltransferase (GGT) may be elevated. An elevation of liver enzymes can also be used as a marker of a return to drinking in a previously abstinent patient (Table 11–11). The following subtypes of alcohol dependence have been described:

a. **Type A:** late onset, mild dependence, few alcohol-related problems, and little psychopathology (sometimes called *type I*).

b. **Type B:** severe dependence, early onset of alcohol-related problems, strong history of family alcohol use, high number of life stressors, severe psychopathology, polysubstance use, and high psychopathology (sometimes called *type II*).

c. **Affiliative drinkers:** tend to drink daily in moderate amounts in social settings.

d. **Schizoid-isolated drinkers:** tend to drink alone and subject to binge drinking.

e. **Gamma alcohol dependence:** persons unable to stop drinking once they start.

Table 11–11
State Markers of Heavy Drinking Useful in Screening for Alcoholism

Test	Relevant Range of Results
γ-Glutamyltransferase (GGT)	>30 U/L
Carbohydrate-deficient transferrin (CDT)	>20 mg/L
Mean corpuscular volume (MCV)	>91 μm^3
Uric acid	>6.4 mg/dL for men
	>5.0 mg/dL for women
Aspartate aminotransferase (AST)	>45 IU/L
Alanine aminotransferase (ALT)	>45 IU/L
Triglycerides	>160 mg/dL

Adapted from Marc A. Schuckitt, M.D.

8. Treatment. The goal is the prolonged maintenance of total sobriety. Relapses are common. Initial treatment requires detoxification, on an inpatient basis if necessary, and treatment of any withdrawal symptoms. Coexisting mental disorders should be treated when the patient is sober.

 CLINICAL HINT:
When doing individual therapy, if the patient comes to a session under the influence of alcohol, the session should not be held. If suicidal ideation is expressed, hospitalization should be obtained.

---

a. **Insight.** Critically necessary but often difficult to achieve. The patient must acknowledge that he or she has a drinking problem. Severe denial may have to be overcome before the patient will cooperate in seeking treatment. Often, this requires the collaboration of family, friends, employers, and others. The patient may need to be confronted with the potential loss of career, family, and health if he or she continues to drink. Individual psychotherapy has been used, but group therapy may be more effective. Group therapy may also be more acceptable to many patients who perceive alcohol dependence as a social problem rather than a personal psychiatric problem.

b. **Alcoholics Anonymous (AA) and Al-Anon.** Supportive organizations, such as AA (for patients) and Al-Anon (for families of patients), can be effective in maintaining sobriety and helping the family to cope. AA emphasizes the inability of the member to cope alone with addiction to alcohol and encourages dependence on the group for support; AA also utilizes many techniques of group therapy. Most experts recommend that a recovered alcohol-dependent patient maintain lifelong sobriety and discourage attempts by recovered patients to learn to drink normally. (A dogma of AA is, "It's the first drink that gets you drunk.")

c. **Psychosocial interventions.** Often necessary and very effective. Family therapy should focus on describing the effects of alcohol use on other family members. Patients must be forced to relinquish the perception of their right to be able to drink and recognize the detrimental effects on the family.

d. **Psychopharmacotherapy**
(1) **Disulfiram (Antabuse).** A daily dosage of 25 to 500 mg of disulfiram may be used if the patient desires enforced sobriety. The usual dosage is 250 mg/day. Patients taking disulfiram have an extremely unpleasant reaction when they ingest even small amounts of alcohol. The reaction, caused by an accumulation of acetaldehyde resulting from the inhibition of aldehyde dehydrogenase, includes flushing, headache, throbbing in the head and neck, dyspnea, hyperventilation, tachycardia, hypotension, sweating, anxiety, weakness, and confusion. Life-threatening complications, although uncommon, can occur. Patients with

preexisting heart disease, cerebral thrombosis, diabetes, and several other conditions cannot take disulfiram because of the risk of a fatal reaction. Disulfiram is useful only temporarily to help establish a long-term pattern of sobriety and to change long-standing alcohol-related coping mechanisms.

 CLINICAL HINT:
Advise patients using Antabuse not to use any after-shave lotions or colognes that contain alcohol. Inhalation of the alcohol can produce a reaction.

---

(2) **Naltrexone (ReVia).** This agent decreases the craving for alcohol, probably by blocking the release of endogenous opioids, thereby aiding the patient to achieve the goal of abstinence by preventing the "high" associated with alcohol consumption. A dosage of 50 mg once daily is recommended for most patients.

(3) **Acamprosate (Campral).** This drug is used with patients who have already achieved abstinence. It helps patients remain abstinent by a yet unexplained mechanism involving neuronal excitation and inhibition. It is taken in a delayed release tablet in dosages of 2 g once a day.

9. **Medical complications.** Alcohol is toxic to numerous organ systems. Complications of chronic alcohol abuse and dependence (or associated nutritional deficiencies) are listed in Table 11–12. Alcohol use during pregnancy is toxic to the developing fetus and can cause congenital defects in addition to fetal alcohol syndrome.

C. **Alcohol intoxication**

1. **Definition.** Alcohol intoxication, also called simple drunkenness, is the recent ingestion of a sufficient amount of alcohol to produce acute maladaptive behavioral changes.

2. **Diagnosis, signs, and symptoms.** Whereas mild intoxication may produce a relaxed, talkative, euphoric, or disinhibited person, severe intoxication often leads to more maladaptive changes, such as aggressiveness, irritability, labile mood, impaired judgment, and impaired social or work functioning, among others.

Persons exhibit at least one of the following: slurred speech, incoordination, unsteady gait, nystagmus, memory impairment, stupor. Severe intoxication can lead to withdrawn behavior, psychomotor retardation, blackouts, and eventually obtundation, coma, and death. Common complications of alcohol intoxication include motor vehicle accidents, head injury, rib fracture, criminal acts, homicide, and suicide. Stages of alcohol intoxication and effects on behavior at different blood alcohol levels is presented in Table 11–13.

3. **Evaluation.** A thorough medical evaluation should be conducted including a physical examination and blood chemistry screen and standard liver function tests; consider a possible subdural hematoma or a concurrent

Table 11–12
Neurological and Medical Complications of Alcohol Use

Alcohol intoxication
  Acute intoxication
  Pathological intoxication (atypical, complicated, unusual)
  Blackouts
Alcohol withdrawal syndromes
  Tremulousness (shakes or jitters)
  Alcoholic hallucinosis (horrors)
  Withdrawal seizures (rum fits)
  Delirium tremens (shakes)
Nutritional diseases of the nervous system secondary to alcohol abuse
  Wernicke–Korsakoff's syndrome
  Cerebellar degeneration
  Peripheral neuropathy
  Optic neuropathy (tobacco–alcohol amblyopia)
  Pellagra
Alcoholic diseases of uncertain pathogenesis
  Central pontine myelinolysis
  Marchiafava-Bignami disease
  Fetal alcohol syndrome
  Myopathy
  Alcoholic dementia (?)
  Alcoholic cerebral atrophy
Systemic diseases due to alcohol with secondary neurological complications
  Liver disease
    Hepatic encephalopathy
    Acquired (nonwilsonian) chronic hepatocerebral degeneration
  Gastrointestinal diseases
    Malabsorption syndromes
    Postgastrectomy syndromes
    Possible pancreatic encephalopathy
  Cardiovascular diseases
    Cardiomyopathy with potential cardiogenic emboli and cerebrovascular disease
    Arrhythmias and abnormal blood pressure leading to cerebrovascular disease
  Hematologic disorders
    Anemia, leukopenia, thrombocytopenia (could possibly lead to hemorrhagic cerebrovascular
      disease)
  Infectious disease, especially meningitis (especially pneumococcal and meningococcal)
  Hypothermia and hyperthermia
  Hypotension and hypertension
  Respiratory depression and associated hypoxia
  Toxic encephalopathies (alcohol and other substances)
  Electrolyte imbalances leading to acute confusional states and rarely focal neurological signs and
    symptoms
    Hypoglycemia
    Hyperglycemia
    Hyponatremia
    Hypercalcemia
    Hypomagnesemia
    Hypophosphatemia
Increased incidence of trauma
  Epidural, subdural, and intracerebral hematoma
  Spinal cord injury
  Posttraumatic seizure disorders
  Compressive neuropathies and brachial plexus injuries (Saturday night palsies)
  Posttraumatic symptomatic hydrocephalus (normal-pressure hydrocephalus)
  Muscle crush injuries and compartment syndromes

Reprinted from Rubino FA. Neurologic complications of alcoholism. *Psychiatr Clin North Am*
1992;15:361, with permission.

Table 11–13
Impairment Likely to Be Seen at Different Blood Alcohol Concentrations

Level	Likely Impairment
20–30 mg/dL	Slowed motor performance and decreased thinking ability
30–80 mg/dL	Increases in motor and cognitive problems
80–200 mg/dL	Increases in incoordination and judgment errors
	Mood lability
	Deterioration in cognition
200–300 mg/dL	Nystagmus, marked slurring of speech, and alcoholic blackouts
>300 mg/dL	Impaired vital signs and possible death

Table from Marc A. Schuckitt, M.D.

infection. Always evaluate for possible intoxication with other substances. Alcohol is frequently used in combination with other central nervous system (CNS) depressants, such as benzodiazepines and barbiturates. The CNS depressant effects of such combinations can be synergistic and potentially fatal. Blood alcohol levels are seldom important in the clinical evaluation (except to determine legal intoxication) because tolerance varies.

   a. A variant of alcohol intoxication is called *alcohol idiosyncratic intoxication.* It is characterized by maladaptive behavior (often aggressive or assaultive) after the ingestion of a small amount of alcohol that would not cause intoxication in most people (i.e., pathological intoxication). The behavior must be atypical for the person when he or she is not drinking. Brain-damaged persons may also be more susceptible to alcohol idiosyncratic intoxication.

   b. Blackouts consist of episodes of intoxication during which the patient exhibits complete anterograde amnesia and appears awake and alert. They occasionally can last for days, during which the intoxicated person performs complex tasks, such as long-distance travel, with no subsequent recollection. Brain-damaged persons may be more susceptible to blackouts.

4. Treatment

   a. Usually only supportive.

   b. May give nutrients (especially thiamine, vitamin B_{12}, folate).

   c. Observation for complications (e.g., combativeness, coma, head injury, falling) may be required.

   d. Alcoholic idiosyncratic intoxication is a medical emergency that requires steps to prevent the patient from harming others or self. Lorazepam (Ativan) 1 to 2 mg by mouth or intramuscularly or haloperidol (Haldol; 2 to 5 mg by mouth or intramuscularly) can be used for agitation. Physical restraints may be necessary.

D. Alcohol-induced psychotic disorder, with hallucinations (previously known as alcohol hallucinosis). Vivid, persistent hallucinations (often visual and auditory), without delirium, following (usually within 2 days) a decrease in alcohol consumption in an alcohol-dependent person. May persist and progress to a more chronic form that is clinically similar to schizophrenia. Rare. The male-to-female ratio is 4:1. The condition usually requires at least 10 years of alcohol dependence. If the patient is agitated, possible treatments include benzodiazepines (e.g., 1 to 2 mg of lorazepam orally or intramuscularly, 5 to 10 mg of diazepam [Valium]), or low doses of a high-potency antipsychotic (e.g., 2 to 5 mg of haloperidol orally or intramuscularly as needed every 4 to 6 hours).

E. Alcohol withdrawal. Begins within several hours after cessation of, or reduction in, prolonged (at least days) heavy alcohol consumption. At least two of the following must be present: autonomic hyperactivity, hand tremor, insomnia, nausea or vomiting, transient illusions or hallucinations, anxiety, grand mal seizures, and psychomotor agitation. May occur with perceptual disturbances (e.g., hallucinations) and intact reality testing.

F. Alcohol withdrawal delirium (delirium tremens [DTs]). Usually occurs only after recent cessation of or reduction in severe, heavy alcohol use in medically compromised patients with a long history of dependence. Less common than uncomplicated alcohol withdrawal. Occurs in 1% to 3% of alcohol-dependent patients.

1. Diagnosis, signs, and symptoms
   a. Delirium.
   b. Marked autonomic hyperactivity—tachycardia, sweating, fever, anxiety, or insomnia.
   c. Associated features—vivid hallucinations that may be visual, tactile, or olfactory; delusions; agitation; tremor; fever; and seizures or so-called rum fits (if seizures develop, they always occur before delirium).
   d. Typical features—paranoid delusions, visual hallucinations of insects or small animals, and tactile hallucinations.

2. Medical workup
   a. Complete history and physical.
   b. Laboratory tests—complete blood cell count with differential; measurement of electrolytes, including calcium and magnesium; blood chemistry panel; liver function tests; measurement of bilirubin, blood urea nitrogen, creatinine, fasting glucose, prothrombin time, albumin, total protein, hepatitis type B surface antigen, vitamin B, folate, and serum amylase; stool guaiac; urinalysis and urine drug screen; electrocardiogram (ECG); and chest roentgenography. Other possible tests include electroencephalogram (EEG), lumbar puncture, computed tomography of the head, and gastrointestinal series.

3. Treatment
   a. Take vital signs every 6 hours.
   b. Observe the patient constantly.
   c. Decrease stimulation.
   d. Correct electrolyte imbalances and treat coexisting medical problems (e.g., infection, head trauma).
   e. If the patient is dehydrated, hydrate.
   f. Chlordiazepoxide (Librium): 25 to 100 mg orally every 6 hours (other sedative–hypnotics can be substituted, but this is the convention). Use

Table 11–14
Drug Therapy for Alcohol Intoxication, and Withdrawal and Maintenance

Clinical Problem	Drug	Route	Dosage[a]	Comment
Tremulousness and mild to moderate agitation	Chlordiaze- poxide	Oral	25–100 mg every 4–6 hours	Initial dose can be repeated every 2 hours until patient is calm; subsequent doses must be individualized and titrated.
	Diazepam	Oral	5–20 mg every 4–6 hours	
Hallucinosis	Lorazepam	Oral	2–10 mg every 4–6 hours	
Extreme agitation	Chlordiaze- poxide	Intravenous	0.5 mg/kg at 12.5 mg/min	Give until patient is calm; subsequent doses must be individualized and titrated.
Withdrawal seizures	Diazepam	Intravenous	0.15 mg/kg at 2.5 mg/min	
Delirium tremens	Lorazepam	Intravenous	0.1 mg/kg at 2.0 mg/min	
Maintenance	Acamprosate	Oral	2 g/day	Only used after patient has achieved abstinence.

[a]Scheduled doses should be held for somnolence.
Adapted from Koch-Weser J, Sellers EM, Kalant J. Alcohol Intoxication and withdrawal. *N Engl J Med* 1976;294:757, with permission.

as needed for agitation, tremor, or increased vital signs (temperature, pulse, blood pressure). In the treatment of alcohol withdrawal delirium in the geriatric patient, lorazepam 1 to 2 mg by mouth, intravenously, or intramuscularly every 4 hours may be used with a 50% decrease in dose on Days 2 and 3. (See Table 11–14.)

g. Thiamine: 100 mg orally one to three times a day.

h. Folic acid: 1 mg orally daily.

i. One multivitamin daily.

j. Magnesium sulfate: 1 g intramuscularly every 6 hours for 2 days (in patients who have had postwithdrawal seizures).

k. After the patient is stabilized, taper chlordiazepoxide by 20% every 5 to 7 days.

l. Provide medication for adequate sleep.

m. Treat malnutrition if present.

n. This regimen allows for a very flexible dosage of chlordiazepoxide. If prescribing a sedative on a standing regimen, be sure that the medication will be held if the patient is asleep or not easily aroused. The necessary total dose of benzodiazepine varies greatly among patients owing to inherent individual differences, differing levels of alcohol intake, and concomitant use of other substances. Because many of these patients have impaired liver function, it also may be difficult to estimate the elimination half-life of the sedative accurately.

o. Generally, antipsychotics should be used cautiously because they can precipitate seizures. If the patient is agitated and psychotic and shows signs of benzodiazepine toxicity (ataxia, slurred speech) despite being agitated, then consider using an antipsychotic such as haloperidol or fluphenazine (Prolixin, Permitil), which is less likely to precipitate seizures.

G. Alcohol-induced persisting amnestic disorder. Disturbance in short-term memory resulting from prolonged heavy use of alcohol; rare in persons under the age of 35. The classic names for the disorder are *Wernicke's encephalopathy* (an acute set of neurologic symptoms) and *Korsakoff's syndrome* (a chronic condition).

1. **Wernicke's encephalopathy** (also known as *alcoholic encephalopathy*). An acute syndrome caused by thiamine deficiency. Characterized by nystagmus, abducens and conjugate gaze palsies, ataxia, and global confusion. Other symptoms may include confabulation, lethargy, indifference, mild delirium, anxious insomnia, and fear of the dark. Thiamine deficiency usually is secondary to chronic alcohol dependence. Treat with 100 to 300 mg of thiamine per day until ophthalmoplegia resolves. The patient may also require magnesium (a cofactor for thiamine metabolism). With treatment, most symptoms resolve except ataxia, nystagmus, and sometimes peripheral neuropathy. The syndrome may clear in a few days or weeks or progress to Korsakoff's syndrome.

2. **Korsakoff's syndrome** (also known as *Korsakoff's psychosis*). A chronic condition, usually related to alcohol dependence, wherein alcohol represents a large portion of the caloric intake for years. Caused by thiamine deficiency. Rare. Characterized by retrograde and anterograde amnesia. The patient also often exhibits confabulation, disorientation, and polyneuritis. In addition to thiamine replacement, clonidine (Catapres) and propranolol (Inderal) may be of some limited use. Often coexists with alcohol-related dementia. Twenty-five percent of patients recover fully, and 50% recover partially with long-term oral administration of 50 to 100 mg of thiamine per day.

H. Substance-induced persisting dementia. This diagnosis should be made when other causes of dementia have been excluded and a history of chronic heavy alcohol abuse is evident. The symptoms persist past intoxication or withdrawal states. The dementia is usually mild. Management is similar to that for dementia of other causes.

I. Opioids

1. **Introduction.** Opiate dependence is resurgent. Opiates have become the fastest growing substance of abuse.

   Opioids include the natural drug opium and its derivatives, in addition to synthetic drugs with similar actions. The natural drugs derived from opium include morphine and codeine; the synthetic opioids include methadone, oxycodone, hydromorphone (Dilaudid), levorphanol (Levo-Dromoran), pentazocine (Talwin), meperidine (Demerol), and propoxyphene (Darvon). Heroin is considered a semisynthetic drug

Table 11–15
DSM-IV-TR Opioid-Related Disorders

Opioid use disorders
Opioid dependence
Opioid abuse
Opioid-induced disorders
Opioid intoxication
   Specify if:
     With perceptual disturbances
Opioid withdrawal
Opioid intoxication delirium
Opioid-induced psychotic disorder, with delusions
   Specify if:
     With onset during intoxication
Opioid-induced psychotic disorder, with hallucinations
   Specify if:
     With onset during intoxication
Opioid-induced mood disorder
   Specify if:
     With onset during intoxication
Opioid-induced sexual dysfunction
   Specify if:
     With onset during intoxication
Opioid-induced sleep disorder
   Specify if:
     With onset during intoxication
     With onset during withdrawal
Opioid-related disorder not otherwise specified

From American Psychiatric Association. *Diagnostic and Statistical Manual of Mental Disorders.* 4th ed. Text rev. Washington, DC: American Psychiatric Association; 2000, with permission.

and has the strongest euphoriant property, thus producing the most craving.

Opioids affect opioid receptors. μ-opioid receptors mediate analgesia, respiratory depression, constipation, and dependence; δ-opioid receptors mediate analgesia, diuresis, and sedation. Opioids also affect dopaminergic and noradrenergic systems. Dopaminergic reward pathways mediate addiction. Heroin is more lipid-soluble than morphine and more potent. It crosses the blood–brain barrier more rapidly, has a faster onset of action, and is more addictive. The *DSM-IV-TR* opioid-related disorders are listed in Table 11–15.

2. **Epidemiology.** In developed countries, the opioid drug most associated with abuse is heroin, with an estimated 1,000,000 heroin users reported in the United States. The lifetime rate of heroin use in the United States is about 2%. Dependence on opioids other than heroin is seen most often in persons who have become dependent in the course of medical treatment. The male-to-female ratio of persons with heroin dependence is about 3:1. Most users are in their 30s and 40s. Heroin is exclusively a drug of abuse and is most commonly used by patients of lower socioeconomic status, who often engage in criminal activities to pay for drugs. However, prescription opiate abuse is also a major public health problem.

3. **Route of administration.** Depends on the drug. Opium is smoked. Heroin is typically injected (intravenously or subcutaneously) or inhaled

(snorted) nasally, and it may be combined with stimulants for intravenous injection (speedball). Heroin snorting and smoking are increasingly popular owing to increased drug purity and concerns about HIV risk. Pharmaceutically available opioids are typically taken orally, but some are also injectable.

CLINICAL HINT:
Look for "track marks" on extremities (including hands and feet), indicating chronic injection of substances.

---

4. **Dose.** Often difficult to determine by history for two reasons. First, the abuser has no way of knowing the concentration of the heroin he or she has bought and may underestimate the amount taken (which can lead to accidental overdose if the person suddenly obtains one bag containing 15% heroin when the typical amount is 5%). Second, the abuser may overstate the dosage in an attempt to get more methadone.

5. **Intoxication.** See Table 11–16.
   a. **Objective signs and symptoms.** CNS depression, decreased gastrointestinal motility, respiratory depression, analgesia, nausea and vomiting, slurred speech, hypotension, bradycardia, pupillary constriction, and seizures (in overdose). Tolerant patients still have pupillary constriction and constipation.
   b. **Subjective signs and symptoms.** Euphoria (heroin intoxication, described as a total-body orgasm), at times anxious dysphoria, tranquility, decreased attention and memory, drowsiness, and psychomotor retardation.

6. **Overdose.** Can be a medical emergency and is usually accidental and often results from combined use with other CNS depressants (e.g.,

---

Table 11–16
***DSM-IV-TR* Diagnostic Criteria for Opioid Intoxication**

A. Recent use of an opioid.
B. Clinically significant maladaptive behavioral or psychological changes (e.g., initial euphoria followed by apathy, dysphoria, psychomotor agitation or retardation, impaired judgment, or impaired social or occupational functioning) that developed during, or shortly after, opioid use.
C. Pupillary constriction (or pupillary dilation due to anoxia from severe overdose) and one (or more) of the following signs, developing during, or shortly after, opioid use:
   1. drowsiness or coma
   2. slurred speech
   3. impairment in attention or memory
D. The symptoms are not due to a general medical condition and are not better accounted for by another mental disorder.
Specify if:
   With perceptual disturbances

From American Psychiatric Association. *Diagnostic and Statistical Manual of Mental Disorders.* 4th ed. Text rev. Washington, DC: American Psychiatric Association; 2000, with permission.

alcohol or sedative–hypnotics). Clinical signs include pinpoint pupils, respiratory depression, and CNS depression.

7. **Treatment**
   a. ICU admission and support of vital functions (e.g., intravenous fluids).
   b. Immediately administer 0.8 mg of naloxone (Narcan) (0.01 mg/kg for neonates), an opioid antagonist, intravenously and wait 15 minutes.
   c. If no response, give 1.6 mg intravenously and wait 15 minutes.
   d. If still no response, give 3.2 mg intravenously and suspect another diagnosis.
   e. If successful, continue at 0.4 mg/hour intravenously.
   f. Always consider possible polysubstance overdose. A patient successfully treated with naloxone may wake up briefly only to succumb to subsequent overdose symptoms from another, slower-acting drug (e.g., sedative–hypnotic) taken simultaneously. Remember that naloxone will precipitate rapid withdrawal symptoms. It has a short half-life and must be administered continuously until the opioid has been cleared (up to 3 days for methadone). Babies born to opioid-abusing mothers may experience intoxication, overdose, or withdrawal.

 CLINICAL HINT:
Consider opiate addiction irrespective of socioeconomic status. Prescription opiate addiction far exceeds heroin use.

8. **Tolerance, dependence, and withdrawal.** Develop rapidly with long-term opioid use, which changes the number and sensitivity of opioid receptors and increases the sensitivity of dopaminergic, cholinergic, and serotonergic receptors. Produce profound effects on noradrenergic systems. Occur after cessation of long-term use or after abrupt cessation, as with administration of an opioid antagonist. Symptoms are primarily related to rebound hyperactivity of noradrenergic neurons of the locus ceruleus. Withdrawal is seldom a medical emergency. See Table 11–17. Clinical signs are flulike and include drug craving, anxiety, lacrimation, rhinorrhea, yawning, sweating, insomnia, hot and cold flashes, muscle aches, abdominal cramping, dilated pupils, piloerection, tremor, restlessness, nausea and vomiting, diarrhea, and increased vital signs. Intensity depends on previous dose and on rate of decrease. Less intense with drugs that have long half-lives, such as methadone; more intense with drugs that have short half-lives, such as meperidine. Patients have severe craving for opioid drugs and will demand and manipulate for opioids. Beware of malingerers and look for piloerection, dilated pupils, tachycardia, and hypertension. If objective signs are absent, do not give opioids for withdrawal.

Table 11–17
DSM-IV-TR Diagnostic Criteria for Opioid Withdrawal

A. Either of the following:
   1. cessation of (or reduction in) opioid use that has been heavy and prolonged (several weeks or longer)
   2. administration of an opioid antagonist after a period of opioid use
B. Three (or more) of the following, developing within minutes to several days after Criterion A:
   1. dysphoric mood
   2. nausea or vomiting
   3. muscle aches
   4. lacrimation or rhinorrhea
   5. pupillary dilation, piloerection, or sweating
   6. diarrhea
   7. yawning
   8. fever
   9. insomnia
C. The symptoms in Criterion B cause clinically significant distress or impairment in social, occupational, or other important areas of functioning.
D. The symptoms are not due to a general medical condition and are not better accounted for by another mental disorder.

From American Psychiatric Association. *Diagnostic and Statistical Manual of Mental Disorders*. 4th ed. Text rev. Washington, DC: American Psychiatric Association; 2000, with permission.

9. **Detoxification.** If objective withdrawal signs are present, give 10 mg of methadone. If withdrawal persists after 4 to 6 hours, give an additional 5 to 10 mg, which may be repeated every 4 to 6 hours. Total dose in 24 hours equals the dose for the second day (seldom >40 mg). Give twice a day or every day and decrease dosage by 5 mg/day for heroin withdrawal; methadone withdrawal may require slower detoxification. Pentazocine-dependent patients should be detoxified on pentazocine because of its mixed opioid receptor agonist and antagonist properties. Many nonopioid drugs have been tried for opioid detoxification, but the only promising one is clonidine (Catapres), which is a centrally acting agent that effectively relieves the nausea, vomiting, and diarrhea associated with opioid withdrawal (it is not effective for most other symptoms). Give 0.1 to 0.2 mg every 3 hours as needed, not to exceed 0.8 mg/day. Titrate dose according to symptoms. When dosage is stabilized, taper over 2 weeks. Hypotension is a side effect. Clonidine is short-acting and not a narcotic.

The general approach in withdrawal is one of support, detoxification, and progression to methadone maintenance or abstinence. Patients dependent on multiple drugs (e.g., an opioid and a sedative–hypnotic) should be maintained on a stable dosage of one drug while being detoxified from the other. Naltrexone (a long-acting oral opioid antagonist) can be used with clonidine to expedite detoxification. It is orally effective, and when given three times a week (100 mg on weekdays and 150 mg on weekends), it blocks the effects of heroin. After detoxification, oral naltrexone has been effective in helping to maintain abstinence for up to 2 months.

Ultrarapid detoxification is the procedure of precipitating withdrawal with opioid antagonists under general anesthesia. Further research is needed to determine whether the use of this expensive and intensive method, which adds anesthetic risk to the detoxification process, is of any benefit.

10. **Opioid substitutes.** The main long-term treatment for opiate dependence, methadone maintenance, is a slow, extended detoxification. Most patients can be maintained on daily doses of 60 mg or less. Although often criticized, methadone maintenance programs do decrease rates of heroin use. A sufficient methadone dosage is necessary; the use of plasma methadone concentrations may help to determine the appropriate dosage.

Levomethadyl (ORLAAM, also known as LAAM) is a longer-acting opioid than methadone. Due to its potential for serious and possibly life-threatening, proarrhythmic effects, LAAM was taken off the market.

Buprenorphine (Buprenex) is a partial μ-opioid receptor agonist that is of use for both detoxification and maintenance treatment. Treatment is given 3 days a week because it is long-acting. A dosage of 8 to 16 mg/day appears to reduce heroin use.

11. **Therapeutic communities.** Residential programs that emphasize abstinence and group therapy in a structured environment (e.g., Phoenix House).

12. **Other interventions.** Education about HIV transmission, free needle-exchange programs, individual and group psychotherapies, self-help groups (e.g., Narcotics Anonymous), and outpatient drug-free programs are also of benefit.

J. Sedatives, hypnotics, and anxiolytics

1. **Introduction.** The drugs associated with this group are the benzodiazepines, for example, diazepam (Valium) and flunitrazepam (Rohypnol); barbiturates, for example, secobarbital (seconal); and the barbituratelike substances, which include methaqualone (formerly know as Quaalude) and meprobamate (Miltown).

Drugs of this class are used to treat insomnia and anxiety. Alcohol and all drugs of this class are cross-tolerant and their effects are additive. They all have agonist effects on the γ-aminobutyric acid type A (GABA$_A$) receptor complex. Sedatives, hypnotics, and anxiolytics are the most commonly prescribed psychoactive drugs and are taken orally. Dependence develops only after at least several months of daily use, but persons vary widely in this respect. Many middle-aged patients begin taking benzodiazepines for insomnia or anxiety, become dependent, and then seek multiple physicians to prescribe them. Sedative–hypnotics are used illicitly for their euphoric effects, to augment the effects of other CNS depressant drugs (e.g., opioids and alcohol), and to temper the excitatory and anxiety-producing effects of stimulants (e.g., cocaine).

Table 11–18
Signs and Symptoms of the Benzodiazepine Discontinuation Syndrome

The following signs and symptoms may be seen when benzodiazepine therapy is discontinued; they
reflect the return of the original anxiety symptoms (recurrence), worsening of the original anxiety
symptoms (rebound), or emergence of new symptoms (true withdrawal):
Disturbances of mood and cognition
  Anxiety, apprehension, dysphoria, pessimism, irritability, obsessive rumination, and paranoid
  ideation
Disturbances of sleep
  Insomnia, altered sleep–wake cycle, and daytime drowsiness
Physical signs and symptoms
  Tachycardia, elevated blood pressure, hyperreflexia, muscle tension, agitation/motor
  restlessness, tremor, myoclonus, muscle and joint pain, nausea, coryza, diaphoresis, ataxia,
  tinnitus, and grand mal seizures
Perceptual disturbances
  Hyperacusis, depersonalization, blurred vision, illusions, and hallucinations

The major complication of sedative, hypnotic, or anxiolytic intoxication is overdose, with associated CNS and respiratory depression. Although mild intoxication is not in itself dangerous (unless the patient is driving or operating machinery), the possibility of a covert overdose must always be considered. The lethality of benzodiazepines is low and overdose has been reduced by the use of the specific benzodiazepine antagonist flumazenil (Romazicon) in emergency department settings.

Sedative, hypnotic, or anxiolytic intoxication is similar to alcohol intoxication, but idiosyncratic aggressive reactions are uncommon. These drugs are often taken with other CNS depressants (e.g., alcohol), which can produce additive effects. Withdrawal is dangerous and can lead to delirium or seizures. See Table 11–18.

2. **Epidemiology.** About 6% of persons have used these drugs illicitly, usually before the age of 40. The highest prevalence of illicit use is between the ages of 26 to 35, with a female-to-male ratio of 3:1 and a white-to-black ratio of 2:1. Barbiturate abuse is more common in those over age 40.

3. **Intoxication.** Intoxication also can cause disinhibition and amnesia. Table 11–19 describes intoxication and withdrawl from substances.

4. **Withdrawal.** Can range from a minor to a potentially life-threatening condition requiring hospitalization. Individual differences in tolerance are large. All sedatives, hypnotics, and anxiolytics are cross-tolerant with each other and with alcohol. Drugs with a short half-life (e.g., alprazolam) may induce a more rapid onset of withdrawal and a more severe withdrawal than drugs with a long half-life (e.g., diazepam). The degree of tolerance can be measured with the pentobarbital challenge test (see Table 11–20), which identifies the dose of pentobarbital needed to prevent withdrawal. True withdrawal, a return of original anxiety symptoms (recurrence) or worsening of original anxiety symptoms (rebound), can be precipitated by drug discontinuation. Guidelines for treatment of benzodiazepine withdrawal are presented in Table 11–21. Dose equivalents are presented in Table 11–22.

Table 11–19
Signs and Symptoms of Substance Intoxication and Withdrawal

Substance	Intoxication	Withdrawal
Opioid	Drowsiness Slurred speech Impaired attention or memory Analgesia Anorexia Decreased sex drive Hypoactivity	Craving for drug Nausea, vomiting Muscle aches Lacrimation, rhinorrhea Pupillary dilation Piloerection Sweating Diarrhea Fever Insomnia Yawning
Amphetamine or cocaine	Perspiration, chills Tachycardia Pupillary dilation Elevated blood pressure Nausea, vomiting Tremor Arrhythmia Fever Convulsions Anorexia, weight loss Dry mouth Impotence Hallucinations Hyperactivity Irritability Aggressiveness Paranoid ideation	Dysphoria Fatigue Sleep disorder Agitation Craving
Sedative, hypnotic, or anxiolytic	Slurred speech Incoordination Unsteady gait Impaired attention or memory	Nausea, vomiting Malaise, weakness Autonomic hyperactivity Anxiety, irritability Increased sensitivity to light and sound Coarse tremor Marked insomnia Seizures

Table 11–20
Pentobarbital^a Challenge Test

1. Give 200 mg of pentobarbital orally.
2. Observe patient for intoxication after 1 hour (e.g., sleepiness, slurred speech, or nystagmus).
3. If patient is not intoxicated, give another 100 mg of pentobarbital every 2 hours (maximum 500 mg over 6 hours).
4. Total dose given to produce mild intoxication is equivalent to daily abuse level of barbiturates.
5. Substitute 30 mg of phenobarbital (longer half-life) for each 100 mg of pentobarbital.
6. Decrease dose by about 10% a day.
7. Adjust rate if signs of intoxication or withdrawal are present.

^{a}Other drugs can also be used.

Table 11–21
Guidelines for Treatment of Benzodiazepine Withdrawal

1. Evaluate and treat concomitant medical and psychiatric conditions.
2. Obtain drug history and urine and blood samples for drug and ethanol assay.
3. Determine required dose of benzodiazepine or barbiturate for stabilization, guided by history, clinical presentation, drug-ethanol assay, and (in some cases) challenge dose.
4. Detoxification from supratherapeutic dosages:
   a. Hospitalize if there are medical or psychiatric indications, poor social supports, or polysubstance dependence or the patient is unreliable.
   b. Some clinicians recommend switching to longer-acting benzodiazepine for withdrawal (e.g., diazepam, clonazepam); others recommend stabilizing on the drug that the patient was taking or on phenobarbital.
   c. After stabilization, reduce dosage by 30% on the second or third day and evaluate the response, keeping in mind that symptoms occur sooner after decreases in benzodiazepines with short elimination half-lives (e.g., lorazepam) than after decreases in those with longer elimination half-lives (e.g., diazepam).
   d. Reduce dosage further by 10% to 25% every few days if tolerated.
   e. Use adjunctive medications if necessary; carbamazepine, β-adrenergic receptor antagonists, valproate, clonidine, and sedative antidepressants have been used, but their efficacy in the treatment of the benzodiazepine abstinence syndrome has not been established.
5. Detoxification from therapeutic dosages:
   a. Initiate 10% to 25% dose reduction and evaluate response.
   b. Dose, duration of therapy, and severity of anxiety influence the rate of taper and need for adjunctive medications.
   c. Most patients taking therapeutic doses have uncomplicated discontinuation.
6. Psychological interventions may assist patients in detoxification from benzodiazepines and in the long-term management of anxiety.

Adapted from Domenic A. Ciraulo M.D., and Ofra Sarid-Segal, M.D.

K. Amphetamines and amphetaminelike substances (stimulants). Amphetaminelike substances exert their major effect by releasing catecholamines, primarily dopamine, from presynaptic stores, particularly in the "reward pathway" of dopaminergic neurons projecting from the ventral tegmentum to the cortex. Legitimate indications include attention-deficit

Table 11–22
Approximate Therapeutic Equivalent Doses of Benzodiazepines

Generic Name	Trade Name	Dose (mg)
Alprazolam	Xanax	1
Chlordiazepoxide	Librium	25
Clonazepam	Klonopin	0.5–1
Clorazepate	Tranxene	15
Diazepam	Valium	10
Estazolam	ProSom	1
Flurazepam	Dalmane	30
Lorazepam	Ativan	2
Oxazepam	Serax	30
Prazepam	Paxipam	80
Temazepam	Restoril	20
Triazolam	Halcion	0.25
Quazepam	Doral	15
Zolpidem[a]	Ambien	10

[a]An imidazopyridine benzodiazepine agonist.

disorders, narcolepsy, and depression. Methylphenidate (Ritalin) appears less addictive than other amphetamines, possibly because it has a different mechanism of action (inhibits dopamine reuptake). Effects are euphoric and anorectic. Amphetamines are usually taken orally but also can be injected, nasally inhaled, or smoked. The clinical syndromes associated with amphetamines are similar to those associated with cocaine, although the oral route of amphetamine administration produces a less rapid euphoria and consequently is less addictive. Intravenous amphetamine abuse is highly addictive.

 CLINICAL HINT:
Amphetamines are commonly abused by students, long-distance truck drivers, and other persons who desire prolonged wakefulness and attentiveness.

Amphetamines can induce a paranoid psychosis similar to paranoid schizophrenia. Intoxication usually resolves in 24 to 48 hours. Amphetamine abuse can cause severe hypertension, cerebrovascular disease, and myocardial infarction and ischemia. Neurologic symptoms range from twitching to tetany to seizures, coma, and death as doses escalate. Tremor, ataxia, bruxism, shortness of breath, headache, fever, and flushing are common but less severe physical effects.

1. **Epidemiology.** In the United States, about 7% of the population used psychostimulants, with the highest use in the 18 to 25 year old age group, followed by the 12 to 17 year old age group. The lifetime prevalence of amphetamine dependence and abuse is 1.5%, with about equal use in men and women.

2. **Drugs**

   a. **Major amphetamines.** Amphetamine, dextroamphetamine (Dexedrine), methamphetamine (Desoxyn, "speed"), methylphenidate, pemoline (Cylert).

   b. **Related substances.** Ephedrine, phenylpropanolamine (PPA), khat, methcathinone ("crank").

   c. **Substituted (designer) amphetamines** (also classified as hallucinogens). Have neurochemical effects on both serotonergic and dopaminergic systems; have both amphetaminelike and hallucinogenlike behavioral effects (e.g., 3,4-methylenedioxymethamphetamine [MDMA, "ecstasy"]; 2.5-dimethoxy-4-methylamphetamine [DOM], also referred to as "STP"; N-ethyl-3,4-methylenedioxyamphetamine [MDEA]; 5-methoxy-3,4-methylenedioxyamphetamine [MMDA]). MDMA use is associated with increased self-confidence and sensory sensitivity, and peaceful feelings with insight, empathy, and a sense of personal closeness with other people. Effects are activating and energizing with a hallucinogenic character but less disorientation and perceptual disturbance than are seen with classic hallucinogens.

Table 11–23
DSM-IV-TR Diagnostic Criteria for Amphetamine Intoxication

A. Recent use of amphetamine or a related substance (e.g., methylphenidate).
B. Clinically significant maladaptive behavioral or psychological changes (e.g., euphoria or affective blunting; changes in sociability; hypervigilance; interpersonal sensitivity; anxiety, tension, or anger; stereotyped behaviors; impaired judgment; or impaired social or occupational functioning) that developed during, or shortly after, use of amphetamine or a related substance.
C. Two (or more) of the following, developing during, or shortly after, use of amphetamine or a related substance:
1. Tachycardia or bradycardia
2. Pupillary dilation
3. Elevated or lowered blood pressure
4. Perspiration or chills
5. Nausea or vomiting
6. Evidence of weight loss
7. Psychomotor agitation or retardation
8. Muscular weakness, respiratory depression, chest pain, or cardiac arrhythmias
9. Confusion, seizures, dyskinesias, dystonias, or coma
D. The symptoms are not due to a general medical condition and are not better accounted for by another mental disorder.
Specify if:
   With perceptual disturbances

From American Psychiatric Association. *Diagnostic and Statistical Manual of Mental Disorders.* 4th ed. Text rev. Washington, DC: American Psychiatric Association; 2000, with permission.

MDMA is associated with hyperthermia, particularly when used in close quarters in combination with increased physical activity, as is common at "raves." Heavy or long-term use may be associated with serotonergic nerve damage.

  d. **"Ice."** Pure form of methamphetamine (inhaled, smoked, injected). Particularly powerful. Psychological effects can last for hours. Synthetic, manufactured domestically.

3. **Intoxication and withdrawal.** Autonomic nervous system hyperactivity and behavioral change. See Tables 11–23 and 11–24.

Table 11–24
DSM-IV-TR Diagnostic Criteria for Amphetamine Withdrawal

A. Cessation of (or reduction in) amphetamine (or a related substance) use that has been heavy and prolonged.
B. Dysphoric mood and two (or more) of the following physiologic changes, developing within a few hours to several days after Criterion A:
1. Fatigue
2. Vivid, unpleasant dreams
3. Insomnia or hypersomnia
4. Increased appetite
5. Psychomotor retardation or agitation
C. The symptoms in Criterion B cause clinically significant distress or impairment in social, occupational, or other important areas of functioning.
D. The symptoms are not due to a general medical condition and are not better accounted for by another mental disorder.

From American Psychiatric Association. *Diagnostic and Statistical Manual of Mental Disorders.* 4th ed. Text rev. Washington, DC: American Psychiatric Association; 2000, with permission.

CLINICAL HINT:

Amphetamine can also produce psychotic symptoms similar to paranoid schizophrenia (amphetamine-induced psychosis); unlike schizophrenia, it clears in a few days and a positive finding in a urine drug screen reveals the correct diagnosis.

4. **Treatment.** Symptomatic. Benzodiazepines for agitation. Fluoxetine (Prozac) or bupropion (Wellbutrin) has been used for maintenance therapy after detoxification.

L. **Cocaine.** One of the most addictive of the commonly abused substances; referred to as *coke, blow, crack,* or *freebase*. The effects of cocaine are pharmacologically similar to those of other stimulants, but its widespread use warrants a separate discussion. Before it was well known that cocaine was highly addictive, it was widely used as a stimulant and euphoriant. Cocaine is usually inhaled but can be smoked or injected.

Crack is smoked, has a rapid onset of action, and is highly addictive. The onset of action of smoked cocaine is comparable with that of intravenously injected cocaine, and the drug is equally addictive in this circumstance. The euphoria is intense, and a risk for dependence develops after only one dose. Like amphetamines, cocaine can be taken in binges lasting up to several days. This phenomenon is partly the result of greater euphoric effects derived from subsequent doses (sensitization). During binges, the abuser takes the cocaine repeatedly until exhausted or out of the drug. There follows a crash of lethargy, hunger, and prolonged sleep, followed by another binge. With repeated use, tolerance develops to the euphoriant, anorectic, hyperthermic, and cardiovascular effects.

Intravenous cocaine use is associated with risks for the same conditions as other forms of intravenous drug abuse, including AIDS, septicemia, and venous thrombus.

 CLINICAL HINT:

Long-term snorting can lead to a rebound rhinitis, which is often self-treated with nasal decongestants; it also causes nosebleeds and eventually may lead to a perforated nasal septum.

Other physical sequelae include cerebral infarctions, seizures, myocardial infarctions, cardiac arrhythmias, and cardiomyopathies.

1. **Epidemiology.** About 10% of the U.S. population has tried cocaine, and the lifetime rate of cocaine abuse or dependence is about 2%. It is most common in persons in the 18 to 25 year old age group, with a male-to-female ratio of 2:1. All races and socioeconomic groups are equally affected.

2. **Cocaine intoxication.** See Table 11–25. Can cause restlessness, agitation, anxiety, talkativeness, pressured speech, paranoid ideation, aggressiveness, increased sexual interest, heightened sense of awareness, grandiosity, hyperactivity, and other manic symptoms. Physical signs include tachycardia, hypertension, pupillary dilation, chills, anorexia,

Table 11–25
DSM-IV-TR Diagnostic Criteria for Cocaine Intoxication

A. Recent use of cocaine.
B. Clinically significant maladaptive behavioral or psychological changes (e.g., euphoria or affective blunting; changes in sociability; hypervigilance; interpersonal sensitivity; anxiety, tension, or anger; stereotyped behaviors; impaired judgment; or impaired social or occupational functioning) that developed during, or shortly after, use of cocaine.
C. Two (or more) of the following, developing during, or shortly after, cocaine use:
  1. Tachycardia or bradycardia
  2. Pupillary dilation
  3. Elevated or lowered blood pressure
  4. Perspiration or chills
  5. Nausea or vomiting
  6. Evidence of weight loss
  7. Psychomotor agitation or retardation
  8. Muscular weakness, respiratory depression, chest pain, or cardiac arrhythmias
  9. Confusion, seizures, dyskinesias, dystonias, or coma
D. The symptoms are not due to a general medical condition and are not better accounted for by another mental disorder.
Specify if:
  With perceptual disturbances

From American Psychiatric Association. *Diagnostic and Statistical Manual of Mental Disorders.* 4th ed. Text rev. Washington, DC: American Psychiatric Association; 2000, with permission.

insomnia, and stereotyped movements. Cocaine use has also been associated with sudden death from cardiac complications and delirium. Delusional disorders are typically paranoid. Delirium may involve tactile or olfactory hallucinations. Delusions and hallucinations may occur in up to 50% of all persons who use cocaine. Delirium may lead to seizures and death.

3. **Withdrawal.** See Table 11–26. The most prominent sign of cocaine withdrawal is the craving for cocaine. The tendency to develop dependence is related to the route of administration (lower with snorting, higher with intravenous injection or smoking freebase cocaine). Withdrawal symptoms include fatigue, lethargy, guilt, anxiety, and feelings of helplessness,

Table 11–26
DSM-IV-TR Diagnostic Criteria for Cocaine Withdrawal

A. Cessation of (or reduction in) cocaine use that has been heavy and prolonged.
B. Dysphoric mood and two (or more) of the following physiologic changes, developing within a few hours to several days after Criterion A:
  1. Fatigue
  2. Vivid, unpleasant dreams
  3. Insomnia or hypersomnia
  4. Increased appetite
  5. Psychomotor retardation or agitation
C. The symptoms in Criterion B cause clinically significant distress or impairment in social, occupational, or other important areas of functioning.
D. The symptoms are not due to a general medical condition and are not better accounted for by another mental disorder.

From American Psychiatric Association. *Diagnostic and Statistical Manual of Mental Disorders.* 4th ed. Text rev. Washington, DC: American Psychiatric Association; 2000, with permission.

hopelessness, and worthlessness. Long-term use can lead to depression, which may require antidepressant treatment. Observe for possible suicidal ideation. Withdrawal symptoms usually peak in several days, but the syndrome (especially depressive symptoms) may last for weeks.

4. **Treatment.** Treatment is largely symptomatic. Agitation can be treated with restraints, benzodiazepines, or, if severe (delirium or psychosis), low doses of high-potency antipsychotics (only as a last resort because the medications lower the seizure threshold). Somatic symptoms (e.g., tachycardia, hypertension) can be treated with β-adrenergic receptor antagonists (β-blockers). Evaluate for possible medical complications.

M. **Cannabis (marijuana).** *Cannabis sativa* is a plant from which cannabis or marijuana is derived. All parts of the plant contain psychoactive cannabinoids of which Δ-9-tetrahydrocannabinol (THC) is the main active euphoriant (many other active cannabinoids are probably responsible for the other varied effects). Sometimes, purified THC also is abused. Cannabinoids usually are smoked but also can be eaten (onset of effect is delayed, but one can eat very large doses).

1. **Epidemiology.** There is a 5% lifetime rate of cannabis abuse or dependence with those aged 18 to 21 being the highest users, but all age groups are affected. Use is highest among whites compared to other ethnic groups.

2. **Cannabis intoxication.** When cannabis is smoked, euphoric effects appear within minutes, peak in 30 minutes, and last 2 to 4 hours. Motor and cognitive effects can last 5 to 12 hours. Symptoms include euphoria or dysphoria, anxiety, suspiciousness, inappropriate laughter, time distortion, social withdrawal, impaired judgment, and the following objective signs: conjunctival injection, increased appetite, dry mouth, and tachycardia. It also causes a dose-dependent hypothermia and mild sedation. Often used with alcohol, cocaine, and other drugs. Can cause depersonalization and, rarely, hallucinations. More commonly causes mild persecutory delusions, which seldom require medication. In very high doses, can cause mild delirium with panic symptoms or a prolonged cannabis psychosis (may last up to 6 weeks). Long-term use can lead to anxiety or depression and an apathetic amotivational syndrome. Chronic respiratory disease and lung cancer are long-term risks secondary to inhalation of carcinogenic hydrocarbons. Results of urinary testing for THC are positive for up to 4 weeks after intoxication.

3. **Cannabis dependence.** Dependence and withdrawal are controversial diagnoses; there are certainly many psychologically dependent abusers, but forced abstinence, even in heavy users, does not consistently cause a characteristic withdrawal syndrome.

4. **Therapeutic uses.** Cannabis and its primary active components (Δ-9-THC) have been used successfully to treat nausea secondary to cancer chemotherapy, to stimulate appetite in patients with AIDS, and in the treatment of glaucoma.

5. **Treatment.** Treatment of intoxication usually is not required. Anxiolytics for anxiety; antipsychotics for hallucinations or delusions.

N. Hallucinogens. Hallucinogens are natural and synthetic substances, also known as psychedelics or psychotomimetics because they produce hallucinations, a loss of contact with reality, and an experience of expanded or heightened consciousness. The classic, naturally occurring hallucinogens are psilocybin (from some mushrooms) and mescaline (from peyote cactus); others are harmine, harmaline, ibogaine, and dimethyltryptamine. The classic substituted amphetamines include MDMA, MDEA, 2,5-dimethoxy-4-methylamphetamine (DOM, STP), dimethyltryptamine (DMT), MMDA, and trimethoxyamphetamine (TMA), which are also commonly classified with amphetamines. See Table 11–27.

1. **General considerations.** Hallucinogens usually are eaten, sucked out of paper (buccally ingested), or smoked. This category includes many different drugs with different effects. Hallucinogens act as sympathomimetics and cause hypertension, tachycardia, hyperthermia, and dilated pupils. Psychological effects range from mild perceptual changes to frank hallucinations; most users experience only mild effects. Usually used sporadically because of tolerance, which develops rapidly and remits within several days of abstinence. Physical dependence or withdrawal does not occur, but psychological dependence can develop. Hallucinogens often are contaminated with anticholinergic drugs. Hallucinogen potency is associated with binding affinity at the serotonin-5-HT$_2$ receptor, where these drugs act as partial agonists.

2. **Epidemiology.** Hallucinogen use is most common among young men (ages 15 to 35), with white men having the highest use compared to women and other ethnic groups. The lifetime use of hallucinogen in the United States is about 12%.

3. **Hallucinogen intoxication (hallucinosis)**

   a. **Diagnosis, signs, and symptoms.** In a state of full wakefulness and alertness, maladaptive behavioral changes (anxiety, depression, ideas of reference, paranoid ideation); changes in perception (hallucinations, illusions, depersonalization); pupillary dilation, tachycardia or palpitations, sweating, blurring of vision, tremors, and incoordination. Panic reactions ("bad trips") can occur even in experienced users. The user typically becomes convinced that the disturbed perceptions are real. In the typical bad trip, the user feels as if he or she is going mad, has damaged his or her brain, and will never recover. See Table 11–28.

   b. **Treatment.** Involves reassurance and keeping the patient in contact with trusted, supportive people (friends, nurses). Diazepam (20 mg orally) can rapidly curtail hallucinogen intoxication and is considered superior to "talking down" the patient, which may take hours. If the patient is psychotic and agitated, high-potency antipsychotics, such as haloperidol (Haldol), fluphenazine (Prolixin), or thiothixene (Navane), may be used (avoid low-potency antipsychotics because of anticholinergic effects). A controlled environment is necessary to prevent possible dangerous actions resulting from grossly impaired judgment. Physical restraints may be required. Prolonged psychosis

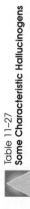

Table 11-27
Some Characteristic Hallucinogens

Agent	Locale	Chemical Classification	Biologic Sources	Common Route	Typical Dose	Duration of Effects
Lysergic acid diethylamine	Global	Indolalkylamine	Lysergic acid, semisynthetic	Oral	75 mcg	6–12 hours
Mescaline	Southwestern United States	Phenethylamine	Peyote cactus, *Lophophora williamsii*, *Lophophora diffusa*	Oral	200–400 mg or 4–6 cactus buttons	10–12 hours
Methylenedioxy-methamphetamine	Global	Phenethylamine	Synthetic	Oral	50–150 mg	4–6 hours
Psilocybin	Southern United States, Mexico, South America	Phosphorylated hydroxylated DMT	Psilocybin mushrooms	Oral	5 mg or 8 g of dried mushroom	4–6 hours
DMT[a]	South America, synthetic	Substituted tryptamine	Leaves of *Virola calophylla*	As a snuff, IV, smoked	0.2 mg/kg IV	30 minutes
Ibogaine	West Central Africa	Indolalkylamine	*Tabernanthe iboga* powdered root	Oral	200–400 mg	8–48 hours
Ayahuasca	South America East Amazon	Harmine, other β carbolines	Bark or leaves of liana vine	Orally as a tea	300–400 mg	4–8 hours
Morning glory seeds	American temperate zones	D-Lysergic acid alkaloids	Seeds of *Ipomoea violacea, Turbina corymbosa*	Orally as a tea	7–13 seeds	3 hours

[a]DMT, dimethyltryptamine.

136

Table 11–28
***DSM-IV-TR* Diagnostic Criteria for Hallucinogen Intoxication**

A. Recent use of a hallucinogen.
B. Clinically significant maladaptive behavioral or psychological changes (e.g., marked anxiety or depression, ideas of reference, fear of losing one's mind, paranoid ideation, impaired judgment, or impaired social or occupational functioning) that developed during, or shortly after, hallucinogen use.
C. Perceptual changes occurring in a state of full wakefulness and alertness (e.g., subjective intensification of perceptions, depersonalization, derealization, illusions, hallucinations, synesthesias) that developed during, or shortly after, hallucinogen use.
D. Two (or more) of the following signs, developing during, or shortly after, hallucinogen use:
1. Pupillary dilation
2. Tachycardia
3. Sweating
4. Palpitations
5. Blurring of vision
6. Tremors
7. Incoordination
E. The symptoms are not due to a general medical condition and are not better accounted for by another mental disorder.

From American Psychiatric Association. *Diagnostic and Statistical Manual of Mental Disorders*. 4th ed. Text rev. Washington, DC: American Psychiatric Association; 2000, with permission.

resembling schizophreniform disorder occasionally develops in vulnerable patients. Delusional syndromes and mood (usually depressive) disorders may also develop.

4. **Hallucinogen persisting perception disorder.** A distressing repeated experience of impaired perception after cessation of hallucinogen use (i.e., a **flashback**). The patient may require low doses of a benzodiazepine (for an acute episode) or antipsychotic drug (if persistent). Anticonvulsants such as valproic acid (Depakene) and carbamazepine (Tegretol) have also been of use. See Table 11–29.

O. **Phencyclidine (PCP) and similarly acting drugs.** Phencyclidine (PCP; 1-1-phenylcyclohexyl-piperidine), also known as *angel dust*, is a dissociative anesthetic with hallucinogenic effects. Similarly acting drugs include ketamine (Ketalar), also referred to as *special K*. PCP commonly causes

Table 11–29
***DSM-IV-TR* Diagnostic Criteria for Hallucinogen Persisting Perception Disorder (Flashbacks)**

A. The reexperiencing, after cessation of use of a hallucinogen, of one or more of the perceptual symptoms that were experienced while intoxicated with the hallucinogen (e.g., geometric hallucinations, false perceptions of movement in the peripheral visual fields, flashes of color, intensified colors, trails of images of moving objects, positive afterimages, halos around objects, macropsia, and micropsia).
B. The symptoms in Criterion A cause clinically significant distress or impairment in social, occupational, or other important areas of functioning.
C. The symptoms are not due to a general medical condition (e.g., anatomic lesions and infections of the brain, visual epilepsies) and are not better accounted for by another mental disorder (e.g., delirium, dementia, schizophrenia) or hypnopompic hallucinations.

From American Psychiatric Association. *Diagnostic and Statistical Manual of Mental Disorders*. 4th ed. Text rev. Washington, DC: American Psychiatric Association; 2000, with permission.

paranoia and unpredictable violence, which often brings abusers to medical attention. The primary pharmacodynamic effect is antagonism of the NMDA subtype of glutamate receptors.

1. **Epidemiology.** About 14% of 18 to 25 year old men and women have used PCP in their lifetime; its use is declining, however. PCP is associated with 3% of substance-abuse deaths and 32% of substance-related disorders.

2. **PCP intoxication**

   a. **Diagnosis, signs, and symptoms.** Belligerence, assaultiveness, agitation, impulsiveness, unpredictability, and the following signs: nystagmus, increased blood pressure or heart rate, numbness or diminished response to pain, ataxia, dysarthria, muscle rigidity, seizures, and hyperacusis.

   Typically, PCP is smoked with marijuana (a laced joint) or tobacco, but it can be eaten, injected, or inhaled nasally. PCP use should be considered in patients who describe unusual experiences with marijuana or LSD. PCP may remain detectable in blood and urine for more than 1 week.

   Effects are dose related. At low doses, PCP acts as a CNS depressant, producing nystagmus, blurred vision, numbness, and incoordination. At moderate doses, PCP produces hypertension, dysarthria, ataxia, increased muscle tone (especially in the face and neck), hyperactive reflexes, and sweating. At higher doses, PCP produces agitation, fever, abnormal movements, rhabdomyolysis, myoglobinuria, and renal failure. Overdose can cause seizures, severe hypertension, diaphoresis, hypersalivation, respiratory depression, stupor (with eyes open), coma, and death. Violent actions are common with intoxication. Because of the analgesic effects of PCP, patients may have no regard for their own bodies and may severely injure themselves while agitated and combative. Psychosis, sometimes persistent (may resemble schizophreniform disorder), may develop. This is especially likely in patients with underlying schizophrenia. Other possible complications include delirium, mood disorder, and delusional disorder. Ketamine, derived from PCP, produces a similar clinical picture.

   b. **Treatment.** Isolate the patient in a nonstimulating environment. Do not try to talk down the intoxicated patient, as you might with a patient with anxiety disorder; wait for the PCP to clear first. Urine acidification may increase drug clearance (ascorbic acid or ammonium chloride), but it may be ineffective and increase the risk for renal failure. Screen for other drugs. If the patient is acutely agitated, use benzodiazepines. If agitated and psychotic, an antipsychotic may be used. Avoid antipsychotics with potent intensive anticholinergic properties, because high-dose PCP has anticholinergic actions. If physical restraint is required, immobilize the patient completely to prevent self-injury. Recovery is usually rapid. Protect the patient and staff. Always evaluate for concomitant medical conditions. Treatment for ketamine intoxication is similar.

P. Inhalants. Inhalant drugs (also called *inhalants* or *volatile substances*) are volatile hydrocarbons that are inhaled for psychotropic effects. They include gasoline, kerosene, plastic and rubber cements, airplane and household glues, paints, lacquers, enamels, paint thinners, aerosols, polishes, fingernail polish remover, nitrous oxide, amyl nitrate, butyl nitrate, and cleaning fluids. Inhalants typically are abused by adolescents in lower socioeconomic groups.

 CLINICAL HINT:

Some persons use "poppers" (amyl nitrate, butyl nitrate) during sex to intensify orgasm through vasodilation, which produces light-headedness, giddiness, and euphoria. With the introduction of sildenafil (Viagra) used to produce penile erections, a special warning must be given to those who use nitrate-containing drugs, because the combination can cause cardiovascular collapse and death.

Symptoms of mild intoxication are similar to intoxication with alcohol or sedative–hypnotics. Psychological effects include mild euphoria, belligerence, assaultiveness, impaired judgment, and impulsiveness. Physical effects include ataxia, confusion, disorientation, slurred speech, dizziness, depressed reflexes, and nystagmus. These can progress to delirium and seizures. Possible toxic effects include brain damage, liver damage, bone marrow depression, peripheral neuropathies, and immunosuppression. See Table 11–30. Rarely a withdrawal syndrome can develop. It is characterized by irritability, sleep disturbances, jitters, sweats, nausea, vomiting,

 Table 11–30
DSM-IV-TR Diagnostic Criteria for Inhalant Intoxication

A. Recent intentional use or short-term, high-dose exposure to volatile inhalants (excluding anesthetic gases and short-acting vasodilators).
B. Clinically significant maladaptive behavioral or psychological changes (e.g., belligerence, assaultiveness, apathy, impaired judgment, impaired social or occupational functioning) that developed during, or shortly after, use of or exposure to volatile inhalants.
C. Two (or more) of the followings signs, developing during, or shortly after, inhalant use or exposure:
 1. Dizziness
 2. Nystagmus
 3. Incoordination
 4. Slurred speech
 5. Unsteady gait
 6. Lethargy
 7. Depressed reflexes
 8. Psychomotor retardation
 9. Tremor
 10. Generalized muscle weakness
 11. Blurred vision or diplopia
 12. Stupor or coma
 13. Euphoria
D. The symptoms are not due to a general medical condition and are not better accounted for by another mental disorder.

From American Psychiatric Association. *Diagnostic and Statistical Manual of Mental Disorders.* 4th ed. Text rev. Washington, DC: American Psychiatric Association; 2000, with permission.

Table 11–31
Typical Caffeine Content of Foods and Medications

Substance	Caffeine Content
Brewed coffee	100 mg/6 oz
Instant coffee	70 mg/6 oz
Decaffeinated coffee	4 mg/6 oz
Leaf or bag tea	40 mg/6 oz
Instant tea	25 mg/6 oz
Caffeinated soda	45 mg/12 oz
Cocoa beverage	5 mg/6 oz
Chocolate milk	4 mg/6 oz
Dark chocolate	20 mg/1 oz
Milk chocolate	6 mg/1 oz
Caffeine-containing cold remedies	25–50 mg/tablet
Caffeine-containing analgesics	25–65 mg/tablet
Stimulants	100–350 mg/tablet
Weight-loss aids	75–200 mg/tablet

Adapted from *DSM-IV-TR* and Barone JJ, Roberts HR. Caffeine consumption. *Food Chem Toxicol* 1996;34:119, with permission.

tachycardia, and sometimes hallucinations and delusions. Short-term treatment is supportive medical care (e.g., fluids and monitoring of blood pressure).

Q. **Caffeine.** Caffeine is present in coffee, tea, chocolate, cola and other carbonated beverages, cocoa, cold medications, and OTC stimulants. (See Table 11–31 for the typical caffeine content of foods and medications.) Intoxication is characterized by restlessness, nervousness, excitement, insomnia, flushed face, diuresis, gastrointestinal disturbance, muscle twitching, rambling flow of thought and speech, tachycardia or cardiac arrhythmia, periods of inexhaustibility, and psychomotor agitation. High doses can increase symptoms of psychiatric disorders (e.g., anxiety, psychosis). Tolerance develops. Withdrawal is usually characterized by headache and lasts 4 to 5 days. Treatment is symptomatic. A short course of a benzodiazepine (diazepam, 15 mg/day for 2 to 5 days) may help alleviate withdrawal agitation and insomnia.

R. **Nicotine.** Nicotine is taken through tobacco smoking and chewing. Nicotine dependence is the most prevalent and deadly substance use disorder. Nicotine activates nicotine acetylcholine receptors in addition to the dopamine reward system and increases multiple stimulatory neurohormones. It is rapidly absorbed when inhaled and reaches the CNS within 15 seconds.

1. **Epidemiology.** About 25% of Americans smoke, 25% are former smokers, and 50% have never smoked. The mean age of onset of smoking is 16 years of age, and few persons start after 20 years of age. Worldwide, about 47% of people smoke.

2. **Nicotine dependence.** Develops rapidly and is strongly affected by environmental conditioning. Often coexists with dependence on other substances (e.g., alcohol, marijuana). Treatments for dependence include hypnosis, aversive therapy, acupuncture, nicotine nasal sprays and gums, transdermal nicotine (nicotine patches), clonidine, and a variety of other nonnicotine psychopharmacologic agents. Bupropion (Zyban) at doses

Table 11–32
Effect of Abstinence from Smoking on Blood Concentrations of Psychiatric Medicines

Abstinence increases blood concentrations			
Clomipramine	Desmethyldiazepam	Haloperidol	Nortriptyline
Clozapine	Doxepin	Imipramine	Propranolol
Desipramine	Fluvoxamine	Oxazepam	
Abstinence does not increase blood concentrations			
Amitriptyline	Ethanol	Midazolam	
Chlordiazepoxide	Lorazepam	Triazolam	
Effects of abstinence unclear			
Alprazolam	Chlorpromazine	Diazepam	

of 300 mg/day may increase the quit rate in smokers with and without depression. The combined use of systemic nicotine administration and behavioral counseling has resulted in sustained abstinence rates of 60%. High relapse rates. *Chantix* (varenicline) is a partial nicotine agonist for $\alpha_4\beta_2$ nicotinic acetylcholine receptor subtypes. It is usually dosed at 1 mg b.i.d. following a 1-week titration beginning at 0.5 mg/day for several days. Psychiatrists should be aware of the effects of abstinence from smoking on blood concentrations of psychotropic drugs (Table 11–32). Smoking is more habit-forming than chewing. Smoking is associated with chronic obstructive pulmonary disease, cancers, coronary heart disease, and peripheral vascular disease. Tobacco chewing is associated with peripheral vascular disease.

   3. Nicotine withdrawal. Characterized by nicotine craving, irritability, frustration, anger, anxiety, difficulty concentrating, restlessness, bradycardia, and increased appetite. The withdrawal syndrome may last for up to several weeks and is often superimposed on withdrawal from other substances.

   4. Treatment. A summary of treatment techniques is given in Table 11–33.

S. Anabolic steroids. Anabolic steroids are a family of drugs comprising the natural male hormone testosterone and a group of more than 50 synthetic analogs of testosterone. They are Drug Enforcement Agency Schedule III

Table 11–33
Scientifically Proven Treatments for Smoking

Psychosocial therapy
  Behavior therapy
Pharmacologic therapies
  Nicotine gum
  Nicotine patch
  Nicotine gum + patch
  Nicotine nasal spray
  Nicotine inhaler
  Bupropion
  Bupropion + nicotine patch
  Clonidine[a]
  Nortriptyline[a]

[a]Not an FDA-approved use.

Table 11–34
Examples of Commonly Used Anabolic Steroids^a

Compounds usually administered orally
Fluoxymesterone (Halotestin, Android-F, Ultandren)
Methandienone (formerly called *methandrostenolone*) (Dianabol)
Methyltestosterone (Android, Testred, Virilon)
Mibolerone (Cheque Drops)^b
Oxandrolone (Anavar)
Oxymetholone (Anadrol, Hemogenin)
Mesterolone (Mestoranum, Proviron)
Stanozolol (Winstrol)
Compounds usually administered intramuscularly
Nandrolone decanoate (Deca-Durabolin)
Nandrolone phenpropionate (Durabolin)
Methenolone enanthate (Primobolan depot)
Boldenone undecylenate (Equipoise)^b
Stanozolol (Winstrol-V)^b
Testosterone esters blends (Sustanon, Sten)
Testosterone cypionate
Testosterone enanthate (Delatestryl)
Testosterone propionate (Testoviron, Androlan)
Testosterone undecanoate (Andriol, Restandol)
Trenbolone acetate (Finajet, Finaplix)^b
Trenbolone hexahydrobencylcarbonate (Parabolan)

^{a}Many of the brand names listed are foreign but are included because of the widespread illicit use of foreign steroid preparations in the United States.
^{b}Veterinary compound.

controlled substances that are illegally used to enhance physical performance and appearance and to increase muscle bulk. Examples of commonly used anabolic steroids are listed in Table 11–34. An estimated 1 million Americans have used illegal steroids at least once. Use has been increasing among male adolescents and young adults.

People drawn to these drugs are usually involved in athletics. Reinforcement occurs when the drugs produce desired results, such as enhanced performance and appearance. Anabolic steroid users typically use a variety of ergogenic (performance-enhancing) drugs to gain muscle, lose fat, or lose water for bodybuilding competitions. These drugs include thyroid hormones and stimulants. Dehydroepiandrosterone (DHEA) and androstenedione are adrenal androgens marketed as food supplements and sold over the counter. Steroids initially produce euphoria and hyperactivity, which can give way to hostility, irritability, anxiety, somatization, depression, manic symptoms, and violent outbursts ("roid rage"). Steroids are addictive. Abstinence can produce depression, anxiety, and worry about physical appearance. Physical complications of abuse include acne, premature balding, gynecomastia, testicular atrophy, yellowing of the skin and eyes, clitoral enlargement, menstrual abnormalities, and hirsutism.

Treatment includes psychotherapy to cope with body image distortions and the profound physical side effects of prolonged steroid use. As with other substances of abuse, abstinence is the goal. Frequent urine testing is indicated.

For a more detailed discussion of this topic, see Substance-Related Disorders, Ch 11, p. 1237, in CTP/IX.
For a more detailed discussion of alcohol, see Alcohol-Related Disorders, Sec. 11.2, p. 1268, in CTP/IX.

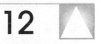
Schizophrenia

I. Definition

Schizophrenia is a syndrome of unknown etiology characterized by disturbances in cognition, emotion, perception, thinking, and behavior. Schizophrenia is well established as a brain disorder, with structural and functional abnormalities visible in neuroimaging studies and a genetic component, as seen in twin studies. The disorder is usually chronic, with a course encompassing a prodromal phase, an active phase, and a residual phase. The active phase has symptoms such as hallucinations, delusions, and disorganized thinking. The prodromal and residual phases are characterized by attenuated forms of active symptoms, such as odd beliefs and magical thinking, as well as deficits in self-care and interpersonal relatedness. Since the 1970s, the number of schizophrenic patients in hospitals has decreased by over 50% (deinstitutionalization). Of those being treated, over 80% are managed as outpatients. Although schizophrenia is discussed as if it is a single disease, it probably comprises a group of disorders of heterogeneous etiology. A brief history of the disorder is to be found in Table 12–1.

II. Epidemiology

A. Incidence and prevalence. In the United States, the lifetime prevalence of the disease is about 1%, which means that 1 in 100 persons will develop the disorder during his or her lifetime. It is found in all societies and in all geographic areas. Worldwide, 2 million new cases appear each year. In the United States, only about 0.05% of the total population is treated for schizophrenia in any single year, and only about half of all patients obtain treatment of any kind. There are over 2 million persons suffering from schizophrenia in the United States.

B. Gender and age. Equally prevalent between men and women; usually onset is earlier in men. Peak age of onset is between 15 and 35 years (50% of cases occur before age 25). Onset before age 10 (called early-onset schizophrenia) or after age 45 (called late-onset schizophrenia) is uncommon.

C. Infection and birth season. Persons born in winter are more likely to develop the disease than those born in spring or summer (applies to both Northern and Southern Hemispheres). Increased in babies born to mothers who have influenza during pregnancy.

D. Race and religion. Jews are affected less often than Protestants and Catholics, and prevalence is higher in nonwhite populations.

E. Medical and mental illness. Higher mortality rate from accidents and natural causes than in general population. Leading cause of death in schizophrenic patients is suicide (10% kill themselves). Over 40% of schizophrenic patients abuse drugs and alcohol. Treatment with antipsychotic

Table 12–1
History of Schizophrenia

1852—Schizophrenia was first formally described by Belgian psychiatrist Benedict Morel, who called it *démence précoce*.
1896—Emil Kraepelin, a German psychiatrist, applied the term *dementia praecox* to a group of illnesses beginning in adolescence that ended in dementia.
1911—Swiss psychiatrist Eugen Bleuler introduced the term *schizophrenia*. No signs or symptoms are pathognomonic; instead, a cluster of characteristic findings indicates the diagnosis. He introduced the concept of the fundamental symptoms, called the *four As*: (1) associational disturbances, (2) affective disturbances, (3) autism, and (4) ambivalence.

agents increase the risk of developing diabetes and the metabolic syndrome.

    F. Socioeconomics. More common among lower rather than higher socioeconomic groups; high prevalence among recent immigrants; most common in cities with over 1 million population. Direct and indirect costs resulting from schizophrenic illness in the United States are over $100 billion per year.

III. Etiology
Owing to the heterogeneity of the symptomatic and prognostic presentations of schizophrenia, no single factor is considered causative. The *stress diathesis model* is most often used, which states that the person in whom schizophrenia develops has a specific biological vulnerability, or diathesis, that is triggered by stress and leads to schizophrenic symptoms. Stressors may be genetic, biological, and psychosocial or environmental.

    A. Genetic. Both single-gene and polygenic theories have been proposed (Table 12–2). Although neither theory has been definitively substantiated, the polygenic theory appears to be more consistent with the presentation of schizophrenia.

        1. Consanguinity. Incidence in families is higher than in the general population, and monozygotic (MZ) twin concordance is greater than dizygotic (DZ) (Table 12–3).

        2. Adoption studies

            a. The prevalence of schizophrenia is greater in the biological parents of schizophrenic adoptees than in adoptive parents.

            b. MZ twins reared apart have the same concordance rate as twins reared together.

Table 12–2
Features Consistent with Polygenic Inheritance[a]

- Disorder can be transmitted with two normal parents.
- Presentation of disorder ranges from very severe to less severe.
- More severely affected persons have a greater number of ill relatives than mildly affected persons do.
- Risk decreases as the number of shared genes decreases.
- Disorder present in both mother's and father's side of family.

[a]The number of affected genes determines a person's risk and symptomatic picture.

Table 12–3
Prevalence of Schizophrenia in Specific Populations

Population	Prevalence
General population	1–1.5
First-degree relative*a*	10–12
Second-degree relative	5–6
Child of two schizophrenic parents	40
Dizygotic twin	12–15
Monozygotic twin	45–50

*a*Schizophrenia is not a sex-linked disorder; it does not matter which parent has the disorder in terms of risk.

    c. Rates of schizophrenia are not increased in children born to unaffected parents but raised by a schizophrenic parent.

B. Biological

    1. Dopamine hypothesis. Schizophrenic symptoms may result from increased limbic dopamine activity (positive symptoms) and decreased frontal dopamine activity (negative symptoms). Dopaminergic pathology may be secondary to abnormal receptor number or sensitivity, or abnormal dopamine release (too much or too little). The theory is based on psychotogenic effects of drugs that increase dopamine levels (e.g., amphetamines, cocaine) and the antipsychotic effects of dopamine receptor antagonists (e.g., haloperidol [Haldol]). Dopamine receptors D_1 through D_5 have been identified. The D_1 receptor may play a role in negative symptoms. Specific D_3 and D_4 receptor agonist and antagonist drugs are under development. Levels of the dopamine metabolite homovanillic acid may correlate with the severity and potential treatment responsiveness of psychotic symptoms. Limitations of the theory include the responsiveness of all types of psychoses to dopamine-blocking agents, which implicates dopaminergic abnormalities in psychoses of multiple causes. The complex interplay of different neurotransmitter systems, including serotonin–dopamine interactions, in addition to the effects of amino acid neurotransmitters on monoamine render single-neurotransmitter theories incomplete.

    2. Norepinephrine hypothesis. Increased norepinephrine levels in schizophrenia lead to increased sensitization to sensory input.

    3. γ-Aminobutyric acid (GABA) hypothesis. Decreased GABA activity results in increased dopamine activity.

    4. Serotonin hypothesis. Serotonin metabolism apparently is abnormal in some chronically schizophrenic patients, with both hyperserotoninemia and hyposerotoninemia being reported. Specifically, antagonism at the serotonin 5-HT_2 receptor has been emphasized as important in reducing psychotic symptoms and the development of movement disorders related to D_2 antagonism. Research on mood disorders has implicated serotonin activity in suicidal and impulsive behavior, which schizophrenic patients can also exhibit.

5. **Glutamate hypothesis.** Hypofunction of the glutamate *N*-methyl-D-aspartate (NMDA)-type receptor is theorized to cause both positive and negative symptoms of schizophrenia based on the observed psychotogenic effects of the NMDA antagonists phencyclidine and ketamine (Ketalar), in addition to the observed therapeutic effects (in research settings) of the NMDA agonists glycine and D-cycloserine.

6. **Neurodevelopmental theories.** There is evidence of abnormal neuronal migration during the second trimester of fetal development. Abnormal neuronal functioning may lead to the emergence of symptoms during adolescence.

C. **Psychosocial and environmental**

1. **Family factors.** Patients whose families have high levels of expressed emotion (EE) have higher relapse rate than those whose families have low EE levels. EE has been defined as any overly involved, intrusive behavior, be it hostile and critical or controlling and infantilizing. Relapse rates are better when family behavior is modified to lower EE. Most observers believe that family dysfunction is a consequence, rather than a cause, of schizophrenia.

2. **Other psychodynamic issues.** Knowing what psychological and environmental stresses are most likely to trigger psychotic decompensation in a patient helps the clinician to address these issues supportively and, in the process, helps the patient to feel and remain more in control.

D. **Infectious theory.** Evidence for a slow virus etiology includes *neuropathological* changes consistent with past infections: gliosis, glial scarring, and antiviral antibodies in the serum and cerebrospinal fluid (CSF) of some schizophrenia patients. Increased frequency of perinatal complications and seasonality of birth data also support an infectious theory.

IV. **Diagnosis, Signs, and Symptoms**

Schizophrenia is a disorder whose diagnosis is based on observation and description of the patient. Abnormalities are often present on most components of the mental status examination. There are no pathognomonic signs or symptoms. According to the text revision of the fourth edition of the *Diagnostic Statistical Manual of Mental Disorders* (*DSM-IV-TR*), at least two of the following five signs or symptoms must be present for at least 1 month: (1) hallucinations, (2) delusions, (3) disorganized speech, (4) disorganized behavior, or (5) negative symptoms (e.g., flat affect, abulia). The signs and symptoms should be present for at least 6 months for the disorder to be confirmed (Table 12–4). Other diagnostic features of schizophrenia are listed below.

A. **Overall functioning.** Level of functioning declines or fails to achieve the expected level.

B. **Thought content.** Abnormal (e.g., delusions, ideas of reference, poverty of content). Delusion and hallucinations are not necessary to make the diagnosis if other signs and symptoms are present.

Table 12–4
DSM-IV-TR Diagnostic Criteria for Schizophrenia

A. *Characteristic symptoms*: Two (or more) of the following, each present for a significant portion of time during a 1-month period (or less if successfully treated):
   1. delusions
   2. hallucinations
   3. disorganized speech (e.g., frequent derailment or incoherence)
   4. grossly disorganized or catatonic behavior
   5. negative symptoms (i.e., affective flattening, alogia, or avolition)
   Note: Only one Criterion A symptom is required if delusions are bizarre or hallucinations consist of a voice keeping up a running commentary on the person's behavior or thoughts, or two or more voices conversing with each other.
B. *Social/occupational dysfunction*: For a significant portion of the time since the onset of the disturbance, one or more major areas of functioning, such as work, interpersonal relations, or self-care, are markedly below the level achieved prior to the onset (or when the onset is in childhood or adolescence, failure to achieve expected level of interpersonal, academic, or occupational achievement).
C. *Duration*: Continuous signs of the disturbance persist for at least 6 months. This 6-month period must include at least 1 month of symptoms (or less if successfully treated) that meet Criterion A (i.e., active-phase symptoms) and may include periods of prodromal or residual symptoms. During these prodromal or residual periods, the signs of the disturbance may be manifested by only negative symptoms or two or more symptoms listed in Criterion A present in attenuated form (e.g., odd beliefs, unusual perceptual experiences).
D. *Schizoaffective and mood disorder exclusion*: Schizoaffective disorder and mood disorder with psychotic features have been ruled out because either (1) no major depressive, manic, or mixed episodes have occurred concurrently with the active-phase symptoms, or (2) if mood episodes have occurred during active-phase symptoms, their total duration has been brief relative to the duration of the active and residual periods.
E. *Substance/general medical condition exclusion*: The disturbance is not due to the direct physiologic effects of a substance (e.g., a drug of abuse, a medication) or a general medical condition.
F. *Relationship to a pervasive developmental disorder*: If there is a history of autistic disorder or another pervasive developmental disorder, the additional diagnosis of schizophrenia is made only if prominent delusions or hallucinations are also present for at least a month (or less if successfully treated.)
Classification of longitudinal course (can be applied only after at least 1 year has elapsed since the initial onset of active-phase symptoms):
   Episodic with interepisode residual symptoms (episodes are defined by the reemergence of prominent psychotic symptoms); *also specify if*: **with prominent negative symptoms.**
   Episodic with no interepisode residual symptoms
   Continuous (prominent psychotic symptoms are present throughout the period of observation); *also specify if*: **with prominent negative symptoms**
   Single episode in partial remission; *also specify if*: **with prominent negative symptoms**
   Single episode in full remission
   Other or unspecified pattern

From American Psychiatric Association. *Diagnostic and Statistical Manual of Mental Disorders*, text revision, 4th ed. Washington, DC: American Psychiatric Association; 2000, with permission.

C. **Form of thought.** Illogical (e.g., derailment, loosening of associations, incoherence, circumstantially, tangentiality, overinclusiveness, neologisms, blocking, echolalia—all incorporated as a thought disorder).
D. **Perception.** Distorted (e.g., hallucinations: visual, olfactory, tactile, and, most frequently, auditory).
E. **Affect.** Abnormal (e.g., flat, blunted, silly, labile, inappropriate).
F. **Sense of self.** Impaired (e.g., loss of ego boundaries, gender confusion, inability to distinguish internal from external reality).

G. Volition. Altered (e.g., inadequate drive or motivation and marked ambivalence).

H. Interpersonal functioning. Impaired (e.g., social withdrawal and emotional detachment, aggressiveness, sexual inappropriateness).

I. Psychomotor behavior. Abnormal or changed (e.g., agitation versus withdrawal, grimacing, posturing, rituals, catatonia).

J. Cognition. Impaired (e.g., concreteness, inattention, impaired information processing).

V. Types

A. Paranoid

1. Characterized mainly by the presence of delusions of persecution or grandeur.
2. Frequent auditory hallucinations related to a single theme, usually persecutory.
3. Patients typically are tense, suspicious, guarded, reserved, and sometimes hostile or aggressive.
4. None of the following: incoherence, loosening of associations, flat or grossly inappropriate affect, catatonic behavior, grossly disorganized behavior. Intelligence remains intact.
5. Age of onset later than catatonic or disorganized type, and the later the onset, the better the prognosis.

B. Disorganized (formerly called hebephrenia)

1. Characterized by marked regression to primitive, disinhibited, and chaotic behavior.
2. Incoherence, marked loosening of associations, flat or grossly inappropriate affect, and pronounced thought disorder.
3. Unkempt appearance, incongruous grinning and grimacing.
4. Early onset, usually before age 25.
5. Does not meet criteria for catatonic type.

C. Catatonic

1. Classic feature is a marked disturbance in motor function called waxy flexibility.
2. May involve rigidity, stupor, posturing, echopraxia; patients may hold awkward positions for long periods of time.
3. Purposeless excitement with risk of injury to self or others may occur.

 CLINICAL HINT:
Patient may emerge from catatonic state suddenly and, without warning, be quite violent.

---

4. Speech disturbances such as echolalia or mutism may occur.
5. May need medical care for associated malnutrition, exhaustion, or hyperpyrexia.

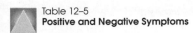

Table 12–5
Positive and Negative Symptoms

Positive Symptoms	Negative Symptoms
Delusions	Affective flattening
Hallucinations	Alogia
Disorganized behavior	Avolition
	Anhedonia

D. Undifferentiated type
1. Prominent delusions, hallucinations, incoherence, or grossly disturbed behavior.
2. Does not meet the criteria for paranoid, catatonic, or disorganized type.

E. Residual type
1. Absence of prominent delusions, hallucinations, incoherence, or grossly disorganized behavior.
2. Continuing evidence of the disturbance through two or more residual symptoms (e.g., emotional blunting, social withdrawal).

F. Other subtypes
1. **Negative and positive symptoms.** Another system classifies schizophrenia into one that is based on the presence of positive or negative symptoms. The negative symptoms include affective flattening or blunting, poverty of speech or speech content, blocking, poor grooming, lack of motivation, anhedonia, social withdrawal, cognitive defects, and attentional deficits. Positive symptoms include loose associations, hallucinations, bizarre behavior, and increased speech (Table 12–5). Patients with positive symptoms have a better prognosis than those with negative symptoms.
2. **Paraphrenia.** Sometimes used as a synonym for *paranoid schizophrenia*. The term also is used for either a progressively deteriorating course of illness or the presence of a well-systematized delusional system. These multiple meanings have reduced the usefulness of the term.
3. **Simple deteriorative schizophrenia (simple schizophrenia).** Characterized by a gradual, insidious loss of drive and ambition. Patients with the disorder are usually not overtly psychotic and do not experience persistent hallucinations or delusions. The primary symptom is the withdrawal of the patient from social and work-related situations.
4. **Early-onset schizophrenia.** Schizophrenia that develops in childhood. Very rare.
5. **Late-onset schizophrenia** Onset after age 45. More common in women, most often of the paranoid type, with good response to medication.

VI. Laboratory and Psychological Tests
A. **EEG.** Most schizophrenic patients have normal EEG findings, but some have decreased alpha and increased theta and delta activity, paroxysmal abnormalities, and increased sensitivity to activation procedures (e.g., sleep deprivation).

B. **Evoked potential studies.** Initial hypersensitivity to sensory stimulation, with later compensatory blunting of information processing at higher cortical levels.

C. **Immunological studies.** In some patients, atypical lymphocytes and decreased numbers of natural killer cells.

D. **Endocrinological studies.** In some patients, decreased levels of luteinizing hormone and follicle-stimulating hormone; diminished release of prolactin and growth hormone following stimulation by gonadotropin-releasing hormone or thyrotropin-releasing hormone.

E. **Neuropsychological testing.** Thematic apperception test and Rorschach test usually reveal bizarre responses. When compared with the parents of normal controls, the parents of schizophrenic patients show more deviation from normal values in projective tests (may be a consequence of living with schizophrenic family member). Halstead–Reitan battery reveals impaired attention and intelligence, decreased retention time, and disturbed problem-solving ability in approximately 20% to 35% of patients. Schizophrenic patients have lower IQs when compared with non-schizophrenic patients, although the range of IQ scores is wide. Decline in IQ occurs with progression of the illness.

VII. **Pathophysiology**
A. **Neuropathology.** No consistent structural defects; changes noted include decreased number of neurons, increased gliosis, and disorganization of neuronal architecture. Degeneration in the limbic system, especially the amygdala, hippocampus, and cingulate cortex, and in the basal ganglia, especially the substantia nigra and dorsolateral prefrontal cortex. Abnormal functioning in basal ganglia and cerebellum may account for movement disorders in schizophrenic patients.

B. **Brain imaging**
1. **Computed tomography (CT).** Cortical atrophy in 10% to 35% of patients; enlargement of the lateral and third ventricle in 10% to 50% of patients; atrophy of the cerebellar vermis and decreased radiodensity of brain parenchyma. Abnormal CT findings may correlate with the presence of negative symptoms (e.g., flattened affect, social withdrawal, psychomotor retardation, lack of motivation, neuropsychiatric impairment, increased frequency of extrapyramidal symptoms, resulting from antipsychotic medications and poor premorbid history).

2. **Magnetic resonance imaging (MRI).** Ventricles in MZ twins with schizophrenia are larger than those of unaffected siblings. Reduced volume of hippocampus, amygdala, and parahippocampal gyrus. Reduced limbic volume correlating with disease severity.

3. **Magnetic resonance spectroscopy.** Decreased metabolism of the dorsolateral prefrontal cortex.

4. **Positron emission tomography (PET).** In some patients, decreased frontal and parietal lobe metabolism, relatively high rate of posterior metabolism, and abnormal laterality.

5. **Cerebral blood flow (CBF).** In some patients, decreased resting levels of frontal blood flow, increased parietal blood flow, and decreased whole-brain blood flow. When PET and CBF studies are considered together with CT findings, dysfunction of the frontal lobe is most clearly implicated. Frontal lobe dysfunction may be secondary, however, to disease elsewhere in the brain.

C. **Physical findings.** Minor (soft) neurological findings occur in 50% to 100% of patients: increased prevalence of primitive reflexes (e.g., grasp reflex), abnormal stereognosis and two-point discrimination, and dysdiadochokinesia (impairment in ability to perform rapidly alternating movements). Paroxysmal saccadic eye movements (inability to follow object through space with smooth eye movements) occur in 50% to 80% of schizophrenic patients and in 40% to 45% of first-degree relatives of schizophrenic patients (compared with an 8% to 10% prevalence in nonschizophrenic persons). This may be a neurophysiological marker of a vulnerability to schizophrenia. Resting heart rates have been found to be higher in schizophrenic patients than in controls and may reflect a hyperaroused state.

VIII. **Psychodynamic Factors**
Understanding a patient's dynamics (or psychological conflicts and issues) is critical for complete understanding of the symbolic meaning of symptoms. A patient's internal experience is usually one of confusion and overwhelming sensory input, and defense mechanisms are the ego's attempt to deal with powerful affects. Three major primitive defenses interfere with reality testing: (1) psychotic projection—attributing inner sensations of aggression, sexuality, chaos, and confusion to the outside world, as opposed to recognizing them as emanating from within; boundaries between inner and outer experience are confused; projection is the major defense underlying paranoid delusions; (2) reaction formation—turning a disturbing idea or impulse into its opposite; and (3) psychotic denial—transforming confusing stimuli into delusions and hallucinations.

IX. **Differential Diagnosis**
A. **Medical and neurological disorders.** Present with impaired memory, orientation, and cognition; visual hallucinations; signs of CNS damage. Many neurological and medical disorders can present with symptoms identical to those of schizophrenia, including substance intoxication (e.g., cocaine, phencyclidine) and substance-induced psychotic disorder, CNS infections (e.g., herpes encephalitis), vascular disorders (e.g., systemic lupus erythematosus), complex partial seizures (e.g., temporal lobe epilepsy), and degenerative disease (e.g., Huntington's disease).

B. **Schizophreniform disorder.** Symptoms may be identical to those of schizophrenia, but last for less than 6 months. Also, deterioration is less pronounced and the prognosis is better.

C. **Brief psychotic disorder.** Symptoms last less than 1 month and proceed from a clearly identifiable psychosocial stress.

D. **Mood disorders.** Both manic episodes and major depressive episodes of bipolar I disorder and major depressive disorder may present with psychotic symptoms. The differential diagnosis is particularly important because of the availability of specific and effective treatments for the mood disorders. *DSM-IV-TR* states that mood symptoms in schizophrenia must be brief relative to the essential criteria. Also, if hallucinations and delusions are present in a mood disorder, they develop in the context of the mood disturbance and do not persist. Other factors that help differentiate mood disorders from schizophrenia include family history, premorbid history, course (e.g., age at onset), prognosis (e.g., absence of residual deterioration following the psychotic episode), and response to treatment. Patients may experience postpsychotic depressive disorder of schizophrenia (i.e., a major depressive episode occurring during the residual phase of schizophrenia). True depression in these patients must be differentiated from medication-induced adverse effects, such as sedation, akinesia, and flattening of affect.

E. **Schizoaffective disorder.** Mood symptoms develop concurrently with symptoms of schizophrenia, but delusions or hallucinations must be present for 2 weeks in the absence of prominent mood symptoms during some phase of the illness. The prognosis of this disorder is better than that expected for schizophrenia and worse than that for mood disorders.

F. **Psychotic disorder not otherwise specified.** An atypical psychosis with a confusing clinical feature (e.g., persistent auditory hallucinations as the only symptom, many culture-bound psychoses).

G. **Delusional disorders.** Nonbizarre, systematized delusions that last at least 6 months in the context of an intact, relatively well-functioning personality in the absence of prominent hallucinations or other schizophrenic symptoms. Onset is in middle to late adult life.

H. **Personality disorders.** Generally no psychotic symptoms, but if present, they tend to be transient and not prominent. The most important personality disorders in this differential diagnosis are schizotypal, schizoid, borderline, and paranoid.

I. **Factitious disorder and malingering.** No laboratory test or biological marker can objectively confirm the diagnosis of schizophrenia. Schizophrenic symptoms are therefore possible to feign for either clear secondary gain (malingering) or deep psychological motivations (factitious disorder).

J. **Pervasive developmental disorders.** Pervasive developmental disorders (e.g., autistic disorder) are usually recognized before 3 years of age. Although behavior may be bizarre and deteriorated, no delusions, hallucinations, or clear formal thought disorder is present (e.g., loosening of associations).

K. **Mental retardation.** Intellectual, behavioral, and mood disturbances that suggest schizophrenia. However, mental retardation involves no overt psychotic symptoms and involves a constant low level of functioning rather than a deterioration. If psychotic symptoms are present, a diagnosis of schizophrenia may be made concurrently.

L. Shared cultural beliefs. Seemingly odd beliefs shared and accepted by a cultural group are not considered psychotic.

X. Course and Prognosis

A. Course. Prodromal symptoms of anxiety, perplexity, terror, or depression generally precede the onset of schizophrenia, which may be acute or insidious. Prodromal symptoms may be present for months before a definitive diagnosis is made. Onset is generally in the late teens and early 20s; women generally are older at onset than men. Precipitating events (e.g., emotional trauma, use of drugs, a separation) may trigger episodes of illness in predisposed persons. Classically, the course of schizophrenia is one of deterioration over time, with acute exacerbations superimposed on a chronic picture. Vulnerability to stress is lifelong. Postpsychotic depressive episodes may occur in the residual phase. Other comorbidities include substance use disorders, obsessive–compulsive disorder, hyponatremia secondary to polydipsia, smoking, and HIV infection.

 CLINICAL HINT:
During the course of the illness, the more florid positive psychotic symptoms, such as bizarre delusions and hallucinations, tend to diminish in intensity, whereas the more residual negative symptoms, such as poor hygiene, flattened emotional response, and various oddities of behavior, tend to increase.

Relapse rates are approximately 40% in 2 years on medication and 80% in 2 years off medication. Suicide is attempted by 50% of patients; 10% are successful. Violence is a risk, particularly in untreated patients. Risk factors include persecutory delusions, a history of violence, and neurological deficits. The risk for sudden death and medical illness is increased, and life expectancy is shortened.

B. Prognosis. See Table 12 6. In terms of overall prognosis, some investigators have described a loose rule of thirds: approximately one third of patients lead somewhat normal lives, one-third continue to experience significant symptoms but can function within society, and the remaining one-third are markedly impaired and require frequent hospitalization. Approximately 10% of this final third of patients require long-term institutionalization. In general, women have a better prognosis than do men.

XI. Treatment

Clinical management of the schizophrenic patient may include hospitalization and antipsychotic medication in addition to psychosocial treatments, such as behavioral, family, group, individual, and social skills and rehabilitation therapies. Any of these treatment modalities can be given on an inpatient or outpatient basis. Indications for hospitalization include posing a danger to others, suicidality, severe symptomatology leading to poor self-care or risk for injury secondary to disorganization, diagnostic evaluation, failure to respond

Table 12–6
Features Weighting Toward Good or Poor Prognosis in Schizophrenia

Good Prognosis	Poor Prognosis
Late onset	Early onset
Obvious precipitating factors	No precipitating factors
Acute onset	Insidious onset
Good premorbid social, sexual, and work histories	Poor premorbid social, sexual, and work histories
Mood disorder symptoms (especially depressive disorders)	Withdrawn, autistic behavior
Married	Single, divorced, or widowed
Family history of mood disorders and family history of schizophrenia	
Good support systems	Poor support systems
Positive symptoms	Negative symptoms
Female sex	Neurological signs and symptoms
	History of perinatal trauma
	No remissions in 3 years
	Many relapses
	History of assaultiveness

to treatment in less restrictive settings, complicating comorbidities, and the need to alter complex drug treatment regimens.

A. **Pharmacologic.** The antipsychotics include the first-generation dopamine receptor antagonists and the second-generation agents such as serotonin–dopamine antagonists (SDAs), such as risperidone (Risperdal) and clozapine (Clozaril). See Table 12–7.

1. **Choice of drug.**

a. **First-generation antipsychotics** (also known as typical antipsychotics, or dopamine receptor antagonists)—the classic antipsychotic drugs, which are often effective in the treatment of positive symptoms of schizophrenia. High-potency agents (e.g., haloperidol) are most likely to cause extrapyramidal side effects such as akathisia, acute dystonia, and pseudoparkinsonism. Low-potency agents (e.g., chlorpromazine [Thorazine]) are more sedating, hypotensive, and anticholinergic. These agents can cause tardive dyskinesia at a rate of roughly 5% per year of exposure. A significant portion of patients are either unresponsive to or intolerant of these drugs. The newer, second-generation antipsychotic drugs—described below—are usually preferred and used more frequently than the first-generation antipsychotics. They are equally if not more effective and with fewer side effects.

b. **Second-generation antipsychotics** (also known as atypical, novel, or serotonin–dopamine antagonists)—the newer-generation antipsychotic drugs that provide potent 5-HT$_2$ receptor blockade and varying degrees of D$_2$-receptor blockade, in addition to other receptor effects. In comparison with the dopamine receptor antagonists, these drugs improve two classes of disabilities typical of schizophrenia: (1) positive symptoms such as hallucinations, delusions, disordered thought, and agitation and (2) negative symptoms such as

Table 12–7
Commonly Used Antipsychotic Medications

| | Chlorpromazine | | |
Antipsychotic Medication	Recommended Dose Range (mg/day)	Equivalents (mg/day)	Half-Life (hours)
First-generation agents (typical)			
Phenothiazines			
Chlorpromazine (Thorazine)	300–1,000	100	5–7
Fluphenazine (Prolixin Decanoate)	5–20	2	32–34
Mesoridazine (Serentil)	150–400	50	35–37
Perphenazine (Trilafon)	16–64	10	9–11
Thioridazine (Mellaril)	300–800	100	23–25
Trifluoperazine (Stelazine)	15–50	5	23–25
Butyrophenone			
Haloperidol (Haldol)	5–20	2	20–22
Others			
Loxapine (Loxitane)	30–100	10	3–5
Molindone (Moban)	30–100	10	23–25
Thiothixene (Navane)	15–50	5	33–35
Second-generation agents (atypical or novel)			
Aripiprazole (Abilify)	10–30	N/A	74–76
Asenapine (Saphris)	5–10	N/A	24
Clozapine (Clozaril)	150–600	N/A	11–13
Iloperidone (Fanapt)	12–24	N/A	18–24
Olanzapine (Zyprexa)	10–30	N/A	32–34
Paliperidone (Invega)	3–6	N/A	24
Quetiapine (Seroquel) (also XR)	300–800	N/A	5–7
Risperidone (Risperdal)	2–8	N/A	23–25
Risperidone (Risperdal Consta)	25–75*	N/A	24
Ziprasidone (Geodon)	120–200	N/A	6–8

*Given once every two weeks

withdrawal, flat affect, anhedonia, poverty of speech, and cognitive impairment. They cause fewer extrapyramidal side effects, do not elevate prolactin levels, and are less likely to cause tardive dyskinesia. Clozapine is the most atypical in that it causes minimal or no extrapyramidal side effects, regardless of dosage; seldom causes tardive dyskinesia; and is extremely effective in treating refractory patients despite weak D_2 receptor blockade. As a group, these agents can be highly sedating and cause weight gain in excess of that associated with the dopamine receptor antagonists (with the exception of risperidone). The second-generation drugs are widely prescribed as first-line treatment for patients with schizophrenia. They include aripiprazole (Abilify), risperidone (Risperdal), olanzapine (Zyprexa), paliperidone (Invega), clozapine (Clozaril), ziprasidone (Geodon), and asenapine (Saphris) which is a new drug that comes in sublingual tablets.

2. **Dosage.** A moderate fixed dose that is maintained for 4 to 6 weeks (or longer in more chronic cases) is recommended for acute psychotic episodes. High dosages of antipsychotics (>1 g of chlorpromazine equivalents) and rapid neuroleptization are no longer recommended,

as they increase side effects without enhancing efficacy. Typical therapeutic dosages are 4 to 6 mg of risperidone a day, 10 to 20 mg of olanzapine (Zyprexa) a day, and 6 to 20 mg of haloperidol a day. First-episode patients may respond well to lower dosages, whereas selected chronic or refractory patients may rarely require higher dosages. An antipsychotic response develops gradually. Agitation can be managed with benzodiazepines (e.g., 1 to 2 mg of lorazepam [Ativan] three or four times daily) on a standing or as-needed basis while an antipsychotic response is awaited. Patients who are noncompliant because of lack of insight may benefit from long-acting injectable antipsychotics (e.g., 25 mg of fluphenazine decanoate [Prolixin] intramuscularly every 2 weeks, 100 to 200 mg of haloperidol decanoate intramuscularly every 4 weeks, Risperdal Consta 25–50 mg IM every 2 weeks). Patients should first be treated with oral preparations of these drugs to establish efficacy and tolerability. Patients who are treated with long-acting haloperidol must be converted to the depot drug via a loading-dose strategy or with oral supplementation until the depot preparation reaches steady-state levels (4 months).

Risperidone (Risperdal Consta) is the only SDA currently available in a depot formulation. It is given as an intramuscular (IM) injection formulation every 2 weeks. The dose may be 25, 50, or 75 mg. Oral risperidone should be coadministered with Risperdal Consta for the first 3 weeks before being discontinued.

3. **Maintenance.** Schizophrenia is usually a chronic illness, and long-term treatment with antipsychotic medication is usually required to decrease the risk for relapse. If a patient has been stable for approximately 1 year, then the medication can be gradually decreased to the minimum effective dosage, possibly at the rate of 10% to 20% per month. During dosage reduction, patients and their families must be educated to recognize and report warning signs of relapse, including insomnia, anxiety, withdrawal, and odd behavior. Strategies for dose reduction must be individualized based on the severity of past episodes, stability of symptoms, and tolerability of medication.

4. **Other drugs.** If standard antipsychotic medication alone is ineffective, several other drugs have been reported to cause varying degrees of improvement. The addition of lithium may be helpful in a significant percentage of patients; propranolol (Inderal), benzodiazepines, valproic acid (Depakene) or divalproex (Depakote), and carbamazepine (Tegretol) have been reported to lead to improvement in some cases.

B. **Electroconvulsive therapy (ECT).** Can be effective for acute psychosis and catatonic subtype. Patients in whom the illness has lasted less than 1 year are most responsive. ECT is a promising treatment for refractory positive symptoms. It has been shown to have synergistic efficacy with antipsychotic drugs.

C. **Psychosocial.** Antipsychotic medication alone is not as effective in treating schizophrenic patients as are drugs coupled with psychosocial interventions.

1. **Behavior therapy.** Desired behaviors are positively reinforced by rewarding them with specific tokens, such as trips or privileges. The intent is to generalize reinforced behavior to the world outside the hospital ward.
2. **Group therapy.** Focus is on support and social skills development (activities of daily living). Groups are especially helpful in decreasing social isolation and increasing reality testing.
3. **Family therapy.** Family therapy techniques can significantly decrease relapse rates for the schizophrenic family member. High-EE family interaction can be diminished through family therapy. Multiple family groups, in which family members of schizophrenic patients discuss and share issues, have been particularly helpful.
4. **Supportive psychotherapy.** Traditional insight-oriented psychotherapy is not usually recommended in treating schizophrenic patients because their egos are too fragile. Supportive therapy, which may include advice, reassurance, education, modeling, limit setting, and reality testing, is generally the therapy of choice. The rule is that as much insight as a patient desires and can tolerate is an acceptable goal. A type of supportive therapy called *personal therapy* involves a heavy reliance on the therapeutic relationship, with instillation of hope and imparting of information.

 CLINICAL HINT:
Even though a patient is in a catatonic or withdrawn state, they are often very aware of the environment and cognizant of what is being said around them.

5. **Social skills training.** Attempts to improve social skills deficits, such as poor eye contact, lack of relatedness, inaccurate perceptions of others, and social inappropriateness, by means of supportive structurally based and sometimes manually based therapies (often in group settings), which utilize homework, videotapes, and role playing.
6. **Case management.** Responsible for the schizophrenic patient's concrete needs and coordination of care. Case managers participate in coordinating treatment planning and communication between various providers. They help patients make appointments, obtain housing and financial benefits, and navigate the health care system (advocacy), and also provide outreach and crisis management to keep patients in treatment.
7. **Support groups.** The National Alliance for the Mentally Ill (NAMI), the National Mental Health Association (NMHA), and similar groups provide support, information, and education for patients and their families. NAMI-sponsored support groups are available in most states.

XII. Interviewing Techniques
A. **Understanding.** The most important task is to understand as well as possible what schizophrenic patients may be feeling and thinking. Schizophrenic

patients are described as having extremely fragile ego structures, which leave them open to an unstable sense of self and others; primitive defenses; and a severely impaired ability to modulate external stress.

B. Other critical tasks. The other critical task for the interviewer is to establish contact with the patient in a manner that allows for a tolerable balance of autonomy and interaction.

1. The patient has both a deep wish for and a terrible fear of interpersonal contact, called the *need–fear dilemma*.

2. The fear of contact may represent the fear of a fundamental intrusion, resulting in delusional fears of personal and world annihilation in addition to loss of control, identity, and self.

3. The wish for contact may represent fears that, without human interaction, the person is dead, nonhuman, mechanical, or permanently trapped.

4. Schizophrenic patients may project their own negative, bizarre, and frightening self-images onto others, leading the interviewer to feel as uncomfortable, scared, or angry as the patient. Aggressive or hostile impulses are particularly frightening to these patients and may lead them to disorganization in thought and behavior.

5. Offers of help may be experienced as coercion, attempts to force the person into helplessness, or a sense of being devoured.

6. There is no one right thing to say to a schizophrenic patient. The most important task of the interviewer is to help to diminish the inner chaos, loneliness, and terror that the schizophrenic patient is feeling. The challenge is to convey empathy without being regarded as dangerously intrusive.

 CLINICAL HINTS:

- *Efforts to convince the patient that a delusion is not real generally lead to more tenacious assertions of delusional ideas.*
- *How patients experience the world (e.g., dangerous, bizarre, overwhelming, invasive) is conveyed through their thought content and process. Listen for the feelings behind the delusional ideas—are they afraid, sad, angry, hopeless? Do they feel as though they have no privacy, no control? What is their image of themselves?*
- *Acknowledge the patient's feelings simply and clearly. For example, when the patient says, "When I walk into a room, people can see inside my head and read my thoughts," the clinician might respond with, "What is that like for you?"*
- *Careful listening can convey that the clinician believes the person is human with something important to say.*

For more detailed discussion of this topic, see Schizophrenia and Other Psychotic Disorders, Ch 12, p. 1432, in CTP/IX.

Schizophreniform, Schizoaffective, Delusional, and Other Psychotic Disorders

I. Schizophreniform Disorder

A. **Definition.** Symptoms similar to those of schizophrenia except that they last at least 1 month and resolve within 6 months and then return to baseline level of functioning.

B. **Epidemiology.** Little is known about the incidence, prevalence, and sex ratio of schizophreniform disorder. The disorder is most common in adolescents and young adults and is less than half as common as schizophrenia. A lifetime prevalence rate of 0.2% and a 1-year prevalence rate of 0.1% have been reported.

C. **Etiology.** In general, schizophreniform patients have more mood symptoms and a better prognosis than schizophrenic patients. Schizophrenia occurs more often in families of patients with mood disorders than in families of patients with schizophreniform disorder. Cause remains unknown.

D. **Diagnosis, signs, and symptoms.** A rapid-onset psychotic disorder with hallucinations, delusions, or both. Although many patients with schizophreniform disorder may experience functional impairment at the time of an episode, they are unlikely to report a progressive decline in social and occupational functioning. See Table 13–1.

E. **Differential diagnosis**

1. **Schizophrenia.** Schizophrenia is diagnosed if the duration of the prodromal, active, and residual phases lasts for more than 6 months.

2. **Brief psychotic disorder.** Symptoms occur for less than 1 month and a major stressor need not be present.

3. **Mood and anxiety disorders.** Can be highly comorbid with schizophrenia and schizophreniform. A thorough longitudinal history is important in elucidating the diagnosis because the presence of psychotic symptoms exclusively during periods of mood disturbance is an indication of a primary mood disorder.

4. **Substance-induced psychosis.** A detailed history of medication use and toxicological screen.

5. **Psychosis due to a medical condition.** A detailed history and physical examination and, when indicated, performing laboratory tests or imaging studies.

F. **Course and prognosis.** Good prognostic features include absence of blunted or flat affect, good premorbid functioning, confusion and disorientation at the height of the psychotic episode, shorter duration, acute onset, and onset of prominent psychotic symptoms within 4 weeks of

Table 13-1
DSM-IV-TR Diagnostic Criteria for Schizophreniform Disorder

A. Criteria A, D, and E of schizophrenia are met.
B. An episode of the disorder (including prodromal, active, and residual phases) lasts at least 1 month but less than 6 months. (When the diagnosis must be made without waiting for recovery, it should be qualified as "provisional.")

Specify if:
Without good prognostic features
With good prognostic features: as evidenced by two (or more) of the following:
1. onset of prominent psychotic symptoms within 4 weeks of the first noticeable change in usual behavior or functioning
2. confusion or perplexity at the height of the psychotic episode
3. good premorbid social and occupational functioning
4. absence of blunted or flat affect

From American Psychiatric Association. *Diagnostic and Statistical Manual of Mental Disorders.* 4th ed. Text rev. Washington, DC: American Psychiatric Association; 2000, with permission.

any first noticeable change in behavior. Most estimates of progression to schizophrenia range between 60% and 80%. Some will have a second or third episode during which they will deteriorate into a more chronic condition of schizophrenia. Others remit and then have periodic recurrences.

G. Treatment. Antipsychotic medications should be used to treat psychotic symptoms. Consideration can be given to withdrawing or tapering the medication if the psychosis has been completely resolved for 6 months. The decision to discontinue medication must be individualized based on treatment response, side effects, and other factors. A trial of lithium (Eskalith), carbamazepine (Tegretol), or valproate (Depakene) may be warranted for treatment and prophylaxis if a patient has a recurrent episode. Psychotherapy is critical in helping patients to understand and deal with their psychotic experiences. Electroconvulsive therapy may be indicated for some patients, especially those with marked catatonic or depressed features.

II. Schizoaffective Disorder

A. Definition. A disorder with concurrent features of both schizophrenia and mood disorder that cannot be diagnosed as either one separately.

B. Epidemiology. Lifetime prevalence is less than 1%. The depressive type of schizoaffective disorder may be more common in older persons than in younger persons, and the bipolar type may be more common in young adults than in older adults. The prevalence of the disorder has been reported to be lower in men than in women, particularly married women; the age of onset for women is later than that for men, as in schizophrenia. Men with schizoaffective disorder are likely to exhibit antisocial behavior and to have a markedly flat or inappropriate affect.

C. Etiology. Some patients may be misdiagnosed; they are actually schizophrenic with prominent mood symptoms or have a mood disorder with prominent psychotic symptoms. The prevalence of schizophrenia is not increased in schizoaffective families, but the prevalence of mood disorders is. Patients with schizoaffective disorder have a better prognosis than

Table 13–2
DSM-IV-TR Diagnostic Criteria for Schizoaffective Disorder

A. An uninterrupted period of illness during which, at some time, there is either a major depressive episode, a manic episode, or a mixed episode concurrent with symptoms that meet Criterion A for schizophrenia.
   Note: The major depressive episode must include Criterion A1: depressed mood.
B. During the same period of illness, there have been delusions or hallucinations for at least 2 weeks in the absence of prominent mood symptoms.
C. Symptoms that meet criteria for a mood episode are present for a substantial portion of the total duration of the active and residual periods of the illness.
D. Tho disturbance is not due to the direct physiologic effects of a substance (e.g., a drug of abuse, a medication) or a general medical condition.
Specify type:
Bipolar type: if the disturbance includes a manic or a mixed episode (or a manic or a mixed episode and major depressive episodes)
Depressive type: if the disturbance only includes major depressive episodes

From American Psychiatric Association. *Diagnostic and Statistical Manual of Mental Disorders.* 4th ed. Text rev. Washington, DC: American Psychiatric Association; 2000, with permission.

patients with schizophrenia and a worse prognosis than patients with mood disorders.

D. Diagnosis, signs, and symptoms. There will be signs and symptoms of schizophrenia coupled with manic or depressive episodes. The disorder is divided into two subtypes: (1) bipolar, if there is both a manic and depressive cycling, and (2) depressive, if the disturbance only includes major depressive episodes. See Table 13–2.

E. Differential diagnosis. Any medical, psychiatric, or drug-related condition that causes psychotic or mood symptoms must be considered.

F. Course and prognosis. Poor prognosis is associated with positive family history of schizophrenia, early and insidious onset without precipitating factors, predominance of psychotic symptoms, and poor premorbid history. Schizoaffective patients have a better prognosis than schizophrenic patients and a worse prognosis than mood disorder patients. Schizoaffective patients respond more often to lithium and are less likely to have a deteriorating course than are schizophrenic patients.

G. Treatment. Antidepressant or antimanic treatments should be used combined with antipsychotic medications to control psychotic signs and symptoms. Selective serotonin reuptake inhibitors (SSRIs, e.g., fluoxetine [Prozac] and sertraline [Zoloft]) are often used as first-line agents. In manic cases, the use of electroconvulsive therapy should be considered. Patients benefit from a combination of family therapy, social skills training, and cognitive rehabilitation.

III. Delusional Disorder

A. Definition. Disorder in which the primary or sole manifestation is a non-bizarre delusion that is fixed and unshakable. The delusions are usually about situations that can occur and are possible in real life, such as being followed, infected, or loved at a distance. Bizarre delusions are considered

Table 13–3
Epidemiological Features of Delusional Disorder

Incidence[a]	0.7–3.0
Prevalence[a]	24–30
Age at onset (range)	18–80 (mean, 34–45 years)
Type of onset	Acute or gradual
Sex ratio	Somewhat more frequently female
Prognosis	Best with early, acute onset
Associated features	Widowhood, celibacy often present, history of substance abuse, head injury not infrequent

[a]Incidence and prevalence figures represent cases per 100,000 population.
Adapted from Kendler KS. Demography of paranoid psychosis (delusional disorder). *Arch Gen Psychiatry.* 1982;39:890, with permission.

impossible, such as being impregnated by an alien being from another planet.

B. Epidemiology. Delusional disorders account for only 1% to 2% of all admissions to inpatient mental health facilities. The mean age of onset is about 40 years, but the range for age of onset runs from 18 years of age to the 90s. A slight preponderance of female patients exists. Men are more likely to develop paranoid delusions than women, who are more likely to develop delusions of erotomania. Many patients are married and employed, but some association is seen with recent immigration and low socioeconomic status. See Table 13–3.

C. Etiology

1. **Genetic.** Genetic studies indicate that delusional disorder is neither a subtype nor an early or prodromal stage of schizophrenia or mood disorder. The risk for schizophrenia or mood disorder is not increased in first-degree relatives; however, there is a slight increase of delusional thinking, particularly suspiciousness, in families of patients with delusional disorder.

2. **Biological.** The neurological conditions most commonly associated with delusions are lesions that affect the limbic system, the basal ganglia, and the parietal lobes. Delusional disorder can also arise as a response to stimuli in the peripheral nervous system (e.g., paresthesias perceived as rays coming from outer space).

3. **Psychosocial.** Delusional disorder is primarily psychosocial in origin. Common background characteristics include a history of physical or emotional abuse; cruel, erratic, and unreliable parenting; and an overly demanding or perfectionistic upbringing. Basic trust (Erik Erikson) does not develop, with the child believing that the environment is consistently hostile and potentially dangerous. Other psychosocial factors include a history of deafness, blindness, social isolation and loneliness, recent immigration or other abrupt environmental changes, and advanced age.

D. Laboratory and psychological tests. No laboratory test can confirm the diagnosis. Projective psychological tests reveal a preoccupation with paranoid or grandiose themes and issues of inferiority, inadequacy, and anxiety.

E. **Pathophysiology.** No known pathophysiology except when patients have discrete anatomic defects of the limbic system or basal ganglia.

F. **Psychodynamic factors.** Defenses used: (1) denial, (2) reaction formation, and (3) projection. Major defense is projection—symptoms are a defense against unacceptable ideas and feelings. Patients deny feelings of shame, humiliation, and inferiority; turn any unacceptable feelings into their opposites through reaction formation (inferiority into grandiosity); and project any unacceptable feelings outward onto others.

G. **Diagnosis, signs, and symptoms.** Delusions last at least 1 month and are well systematized and nonbizarre, as opposed to fragmented and bizarre. The patient's emotional response to the delusional system is congruent with and appropriate to the content of the delusion. The personality remains intact or deteriorates minimally. The fact that patients often are hypersensitive and hypervigilant may lead to social isolation despite their high-level functioning capacities. Under nonstressful circumstances, patients may be judged to be without evidence of mental illness. See Table 13–4.

1. **Persecutory.** Patients with this subtype are convinced that they are being persecuted or harmed. The persecutory beliefs are often associated with querulousness, irritability, and anger. Most common type.

2. **Jealous (also called conjugal paranoia, pathological jealousy).** Delusional disorder with delusions of infidelity has been called *conjugal paranoia* when it is limited to the delusion that a spouse has been

Table 13–4
***DSM-IV-TR* Diagnostic Criteria for Delusional Disorder**

A. Nonbizarre delusions (i.e., involving situations that occur in real life, such as being followed, poisoned, infected, loved at a distance, or deceived by spouse or lover, or having a disease) of at least 1 month's duration.

B. Criterion A for schizophrenia has never been met. **Note:** Tactile and olfactory hallucinations may be present in delusional disorder if they are related to the delusional theme.

C. Apart from the impact of the delusion(s) or its ramifications, functioning is not markedly impaired and behavior is not obviously odd or bizarre.

D. If mood episodes have occurred concurrently with delusions, their total duration has been brief relative to the duration of the delusional periods.

E. The disturbance is not due to the direct physiologic effects of a substance (e.g., a drug of abuse, a medication) or a general medical condition.

Specify type (the following types are assigned based on the predominant delusional theme):

Erotomanic type: delusions that another person, usually of higher status, is in love with the individual

Grandiose type: delusions of inflated worth, power, knowledge, identity, or special relationship to a deity or famous person

Jealous type: delusions that the individual's sexual partner is unfaithful

Persecutory type: delusions that the person (or someone to whom the person is close) is being malevolently treated in some way

Somatic type: delusions that the person has some physical defect or general medical condition

Mixed type: delusions characteristic of more than one of the above types, but no one theme predominates

Unspecified type

From American Psychiatric Association. *Diagnostic and Statistical Manual of Mental Disorders.* 4th ed. Text rev. Washington, DC: American Psychiatric Association; 2000, with permission.

unfaithful. The eponym *Othello syndrome* has been used to describe morbid jealousy that can arise from multiple concerns. The delusion usually afflicts men, often those with no prior psychiatric illness. May be associated with violence, including homicide.

3. **Erotomanic.** Patient believes that someone, usually of higher socioeconomic status, is in love with him or her. Criteria can include (1) a delusional conviction of amorous communication, (2) object of much higher rank, (3) object being the first to fall in love, (4) object being the first to make advances, (5) sudden onset (within a 7-day period), (6) object remains unchanged, (7) patient rationalizes paradoxical behavior of the object, (8) chronic course, and (9) absence of hallucinations. More common in women. Accounts for stalking behavior.

4. **Somatic.** Belief that patient is suffering from an illness; common delusions are of parasites, foul odors coming from the body, misshapen body parts (dysmorphophobia), or of fatal illness.

5. **Grandiose.** Persons think they have special powers or are deities.

6. **Shared delusional disorder** (also known as *folie à deux*). Two people have the same delusional belief. Most common in mother–daughter relationships.

H. Differential diagnosis

1. **Psychotic disorder resulting from a general medical condition with delusions.** Conditions that may mimic delusional disorder include hypothyroidism and hyperthyroidism, Parkinson's disease, multiple sclerosis, Alzheimer's disease, tumors, and trauma to the basal ganglia. Many medical and neurological illnesses can be present with delusions (Table 13–5). The most common sites for lesions are the basal ganglia and the limbic system.

2. **Substance-induced psychotic disorder with delusions.** Intoxication with sympathomimetics (e.g., amphetamines, marijuana, or levodopa [Larodopa]) is likely to result in delusional symptoms.

3. **Paranoid personality disorder.** No true delusions are present, although overvalued ideas that verge on being delusional may be present. Patients are predisposed to delusional disorders.

Table 13–5
Neurological and Medical Conditions that can Present with Delusions

Basal ganglia disorders—Parkinson's disease, Huntington's disease
Deficiency states—B_{12}, folate, thiamine, niacin
Delirium
Dementia—Alzheimer's disease, Pick's disease
Drug induced—amphetamines, anticholinergics, antidepressants, antihypertensives, antituberculosis drugs, anti-Parkinson agents, cimetidine, cocaine, disulfiram (Antabuse), hallucinogens
Endocrinopathies—adrenal, thyroid, parathyroid
Limbic system disorders—epilepsy, cerebrovascular diseases, tumors
Systemic—hepatic encephalopathy, hypercalcemia, hypoglycemia, porphyria, uremia

4. **Paranoid schizophrenia.** More likely to present with prominent auditory hallucinations, personality deterioration, and more marked disturbance in role functioning. Age at onset tends to be younger in schizophrenia than in delusional disorder. Delusions are more bizarre.

5. **Major depressive disorder.** Depressed patients may have paranoid delusions secondary to major depressive disorder, but the mood symptoms and associated characteristics (e.g., vegetative symptoms, positive family history, response to antidepressants) are prominent.

6. **Bipolar I disorder.** Manic patients may have grandiose or paranoid delusions that are clearly secondary to the primary and prominent mood disorder; associated with such characteristics as euphoric and labile mood, positive family history, and response to lithium.

I. **Course and prognosis.** Delusional disorder is considered a fairly stable diagnosis. About 50% of patients have recovered at long-term follow-up, 20% show decreased symptoms, and 30% exhibit no change. A good prognosis is associated with high levels of occupational, social, and functional adjustments; female sex; onset before age 30 years; sudden onset; short duration of illness; and the presence of precipitating factors. Although reliable data are limited, patients with persecutory, somatic, and erotic delusions are thought to have a better prognosis than patients with grandiose and jealous delusions.

J. **Treatment.** Patients rarely enter therapy voluntarily; rather, they are brought by concerned friends and relatives. Establishing rapport is difficult; patient's hostility is fear motivated.

1. **Hospitalization.** Hospitalization is necessary if the patient is unable to control suicidal or homicidal impulses, if impairment is extreme (e.g., refusal to eat because of a delusion about food poisoning), or if a thorough medical workup is indicated.

2. **Psychopharmacotherapy.** Patients tend to refuse medications because of suspicion. Severely agitated patients may require intramuscular antipsychotic medication. Otherwise, oral antipsychotics may be tried. Delusional disorder may preferentially respond to pimozide (Orap). Delusional patients are more likely to react to drug side effects with delusional ideas; thus, a very gradual increase in dose is recommended to diminish the likelihood of disturbing adverse effects. Antidepressants may be of use with severe depression. SSRIs may be helpful in somatic type.

3. **Psychotherapy.** Individual therapy seems to be more effective than group therapy; insight-oriented, supportive, cognitive, and behavioral therapies are often effective. A good therapeutic outcome depends on a psychiatrist's ability to respond to the patient's mistrust of others and the resulting interpersonal conflicts, frustrations, and failures. The mark of successful treatment may be a satisfactory social adjustment rather than abatement of the patient's delusions.

CLINICAL HINTS: PSYCHOTHERAPY

- *Do not argue with or challenge the patient's delusions. A delusion may become even more entrenched if the patient feels that it must be defended.*
- *Do not pretend that the delusion is true. However, do listen to the patient's concerns about the delusion and try to understand what the delusion may mean, specifically in terms of the patient's self-esteem.*
- *Respond sympathetically to the fact that the delusion is disturbing and intrusive in the patient's life.*
- *Understand that the delusional system may be a means of grappling with profound feelings of shame and inadequacy, and that the patient may be hypersensitive to any imagined slights or condescension.*
- *Be straightforward and honest in all dealings with the patient, as these patients are hypervigilant about being tricked or deceived. Explain side effects of medications and reasons for prescribing (e.g., to help with anxiety, irritability, insomnia, anorexia); be reliable and on time for appointments; schedule regular appointments.*
- *Examine what triggered the first appearance of the delusion. Similar stresses or experiences in the patient's life may exacerbate delusional symptoms. Help the patient develop alternative means of responding to stressful situations.*

IV. **Brief Psychotic Disorder**
   A. **Definition.** This is a transient psychotic syndrome in which symptoms last for less than 1 month and follow a severe and obvious stress in the patient's life.
   B. **Epidemiology.** No definitive data are available. More frequent in persons with pre-existing personality disorders or who have previously experienced major stressors, such as disasters or dramatic cultural changes. Onset is usually between 20 and 35 years of age, with a slightly higher incidence in women.
   C. **Etiology.** Mood disorders are more common in the families of these patients. Psychosocial stress triggers the psychotic episode. Psychosis is understood as a defensive response in a person with inadequate coping mechanisms.
   D. **Diagnosis, signs, and symptoms.** Similar to those of other psychotic disorders, with an increase in emotional volatility, strange or bizarre behavior, confusion, disorientation, and lability in mood ranging from elation to suicidality. See Table 13–6.
   E. **Differential diagnosis.** Medical causes must be ruled out—in particular, drug intoxication and withdrawal. Seizure disorders must also be considered. Factitious disorders, malingering, schizophrenia, mood disorders, and transient psychotic episodes associated with borderline and schizotypal personality disorders must be ruled out.
   F. **Course and prognosis.** By definition, course of the disorder is less than 1 month. Recovery is up to 80% with treatment. See Table 13–7.

Table 13–6
***DSM-IV-TR* Diagnostic Criteria for Brief Psychotic Disorder**

A. Presence of one (or more) of the following symptoms:
   1. delusions
   2. hallucinations
   3. disorganized speech (e.g., frequent derailment or incoherence)
   Note: Do not include a symptom if it is a culturally sanctioned response pattern.
B. Duration of an episode of the disturbance is at least 1 day but less than 1 month, with eventual full return to premorbid level of functioning.
C. The disturbance is not better accounted for by a mood disorder with psychotic features, schizoaffective disorder, or schizophrenia and is not due to the direct physiologic effects of a substance (e.g., a drug of abuse, a medication) or a general medical condition.
Specify if:
   With marked stressor(s) (brief reactive psychosis): if symptoms occur shortly after and apparently in response to events that, singly or together, would be markedly stressful to almost anyone in similar circumstances in the person's culture
   Without marked stressor(s): if psychotic symptoms do not occur shortly after, or are not apparently in response to, events that, singly or together, would be markedly stressful to almost anyone in similar circumstances in the person's culture
   With postpartum onset: if onset within 4 weeks postpartum

From American Psychiatric Association. *Diagnostic and Statistical Manual of Mental Disorders.* 4th ed. Text rev. Washington, DC: American Psychiatric Association; 2000, with permission.

G. Treatment

1. **Hospitalization.** A patient who is acutely psychotic may need brief hospitalization for both evaluation and protection. Seclusion, physical restraints, or one-to-one monitoring of the patient may be necessary.

2. **Pharmacotherapy.** The two major classes of drugs to be considered in the treatment of brief psychotic disorder are the antipsychotic drugs (i.e., haloperidol or ziprasidone) and the benzodiazepines. Anxiolytic medications are often used during the first 2 to 3 weeks after the resolution of the psychotic episode. Long-term use of any medication should be avoided.

3. **Psychotherapy.** Psychotherapy is of use in providing an opportunity to discuss the stressors and the psychotic episode. An individualized treatment strategy based on increasing problem-solving skills while strengthening the ego structure through psychotherapy appears to be the most efficacious. Family involvement in the treatment process may be crucial to a successful outcome.

Table 13–7
Good Prognostic Features for Brief Psychotic Disorder

Good premorbid adjustment
Few premorbid schizoid traits
Severe precipitating stressor
Sudden onset of symptoms
Affective symptoms
Confusion and perplexity during psychosis
Little affective blunting
Short duration of symptoms
Absence of schizophrenic relatives

V. Shared Psychotic Disorder

A. Definition. Delusional system shared by two or more persons; previously called *induced paranoid disorder* and *folie à deux*.

B. Epidemiology. The disorder is rare; more common in women and in persons with physical disabilities that make them dependent on another person. Family members are involved in 95% of cases.

C. Etiology. The cause is primarily psychological; however, a genetic influence is possible because the disorder most often affects members of the same family. The families of persons with this disorder are at risk for schizophrenia. Psychological or psychosocial factors include a socially isolated relationship in which one person is submissive and dependent and the other is dominant with an established psychotic system.

D. Psychodynamic factors. The dominant psychotic personality maintains some contact with reality through the submissive person, whereas the submissive personality is desperately anxious to be cared for and accepted by the dominant person. The two often have a strongly ambivalent relationship.

E. Diagnosis, signs, and symptoms. Persecutory delusions are most common, and the key presentation is the sharing and blind acceptance of these delusions between two people. Suicide or homicide pacts may be present. See Table 13–8.

F. Differential diagnosis. Rule out personality disorders, malingering, and factitious disorders in the submissive patient. Medical causes must always be considered.

G. Course and prognosis. Recovery rates vary; some are as low as 10% to 40%. Traditionally, the submissive partner is separated from the dominant, psychotic partner, with the ideal outcome being a rapid diminution in the psychotic symptoms. If symptoms do not remit, the submissive person may meet the criteria for another psychotic disorder, such as schizophrenia or delusional disorder.

H. Treatment. Separate the persons and help the more submissive, dependent partner develop other means of support to compensate for the loss of the relationship. Antipsychotic medications are beneficial for both persons.

Table 13–8
***DSM-IV-TR* Diagnostic Criteria for Shared Psychotic Disorder**

A. A delusion develops in an individual in the context of a close relationship with another person(s), who has an already-established delusion.
B. The delusion is similar in content to that of the person who already has the established delusion.
C. The disturbance is not better accounted for by another psychotic disorder (e.g., schizophrenia) or a mood disorder with psychotic features and is not due to the direct physiologic effects of a substance (e.g., a drug of abuse, a medication) or a general medical condition.

From American Psychiatric Association. *Diagnostic and Statistical Manual of Mental Disorders.* 4th ed. Text rev. Washington, DC: American Psychiatric Association; 2000, with permission.

VI. Postpartum Psychosis

A. **Definition.** Syndrome occurring after childbirth and characterized by severe depression and delusions. Most data suggest a close relation between postpartum psychosis and mood disorders.

B. **Epidemiology.** Incidence is about 1 to 2 per 1,000 childbirths. About 50% to 60% of affected women have just had their first child, and about 50% of cases involve deliveries associated with nonpsychiatric perinatal complications. About 50% of the affected women have a family history of mood disorders.

C. **Etiology.** Usually secondary to underlying mental illness (e.g., schizophrenia, bipolar disorder).

1. Sudden change in hormonal levels after parturition may contribute.

2. Psychodynamic conflicts about motherhood—unwanted pregnancy, entrapment in unhappy marriage, and fears of mothering.

D. **Diagnosis, signs, and symptoms.** Most cases occur 2 to 3 days postpartum. Initial complaints of insomnia, restlessness, and emotional lability progress to confusion, irrationality, delusions, and obsessive concerns about the infant. Thoughts of wanting to harm the baby or self are characteristic.

E. **Differential diagnosis**

1. **Postpartum blues.** Most women experience postpartum emotional lability. Clears spontaneously. No evidence of psychotic thinking.

2. **Substance-induced mood disorder.** Depression associated with postanesthetic states, such as after cesarean section or meperidine (Demerol)–scopolamine analgesia (twilight sleep).

3. **Psychotic disorder resulting from a general medical condition.** Rule out infection, hormonal imbalance (e.g., hypothyroidism), encephalopathy associated with toxemia of pregnancy, and preeclampsia.

F. **Course and prognosis.** Risk for infanticide, suicide, or both is high in untreated cases. Supportive family network, good premorbid personality, and appropriate treatment are associated with good to excellent prognosis. Subsequent pregnancies are associated with an increased risk of another episode, sometimes as high as 50%.

G. **Treatment.** Suicidal precautions in presence of suicidal ideation. Do not leave the infant alone with the mother if she has delusions or ruminates about the infant's health.

1. **Pharmacologic.** Medication for primary symptoms: antidepressants for suicidal ideation and depression, antianxiety agents for agitation and insomnia (e.g., 0.5 mg of lorazepam [Ativan] every 4 to 6 hours), lithium for manic behavior, and antipsychotic agents for delusions (e.g., 0.5 mg of haloperidol every 6 hours). Since these patients rarely breastfeed, maternal drug–infant transmission is not a factor.

2. **Psychological.** Psychotherapy, both individual and marital therapy, to deal with intrapsychic or interpersonal conflicts. Consider discharging mother and infant to home only after arrangements for temporary homemaker are in place to reduce environmental stresses associated with care of the newborn.

CLINICAL HINT:

The risk of infanticide remains high even if caregivers are in the home. Careful supervision of mother–infant interaction can provide important clues about hostile or loving feelings.

VII. **Psychotic Disorder Not Otherwise Specified**
   A. **Definition.** Patients whose psychotic presentation does not meet the diagnostic criteria for any established psychotic disorder; also known as *atypical psychosis.*
   B. **Diagnosis, signs, and symptoms.** This diagnostic category includes disorders that present with various psychotic features (e.g., delusions, hallucinations, loosening of associations, catatonic behaviors) but that cannot be delineated as any specific disorder. The disorders may include postpartum psychoses and rare or exotic syndromes (e.g., specific culture-bound syndromes). See Table 13–9.
      1. **Autoscopic psychosis.** Rare hallucinatory psychosis during which the patient sees a phantom or specter of his or her own body. May be psychogenic in origin, but consider lesion of temporoparietal lobe. Responds to antipsychotic medications.
      2. **Capgras' syndrome.** Delusion that persons in the environment are not their real selves but are doubles imitating the patient or impostors imitating someone else. May be part of schizophrenia or cerebral lesions. Treat with antipsychotic medication. Psychotherapy is useful in understanding the dynamics of the delusional belief (e.g., distrust of certain real persons in the environment).
      3. **Cotard's syndrome.** Delusions of nihilism (e.g., nothing exists, the body has disintegrated, the world is coming to an end). Usually seen

 Table 13–9
DSM-IV-TR Diagnostic Criteria for Psychotic Disorder Not Otherwise Specified

This category includes psychotic symptomatology (i.e., delusions, hallucinations, disorganized speech, grossly disorganized or catatonic behavior) about which there is inadequate information to make a specific diagnosis or about which there is contradictory information, or disorders with psychotic symptoms that do not meet the criteria for any specific psychotic disorder.
Examples include:
   1. Postpartum psychosis that does not meet criteria for mood disorder with psychotic features, brief psychotic disorder, psychotic disorder due to a general medical condition, or substance-induced psychotic disorder
   2. Psychotic symptoms that have lasted for less than 1 month but that have not yet remitted, so that the criteria for brief psychotic disorder are not met
   3. Persistent auditory hallucinations in the absence of any other features
   4. Persistent nonbizarre delusions with periods of overlapping mood episodes that have been present for a substantial portion of the delusional disturbance
   5. Situations in which the clinician has concluded that a psychotic disorder is present, but is unable to determine whether it is primary, due to a general medical condition, or substance induced

From American Psychiatric Association. *Diagnostic and Statistical Manual of Mental Disorders.* 4th ed. Text rev. Washington, DC: American Psychiatric Association; 2000, with permission.

as part of schizophrenia or severe bipolar disorder. May be an early sign of Alzheimer's disease or other cerebral lesion. May respond to antipsychotic or antidepressant medication.

VIII. Culture-Bound Syndromes
See Table 13–10.

Table 13–10
Examples of Culture-Bound Syndromes

amok A dissociative episode characterized by a period of brooding followed by an outburst of violent, aggressive, or homicidal behavior directed at persons and objects. The episode tends to be precipitated by a perceived slight or insult and seems to be prevalent only among men. The episode is often accompanied by persecutory ideas, automatism, amnesia, exhaustion, and a return to premorbid state following the episode. Some instances of amok may occur during a brief psychotic episode or constitute the onset or an exacerbation of a chronic psychotic process. The original reports that used this term were from Malaysia. A similar behavior pattern is found in Laos, Philippines, Polynesia (*cafard* or *cathard*), Papua New Guinea, Puerto Rico (*mal de pelea*), and among the Navajo (*iich'aa*).

ataques de nervios An idiom of distress principally reported among Latinos from the Caribbean, but recognized among many Latin American and Latin Mediterranean groups. Commonly reported symptoms include uncontrollable shouting, attacks of crying, trembling, heat in the chest rising into the head, and verbal or physical aggression. Dissociative experiences, seizurelike or fainting episodes, and suicidal gestures are prominent in some attacks but absent in others. A general feature of an *ataque de nervios* is a sense of being out of control. *Ataques de nervios* frequently occur as a direct result of a stressful event relating to the family (e.g., death of a close relative, separation or divorce from a spouse, conflicts with a spouse or children, or witnessing an accident involving a family member). Persons may experience amnesia for what occurred during the *ataque de nervios*, but they otherwise return rapidly to their usual level of functioning. Although descriptions of some *ataques de nervios* most closely fit the *DSM-IV* description of panic attacks, the association of most *ataques* with a precipitating event and the frequent absence of the hallmark symptoms of acute fear or apprehension distinguish them from panic disorder. *Ataques* span the range from normal expressions of distress not associated with a mental disorder to symptom presentations associated with anxiety, mood, dissociative, or somatoform disorders.

bilis and colera (also referred to as *muina*) The underlying cause is thought to be strongly experienced anger or rage. Anger is viewed among many Latino groups as a particularly powerful emotion that can have direct effects on the body and exacerbate existing symptoms. The major effect of anger is to disturb core body balances (which are understood as a balance between hot and cold valences in the body and between the material and spiritual aspects of the body). Symptoms can include acute nervous tension, headache, trembling, screaming, stomach disturbances, and, in more severe cases, loss of consciousness. Chronic fatigue may result from an acute episode.

boufée délirante A syndrome observed in West Africa and Haiti. The French term refers to a sudden outburst of agitated and aggressive behavior, marked confusion, and psychomotor excitement. It may sometimes be accompanied by visual and auditory hallucinations or paranoid ideation. The episodes may resemble an episode of brief psychotic disorder.

brain fag A term initially used in West Africa to refer to a condition experienced by high school or university students in response to the challenges of schooling. Symptoms include difficulties in concentrating, remembering, and thinking. Students often state that their brains are "fatigued." Additional somatic symptoms are usually centered around the head and neck and include pain, pressure or tightness, blurring of vision, heat, or burning. "Brain tiredness" or fatigue from "too much thinking" is an idiom of distress in many cultures, and resulting syndromes can resemble certain anxiety, depressive, and somatoform disorders.

dhat A folk diagnostic term used in India to refer to severe anxiety and hypochondriacal concerns associated with the discharge of semen, whitish discoloration of the urine, and feelings of weakness and exhaustion. Similar to *jiryan* (India), *sukra prameha* (Sri Lanka), and *shen-K'uei* (China).

(continued)

Table 13–10—*continued*
Examples of Culture-Bound Syndromes

falling-out or blackout Episodes that occur primarily in southern United States and Caribbean groups. They are characterized by a sudden collapse, which sometimes occurs without warning but is sometimes preceded by feelings of dizziness or "swimming" in the head. The person's eyes are usually open, but the person claims an inability to see. Those affected usually hear and understand what is occurring around them but feel powerless to move. This may correspond to a diagnosis of conversion disorder or a dissociative disorder.

ghost sickness A preoccupation with death and the deceased (sometimes associated with witchcraft), frequently observed among members of many American Indian tribes. Various symptoms can be attributed to ghost sickness, including bad dreams, weakness, feeling of danger, loss of appetite, fainting, dizziness, fear, anxiety, hallucinations, loss of consciousness, confusion, feelings of futility, and a sense of suffocation.

hwa-byung (also known as *wool-hwa-byung*) A Korean folk syndrome literally translated into English as "anger syndrome" and attributed to the suppression of anger. The symptoms include insomnia, fatigue, panic, fear of impending death, dysphoric affect, indigestion, anorexia, dyspnea, palpitations, generalized aches and pains, and a feeling of a mass in the epigastrium.

koro A term probably of Malaysian origin, that refers to an episode of sudden and intense anxiety that the penis (or, in women, the vulva and nipples) will recede into the body and possibly cause death. The syndrome is reported in South and East Asia, where it is known by a variety of local terms, such as *shuk yang, shook yong,* and *suo yang* (Chinese); *jinjinia bemar* (Assam); or *rok-joo* (Thailand). It is occasionally found in the West. *Koro* at times occurs in localized epidemic form in East Asian areas. The diagnosis is included in the second edition of *Chinese Classification of Mental Disorders (CCMD-2).*

latah Hypersensitivity to sudden fright, often with echopraxia, echolalia, command obedience, and dissociative or trancelike behavior. The term *latah* is of Malaysian or Indonesian origin, but the syndrome has been found in many parts of the world. Other terms for the condition are *amurakh, irkunil, ikota, olan, myriachit,* and *menkeiti* (Siberian groups); *bah tschi, bah-tsi, baah-ji* (Thailand); *imu* (Ainu, Sakhalin, Japan); and *mali-mali* and *silok* (Philippines). In Malaysia, it is more frequent in middle-aged women.

locura A term used by Latinos in the United States and Latin America to refer to a severe form of chronic psychosis. The condition is attributed to an inherited vulnerability, to the effect of multiple life difficulties, or to a combination of both factors. Symptoms exhibited by persons with *locura* include incoherence, agitation, auditory and visual hallucinations, inability to follow rules of social interaction, unpredictability, and possibly violence.

mal de ojo A concept widely found in Mediterranean cultures and elsewhere in the world. *Mal de ojo* is a Spanish phrase translated into English as "evil eye." Children are especially at risk. Symptoms include fitful sleep, crying without apparent cause, diarrhea, vomiting, and fever in a child or infant. Sometimes adults (especially women) have the condition.

nervios A common idiom of distress among Latinos in the United States and Latin America. A number of other ethnic groups have related, though often somewhat distinctive, ideas of nerves (such as *nerva* among Greeks in North America). *Nervios* refers to a general state of vulnerability to stressful life experiences and to a syndrome brought on by difficult life circumstances. The term *nervios* includes a wide range of symptoms of emotional distress, somatic disturbance, and inability to function. Common symptoms include headaches and brain aches, irritability, stomach disturbances, sleep difficulties, nervousness, easy tearfulness, inability to concentrate, trembling, tingling sensations, and *mareos* (dizziness with occasional vertigolike exacerbations). *Nervios* tends to be an ongoing problem, although variable in the degree of disability that is manifest. *Nervios* is a very broad syndrome that spans the range from patients free of a mental disorder to presentations resembling adjustment, anxiety, depressive, dissociative, somatoform, or psychotic disorders. Differential diagnosis depends on the constellation of symptoms experienced, the kinds of social events that are associated with the onset and progress of *nervios,* and the level of disability experienced.

piblokto An abrupt dissociative episode accompanied by extreme excitement of up to 30 minutes' duration and frequently followed by convulsive seizures and coma lasting up to 12 hours. It is observed primarily in Arctic and subarctic Eskimo communities, although regional variations in name exist. The person may be withdrawn or mildly irritable for a period of hours or days before the attack and typically reports complete amnesia for the attack. During the attack, persons may tear off their clothing, break furniture, shout obscenities, eat feces, flee from protective shelters, or perform other irrational or dangerous acts.

(continued)

Table 13–10—*continued*
Examples of Culture-Bound Syndromes

qi-gong psychotic reactions Acute, time-limited episodes characterized by dissociative, paranoid, or other psychotic or nonpsychotic symptoms that may occur after participation in the Chinese folk health-enhancing practice of *qi-gong* (exercise of vital energy). Especially vulnerable are persons who become overly involved in the practice. This diagnosis is included in *CCMD-2*.

rootwork A set of cultural interpretations that ascribe illness to hexing, witchcraft, sorcery, or evil influence of another person. Symptoms may include generalized anxiety and gastrointestinal complaints (e.g., nausea, vomiting, diarrhea), weakness, dizziness, the fear of being poisoned, and sometimes fear of being killed (voodoo death). Roots, spells, or hexes can be put or placed on other person, causing a variety of emotional and psychological problems. The hexed person may even fear death until the root has been taken off (eliminated), usually through the work of a root doctor (a healer in this tradition), who can also be called on to bewitch an enemy. Rootwork is found in the southern United States among both African-American and European-American populations and in Caribbean societies. It is also known as *mal puesto* or *brujeria* in Latino societies.

sangue dormido ("sleeping blood") A syndrome found among Portuguese Cape Verde Islanders (and immigrants from there to the United States). It includes pain, numbness, tremor, paralysis, convulsions, stroke, blindness, heart attack, infection, and miscarriages.

Shenjing shuariuo ("neurasthenia") In China, a condition characterized by physical and mental fatigue, dizziness, headaches, other pains, concentration difficulties, sleep disturbance, and memory loss. Other symptoms include gastrointestinal problems, sexual dysfunction, irritability, excitability, and various signs suggesting disturbance of the autonomic nervous system. In many cases, the symptoms would meet the criteria for a *DSM-IV* mood or anxiety disorder. The diagnosis is included in *CCMD-2*.

shen-k'uei (Taiwan); *shenkui* (China) A Chinese folk label describing marked anxiety or panic symptoms with accompanying somatic complaints for which no physical cause can be demonstrated. Symptoms include dizziness, backache, fatigability, general weakness, insomnia, frequent dreams, and complaints of sexual dysfunction, such as premature ejaculation and impotence. Symptoms are attributed to excessive semen loss from frequent intercourse, masturbation, nocturnal emission, or passing of white turbid urine believed to contain semen. Excessive semen loss is feared because of the belief that it represents the loss of one's vital essence and can therefore be life threatening.

shin-byung A Korean folk label for a syndrome in which initial phases are characterized by anxiety and somatic complaints (general weakness, dizziness, fear, anorexia, insomnia, gastrointestinal problems), with subsequent dissociation and possession by ancestral spirits.

spell A trance state in which persons "communicate" with deceased relatives or spirits. At times, the state is associated with brief periods of personality change. The culture-specific syndrome is seen among African Americans and European Americans from the southern United States. Spells are not considered to be medical events in the folk tradition, but may be misconstrued as psychotic episodes in clinical settings.

susto (*trigh* or "soul loss") A folk illness prevalent among some Latinos in the United States and among people in Mexico, Central America, and South America. *Susto* is also referred to as *espanto, pasmo, tripa ida, perdida del alma*, or *chibih*. *Susto* is an illness attributed to a frightening event that causes the soul to leave the body and results in unhappiness and sickness. Persons with *susto* also experience significant strains in key social roles. Symptoms may appear any time from days to years after the fright is experienced. It is believed that in extreme cases, *susto* may result in death. Typical symptoms include appetite disturbances, inadequate or excessive sleep, troubled sleep or dreams, feelings of sadness, lack of motivation to do anything, and feelings of low self-worth or dirtiness. Somatic symptoms accompanying *susto* include muscle aches and pains, headache, stomachache, and diarrhea. Ritual healings are focused on calling the soul back to the body and cleansing the person to restore bodily and spiritual balance. Different experiences of *susto* may be related to major depressive disorder, posttraumatic stress disorders, and somatoform disorders. Similar etiologic beliefs and symptom configurations are found in many parts of the world.

taijin kyofu sho A culturally distinctive phobia in Japan, in some ways resembling social phobia in *DSM*. The syndrome refers to an intense fear that one's body, its parts, or its functions, displease, embarrass, or are offensive to other people in appearance, odor, facial expressions, or movements. The syndrome is included in the official Japanese diagnostic system for mental disorders.

(continued)

Table 13–10—*continued*
Examples of Culture-Bound Syndromes

zar A general term applied in Ethiopia, Somalia, Egypt, Sudan, Iran, and other North African and Middle Eastern societies to the experience of spirits possessing a person. Persons possessed by a spirit may experience dissociative episodes that may include shouting, laughing, hitting the head against a wall, singing, or weeping. They may show apathy and withdrawal, refusing to eat or carry out daily tasks or may develop a long-term relationship with the possessing spirit. Such behavior is not considered pathological locally.

From American Psychiatric Association. *Diagnostic and Statistical Manual of Mental Disorders.* 4th ed. Text rev. Washington, DC: American Psychiatric Association; 2000, with permission.

For more detailed discussion of this topic, see Other Psychotic Disorders, Sec 12.17, p. 1605, and Culture-Bound Syndromes, Ch 27, p. 2519, in CTP/IX.

14

Mood Disorders

I. Introduction

Mood is a pervasive and sustained feeling tone that is experienced internally and that influences a person's behavior and perception of the world. Affect is the external expression of mood. Mood can be normal, elevated, or depressed. Healthy persons experience a wide range of moods and have an equally large repertoire of affective expressions; they feel in control of their moods and affects.

Mood disorders encompass a large spectrum of disorders in which pathological mood disturbances dominate the clinical picture. They include the following 7 disorders:

- Major depressive disorders
- Bipolar disorders (types I and II)
- Dysthymic disorder
- Cyclothymic disorder
- Mood disorders due to a general medical condition
- Substance-induced mood disorder
- The general category of depressive and bipolar disorders not otherwise specified.

II. Epidemiology

A. Incidence and prevalence. Mood disorders are common. In the most recent surveys, major depressive disorder has the highest lifetime prevalence (almost 17%) of any psychiatric disorder. The annual incidence (number of new cases) of a major depressive episode is 1.59% (women, 1.89%; men, 1.10%). The annual incidence of bipolar illness is less than 1%, but it is difficult to estimate because milder forms of bipolar disorder are often missed (Table 14–1).

B. Sex. Major depression is more common in women; bipolar I disorder is equal in women and men. Manic episodes are more common in women, and depressive episodes are more common in men.

C. Age. The age of onset for bipolar I disorder is usually about age 30. However, the disorder also occurs in young children, as well as older adults.

D. Sociocultural. Depressive disorders are more common among single and divorced persons compared to married persons. No correlation with socioeconomic status. No difference between races or religious groups.

III. Etiology

A. Neurotransmitters

1. Serotonin. Serotonin has become the biogenic amine neurotransmitter most commonly associated with depression. Serotonin depletion

Table 14–1
Lifetime Prevalence of Some *DSM-IV-TR* Mood Disorders

Mood Disorder	Lifetime Prevalence
Depressive disorders	
Major depressive disorder (MDD)	10%–25% for women; 5%–12% for men
Recurrent, with full interepisode recovery, superimposed on dysthymic disorder	Approximately 3% of persons with MDD
Recurrent, without full interepisode recovery, superimposed on dysthymic disorder (double depression)	Approximately 25% of persons with MDD
Dysthymic disorder	Approximately 6%
Bipolar disorders	
Bipolar I disorder	0.4%–1.6%
Bipolar II disorder	Approximately 0.5%
Bipolar I disorder or bipolar II disorder, with rapid cycling	5%–15% of persons with bipolar disorder
Cyclothymic disorder	0.4%–1.0%

Data from American Psychiatric Association. *Diagnostic and Statistical Manual of Mental Disorders,* 4th ed. Text rev. Washington, DC: American Psychiatric Association; 2000, with permission.

occurs in depression; thus, serotonergic agents are effective treatments. The identification of multiple serotonin receptor subtypes may lead to even more specific treatments for depression. Some patients with suicidal impulses have low cerebrospinal fluid (CSF) concentrations of serotonin metabolites (5-hydroxyindole acetic acid [5-HIAA]) and low concentrations of serotonin uptake sites on platelets. This may prove to be a marker for depression with a high risk of suicide.

2. **Norepinephrine.** Abnormal levels (usually low) of norepinephrine metabolites (3-methoxy-4-hydroxyphenylglycol [MHPG]) are found in blood, urine, and CSF of depressed patients. Venlafaxine (Effexor) increases both serotonin and norepinephrine levels and is used in depression for that reason.

3. **Dopamine.** Dopamine activity may be reduced in depression and increased in mania. Drugs that reduce dopamine concentrations (e.g., reserpine [Serpasil]) and diseases that reduce dopamine concentrations (e.g., Parkinson's disease) are associated with depressive symptoms. Drugs that increase dopamine concentrations, such as tyrosine, amphetamine, and bupropion (Wellbutrin), reduce the symptoms of depression. Two recent theories about dopamine and depression are that the mesolimbic dopamine pathway may be dysfunctional in depression and that the dopamine D_1 receptor may be hypoactive in depression.

B. **Psychosocial**

1. **Psychoanalytic.** Freud described internalized ambivalence toward a love object (person), which can produce a pathological form of mourning if the object is lost or perceived as lost. This mourning takes the form of severe depression with feelings of guilt, worthlessness, and suicidal ideation. Symbolic or real loss of love object is perceived as rejection. Mania and elation are viewed as defense against underlying

depression. Rigid superego serves to punish a person with feelings of guilt about unconscious sexual or aggressive impulses. Suicide has been called "inverted homicide."

2. **Psychodynamics.** In depression, introjection of ambivalently viewed lost objects leads to an inner sense of conflict, guilt, rage, pain, and loathing; a pathological mourning becomes depression as ambivalent feelings meant for the introjected object are directed at the self. In mania, feelings of inadequacy and worthlessness are converted by means of denial, reaction formation, and projection to grandiose delusions.

3. **Cognitive.** Cognitive triad of Aaron Beck: (1) negative self-view ("things are bad because I'm bad"), (2) negative interpretation of experience ("everything has always been bad"), and (3) negative view of future (anticipation of failure). Challenging these cognitive schemas can improve mood.

4. **Learned helplessness.** A theory that attributes depression to a person's inability to control events. Theory is derived from observed behavior of animals experimentally given unexpected random shocks from which they cannot escape.

5. **Stressful life events.** Often precede first episodes of mood disorders. Such events may cause permanent neuronal changes that predispose a person to subsequent episodes of a mood disorder. Losing a parent before age 11 is the life event most associated with later development of depression.

IV. Laboratory, Brain Imaging, and Psychological Tests

A. **Dexamethasone suppression test.** Nonsuppression (positive test result) represents hypersecretion of cortisol secondary to hyperactivity of hypothalamic–pituitary–adrenal axis. Abnormal in 50% of patients with major depression. Of limited clinical usefulness owing to frequency of false-positive and false-negative results. Diminished release of TSH in response to thyrotropin-releasing hormone (TRH) reported in both depression and mania. Prolactin release decreased in response to tryptophan. Tests are not definitive.

B. **Brain imaging.** No gross brain changes. Enlarged cerebral ventricles on computed tomography (CT) in some patients with mania or psychotic depression; diminished basal ganglia blood flow in some depressive patients. Magnetic resonance imaging (MRI) studies have also indicated that patients with major depressive disorder have smaller caudate nuclei and smaller frontal lobes than do control subjects. Magnetic resonance spectroscopy (MRS) studies of patients with bipolar I disorder have produced data consistent with the hypothesis that the pathophysiology of the disorder may involve an abnormal regulation of membrane phospholipid metabolism.

C. **Psychological tests**

1. **Rating scales.** Can be used to assist in diagnosis and assessment of treatment efficacy. The Beck Depression Inventory (BDI) and Zung

Self-rating Scale are scored by patients. The Hamilton Rating Scale for Depression (HAM-D), Montgomery Asberg Depression Rating Scale (MADRS), and Young Manic Rating Scale are scored by the examiner.

2. **Rorschach test.** Standardized set of ten inkblots scored by examiner— few associations, slow response time in depression.
3. **Thematic apperception test (TAT).** Series of 30 pictures depicting ambiguous situations and interpersonal events. Patient creates a story about each scene. Depressives will create depressed stories, manics more grandiose and dramatic ones.

V. Bipolar Disorder
There are two types of bipolar disorder: bipolar I characterized by the occurrence of manic episodes with or without a major depressive episode and bipolar II characterized by at least one depressive episode with or without a hypomanic episode.

 CLINICAL HINT:
If there is a history of a single full-blown manic episode, the diagnosis will always be bipolar I; a history of a major depressive episode is always present in bipolar II.

A. **Depression (major depressive episode).** See Table 14–2.
 1. **Information obtained from history**
    a. Depressed mood: subjective sense of sadness, feeling "blue" or "down in the dumps" for a prolonged period of time.
    b. Anhedonia: inability to experience pleasure.
    c. Social withdrawal.
    d. Lack of motivation, little tolerance of frustration.
    e. Vegetative signs.
       (1) Loss of libido.
       (2) Weight loss and anorexia.
       (3) Weight gain and hyperphagia.
       (4) Low energy level; fatigability.
       (5) Abnormal menses.
       (6) Early morning awakening (terminal insomnia); approximately 75% of depressed patients have sleep difficulties, either insomnia or hypersomnia.
       (7) Diurnal variation (symptoms worse in morning).
    f. Constipation.
    g. Dry mouth.
    h. Headache.
 2. **Information obtained from mental status examination**
    a. **General appearance and behavior:** psychomotor retardation or agitation, poor eye contact, tearful, downcast, inattentive to personal appearance.

Table 14–2
DSM-IV-TR Diagnostic Criteria for Major Depressive Episode

A. Five (or more) of the following symptoms have been present during the same 2-week period and represent a change from previous functioning; at least one of the symptoms is either (1) depressed mood or (2) loss of interest or pleasure
Note: Do not include symptoms that are clearly due to a general medical condition, or mood-incongruent delusions or hallucinations.
1. depressed mood most of the day, nearly every day, as indicated by either subjective report (e.g., feels sad or empty) or observation made by others (e.g., appears fearful).
Note: in children and adolescents, can be irritable mood
2. markedly diminished interest or pleasure in all, or almost all, activities most of the day, nearly every day (as indicated by either subjective account or observation made by others)
3. significant weight loss when not dieting or weight gain (e.g., a change of more than 5% of body weight in a month), or decrease or increase in appetite nearly every day.
Note: in children, consider failure to make expected weight gains
4. insomnia or hypersomnia nearly every day
5. psychomotor agitation or retardation nearly every day (observable by others, not merely subjective feelings of restlessness or being slowed down)
6. fatigue or loss of energy nearly every day
7. feelings of worthlessness or excessive or inappropriate guilt (which may be delusional) nearly every day (not merely self-reproach or guilt about being sick)
8. diminished ability to think or concentrate, or indecisiveness, nearly every day (either by subjective account or as observed by others)
9. recurrent thoughts of death (not just fear of dying), recurrent suicidal ideation without a specific plan, or a suicide attempt or a specific plan for committing suicide
B. The symptoms do not meet criteria for a mixed episode.
C. The symptoms cause clinically significant distress or impairment in social, occupational, or other important areas of functioning.
D. The symptoms are not due to the direct physiologic effects of a substance (e.g., a drug of abuse, a medication) or a general medical condition (e.g., hypothyroidism).
E. The symptoms are not better accounted for by bereavement (i.e., after the loss of a loved one), or the symptoms persist for longer than 2 months or are characterized by marked functional impairment, morbid preoccupation with worthlessness, suicidal ideation, psychotic symptoms, or psychomotor retardation.

From American Psychiatric Association. *Diagnostic and Statistical Manual of Mental Disorders*, 4th ed. Text rev. Washington, DC: American Psychiatric Association; 2000, with permission.

    b. Affect: constricted or labile.

    c. Mood: depressed, irritable, frustrated, or sad.

    d. Speech: little or no spontaneity; monosyllabic; long pauses; soft, low monotone.

    e. Thought content: suicidal ideation affects 60% of depressed patients, and 15% commit suicide; obsessive rumination; pervasive feelings of hopelessness, worthlessness, and guilt; somatic preoccupation; indecisiveness; poverty of thought content and paucity of speech; mood-congruent hallucinations and delusions.

    f. Cognition: distractible, difficulty concentrating, complaints of poor memory, apparent disorientation; abstract thought may be impaired.

    g. Insight and judgment: impaired because of cognitive distortions of personal worthlessness.

  3. Associated features

    a. Somatic complaints may mask depression: in particular, cardiac, gastrointestinal, and genitourinary symptoms; low back pain and other orthopedic complaints.

    b. Content of delusions and hallucinations, when present, tends to be congruent with depressed mood; most common are delusions of guilt, poverty, and deserved persecution, in addition to somatic and nihilistic (end of the world) delusions. Mood-incongruent delusions are those with content not apparently related to the predominant mood (e.g., delusions of thought insertion, broadcasting, and control, or persecutory delusions unrelated to depressive themes).

  4. Age-specific features. Depression can present differently at different ages.

    a. Prepubertal: somatic complaints, agitation, single-voice auditory hallucinations, anxiety disorders, and phobias.

    b. Adolescence: substance abuse, antisocial behavior, restlessness, truancy, school difficulties, promiscuity, increased sensitivity to rejection, and poor hygiene.

    c. Elderly: cognitive deficits (memory loss, disorientation, confusion); pseudodementia or the dementia syndrome of depression, apathy, and distractibility.

B. Mania (manic episode). Persistent elevated expansive mood. See Table 14–3.

  1. Information obtained from history

    a. Erratic and disinhibited behavior.

      (1) Excessive spending or gambling.

Table 14–3
***DSM-IV-TR* Diagnostic Criteria for Manic Episode**

A. A distinct period of abnormally and persistently elevated, expansive, or irritable mood, lasting at least 1 week (or any duration if hospitalization is necessary).
B. During the period of mood disturbance, three (or more) of the following symptoms have persisted (four if the mood is only irritable) and have been present to a significant degree: 1. inflated self-esteem or grandiosity   2. decreased need for sleep (e.g., feels rested after only 3 hours of sleep)   3. more talkative than usual or pressure to keep talking   4. flight of ideas or subjective experience that thoughts are racing   5. distractibility (i.e., attention too easily drawn to unimportant or irrelevant external stimuli)   6. increase in goal-directed activity (either socially, at work or school, or sexually) or psychomotor agitation   7. excessive involvement in pleasurable activities that have a high potential for painful consequences (e.g., engaging in unrestrained buying sprees, sexual indiscretions, or foolish business investments)
C. The symptoms do not meet criteria for a mixed episode.
D. The mood disturbance is sufficiently severe to cause marked impairment in occupational functioning or in usual social activities or relationships with others, or to necessitate hospitalization to prevent harm to self or others, or there are psychotic features.
E. The symptoms are not due to the direct physiologic effects of a substance (e.g., a drug of abuse, a medication, or other treatment) or a general medical condition (e.g., hyperthyroidism).
Note: Maniclike episodes that are clearly caused by somatic antidepressant treatment (e.g., medication, electroconvulsive therapy, light therapy) should not count toward a diagnosis of bipolar I disorder.

From American Psychiatric Association. *Diagnostic and Statistical Manual of Mental Disorders*, 4th ed. Text rev. Washington, DC: American Psychiatric Association; 2000, with permission.

    (2) Impulsive travel.

    (3) Hypersexuality, promiscuity.

  b. Overextended in activities and responsibilities.

  c. Low frustration tolerance with irritability and outbursts of anger.

  d. Vegetative signs.

    (1) Increased libido.

    (2) Weight loss, anorexia.

    (3) Insomnia (expressed as no need to sleep).

    (4) Excessive energy.

2. Information obtained from mental status examination

  a. General appearance and behavior: psychomotor agitation; seductive, colorful clothing; excessive makeup; inattention to personal appearance or bizarre combinations of clothes; intrusive; entertaining; threatening; and hyperexcited.

  b. Affect: labile, intense (may have rapid depressive shifts).

  c. Mood: euphoric, expansive, irritable, demanding, and flirtatious.

  d. Speech: pressured, loud, dramatic, exaggerated; may become incoherent.

  e. Thought content: highly elevated self-esteem, grandiose, extremely egocentric; delusions and less frequently hallucinations (mood-congruent themes of inflated self-worth and power, most often grandiose and paranoid).

  f. Thought process: flight of ideas (if severe, can lead to incoherence); racing thoughts, neologisms, clang associations, circumstantiality, tangentially.

  g. Sensorium: highly distractible, difficulty concentrating; memory, if not too distracted, generally intact; abstract thinking generally intact.

  h. Insight and judgment: extremely impaired; often total denial of illness and inability to make any organized or rational decisions.

C. Other types of bipolar disorders

  1. Rapid-cycling bipolar disorder. Four or more depressive, manic, or mixed episodes within 12 months. Bipolar disorder with mixed or rapid-cycling episodes appears to be more chronic than bipolar disorder without alternating episodes.

  2. Hypomania. Elevated mood associated with decreased need for sleep, hypoactivity, and hedonic pursuits. Less severe than mania with no psychotic features (see Table 14–4).

D. Depressive disorders

  1. Major depressive disorder. Can occur alone or as part of bipolar disorder. When it occurs alone, it is also known as *unipolar depression*. Symptoms must be present for at least 2 weeks and represent a change from previous functioning. More common in women than in men by 2:1. Precipitating event occurs in at least 25% of patients. Diurnal variation, with symptoms worse early in the morning. Psychomotor retardation or agitation is present. Associated with vegetative signs. Mood-congruent

Table 14–4
***DSM-IV-TR* Criteria for Hypomanic Episode**

A. A distinct period of persistently elevated, expansive, or irritable mood, lasting throughout 4 days, that is clearly different from the usual nondepressed mood.
B. During the period of mood disturbance, three (or more) of the following symptoms have persisted (four if the mood is only irritable) and have been present to a significant degree:
  1. inflated self-esteem or grandiosity
  2. decreased need for sleep (e.g., feels rested after only 3 hours of sleep)
  3. more talkative than usual or pressure to keep talking
  4. flight of ideas or subjective experience that thoughts are racing
  5. distractibility (i.e., attention too easily drawn to unimportant or irrelevant external stimuli)
  6. increase in goal-directed activity (either socially, at work or school, or sexually) or psychomotor agitation
  7. excessive involvement in pleasurable activities that have a high potential for painful consequences (e.g., the person engages in unrestrained buying sprees, sexual indiscretions, or foolish business investments)
C. The episode is associated with an unequivocal change in functioning that is uncharacteristic of the person when not symptomatic.
D. The disturbance in mood and the change in functioning are observable by others.
E. The episode is not severe enough to cause marked impairment in social or occupational functioning, or to necessitate hospitalization, and there are no psychotic features.
F. The symptoms are not due to the direct physiologic effects of a substance (e.g., a drug of abuse, a medication, or other treatment) or a general medical condition (e.g., hyperthyroidism).

From American Psychiatric Association. *Diagnostic and Statistical Manual of Mental Disorders,* 4th ed. Text rev. Washington, DC: American Psychiatric Association; 2000, with permission.

delusions and hallucinations may be present. Median age of onset is 40 years, but can occur at any time. Genetic factor is present. Major depressive disorder may occur as a single episode in a person's life or may be recurrent.

2. **Other types of major depressive disorder**
   a. **Melancholic:** severe and responsive to biological intervention. See Table 14–5.

Table 14–5
***DSM-IV-TR* Diagnostic Criteria for Melancholic Features Specified**

Specify if:
  With melancholic features (can be applied to the current or most recent major depressive episode in major depressive disorder and to a major depressive episode in bipolar I or bipolar II disorder only if it is the most recent type of mood episode)
A. Either of the following, occurring during the most severe period of the current episode:
  1. loss of pleasure in all, or almost all, activities
  2. lack of reactivity to usually pleasurable stimuli (does not feel much better, even temporarily, when something good happens)
B. Three (or more) of the following:
  1. distinct quality of depressed mood (i.e., the depressed mood is experienced as distinctly different from the kind of feeling experienced after the death of a loved one)
  2. depression regularly worse in the morning
  3. early morning awakening (at least 2 hours before usual time of awakening)
  4. marked psychomotor retardation or agitation
  5. significant anorexia or weight loss
  6. excessive or inappropriate guilt

From American Psychiatric Association. *Diagnostic and Statistical Manual of Mental Disorders,* 4th ed. Text rev. Washington, DC: American Psychiatric Association; 2000, with permission.

b. **Chronic:** present for at least 2 years; more common in elderly men, especially alcohol and substance abusers, and responds poorly to medications. Accounts for the condition of 10% to 15% of those with major depressive disorder. Can also occur as part of depression in bipolar I and II disorders.

c. **Seasonal pattern:** depression that develops with shortened daylight in winter and fall and disappears during spring and summer; also known as *seasonal affective disorder*. Characterized by hypersomnia, hyperphagia, and psychomotor slowing. Related to abnormal melatonin metabolism. Treated with exposure to bright, artificial light for 2 to 6 hours each day. May also occur as part of bipolar I and II disorders.

d. **Postpartum onset:** severe depression beginning within 4 weeks of giving birth. Most often occurs in women with underlying or preexisting mood or other psychiatric disorder. Symptoms range from marked insomnia, lability, and fatigue to suicide. Homicidal and delusional beliefs about the baby may be present. Can be psychiatric emergency, with both mother and baby at risk. Also applies to manic or mixed episodes or to brief psychotic disorder (Chapter 13).

e. **Atypical features:** sometimes called *hysterical dysphoria*. Major depressive episode characterized by weight gain and hypersomnia, rather than weight loss and insomnia. More common in women than in men by 2:1 to 3:1. Common in major depressive disorder with seasonal pattern. May also occur as part of depression in bipolar I or II disorder and dysthymic disorder. (See Table 14 6.)

f. **Catatonic:** stuporous, blunted affect, extreme withdrawal, negativism, and psychomotor retardation with posturing and waxy flexibility. Responds to electroconvulsive therapy (ECT).

Table 14 6
DSM-IV-TR **Criteria for Atypical Features Specifier**

Specify if:
With atypical features (can be applied when these features predominate during the most recent 2 weeks of a current major depressive episode in major depressive disorder or in bipolar I or bipolar II disorder when a current major depressive episode is the most recent type of mood episode, or when these features predominate during the most recent 2 years of dysthymic disorder; if the major depressive episode is not current, it applies if the feature predominates during any 2-week period)

A. Mood reactivity (i.e., mood brightens in response to actual or potential positive events)
B. Two (or more) of the following features:
    1. significant weight gain or increase in appetite
    2. hypersomnia
    3. leaden paralysis (i.e., heavy, leaden feelings in arms or legs)
    4. long-standing pattern of interpersonal rejection sensitivity (not limited to episodes of mood disturbance) that results in significant social or occupational impairment
C. Criteria are not met for with melancholic features or with catatonic features during the same episode.

From American Psychiatric Association. *Diagnostic and Statistical Manual of Mental Disorders,* 4th ed. Text rev. Washington, DC: American Psychiatric Association; 2000, with permission.

g. **Pseudodementia:** major depressive disorder presenting as cognitive dysfunction resembling dementia. Occurs in elderly persons, and more often in patients with previous history of mood disorder. Depression is primary and preeminent, antedating cognitive deficits. Responsive to electroconvulsive therapy (ECT) or antidepressant medication.

h. **Depression in children:** not uncommon. Signs and symptoms similar to those in adults. Masked depression seen in somatic symptoms, running away from home, school phobia, and substance abuse. Suicide may occur.

i. **Double depression:** development of superimposed major depressive disorder in dysthymic patients (about 10%–15%).

j. **Depressive disorder not otherwise specified:** depressive features that do not meet the criteria for a specific mood disorder (e.g., minor depressive disorder, recurrent brief depressive disorder, and premenstrual dysphoric disorder).

k. **Psychotic features:** hallucinations or delusions associated with depression.

 CLINICAL HINT:
If delusions are mood incongruent, diagnosis is more likely to be schizophrenia.

---

3. **Dysthymic disorder** (previously known as *depressive neurosis*). Less severe than major depressive disorder. More common and chronic in women than in men. Insidious onset. Occurs more often in persons with history of long-term stress or sudden losses; often coexists with other psychiatric disorders (e.g., substance abuse, personality disorders, obsessive–compulsive disorder). Symptoms tend to be worse later in the day. Onset generally between ages of 20 and 35, although an early-onset type begins before age 21. More common among first-degree relatives with major depressive disorder. Symptoms should include at least two of the following: poor appetite, overeating, sleep problems, fatigue, low self-esteem, poor concentration or difficulty making decisions, and feelings of hopelessness. (See Table 14–7.)

4. **Cyclothymic disorder.** Less severe disorder, with alternating periods of hypomania and moderate depression. The condition is chronic and nonpsychotic. Symptoms must be present for at least 2 years. Equally common in men and women. Onset usually is insidious and occurs in late adolescence or early adulthood. Substance abuse is common. Major depressive disorder and bipolar disorder are more common among first-degree relatives than among the general population. Recurrent mood swings may lead to social and professional difficulties. May respond to lithium. (See Table 14–8.)

Table 14–7
***DSM-IV-TR* Diagnostic Criteria for Dysthymic Disorder**

A. Depressed mood for most of the day, for more days than not, as indicated either by subjective account or observation by others, for at least 2 years. **Note:** In children and adolescents, mood can be irritable and duration must be at least 1 year.

B. Presence, while depressed, of two (or more) of the following:
   1. poor appetite or overeating
   2. insomnia or hypersomnia
   3. low energy or fatigue
   4. low self-esteem
   5. poor concentration or difficulty making decisions
   6. feelings of hopelessness

C. During the 2-year period (1 year for children or adolescents) of the disturbance, the person has never been without the symptoms in Criteria A and B for more than 2 months at a time.

D. No major depressive episode has been present during the first 2 years of the disturbance (1 year for children and adolescents); i.e., the disturbance is not better accounted for by chronic major depressive disorder, or major depressive disorder, in partial remission.
   Note: There may have been a previous major depressive episode provided there was a full remission (no significant signs or symptoms for 2 months) before development of the dysthymic disorder. In addition, after the initial 2 years (1 year in children or adolescents) of dysthymic disorder, there may be superimposed episodes of major depressive disorder, in which case both diagnoses may be given when the criteria are met for a major depressive episode.

E. There has never been a manic episode, a mixed episode, or a hypomanic episode, and criteria have never been met for cyclothymic disorder.

F. The disturbance does not occur exclusively during the course of a chronic psychotic disorder, such as schizophrenia or delusional disorder.

G. The symptoms are not due to the direct physiologic effects of a substance (e.g., a drug of abuse, a medication) or a general medical condition (e.g., hypothyroidism).

H. The symptoms cause clinically significant distress or impairment in social, occupational, or other important areas of functioning.

Specify if:
   Early onset: if onset is before age 21 years
   Late onset: if onset is age 21 years or older
Specify (for most recent 2 years of dysthymic disorder):
   With atypical features

From American Psychiatric Association. *Diagnostic and Statistical Manual of Mental Disorders*, 4th ed. Text rev. Washington, DC: American Psychiatric Association; 2000, with permission.

VI. Differential diagnosis

Table 14–9 lists the clinical differences between depression and mania.

A. **Mood disorder resulting from general medical condition.** Depressive, manic, or mixed features or major depressivelike episode secondary to medical illness (e.g., brain tumor, metabolic illness, HIV disease, Parkinson's disease, Cushing's syndrome) (Table 14–10). Cognitive deficits are common.

   1. **Hypothyroidism.** Hypothyroidism associated with fatigability, depression, and suicidal impulses. May mimic schizophrenia, with thought disorder, delusions, hallucinations, paranoia, and agitation. More common in women. Was called myxedema madness.

   2. **Mercury.** Chronic mercury intoxication (poisoning) produces manic (and sometimes depressive) symptoms. Was called mad hatter's syndrome.

Table 14–8
DSM-IV-TR Diagnostic Criteria for Cyclothymic Disorder

A. For at least 2 years, the presence of numerous periods with hypomanic symptoms and numerous periods with depressive symptoms that do not meet criteria for a major depressive episode. **Note:** In children and adolescents, the duration must be at least 1 year.
B. During the above 2-year period (1 year in children and adolescents), the person has not been without the symptoms in Criterion A for more than 2 months at a time.
C. No major depressive episode, manic episode, or mixed episode has been present during the first 2 years of the disturbance.
   Note: After the initial 2 years (1 year in children and adolescents) of cyclothymic disorder, there may be superimposed manic or mixed episodes (in which case both bipolar I disorder and cyclothymic disorder may be diagnosed) or major depressive episodes (in which case both bipolar II disorder and cyclothymic disorder may be diagnosed).
D. The symptoms in Criterion A are not better accounted for by schizoaffective disorder and are not superimposed on schizophrenia, schizophreniform disorder, delusional disorder, or psychotic disorder not otherwise specified.
E. The symptoms are not due to the direct physiologic effects of a substance (e.g., a drug of abuse, a medication) or a general medical condition (e.g., hyperthyroidism).
F. The symptoms cause clinically significant distress or impairment in social, occupational, or other important areas of functioning.

From American Psychiatric Association. *Diagnostic and Statistical Manual of Mental Disorders,* 4th ed. Text rev. Washington, DC: American Psychiatric Association; 2000, with permission.

B. Substance-induced mood disorder. See Table 14–11. Mood disorders caused by a drug or toxin (e.g., cocaine, amphetamine, propranolol [Inderal], steroids). Must always be ruled out when patient presents with depressive or manic symptoms. Mood disorders often occur simultaneously with substance abuse and dependence.

C. Schizophrenia. Schizophrenia can look like a manic, major depressive, or mixed episode with psychotic features. To differentiate, rely on such factors as family history, course, premorbid history, and response to medication. Depressivelike or maniclike episode with presence of mood-incongruent psychotic features suggests schizophrenia. Thought insertion and broadcasting, loose associations, poor reality testing, or bizarre behavior may also suggest schizophrenia. Bipolar disorder with depression or mania more often is associated with mood-congruent hallucinations or delusions.

D. Grief. Though recent research disputes if it is different in course and severity from major depression. Known as *bereavement* in *Diagnostic and Statistical Manual of Mental Disorders,* fourth edition, text revision (*DSM-IV-TR*). Profound sadness secondary to major loss. Presentation may be similar to that of major depressive disorder, with anhedonia, withdrawal, and vegetative signs. Remits with time. Differentiated from major depressive disorder by absence of suicidal ideation or profound feelings of hopelessness and worthlessness. Usually resolves within a year. May develop into major depressive episode in predisposed persons.

E. Personality disorders. Lifelong behavioral pattern associated with rigid defensive style; depression may occur more readily after stressful life event because of inflexibility of coping mechanisms. Manic episode may also occur more readily in predisposed people with pre-existing personality

Table 14–9
Clinical Differences Between Depression and Mania

	Depressive Syndrome	Mania Syndrome
Mood	Depressed, irritable, or anxious (the patient may, however, smile or deny subjective mood change and instead complain of pain or other somatic distress)	Elated, irritable, or hostile
	Crying spells (the patient may, however, complain of inability to cry or experience emotions)	Momentary tearfulness (as part of mixed state)
Associated psychological manifestations	Lack of self-confidence; low self-esteem; self-reproach	Inflated self-esteem; boasting; grandiosity
	Poor concentration; indecisiveness	Racing thoughts; clang associations (new thoughts triggered by word sounds rather than meaning); distractibility
	Reduction in gratification; loss of interest in usual activities; loss of attachments; social withdrawal	Heightened interest in new activities, people, creative pursuits; increased involvement with people (who are often alienated because of the patient's intrusive and meddlesome behavior); buying sprees; sexual indiscretions; foolish business investment
	Negative expectations; hopelessness; helplessness; increased dependency	
	Recurrent thoughts of death and suicide	
Somatic manifestations	Psychomotor retardation; fatigue	Psychomotor acceleration, eutonia (increased sense of physical well-being)
	Agitation	
	Anorexia and weight loss, or weight gain	Possible weight loss from increased activity and inattention to proper dietary habits
	Insomnia, or hypersomnia	Decreased need for sleep
	Menstrual irregularities; amenorrhea	
	Anhedonia; loss of sexual desire	Increased sexual desire
Psychotic symptoms	Delusions of worthlessness and sinfulness	Grandiose delusions of exceptional talent
	Delusions of reference and persecution	Delusions of assistance; delusions of reference and persecution
	Delusion of ill health (nihilistic, somatic, or hypochondriacal)	Delusions of exceptional mental and physical fitness
	Delusions of poverty	Delusions of wealth, aristocratic ancestry, or other grandiose identity
	Depressive hallucinations in the auditory, visual, and (rarely) olfactory spheres	Fleeting auditory or visual hallucinations

From Berkow R, ed. *Merck Manual*, 15th ed. Rahway, NJ: Merck Sharp & Dohme Research Laboratories, 1987:1518, with permission.

Table 14–10
Neurological and Medical Causes of Depressive (and Manic) Symptoms

Neurological	Parathyroid disorders (hyper- and hypo-)
Cerebrovascular diseases	Postpartum[a]
Dementias (including dementia of the Alzheimer's type with depressed mood)	Thyroid disorders (hypothyroidism and apathetic hyperthyroidism)[a]
Epilepsy[a]	**Infectious and inflammatory**
Fahr's disease[a]	AIDS[a]
Huntington's disease[a]	Chronic fatigue syndrome
Hydrocephalus	Mononucleosis
Infections (including HIV and neurosyphilis)[a]	Pneumonia—viral and bacterial
Migraines[a]	Rheumatoid arthritis
Multiple sclerosis[a]	Sjögren's arteritis
Narcolepsy	Systemic lupus erythematosus[a]
Neoplasms[a]	Temporal arthritis
Parkinson's disease	Tuberculosis
Progressive supranuclear palsy	**Miscellaneous medical**
Sleep apnea	Cancer (especially pancreatic and other gastrointestinal)
Trauma[a]	Cardiopulmonary disease
Wilson's disease[a]	Porphyria
Endocrine	Uremia (and other renal diseases)[a]
Adrenal (Cushing's, Addison's diseases)	Vitamin deficiencies (B$_{12}$, folate, niacin, thiamine)[a]
Hyperaldosteronism	
Menses-related[a]	

[a]These conditions are also associated with manic symptoms.

disorder. A mood disorder may be diagnosed on Axis I simultaneously with a personality disorder on Axis II.

  F. **Schizoaffective disorder.** Signs and symptoms of schizophrenia accompany prominent mood symptoms. Course and prognosis are between those of schizophrenia and mood disorders.

  G. **Adjustment disorder with depressed mood.** Moderate depression in response to clearly identifiable stress, which resolves as stress diminishes. Considered a maladaptive response resulting from either impairment in functioning or excessive and disproportionate intensity of symptoms. Persons with personality disorders or cognitive deficits may be more vulnerable.

  H. **Primary sleep disorders.** Can cause anergy, dyssomnia, and irritability. Distinguish from major depression by assessing for typical signs and symptoms of depression and occurrence of sleep abnormalities only in the context of depressive episodes. Consider obtaining a sleep laboratory evaluation in cases of refractory depression.

  I. **Other mental disorders.** Eating disorders, somatoform disorders, and anxiety disorders are all commonly associated with depressive symptoms and must be considered in the differential diagnosis of a patient with depressive symptoms. Perhaps the most difficult differential is that between anxiety disorders with depression and depressive disorders with marked anxiety. The difficulty of making this differentiation is reflected in the inclusion of the research category of mixed anxiety–depressive disorder in *DSM-IV-TR* (Chapter 15).

Table 14–11
Pharmacological Causes of Depression and Mania

Pharmacological Causes of Depression		Pharmacological Causes of Mania
Cardiac and antihypertensive drugs		Amphetamines
Bethanidine	Digitalis	Antidepressants
Clonidine	Prazosin	Baclofen
Guanethidine	Procainamide	Bromide
Hydralazine	Veratrum	Bromocriptine
Methyldopa	Lidocaine	Captopril
Propranolol	Oxprenolol	Cimetidine
Reserpine	Methoserpidine	Cocaine
Sedatives and hypnotics		Corticosteroids (including corticotropin)
Barbiturates	Benzodiazepines	Cyclosporine
Chloral hydrate	Chlormethiazole	Disulfiram
Ethanol	Clorazepate	Hallucinogens (intoxication and flashbacks)
Steroids and hormones		Hydralazine
Corticosteroids	Triamcinolone	Isoniazid
Oral contraceptives	Norethisterone	Levodopa
Prednisone	Danazol	Methylphenidate
Stimulants and appetite suppressants		Metrizamide (following myelography)
Amphetamine	Diethylpropion	Opioids
Fenfluramine	Phenmetrazine	Phencyclidine
Psychotropic drugs		Procarbazine
Butyrophenones	Phenothiazines	Procyclidine
Neurological agents		Yohimbine
Amantadine	Baclofen	
Bromocriptine	Carbamazepine	
Levodopa	Methsuximide	
Tetrabenazine	Phenytoin	
Analgesics and anti-inflammatory drugs		
Fenoprofen	Phenacetin	
Ibuprofen	Phenylbutazone	
Indomethacin	Pentazocine	
Opioids	Benzydamine	
Antibacterial and antifungal drugs		
Ampicillin	Griseofulvin	
Sulfamethoxazole	Metronidazole	
Clotrimazole	Nitrofurantoin	
Cycloserine	Nalidixic acid	
Dapsone	Sulfonamides	
Ethionamide	Streptomycin	
Tetracycline	Thiocarbanilide	
Antineoplastic drugs		
C-Asparaginase	6-Azauridine	
Mithramycin	Bleomycin	
Vincristine	Trimethoprim	
	Zidovudine	
Miscellaneous drugs		
Acetazolamide	Anticholinesterases	
Choline	Cimetidine	
Cyproheptadine	Diphenoxylate	
Disulfiram	Lysergide	
Methysergide	Mebeverine	
Meclizine	Metoclopramide	
Pizotifen	Salbutamol	

Adapted from Cummings JL. *Clinical Neuropsychiatry.* Orlando, FL: Grune & Stratton, 1985:187, with permission.

VII. Course and Prognosis

Fifteen percent of depressed patients eventually commit suicide. An untreated, average depressed episode lasts about 10 months. At least 75% of affected patients have a second episode of depression, usually within the first 6 months after the initial episode. The average number of depressive episodes in a lifetime is five. The prognosis generally is good: 50% recover, 30% partially recover, 20% have a chronic course. About 20% to 30% of dysthymic patients develop, in descending order of frequency, major depressive disorder (called *double depression*), bipolar II disorder, or bipolar I disorder. A major mood disorder, usually bipolar II disorder, develops in about 30% of patients with cyclothymic disorder. Forty-five percent of manic episodes recur. Untreated, manic episodes last 3 to 6 months, with a high rate of recurrence (average of 10 recurrences). Some 80% to 90% of manic patients eventually experience a full depressive episode. The long-term prognosis for mania is fair: 15% recover, 50% to 60% partially recover (multiple relapses with good interepisodic functioning), and one-third have some evidence of chronic symptoms and social deterioration.

 CLINICAL HINT:
Depressed patients with suicidal ideation should be hospitalized if there is any doubt in the clinician's mind about the risk. If the clinician cannot sleep because of worry about a patient, that patient belongs in a hospital.

VIII. Treatment

A. **Depressive disorders.** Major depressive episodes are treatable in 70% to 80% of patients. The most effective approach is to integrate pharmacotherapy with psychotherapeutic interventions.

1. **Psychopharmacological.**

a. Most clinicians begin treatment with a selective serotonin reuptake inhibitor (SSRI). Early transient side effects include anxiety, gastrointestinal upset, and headache. Educating patients about the self-limited nature of these effects can enhance compliance. Sexual dysfunction is often a persistent, common side effect that may respond to a change in drug or dosage, or adjunctive therapy with an agent such as bupropion (Wellbutrin) or buspirone (BuSpar). The early anxiogenic effects of SSRIs may aggravate suicidal ideation and can be managed by either reducing the dose or adding an anxiolytic (e.g., 0.5 mg of clonazepam [Klonopin] in the morning and at night). Insomnia can be managed with a benzodiazepine, zolpidem (Ambien), trazodone (Desyrel), or mirtazapine (Remeron). Patients who do not respond to or who cannot tolerate one SSRI may respond to another. Some clinicians switch to an agent with a different mechanism of action, such as bupropion, venlafaxine (Effexor), duloxetine (Cymbalta), mirtazapine (Remeron), a tricyclic, or a monoamine oxidase inhibitor (MAOI). The tricyclics and MAOIs are generally considered as second- or third-line agents because of their side effects and potential lethality in overdose.

 CLINICAL HINT:
There is an increased risk of suicide as suicidally depressed patients begin to improve. They have the physical energy to carry out the act, whereas before, they lacked the will to do so. Known as paradoxical suicide.

---

   b. Bupropion is a noradrenergic, dopaminergic drug with stimulantlike properties. It is generally well tolerated and may be particularly useful for depression marked by anergy and psychomotor retardation. It is also devoid of sexual side effects. It may exacerbate anxiety and agitation. Its dopaminergic properties have the potential to exacerbate psychosis. Prior concerns about its tendency to cause seizures have been mitigated because it carries the same risk for seizure as the SSRIs (0.1%). The average dose is 150 to 300 mg/day. In eating disorders caution should be used.

   c. Venlafaxine and duloxetine are serotonin–norepinephrine reuptake inhibitors that may be particularly effective in severe or refractory cases of depression. Response rates increase with higher doses. Side effects are similar to those of SSRIs. The average dose of venlafaxine is 75 to 375 mg/day and of duloxetine 20 to 60 mg/day.

   d. Nefazodone is a drug with serotoninergic properties. Its main mechanism of action is postsynaptic $5-HT_2$ blockade. As a result, it produces beneficial effects on sleep and has a low rate of sexual side effects. It has been associated with liver toxicity and should be used with caution in patients with suspected liver damage. The average dose is 300 to 600 mg/day. It is available only as a generic preparation.

   e. Mirtazapine has antihistamine, noradrenergic, and serotoninergic actions. It specifically blocks $5-HT_2$ and $5-HT_3$ receptors, so that the anxiogenic, sexual, and gastrointestinal side effects of serotoninergic drugs are avoided. At low doses, it can be highly sedating and cause weight gain. At higher dosages, it becomes more noradrenergic relative to its antihistamine effects and so is a more activating drug. Average dose is 15 to 30 mg/day.

   f. The tricyclics are highly effective but require dose titration. Side effects include anticholinergic effects in addition to potential cardiac conduction delay and orthostasis. The secondary amines, such as nortriptyline, are often better tolerated than the tertiary amines, such as amitriptyline (Elavil). Blood levels can be helpful in determining optimal dosage and adequacy of a therapeutic trial. Lethality in overdose remains a concern.

g. Augmentation strategies in treatment-resistant or partially responsive patients include liothyronine (Cytomel), lithium, amphetamines, buspirone, or antidepressant combinations such as bupropion added to an SSRI.

h. If symptoms still do not improve, try an MAOI. An MAOI is safe with reasonable dietary restriction of tyramine-containing substances. Major depressive episodes that have atypical features or psychotic features or that are related to bipolar I disorder may preferentially respond to MAOIs. MAOIs must not be administered for 2 to 5 weeks after discontinuation of an SSRI or other serotoninergic drugs (e.g., 5 weeks for fluoxetine [Prozac], 2 weeks for paroxetine [Paxil]). An SSRI or other serotoninergic drug (e.g., clomipramine [Anafranil]) must not be administered for 2 weeks after discontinuation of an MAOI. Serotoninergic–dopamine antagonists are also of use in depression with psychotic features.

i. Maintenance treatment for at least 5 months with antidepressants helps to prevent relapse. Long-term treatment may be indicated in patients with recurrent major depressive disorder. The antidepressant dosage required to achieve remission should be continued during maintenance treatment.

 CLINICAL HINT:
An extensive NIH study (Star*D) developed a pharmacological protocol for treatment of depression. Clinicians can follow the protocol or vary it depending on the clinical situation and their experience. See Table 14–12.

---

j. ECT is useful in refractory major depressive disorder and major depressive episodes with psychotic features; ECT also is indicated when a rapid therapeutic response is desired or when side effects of antidepressant medications must be avoided. (ECT is underused as a first-line antidepressant treatment.)

k. Lithium can be a first-line antidepressant in treating the depression of bipolar disorder. A heterocyclic antidepressant or MAOI may be added as necessary, but monitor the patient carefully for emergence of manic symptoms.

l. Repetitive transcranial magnetic stimulation (rTMS) shows promise as a treatment for depression. rTMS uses magnetic fields to stimulate specific brain regions (e.g., left prefrontal cortex) believed to be involved in the pathophysiology of specific disorders.

m. Vagus nerve stimulation with implanted electrodes has been successful in some cases of depression and is being studied.

2. Psychological. Psychotherapy in conjunction with antidepressants is more effective than either treatment alone in the management of major depressive disorder.

Table 14–12
Treatment Choices Throughout STAR*D

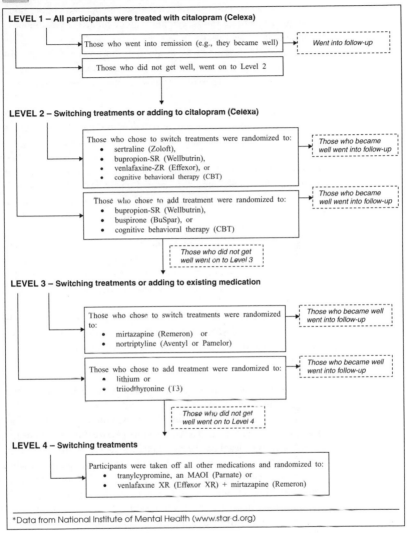

LEVEL 1 – All participants were treated with citalopram (Celexa)

> Those who went into remission (e.g., they became well) ⟶ *Went into follow-up*

> Those who did not get well, went on to Level 2

LEVEL 2 – Switching treatments or adding to citalopram (Celexa)

> Those who chose to switch treatments were randomized to:
> - sertraline (Zoloft),
> - bupropion-SR (Wellbutrin),
> - venlafaxine-ZR (Effexor), or
> - cognitive behavioral therapy (CBT)

Those who became well went into follow-up

> Those who chose to add treatment were randomized to:
> - bupropion-SR (Wellbutrin),
> - buspirone (BuSpar), or
> - cognitive behavioral therapy (CBT)

Those who became well went into follow-up

Those who did not get well went on to Level 3

LEVEL 3 – Switching treatments or adding to existing medication

> Those who chose to switch treatments were randomized to:
> - mirtazapine (Remeron) or
> - nortriptyline (Aventyl or Pamelor)

Those who became well went into follow-up

> Those who chose to add treatment were randomized to:
> - lithium or
> - triiodthyronine (T3)

Those who became well went into follow-up

Those who did not get well went on to Level 4

LEVEL 4 – Switching treatments

> Participants were taken off all other medications and randomized to:
> - tranylcypromine, an MAOI (Parnate) or
> - venlafaxine XR (Effexor XR) + mirtazapine (Remeron)

*Data from National Institute of Mental Health (www.star-d.org)

a. **Cognitive:** short-term treatment with interactive therapist and assigned homework aimed at testing and correcting negative cognitions and the unconscious assumptions that underlie them; based on correcting chronic distortions in thinking that lead to depression, in particular the cognitive triad of feelings of helplessness and hopelessness about one's self, one's future, and one's past.

b. **Behavioral:** based on learning theory (classic and operant conditioning). Generally short-term and highly structured; aimed at specific, circumscribed undesired behaviors. The operant conditioning technique of positive reinforcement may be an effective adjunct in the treatment of depression.

c. **Interpersonal:** developed as a specific short-term treatment for nonbipolar, nonpsychotic depression in outpatients. Emphasis on ongoing, current interpersonal issues as opposed to unconscious, intrapsychic dynamics.

d. **Psychoanalytically oriented:** insight-oriented therapy of indeterminate length aimed at achieving understanding of unconscious conflicts and motivations that may be fueling and sustaining depression.

e. **Supportive:** therapy of indeterminate length with the primary aim of providing emotional support. Indicated particularly in acute crisis, such as grief, or when the patient is beginning to recover from a major depressive episode but cannot yet engage in more demanding, interactive therapy.

f. **Group:** not indicated for acutely suicidal patients. Other depressed patients may benefit from support, ventilation, and positive reinforcement of groups, and from interpersonal interaction and immediate correction of cognitive and transference distortions by other group members.

g. **Family:** particularly indicated when patient's depression is disrupting family stability, when depression is related to family events, or when it is supported or maintained by family patterns.

B. **Bipolar disorders**
   1. **Biological**
      a. Mood stabilizers such as lithium and divalproex (Depakote) are the first choice of drugs used for bipolar disorder but second generation antipsychotics such as olanzapine (Zyprexa) are also used. Carbamazepine (Tegretol) is also a well-established treatment. Lamotrigine (Lamictal) is used in the maintenance phase of bipolar disorder. Topiramate (Topamax) is another anticonvulsant used in bipolar patients. ECT is highly effective in all phases of bipolar disorder. Carbamazepine, divalproex, and valproic acid (Depakene) may be more effective than lithium in the treatment of mixed or dysphoric mania, rapid cycling, and psychotic mania, and in the treatment of patients with a history of multiple manic episodes or comorbid substance abuse.

      b. Treatment of acute manic episodes often requires adjunctive use of potent sedative drugs. Drugs commonly used at the start of treatment include clonazepam (1 mg every 4 to 6 hours) and lorazepam (Ativan) (2 mg every 4 to 6 hours). Physicians should attempt to taper these adjunctive agents when the patient stabilizes. Bipolar patients may be particularly sensitive to the side effects of typical antipsychotics. The atypical antipsychotics (e.g., olanzapine [Zyprexa] [10 to 15 mg/day]) are often used as monotherapy for acute control and has intrinsic antimanic properties.

c. Lithium remains a mainstay of treatment in bipolar disorders. A blood level of 0.8 to 1.2 mEq/L is usually needed to control acute symptoms. A complete trial should last at least 4 weeks, with 2 weeks at therapeutic levels. Prelithium workup includes a complete blood cell count, electrocardiogram (ECG), thyroid function tests, measurement of blood urea nitrogen and serum creatinine, and a pregnancy test. Lithium has a narrow therapeutic index, and levels can become toxic quickly when a patient is dehydrated. A level of 2.0 mEq or higher is toxic. Lithium treatment can be initiated at 300 mg three times per day. A level should be checked after 5 days and the dose titrated accordingly. The clinical response may take 4 days after a therapeutic level has been achieved. Typical side effects include thirst, polyuria, tremor, metallic taste, cognitive dulling, and gastrointestinal upset. Lithium can induce hypothyroidism and, in rare cases, renal toxicity. Lithium achieves an antidepressant response in 50% of patients. Lithium is most effective for prophylaxis of further mood episodes at levels of 0.8 to 1.2 mEq/L. However, in many patients, remission can be maintained at lower levels, which are better tolerated and thereby promote enhanced compliance. Patients with depressive breakthrough on lithium should be assessed for lithium-induced hypothyroidism. Lithium is excreted unchanged by the kidneys and must be used with caution in patients with renal disease. Because lithium is not metabolized by the liver, it may be the best choice for treating bipolar disorder in patients with hepatic impairment.

d. Valproic acid and divalproex have a broad therapeutic index and appear effective at levels of 50 to 125 mcg/mL. Pretreatment workup includes a complete blood cell count and liver function tests. A pregnancy test is needed because this drug can cause neural tube defects in developing fetuses. It can cause thrombocytopenia and increased transaminase levels, both of which are usually benign and self-limited but require increased blood monitoring. Fatal hepatic toxicity has been reported only in children under age 10 who received multiple anticonvulsants.

Typical side effects include hair loss (which can be treated with zinc and selenium), tremor, weight gain, and sedation. Gastrointestinal upset is common but can be minimized by using enteric-coated tablets (Depakote) and titrating gradually. Valproic acid can be loaded for acute symptom control by administering at 20 mg/kg in divided doses. This strategy also produces a therapeutic level and may improve symptoms within 7 days. For outpatients, more physically brittle patients, or less severely ill patients, medication can be started at 250 to 750 mg/day and gradually titrated to a therapeutic level. Blood levels can be checked after 3 days at a particular dosage.

e. Carbamazepine is usually titrated to response rather than blood level, although many clinicians titrate to reach levels of 4 to 12 mcg/mL. Pretreatment evaluation should include liver function tests and a complete blood cell count as well as ECG, electrolytes, reticulocytes, and pregnancy test. Side effects include nausea, sedation, and ataxia. Hepatic toxicity, hyponatremia, or bone marrow suppression may rarely occur. Rash occurs in 10% of patients. Exfoliative rashes (Stevens–Johnson syndrome) are rare but potentially fatal. The drug can be started at 200 to 600 mg/day, with adjustments every 5 days based on clinical response. Improvement may be seen 7 to 14 days after a therapeutic dose has been achieved. Drug interactions complicate carbamazepine use and probably relegate it to second-line status. It is a potent enzyme inducer and can lower levels of other psychotropics, such as haloperidol. Carbamazepine induces its own metabolism (autoinduction), and the dosage often needs to be increased during the first few months of treatment to maintain a therapeutic level and clinical response.

f. Lamotrigine is an anticonvulsant that may have antidepressant, antimanic, and mood-stabilizing properties and does not require blood monitoring. Lamotrigine requires gradual titration to decrease the risk for rash, which occurs in 10% of patients. Stevens–Johnson syndrome occurs in 0.1% of patients treated with lamotrigine. Other side effects include nausea, sedation, ataxia, and insomnia. Dosage can be initiated at 25 to 50 mg/day for 2 weeks and then increased slowly to 150 to 250 mg twice daily. Valproate raises lamotrigine levels. In the presence of valproate, lamotrigine titration should be slower and dosages lower (e.g., 25 mg orally four times daily for 2 weeks, with 25-mg increases every 2 weeks to a maximum of 150 mg/day).

g. Maintenance treatment is required in patients with recurrent illness. During long-term treatment, laboratory monitoring is required for lithium, valproic acid, and carbamazepine.

h. Patients who do not respond adequately to one mood stabilizer may do well with combination treatment. Lithium and valproic acid are commonly used together. Increased neurotoxicity is a risk, but the combination is safe. Other combinations include lithium plus carbamazepine, carbamazepine plus valproic acid (requires increased laboratory monitoring for drug interactions and hepatic toxicity), and combinations with the newer anticonvulsants.

i. Other agents used in bipolar disorder include verapamil (Isoptin, Calan), nimodipine (Nimotop), clonidine (Catapres), clonazepam, and levothyroxine (Levoxyl, Levothroid, Synthroid). Clozapine (Clozaril) has been shown to have antimanic and mood-stabilizing properties and is used if and when patients do not respond to conventional mood stabilizers. Table 14–13 lists the drugs used in the treatment of depression, and Table 14–14 lists commonly used mood stabilizers in the treatment of mania.

Text continues on page 200.

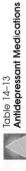

Table 14–13
Antidepressant Medications

Generic (Brand) Name NE Reuptake inhibitors	Usual Daily Dose (mg)	Common Side Effects	Clinical Hints
Desipramine (Norpramin, Pertofrane)	75–300	Drowsiness, insomnia, hypotension, agitation, cardiac, weight gain, anticholinergic[a]	Overdose may be fatal. Dose titration is needed.
Protriptyline (Vivactil)	20–60	Drowsiness, insomnia, agitation, anticholinergic[a]	Overdose may be fatal. Dose titration is needed.
Nortriptyline (Aventyl, Pamelor)	40–200	Drowsiness, weight ↑, anticholinergic[a]	Overdose may be fatal. Dose titration is needed.
Maprotiline (Ludiomil)	100–225	Drowsiness, weight ↑, anticholinergic[a]	Overdose may be fatal. Dose titration is needed.
5-HT Reuptake inhibitors			
Citalopram (Celexa)	20–60	All SSRIs may cause insomnia, agitation, sedation, GI distress, and sexual dysfunction.	Many SSRIs inhibit various cytochrome P450 isoenzymes. They are better tolerated than tricyclics and have high safety in overdose. Shorter half-life SSRIs may be associated with discontinuation symptoms when abruptly stopped.
Escitalopram (Lexapro)	10–20		
Fluoxetine (Prozac)	10–40		
Fluvoxamine (Luvox)[b]	100–300		
Paroxetine (Paxil)	20–50		
Sertraline (Zoloft)	50–150		
NE and 5-HT Reuptake inhibitors			
Amitriptyline (Elavil, Endep)	75–300	Drowsiness, weight ↑, anticholinergic[a]	Overdose may be fatal. Dose titration is needed.
Doxepin (Triadapin, Sinequan)	75–300	Drowsiness, weight ↑, anticholinergic[a]	Overdose may be fatal.
Duloxetine (Cymbalta)	40–60	Drowsiness, hypertension, anticholinergic	Mydriasis, therefore, use with caution in glaucoma.
Imipramine (Tofranil)	75–300	Drowsiness, insomnia and agitation, GI distress, weight ↑, anticholinergic[a]	Overdose may be fatal. Dose titration needed.
Trimipramine (Surmontil)	75–300	Drowsiness, weight ↑, anticholinergic[a]	—
Venlafaxine (Effexor)	150–375	Sleep changes, GI distress	Higher doses may cause hypertension. Dose titration is needed. Abrupt discontinuation may result in discontinuation symptoms.
Desvenlafaxine (Pristiq)	50–150	Sleep changes	—

(continued)

Table 14–13—*continued*
Antidepressant Medications

Generic (Brand) Name	NE Reuptake inhibitors	Usual Daily Dose (mg)	Common Side Effects	Clinical Hints
Pre- and postsynaptic active agents				
Nefazodone (Serzone)		300–600	Sedation	Dose titration is needed. No sexual dysfunction.
Mirtazapine (Remeron)		15–30	Sedation, weight ↑	No sexual dysfunction.
Dopamine reuptake inhibitor				
Bupropion (Wellbutrin)		200–400	Insomnia/agitation, GI distress	Twice-a-day dosing with sustained release. XL dosing is once a day. No sexual dysfunction or weight ↑.
Mixed action agents				
Amoxapine (Asendin)		100–600	Drowsiness, insomnia/ agitation, weight ↑, anticholinergic[a]	Movement disorders may occur. Dose titration is needed.
Clomipramine (Anafranil)		75–300	Drowsiness, weight ↑	Dose titration is needed.
Trazodone (Desyrel)		150–600	Drowsiness, GI distress, weight ↑	Priapism is possible.

Note: Dose ranges are for adults in good general medical health, taking no other medications, aged 18 to 60 years of age. Doses vary depending on the agent, concomitant medications, the presence of general medical or surgical conditions, age, genetic constitution, and other factors. Brand names are those used in the United States. NE, norepinephrine; SSRI, selective serotonin reuptake inhibitor.

[a] Dry mouth, blurred vision, urinary hesitancy, and constipation.

[b] Not approved as an antidepressant in the United States by the U.S. Food and Drug Administration.

Adapted from Rush AJ. Mood disorders: Treatment of depression. In Sadock BJ, Sadock VA, eds: *Comprehensive Textbook of Psychiatry*, 8th ed. Philadelphia: Lippincott Williams & Wilkins; 2005.

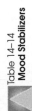

Table 14-14
Mood Stabilizers

This table lists medications for which there are data supporting their use in the treatment of acute mania

Drug	Usual Adult Daily Dose	Starting Dose and Titration	Maximum Recommended Dose or Blood Level	Common Side Effects	Monitoring	Warnings
Lithium and anticonvulsants						
Lithium	Target level 0.6–1.2 mEq/L	300–900 mg; increase by 300 mg/day	1.2 mEq/L plasma level	Nausea, vomiting, diarrhea, sedation, tremor, polyuria, polydipsia, weight ↑, acne, cognitive slowing	Lithium level 12 hours after last dose and every week while titrating, then every 2 months	Lithium toxicity
Carbamazepine	800–1,000 mg; titrate to clinical response (target level 4–12 mcg/mL)	Start 200 mg at night, b.i.d. or t.i.d.; increase by 200 mg/day	1,600 mg/day; Level of 12 mcg/mL	Sedation, dizziness, nausea, cognitive impairment, LFT elevation, dyspepsia, ataxia	CBC, LFT, drug level every 7–14 days while titrating, then monthly for 4 months, then every 6–12 months	Aplastic anemia, agranulocytosis, seizures, myocarditis
Carbamazepine Extended Release	800–1,000 mg; titrate to clinical response (target level 4–12 mcg/mL)	400 mg/day	1,600 mg/day; Level of 12 mcg/mL	Sedation, dizziness, nausea, cognitive impairment, LFT elevation, dyspepsia, ataxia	CBC, LFT, drug level every 7–14 days while titrating, then monthly for 4 months, then every 6–12 months	Aplastic anemia, agranulocytosis, seizures, myocarditis
Divalproex	Titrate to 50–150 mg	Start 250–500 mg at night for 2 days; increase by 250 mg/day. Alternative: orally load 20–30 mg/kg/day to start	Level of 150 mEq/L	Nausea, vomiting, sedation, weight ↑, hair loss	CBC with increased platelets, LFT level weekly until stable, then monthly for 6 months, then every 6–12 months	Hepatoxicity, teratogenicity, pancreatitis
Oxcarbazepine	600–2,400 mg dosed b.i.d. or t.i.d.	Start 300 mg b.i.d.; increase by 300 mg QOD	2,500 mg	Fatigue, nausea/vomiting, dizziness, sedation diplopia, hyponatremia	Electrolytes (sodium)	None

    j. ECT should be considered in refractory or emergent cases. See Chapter 30 for further discussion.

2. **Psychological.** Psychotherapy in conjunction with antimanic drugs (e.g., lithium) is more effective than either treatment alone. Psychotherapy is not indicated when a patient is experiencing a manic episode. In this situation, the safety of the patient and others must be paramount, and pharmacological and physical steps must be taken to protect and calm the patient.

    a. Cognitive: has been studied in relation to increasing compliance with lithium therapy among patients with bipolar disorder.

    b. Behavioral: can be most effective during inpatient treatment of manic patients. Helps to set limits on impulsive or inappropriate behavior through such techniques as positive and negative reinforcement and token economies.

    c. Psychoanalytically oriented: can be beneficial in the recovery and stabilization of manic patients if patient is capable of and desires insight into underlying conflicts that may trigger and fuel manic episodes. Can also help patients understand resistance to medication and thus increase compliance.

    d. Supportive: indicated particularly during acute phases and in early recompensation. Some patients can tolerate only supportive therapy, whereas others can tolerate insight-oriented therapy. Supportive therapy more often is indicated for patients with chronic bipolar disorder, who may have significant interepisodic residual symptoms and experience social deterioration.

    e. Group: can be helpful in challenging denial and defensive grandiosity of manic patients. Useful in addressing such common issues among manic patients as loneliness, shame, inadequacy, fear of mental illness, and loss of control. Helpful in reintegrating patients socially.

    f. Family: particularly important with bipolar patients because their disorder is strongly familial (22%–25% of first-degree relatives) and because manic episodes are so disruptive to patients' interpersonal relationships and jobs. During manic episodes, patients may spend huge amounts of family money or act with sexual inappropriateness; residual feelings of anger, guilt, and shame among family members must be addressed. Ways to help with compliance and recognizing triggering events can be explored.

For more detailed discussion of this topic, see Mood Disorders, Ch. 13, p. 1629, in CTP/IX.

15
Anxiety Disorders

I. Definition
Anxiety is a state that has many effects: It influences cognition and tends to produce distortions of perception. It is differentiated from fear, which is an appropriate response to a known threat; anxiety is a response to a threat that is unknown, vague, or conflictual. Table 15–1 lists the signs and symptoms of anxiety disorders. Most of the effects of anxiety are dread accompanied by somatic complaints that indicate a hyperactive autonomic nervous system such as palpitations and sweating.

II. Classification
There are 11 diagnostic types of anxiety disorders in *Diagnostic Statistical Manual of Mental Disorders, Text Revision,* fourth edition, (*DSM-IV-TR*), ranging from panic disorder with and without agoraphobia to generalized anxiety disorder of unknown or known etiology (e.g., due to a medical condition or to substance abuse). They are among the most common groups of psychiatric disorders. Each disorder is discussed separately below.

A. **Panic disorder with and without agoraphobia.** Panic disorder is characterized by spontaneous panic attacks (Table 15–2). It may occur alone or be associated with agoraphobia (fear of being in open spaces, outside the home alone, or in a crowd). Panic may evolve in stages: subclinical attacks, full panic attacks, anticipatory anxiety, phobic avoidance of specific situations, and agoraphobia. It can lead to alcohol or drug abuse, depression, and occupational and social restrictions. Agoraphobia can occur alone, although patients usually have associated panic attacks. Anticipatory anxiety is characterized by the fear that panic, with helplessness or humiliation, will occur. Patients with panic disorder often have multiple somatic complaints related to autonomic nervous system dysfunction, with a higher risk in females. See Table 15–3.

B. **Agoraphobia without history of panic disorder.** Anxiety about being in places or situations such as in a crowd or in open spaces, outside the home, from which escape or egress is feared to be impossible. The situation is avoided or endured with marked distress, sometimes including the fear of having a panic attack. Agoraphobic patients may become housebound and never leave the home or go outside only with a companion.

C. **Generalized anxiety disorder.** Involves excessive worry about everyday life circumstances, events, or conflicts. The symptoms may fluctuate and overlap with other medical and psychiatric disorders (depressive and other anxiety disorders). The anxiety is difficult to control, is subjectively distressing, and produces impairments in important areas of a person's life. Occurs in children and adults with a lifetime prevalence of 45%. Ratio of women to men is 2:1. See Table 15–4.

Table 15–1
Signs and Symptoms of Anxiety Disorders

Physical Signs	Psychological Symptoms
Trembling, twitching, feeling shaky	Feeling of dread
Backache, headache	Difficulty concentrating
Muscle tension	Hypervigilance
Shortness of breath, hyperventilation	Insomnia
Fatigability	Decreased libido
Startle response	"Lump in the throat"
Autonomic hyperactivity	Upset stomach ("butterflies")
Flushing and pallor	
Tachycardia, palpitations	
Sweating	
Cold hands	
Diarrhea	
Dry mouth (xerostomia)	
Urinary frequency	
Paresthesia	
Difficulty swallowing	

   D. Specific phobia. A phobia is an irrational fear of an object (e.g., horses, heights, needles). The person experiences massive anxiety when exposed to the feared object and tries to avoid it at all costs. Up to 25% of the population have specific phobias. More common in females. See Table 15–5.
   E. Social phobia. Social phobia is an irrational fear of public situations (e.g., speaking in public, eating in public, using public bathrooms [shy bladder]). May be associated with panic attacks. It usually occurs during early teens but can develop during childhood. Affects up to 13% of persons. Equally common in men and women. See Table 15–6.

Table 15–2
***DSM-IV-TR* Diagnostic Criteria for Panic Attack**

Note: A panic attack is not a codable disorder. Code the specific diagnosis in which the panic attack occurs (e.g., panic disorder with agoraphobia).
A discrete period of intense fear or discomfort, in which four (or more) of the following symptoms developed abruptly and reached a peak within 10 minutes:
   1. palpitations, pounding heart, or accelerated heart rate
   2. sweating
   3. trembling or shaking
   4. sensations of shortness of breath or smothering
   5. feeling of choking
   6. chest pain or discomfort
   7. nausea or abdominal distress
   8. feeling dizzy, unsteady, lightheaded, or faint
   9. derealization (feelings of unreality) or depersonalization (being detached from oneself)
   10. fear of losing control or going crazy
   11. fear of dying
   12. paresthesias (numbness or tingling sensations)
   13. chills or hot flushes

From American Psychiatric Association. *Diagnostic and Statistical Manual of Mental Disorders*, 4th ed. Text rev. Washington, DC: American Psychiatric Association; 2000, with permission.

Table 15–3
DSM-IV-TR Diagnostic Criteria for Panic Disorder without Agoraphobia

A. Both 1 and 2:
1. recurrent unexpected panic attacks
2. at least one of the attacks has been followed by 1 month (or more) of one (or more) of the following:
   a. persistent concern about having additional attacks
   b. worry about the implications of the attack or its consequences (e.g., losing control, having a heart attack, "going crazy")
   c. a significant change in behavior related to the attacks
B. Absence of agoraphobia
C. The panic attacks are not due to the direct physiologic effects of a substance (e.g., a drug of abuse, a medication) or a general medical condition (e.g., hyperthyroidism).
D. The panic attacks are not better accounted for by another mental disorder, such as social phobia (e.g., occurring on exposure to feared social situations), specific phobia (e.g., on exposure to a specific phobic situation), obsessive-compulsive disorder (e.g., on exposure to dirt in someone with an obsession about contamination), posttraumatic stress disorder (e.g., in response to stimuli associated with a severe stressor), or separation anxiety disorder (e.g., in response to being away from home or close relatives).

From American Psychiatric Association. _Diagnostic and Statistical Manual of Mental Disorders_, 4th ed. Text rev. Washington, DC: American Psychiatric Association; 2000, with permission.

Table 15–4
DSM-IV-TR Diagnostic Criteria for Generalized Anxiety Disorder

A. Excessive anxiety and worry (apprehensive expectation), occurring more days than not for at least 6 months, about a number of events or activities (such as work or school performance).
B. The person finds it difficult to control the worry.
C. The anxiety and worry are associated with three (or more) of the following six symptoms (with at least some symptoms present for more days than not for the past 6 months). **Note:** Only one item is required in children.
1. restlessness or feeling keyed up or on edge
2. being easily fatigued
3. difficulty concentrating or mind going blank
4. irritability
5. muscle tension
6. sleep disturbance (difficulty falling or staying asleep, or restless, unsatisfying sleep)
D. The focus of the anxiety and worry is not confined to features of an Axis I disorder, for example, the anxiety or worry is not about having a panic attack (as in panic disorder), being embarrassed in public (as in social phobia), being contaminated (as in obsessive-compulsive disorder), being away from home or close relatives (as in separation anxiety disorder), gaining weight (as in anorexia nervosa), having multiple physical complaints (as in somatization disorder), or having a serious illness (as in hypochondriasis), and the anxiety and worry do not occur exclusively during posttraumatic stress disorder.
E. The anxiety, worry, or physical symptoms cause clinically significant distress or impairment in social, occupational, or other important areas of functioning.
F. The disturbance is not due to the direct physiologic effects of a substance (e.g., a drug of abuse, a medication) or a general medical condition (e.g., hyperthyroidism) and does not occur exclusively during a mood disorder, a psychotic disorder, or a pervasive development disorder.

From American Psychiatric Association. _Diagnostic and Statistical Manual of Mental Disorders_, 4th ed. Text rev. Washington, DC: American Psychiatric Association; 2000, with permission.

Table 15–5
DSM-IV-TR Diagnostic Criteria for Specific Phobia

A. Marked and persistent fear that is excessive or unreasonable, cued by the presence or anticipation of a specific object or situation (e.g., flying, heights, animals, receiving an injection, seeing blood).
B. Exposure to the phobic stimulus almost invariably provokes an immediate anxiety response, which may take the form of a situationally bound or situationally predisposed panic attack. **Note:** in children, the anxiety may be expressed by crying, tantrums, freezing, or clinging.
C. The person recognizes that the fear is excessive or unreasonable. **Note:** In children, this feature may be absent.
D. The phobic situation(s) is avoided or else is endured with intense anxiety or distress.
E. The avoidance, anxious anticipation, or distress in the feared situation(s) interferes significantly with the person's normal routine, occupational (or academic) functioning, or social activities or relationships, or there is marked distress about having the phobia.
F. In individuals under age 18 years, the duration is at least 6 months.
G. The anxiety, panic attacks, or phobic avoidance associated with the specific object or situation is not better accounted for by another mental disorder, such as obsessive-compulsive disorder (e.g., fear of dirt in someone with an obsession about contamination), posttraumatic stress disorder (e.g., avoidance of stimuli associated with a severe stressor), separation anxiety disorder (e.g., avoidance of school), social phobia (e.g., avoidance of social situations because of fear of embarrassment), panic disorder with agoraphobia, or agoraphobia without history of panic disorder.
Specify type:
    Animal type
    Natural environment type (e.g., heights, storms, water)
    Blood-injection-injury type
    Situational type (e.g., airplanes, elevators, enclosed places)
    Other type (e.g., phobic avoidance of situations that may lead to choking, vomiting, or contracting an illness; in children, avoidance of loud sounds or costumed characters)

From American Psychiatric Association. *Diagnostic and Statistical Manual of Mental Disorders*, 4th ed. Text rev. Washington, DC: American Psychiatric Association; 2000, with permission.

Table 15–6
DSM-IV-TR Diagnostic Criteria for Social Phobia

A. A marked and persistent fear of one or more social or performance situations in which the person is exposed to unfamiliar people or to possible scrutiny by others. The individual fears that he or she will act in a way (or show anxiety symptoms) that will be humiliating or embarrassing. **Note:** In children, there must be evidence of the capacity for age-appropriate social relationships with familiar people and the anxiety must occur in peer settings, not just in interactions with adults.
B. Exposure to the feared social situation almost invariably provokes anxiety, which may take the form of a situationally bound or situationally predisposed panic attack. **Note:** In children, the anxiety may be expressed by crying, tantrums, freezing, or shrinking from social situations with unfamiliar people.
C. The person recognizes that the fear is excessive or unreasonable. **Note:** In children, this feature may be absent.
D. The feared social or performance situations are avoided or else are endured with intense anxiety or distress.
E. The avoidance, anxious anticipation, or distress in the feared social or performance situation(s) interferes significantly with the person's normal routine, occupational (academic) functioning, or social activities or relationships, or there is marked distress about having the phobia.
F. In individuals under age 18 years, the duration is at least 6 months.
G. The fear or avoidance is not due to the direct physiologic effects of a substance (e.g., a drug of abuse, a medication) or a general medical condition and is not better accounted for by another mental disorder (e.g., panic disorder with or without agoraphobia, separation anxiety disorder, body dysmorphic disorder, a pervasive developmental disorder, or schizoid personality disorder).
H. If a general medical condition or another mental disorder is present, the fear in Criterion A is unrelated to it (e.g., the fear is not of stuttering, trembling in Parkinson's disease, or exhibiting abnormal eating behavior in anorexia nervosa or bulimia nervosa).
Specify if:
    Generalized: if the fears include most social situations (also consider the additional diagnosis of avoidant personality disorder).

From American Psychiatric Association. *Diagnostic and Statistical Manual of Mental Disorders*, 4th ed. Text rev. Washington, DC: American Psychiatric Association; 2000, with permission.

Table 15–7
DSM-IV-TR Diagnostic Criteria for Obsessive–Compulsive Disorder

A. Other obsessions or compulsions:
   Obsessions as defined by 1, 2, 3, and 4:
   1. recurrent and persistent thoughts, impulses, or images that are experienced, at some time during the disturbance, as intrusive and inappropriate and that cause marked anxiety or distress
   2. the thoughts, impulses, or images are not simply excessive worries about real-life problems
   3. the person attempts to ignore or suppress such thoughts, impulses, or images, or to neutralize them with some other thought or action
   4. the person recognizes that the obsessional thoughts, impulses, or images are a product of his or her own mind (not imposed from without, as in thought insertion)
   Compulsions as defined by 1 and 2:
   1. repetitive behaviors (e.g., hand washing, ordering, checking) or mental acts (e.g., praying, counting, repeating words silently) that the person feels driven to perform in response to an obsession, or according to rules that must be applied rigidly
   2. the behaviors or mental acts are aimed at preventing or reducing distress or preventing some dreaded event or situation; however, these behaviors or mental acts either are not connected in a realistic way with what they are designed to neutralize or prevent or are clearly excessive
B. At some point during the course of the disorder, the person has recognized that the obsessions or compulsions are excessive or unreasonable. **Note:** This does not apply to children.
C. The obsessions or compulsions cause marked distress, are time consuming (take more than 1 hour a day), or significantly interfere with the person's normal routine, occupational (or academic) functioning, or usual social activities or relationships.
D. If another Axis I disorder is present, the content of the obsessions or compulsions is not restricted to it (e.g., preoccupation with food in the presence of an eating disorder, hair pulling in the presence of trichotillomania, concern with appearance in the presence of body dysmorphic disorder, preoccupation with drugs in the presence of a substance use disorder, preoccupation with having a serious illness in the presence of hypochondriasis, preoccupations with sexual urges or fantasies in the presence of a paraphilia, or guilty ruminations in the presence of major depressive disorder).
E. The disturbance is not caused by the direct physiologic effects of a substance (e.g., a drug of abuse, a medication) or a general medical condition.
Specify if:
   With poor insight: If, for most of the time during the current episode, the person does not recognize that the obsessions and compulsions are excessive or unreasonable

From American Psychiatric Association. *Diagnostic and Statistical Manual of Mental Disorders*, 4th ed. Text rev. Washington, DC: American Psychiatric Association; 2000, with permission.

F. Obsessive–compulsive disorder. Obsessive–compulsive disorder involves recurrent intrusive ideas, images, ruminations, impulses, thoughts (obsessions), or repetitive patterns of behavior or actions (compulsions). Both obsessions and compulsions are ego-alien and produce anxiety if resisted. Lifetime prevalence is 2% to 3%. Men and women are equally affected. Mean age of onset is 22 years. See Table 15–7.

G. Posttraumatic and acute stress disorders. In these disorders, anxiety is produced by an extraordinarily stressful event. The event is relived in dreams and waking thoughts (flashbacks). The symptoms of repeated experience, avoidance, and hyperarousal last more than 1 month. For patients in whom symptoms have been present less than 1 month, the appropriate diagnosis is acute stress disorder. It occurs twice as often in women, has a chronic course, and can be associated with substance abuse and depression. See Table 15–8.

Table 15–8
***DSM-IV-TR* Diagnostic Criteria for Posttraumatic Stress Disorder**

A. The person has been exposed to a traumatic event in which both of the following were present:
  1. the person experienced, witnessed, or was confronted with an event or events that involved actual or threatened death or serious injury, or a threat to the physical integrity of self or others
  2. the person's response involved intense fear, helplessness, or horror. **Note:** In children, this may be expressed instead by disorganized or agitated behavior.
B. The traumatic event is persistently reexperienced in one (or more) of the following ways:
  1. recurrent and intrusive distressing recollections of the event, including images, thoughts, or perceptions. **Note:** In young children, repetitive play may occur in which themes or aspects of the trauma are expressed.
  2. recurrent distressing dreams of the event. **Note:** In children, there may be frightening dreams without recognizable content.
  3. acting or feeling as if the traumatic event were recurring (includes a sense of reliving the experience, illusions, hallucinations, and dissociative flashback episodes, including those that occur on awakening or when intoxicated). **Note:** In young children, trauma-specific reenactment may occur.
  4. Intense psychological distress at exposure to internal or external cues that symbolize or resemble an aspect of the traumatic event
  5. physiologic reactivity on exposure to internal or external cues that symbolize or resemble an aspect of the traumatic event
C. Persistent avoidance of stimuli associated with the trauma and numbing of general responsiveness (not present before the trauma), as indicated by three (or more) of the following:
  1. efforts to avoid thoughts, feelings, or conversations associated with the trauma
  2. efforts to avoid activities, places, or people that arouse recollections of the trauma
  3. inability to recall an important aspect of the trauma
  4. markedly diminished interest or participation in significant activities
  5. feeling of detachment or estrangement from others
  6. restricted range of affect (e.g., unable to have loving feelings)
  7. sense of a foreshortened future (e.g., does not expect to have a career, marriage, children, or a normal life span)
D. Persistent symptoms of increased arousal (not present before the trauma), as indicated by two (or more) of the following:
  1. difficulty falling or staying asleep
  2. irritability or outbursts of anger
  3. difficulty concentrating
  4. hypervigilance
  5. exaggerated startle response
E. Duration of the disturbance (symptoms in Criteria B, C, and D) is more than 1 month.
F. The disturbance causes clinically significant distress or impairment in social, occupational, or other important areas of functioning.
Specify if:
  Acute: if symptoms last less than 3 months
  Chronic: if symptoms last 3 months or more
Specify if:
  With delayed onset: if symptoms begin at least 6 months after the stressor

From American Psychiatric Association. *Diagnostic and Statistical Manual of Mental Disorders*, 4th ed. Text rev. Washington, DC: American Psychiatric Association; 2000, with permission.

H. **Anxiety disorder due to a general medical condition.** A wide range of medical and neurological conditions can cause anxiety symptoms. See Table 15–9.

I. **Substance-induced anxiety disorder.** A wide range of substances can cause anxiety symptoms that are often associated with intoxication or withdrawal states. See Table 15–10.

J. **Mixed anxiety–depressive disorder.** This disorder describes patients with both anxiety and depressive symptoms that do not meet the diagnostic

Table 15–9
Medical and Neurological Causes of Anxiety

Neurological disorders	Deficiency states
Cerebral neoplasms	Vitamin B_{12} deficiency
Cerebral trauma and postconcussive syndromes	Pellagra
Cerebrovascular disease	**Miscellaneous conditions**
Subarachnoid hemorrhage	Hypoglycemia
Migraine	Carcinoid syndrome
Encephalitis	Systemic malignancies
Cerebral syphilis	Premenstrual syndrome
Multiple sclerosis	Febrile illnesses and chronic infections
Wilson's disease	Porphyria
Huntington's disease	Infectious mononucleosis
Epilepsy	Posthepatitis syndrome
Systemic conditions	Uremia
Hypoxia	**Toxic conditions**
Cardiovascular disease	Alcohol and drug withdrawal
Pulmonary insufficiency	Vasopressor agents
Anemia	Penicillin
Endocrine disturbances	Sulfonamides
Pituitary dysfunction	Mercury
Thyroid dysfunction	Arsenic
Parathyroid dysfunction	Phosphorus
Adrenal dysfunction	Organophosphates
Pheochromocytoma	Carbon disulfide
Female virilization disorders	Benzene
Inflammatory disorders	Aspirin intolerance
Lupus erythematosus	
Rheumatoid arthritis	
Polyarteritis nodosa	
Temporal arteritis	

Adapted from Cummings JL. *Clinical Neuropsychiatry.* Orlando, FL: Grune & Stratton, 1985:214, with permission.

criteria for either an anxiety disorder or a mood disorder. The diagnosis is sometimes used in primary care settings and is used in Europe; sometimes called *neurasthenia*.

K. Anxiety disorder not otherwise specified

    1. Adjustment disorder with anxiety. This applies to the patient with an obvious stressor in whom excessive anxiety develops within 3 months

Table 15–10
Some Substances That May Cause Anxiety

Intoxication	Withdrawal
Amphetamines and other sympathomimetics	Alcohol
Amyl nitrite	Antihypertensives
Anticholinergics	Caffeine
Caffeine	Opioids
Cannabis	
Sedative–hypnotics	
Cocaine	
Hallucinogens	
Theophylline	
Yohimbine	

and is expected to last no longer than 6 months. It may occur as a reaction to illness, rejection, or loss of a job, especially if it is experienced as a defeat or failure.

2. **Anxiety secondary to another psychiatric disorder.** Seventy percent of depressed patients have anxiety. Patients with psychoses—schizophrenia, mania, or brief psychotic disorder—often exhibit anxiety (psychotic anxiety). Anxiety is common in delirium and in dementia (catastrophic reaction).

3. **Situational anxiety.** Effects of a stressful situation temporarily overwhelm the ability to cope. This may occur in minor situations if it brings to mind past overwhelming stress.

4. **Existential anxiety.** This involves fears of helplessness, aging, loss of control, and loss of others in addition to the fear of death and dying.

5. **Separation anxiety and stranger anxiety.** Regressed adults, including some who are medically ill, may manifest anxiety when separated from loved ones or when having to react to staff in a hospital. Separation anxiety disorder occurs in some young children when going to school for the first time. It is a normal reaction in infants and children until about 2.5 years of age.

6. **Anxiety related to loss of self-control.** In circumstances in which control must be surrendered, such as medical illness or hospitalization, patients with a need to feel in control may be very threatened. Loss of autonomy at work can precipitate anxiety.

7. **Anxiety related to dependence or intimacy.** If past dependency needs were not met or resolved, a patient can be anxious being in a close relationship, which involves some dependence, or being a patient in a hospital, which involves giving up control.

8. **Anxiety related to guilt and punishment.** If a patient expects punishment for imagined or real misdeeds, he or she may feel anxiety and the punishment may be actively sought or even self-inflicted.

III. Epidemiology

The anxiety disorders make up the most common group of psychiatric disorders. One in four persons has met the diagnostic criteria for at least one of the above listed anxiety disorders, and there is a 12-month prevalence rate of about 17%. Women are more likely to have an anxiety disorder than are men. The prevalence of anxiety disorders decreases with higher socioeconomic status. An epidemiological overview of anxiety disorders is given in Table 15–11.

IV. Etiology

A. Biological

1. Anxiety involves an excessive autonomic reaction with increased sympathetic tone.

2. The release of catecholamines is increased with increased production of norepinephrine metabolites (e.g., 3-methoxy-4-hydroxyphenylglycol).

Table 15-11
Epidemiology of Anxiety Disorders

	Panic Disorder	Phobia	Obsessive-Compulsive Disorder	Generalized Anxiety Disorder	Posttraumatic Stress Disorder
Lifetime prevalence	1.5%–4% of population	Most common anxiety disorder: 10% of population	2%–3% of population	3%–8% of population	1%–3% of population: 30% of Vietnam veterans
Male-to-female ratio	1:1 (without agoraphobia) 1:2 (with agoraphobia)	1:2	1:1	1:2	1:2
Age of onset	Late 20s	Late childhood	Adolescence or early adulthood	Variable: early adulthood	Any age, including childhood
Family history	20% of first-degree relatives of agoraphobic patients have agoraphobia	May run in families, especially blood injection, injury type	35% in first-degree relatives	25% of first-degree relatives affected	—
Twin studies	Higher concordance in monozygotic (MZ) twins than in dizygotic (DZ) twins	—	Higher concordance in MZ twins than in DZ twins	80%–90% concordance in MZ twins; 10%–15% in DZ twins	—

3. Decreased rapid eye movement (REM), latency, and stage IV sleep (similar to depression) may develop.
4. Decreased levels of γ-aminobutyric acid (GABA) cause central nervous system (CNS) hyperactivity (GABA inhibits CNS irritability and is widespread throughout the brain).
5. Alterations in serotonergic system and increased dopaminergic activity are associated with anxiety.
6. Activity in the temporal cerebral cortex is increased.
7. The locus ceruleus, a brain center of noradrenergic neurons, is hyperactive in anxiety states, especially panic attacks.
8. Recent studies also suggest a role for neuropeptides (substance P, CRF, and cholecystokinin).
9. Hyperactivity and dysregulation in the amygdala may be associated with social anxiety.

B. Psychoanalytic. According to Freud, unconscious impulses (e.g., sex or aggression) threaten to burst into consciousness and produce anxiety. Anxiety is related developmentally to childhood fears of disintegration that derive from the fear of an actual or imagined loss of a love object or the fear of bodily harm (e.g., castration). Freud used the term *signal anxiety* to describe anxiety not consciously experienced but that triggers defense mechanisms used by the person to deal with a potentially threatening situation. See Table 15–12 for an overview of the psychodynamics of anxiety disorders.

C. Learning theory

1. Anxiety is produced by continued or severe frustration or stress. The anxiety then becomes a conditioned response to other situations that are less severely frustrating or stressful.

Table 15–12
Psychodynamics of Anxiety Disorders

Disorder	Defense	Comment
Phobia	Displacement Symbolization	Anxiety detached from idea or situation and displaced on some other symbolic object or situation.
Agoraphobia	Projection Displacement	Repressed hostility, rage, or sexuality projected on environment, which is seen as dangerous.
Obsessive–compulsive disorder	Undoing Isolation Reaction formation	Severe superego acts against impulses about which patient feels guilty; anxiety controlled by repetitious act or thought.
Anxiety	Regression	Repression of forbidden sexual, aggressive, or dependency strivings breaks down.
Panic	Regression	Anxiety overwhelms personality and is discharged in panic state. Total breakdown of repressive defense and regression occurs.
Posttraumatic stress disorder	Regression Repression Denial Undoing	Trauma reactivates unconscious conflicts: ego relives anxiety and tries to master it.

2. It may be learned through identification and imitation of anxiety patterns in parents (social learning theory).
3. Anxiety is associated with a naturally frightening stimulus (e.g., accident). Subsequent displacement or transference to another stimulus through conditioning produces a phobia to a new and different object or situation.
4. Anxiety disorders involve faulty, distorted, or counterproductive patterns of cognitive thinking.

D. Genetic studies
1. Half of patients with panic disorder have one affected relative.
2. About 5% of persons with high levels of anxiety have a polymorphic variant of the gene associated with serotonin transporter metabolism.

V. Psychological Tests
A. Rorschach test
1. Anxiety responses include animal movements, unstructured forms, and heightened color.
2. Phobic responses include anatomic forms or bodily harm.
3. Obsessive–compulsive responses include overattention to detail.

B. Thematic apperception test
1. Increased fantasy productions may be present.
2. Themes of aggression and sexuality may be prominent.
3. Feelings of tension may be evident.

C. Bender-Gestalt
1. No changes indicative of brain damage are apparent.
2. Use of small area may be manifested in obsessive–compulsive disorder.
3. Productions may spread out on the page in anxiety states.

D. Draw-a-Person
1. Attention to head and general detailing may be noted in obsessive–compulsive disorder
2. Body image distortions may be present in phobias.
3. Rapid drawing may be evident in anxiety disorders.

E. Minnesota Multiphasic Personality Inventory-2. High hypochondriasis, psychasthenia, hysteria scales in anxiety.

VI. Laboratory Tests
A. No specific laboratory tests for anxiety.
B. Experimental infusion of lactate increases norepinephrine levels and produces anxiety in patients with panic disorder.

VII. Pathophysiology and Brain-Imaging Studies
A. No consistent pathognomonic changes.
B. In obsessive–compulsive disorder, positron emission tomography (PET) reveals decreased metabolism in the orbital gyrus, caudate nuclei, and cingulate gyrus.

C. In generalized anxiety disorder and panic states, PET reveals increased blood flow in the right parahippocampus in the frontal lobe.

D. Magnetic resonance imaging (MRI) has shown increased ventricular size in some cases, but findings are not consistent.

E. Right temporal atrophy is seen in some panic disorder patients, and cerebral vasoconstriction is often present in anxiety.

F. Mitral valve prolapse is present in 50% of patients with panic disorder, but clinical significance is unknown.

G. Nonspecific electroencephalogram (EEG) changes may be noted.

H. Dexamethasone suppression test does not suppress cortisol in some obsessive–compulsive patients.

I. Panic-inducing substances include carbon dioxide, sodium lactate, methyl-chlorophenylpiperazine (mCPP), carbolines, $GABA_B$ receptor antagonists, caffeine, isoproterenol, and yohimbine (Yocon).

VIII. Differential Diagnosis

A. **Depressive disorders.** Fifty percent to 70% of depressed patients exhibit anxiety or obsessive brooding; 20% to 30% of primarily anxious patients also experience depression.

B. **Schizophrenia.** Schizophrenic patients may be anxious and have severe obsessions in addition to or preceding the outbreak of hallucinations or delusions.

C. **Bipolar I disorder.** Massive anxiety may occur during a manic episode.

D. **Atypical psychosis (psychotic disorder not otherwise specified).** Massive anxiety is present, in addition to psychotic features.

E. **Adjustment disorder with anxiety.** Patient has a history of a psychosocial stressor within 3 months of onset.

F. **Medical and neurological conditions.** A secondary anxiety disorder is caused by a specific medical or biological factor. Undiagnosed hyperthyroidism is a frequent cause. Other causes are listed in Tables 15–9 and 15–13.

Table 15–13
Differential Diagnosis of Common Medical Conditions Mimicking Anxiety

Angina pectoris/myocardial infarction (MI)	Electrocardiogram with ST depression in angina; cardiac enzymes in MI. Crushing chest pain usually associated with angina/MI. Anxiety pains usually sharp and more superficial.
Hyperventilation syndrome	History of rapid, deep respirations; circumoral pallor; carpopedal spasm; responds to rebreathing in paper bag.
Hypoglycemia	Fasting blood sugar usually under 50 mg/dL; signs of diabetes mellitus—polyuria, polydipsia, polyphagia.
Hyperthyroidism	Elevated triiodothyronine (T_1), thyroxine (T_4); exophthalmos in severe cases.
Carcinoid syndrome	Hypertension accompanies anxiety; elevated urinary catecholamines (5-hydroxyindoleacetic acid [5-HIAA]).

G. **Substance-related disorders.** Panic or anxiety is often associated with intoxication (especially caffeine, cocaine, amphetamines, hallucinogens) and withdrawal states (Table 15–10).

H. **Cognitive disorder.** Severe anxiety may interfere with cognition and impairments may occur; however, they remit when the anxiety is diminished, unlike the cognitive defects in dementia.

IX. **Course And Prognosis**
A. **Panic disorder**
1. The course is chronic, with remissions and exacerbations.
2. Panic attacks tend to recur two to three times a week.
3. Patients with panic disorder may be at increased risk for committing suicide.
4. The prognosis is good with combined pharmacotherapy and psychotherapy.
B. **Phobic disorder**
1. The course tends to be chronic.
2. Phobias may worsen or spread if untreated.
3. Agoraphobia is the most resistant of all phobias.
4. Prognosis is good to excellent with therapy.
C. **Obsessive–compulsive disorder**
1. Course is chronic, with waxing and waning of symptoms.
2. Pharmacotherapy is more effective than psychotherapy, but most effective when combined with cognitive-behavioral therapy (CBT).
3. Prognosis with therapy is fair, but some cases are intractable.
D. **Generalized anxiety disorder**
1. Course is chronic; symptoms may diminish as the patient gets older.
2. With time, secondary depression may develop. This is not uncommon if the condition is left untreated.
3. With treatment, prognosis is good; over 70% of patients improve with pharmacological therapy; best when combined with psychotherapy.
E. **Posttraumatic stress disorder**
1. Course is chronic.
2. The trauma is reexperienced periodically for several years.
3. The prognosis is worse with pre-existing psychopathology.

X. **Treatment**
The treatment of anxiety disorders involves both a psychopharmacological approach as well as psychotherapy (CBT, psychodynamic, time limited, group and family therapies).
A. **Pharmacological**
1. **Benzodiazepines.** These drugs are generally effective in reducing anxiety. In panic disorder, they reduce both the number and intensity of attacks. They are also useful in social and specific phobia. Because of concern about physical dependence, physicians do not prescribe

benzodiazepines as often as they should. With proper psychotherapeutic monitoring, however, they can be used safely for long periods of time without being abused. Discontinuation (withdrawal) syndromes may occur in patients who use these drugs for long periods, but if the medication is properly withdrawn, signs and symptoms of withdrawal are easily managed. Commonly used drugs in this class include alprazolam (Xanax), clonazepam (Klonopin), diazepam (Valium), and lorazepam (Ativan). Alprazolam is effective in panic disorder and anxiety associated with depression. Alprazolam has been associated with a discontinuation syndrome after as little as 6 to 8 weeks of treatment.

2. **Selective serotonin reuptake inhibitors (SSRIs).** There are five SSRIs available in the United States that are effective in anxiety disorder: citalopram (Celexa), escitalopram (Lexapro), paroxetine (Paxil), sertraline (Zoloft), and venlafaxine (Effexor). Paroxetine is especially useful for the treatment of panic disorder. SSRIs are safer than the tricyclic drugs because they lack anticholinergic effects and are not as lethal if taken in overdose. The most common side effects are transient nausea, headache, and sexual dysfunction. Some patients, especially those with panic disorder, report an initial increase in anxiety after starting these drugs, which can be controlled with benzodiazepines until the full SSRI effect is felt, usually within 2 to 4 weeks. SSRIs are used with extreme caution in children and adolescents because of reports of agitation and impulsive suicidal acts as side effects of the medication in that population.

3. **Tricyclics.** Drugs in this class reduce the intensity of anxiety in all the anxiety disorders, especially in obsessive–compulsive states. Because of their side effect profile (e.g., anticholinergic effects, cardiotoxicity, and potential lethality in overdose [10 times the daily recommended dose can be fatal]), they are not first-line agents. Typical drugs in this class include imipramine (Tofranil), nortriptyline (Aventyl, Pamelor), and clomipramine (Anafranil).

4. **Monoamine oxidase inhibitors (MAOIs).** MAOIs are effective for the treatment of panic and other anxiety disorders; however, they are not first-line agents because of a major adverse side effect, which is the occurrence of a hypertensive crisis secondary to ingestion of foods containing tyramine. Certain medications such as sympathomimetics and opioids (especially meperidine [Demerol]) must be avoided because if combined with MAOIs, death may ensue. Common drugs in this class include phenelzine (Nardil) and tranylcypromine (Parnate).

5. **Other drugs used in anxiety disorders**

   a. *β*-**Adrenergic receptor antagonists (beta-blockers):** Drugs in this class include propranolol (Inderal) and atenolol (Tenormin), which act to suppress the somatic signs of anxiety, particularly panic attacks. They have been reported to be particularly effective in blocking the anxiety of social phobia (e.g., public speaking) when taken as a single dose about 1 hour before the phobic event. Adverse effects include bradycardia, hypotension, and drowsiness. They are not useful in chronic anxiety, unless it is caused by a hypersensitive adrenergic state.

 CLINICAL HINT:
Do not use beta-blockers if the patient has a history of asthma, congestive heart failure, or diabetes.

  b. **Venlafaxine (Effexor):** This drug has been found to be effective in the treatment of both generalized anxiety disorder and panic disorder. Because it also acts as an antidepressant, it is of use in mixed states. Its major indication is for the treatment of depression.
  c. **Buspirone (BuSpar):** This drug has mild serotonergic effects and is most effective in generalized anxiety disorder rather than in acute states. It is not cross-tolerant with benzodiazepines and cannot be used to treat discontinuation syndromes. It has a slow level of onset and may produce dizziness and headache in some patients.
  d. **Anticonvulsant anxiolytics:** Typical drugs in this class used in the treatment of anxiety disorders include gabapentin (Neurontin), tiagabine (Gabitril), and valproate (Depakene, Depakote). Reports of their efficacy are few and anecdotal; however, they deserve consideration in the treatment of these disorders, especially if panic attacks are present.

Table 15–14 summarizes dosages for drugs used in anxiety disorders.
B. **Psychological**
  1. **Supportive psychotherapy.** This approach involves the use of psychodynamic concepts and a therapeutic alliance to promote adaptive coping. Adaptive defenses are encouraged and strengthened, and maladaptive ones are discouraged. The therapist assists in reality testing and may offer advice regarding behavior.
  2. **Insight-oriented psychotherapy.** The goal is to increase the patient's development of insight into psychological conflicts that, if unresolved, can manifest as symptomatic behavior (e.g., anxiety, phobias, obsessions and compulsions, and posttraumatic stress reactions). This modality is particularly indicated if (1) anxiety symptoms are clearly secondary to an underlying unconscious conflict, (2) anxiety continues after behavioral or pharmacological treatments are instituted, (3) new anxiety symptoms develop after the original symptoms have resolved (symptom substitution), or (4) the anxieties are more generalized and less specific.
  3. **Behavior therapy** The basic assumption is that change can occur without the development of psychological insight into underlying causes. Techniques include positive and negative reinforcement, systematic

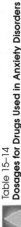

Table 15-14
Dosages for Drugs Used in Anxiety Disorders

	Starting (mg)	Maintenance (mg)	High dosage (mg)	Side Effects
SSRIs				
Paroxetine	5–10	20–60	>60	Nausea, vomiting, dry mouth, headache, somnolence, insomnia, sweating, tremor, diarrhea, sexual dysfunction, syndrome of inappropriate antidiuretic hormone, cytochrome P-450 2D6 substrate elevation due to enzyme inhibition (paroxetine especially; citalopram and escitalopram are not significant inhibitors), discontinuation effects (fatigue, dysphoria, psychomotor changes)
Fluoxetine	2–5	20–60	>80	
Sertraline	12.5–25	50–200	>300	
Citalopram	10	20–40	>60	
Escitalopram	5	10–30	>30	
Tricyclic antidepressants				
Clomipramine	5–12.5	50–125	>200	Orthostasis, conduction defects, ventricular arrhythmias, reflex tachycardia, anticholinergic effects, weight ↑, potential lethality in overdose
Imipramine	10–25	150–500	>300	
Desipramine	10–25	150–200	>300	
Benzodiazepines				
Alprazolam	0.25–0.5 t.i.d.	0.5–2 t.i.d.	>8	Orthostasis, conduction defects, ventricular arrhythmias, reflex tachycardia, anticholinergic effects, weight ↑, potential lethality in overdose
Clonazepam	0.25–0.5 b.i.d.	0.5–2 b.i.d.	>4	
Diazepam	2–5 b.i.d.	5–30 b.i.d.	>80	
Lorazepam	0.25–0.5 b.i.d.	0.5–2 b.i.d.	>8	
MAOIs				
Phenelzine	15 b.i.d.	15–45 b.i.d.	>15	Orthostatic hypotension, insomnia, weight ↑, edema, sexual dysfunction, hypertensive crisis with tyramine-containing foods
Tranylcypromine	10 b.i.d.	10–30 b.i.d.	>70	
SNRIs				
Venlafaxine (Effexor)	6.25–25	50–150	>375	Nausea, somnolence, dizziness, dry mouth, nervousness, tremor, insomnia, constipation, sexual dysfunction, sweating, anorexia, blood pressure elevation, orthostasis, conduction defects, ventricular arrhythmias, discontinuation effects (fatigue, dysphoria, psychomotor changes); half usual dose used in moderate hepatic or renal impairment
Venlafaxine XR (Effexor XR)	37.5	37.5	>225	
Desvenlafaxine (Pristiq)	50–150	100	>375	
Other agents				
Valproic acid	125 b.i.d.	500–750 b.i.d.	>2,000	Nausea, vomiting, indigestion
Gabapentin	100–200	600–3,400	>3,400	Somnolence, ataxia, nausea
BuSpar	5–10	10	>60	Dizziness, fatigue, nausea

desensitization, flooding, implosion, graded exposure, response prevention, stop thought, relaxation techniques, panic control therapy, self-monitoring, and hypnosis.

 CLINICAL HINT:
Some patients may carry a single anxiolytic pill such as 5 mg of diazepam to use if they think they are going to have an anxiety attack. Knowing they have the pill to use in that situation often aborts the attack because they have become conditioned to associate the pill with anxiety reduction.

---

    a. Behavior therapy is indicated for clearly delineated, circumscribed, maladaptive behaviors (e.g., panic attacks, phobias, compulsions, obsessions). Compulsive behavior generally is more responsive than obsessional thinking.

    b. Most current strategies for the treatment of anxiety disorders include a combination of pharmacological and behavioral interventions.

    c. Although drugs can reduce anxiety early, treatment with drugs alone leads to equally early relapse. The response of patients who are also treated with cognitive and behavioral therapies appears to be significantly and consistently better than the response of those who receive drugs alone.

4. Cognitive therapy. This is based on the premise that maladaptive behavior is secondary to distortions in how people perceive themselves and in how others perceive them. Treatment is short-term and interactive, with assigned homework and tasks to be performed between sessions that focus on correcting distorted assumptions and cognitions. The emphasis is on confronting and examining situations that elicit interpersonal anxiety and associated mild depression.

5. Group therapy. Groups range from those that provide only support and an increase in social skills to those that focus on relief of specific symptoms to those that are primarily insight oriented. Groups may be heterogeneous or homogeneous in terms of diagnosis. Homogeneous groups are commonly used in the treatment of such diagnoses as post-traumatic stress disorder, in which therapy is aimed at education about dealing with stress.

For more detailed discussion of this topic, see Anxiety Disorders, Ch 14, p. 1839, in CTP/IX.

16

Somatoform Disorders, Factitious Disorders, and Malingering

I. Introduction

These disorders involve the appearance of symptoms of disease or belief one has a disease or deformity, despite the absence of one. They are often a challenge to detect and treat. They capture a range of both manipulative and unconscious production of symptoms to fulfill various psychological needs, as well as intrusive, focused, worry with respect to the appearance, health, or physical condition of one's body.

II. Somatoform Disorders

The term somatoform disorder is derived from the Greek *soma* for body, and these disorders are distinguished by physical signs and symptoms that suggest a medical condition; however, on examination, they cannot be fully explained by any known medical illness. The symptoms are severe enough to cause the patient significant distress or functional impairment. These tend to be chronic and respond to a consistent psychotherapeutic treatment alliance and support.

Five specific somatoform disorders are recognized in *Diagnostic and Statistical Manual of Mental Disorders,* fourth edition, text revision *(DSM-IV-TR)*: somatization disorder, conversion disorder, hypochondriasis, body dysmorphic disorder, and pain disorder. Two residual diagnostic categories in *DSM-IV-TR* are undifferentiated somatoform disorder and somatoform disorder not otherwise specified. Table 16–1 summarizes the clinical features of the different somatoform disorders, which are discussed separately below.

A. Somatization disorder. Somatization disorder is characterized by ongoing reporting and experience of a range of physical symptoms that are not medically well explained and yet cause significant impairment and/or result in multiple attempts at medical intervention.

   1. Epidemiology
   a. Lifetime prevalence in the general population is 0.1% to 0.5%.
   b. Women outnumber men by a 5:1 ratio.
   c. Lifetime prevalence is 1% to 2% of all women.
   d. More common in less well-educated persons and persons of low socioeconomic status.
   e. Usual onset is in adolescence and young adulthood.

   2. Etiology
   a. Psychological—suppression or repression of anger toward others, with the turning of anger toward self, can account for symptoms. Low self-esteem is common. Identification with parent who models sick role. Some dynamic similarity to depression.

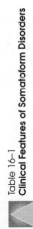

Table 16–1
Clinical Features of Somatoform Disorders

Diagnosis	Clinical Diagnostic Presentation	Demographic and Epidemiological Management Features	Features	Associated Strategy	Differential Prognosis	Contributing Disturbances	Primary for Symptom Presentation	Psychological Processes to Symptoms	Motivation Production
Somatization disorder	Polysymptomatic Recurrent and chronic Sickly by history	Young age Female predominance 20:1 Familial pattern 5%–10% incidence in primary care populations	Review of systems profusely Positive Multiple clinical contacts Polysurgical	Therapeutic alliance Regular appointments Crisis intervention	Poor to fair	Histrionic personality disorder Antisocial personality disorder Alcohol and other substance abuse Many life problems Conversion disorder	Physical disease Depression	Unconscious Cultural and developmental	Unconscious psychological factors
Conversion disorder	Monosymptomatic Mostly acute Simulates disease	Highly prevalent Female predominance Young age Rural and low social class Little-educated and psychologically unsophisticated	Simulation incompatible with known physiological mechanisms or anatomy	Suggestion and persuasion Multiple techniques	Excellent except in chronic conversion disorder	Alcohol and other substance dependence Antisocial personality disorder Somatization disorder Histrionic personality disorder	Depression Schizophrenia Neurological disease	Unconscious Psychological stress or conflict may be present	Unconscious psychological factors
Hypochondriasis	Disease concern or preoccupation	Previous physical disease Middle or old age Male to female ratio equal	Disease conviction amplifies symptoms Obsessional	Document symptoms Psychosocial review Psychotherapeutic	Fair to good Waxes and wanes	Obsessive-compulsive personality disorder Depressive and anxiety disorders	Depression Physical disease Personality disorder Delusional disorder	Unconscious Stress—bereavement Developmental factors	Unconscious psychological factors

(continued)

Table 16-1—*continued*
Clinical Features of Somatoform Disorders

Diagnosis	Clinical Diagnostic Presentation	Demographic and Epidemiological Management Features	Features	Associated Strategy	Differential Prognosis	Contributing Disturbances	Primary for Symptom Presentation	Psychological Processes to Symptoms	Motivation Production
Body dysmorphic disorder	Subjective feelings of ugliness or concern with body defect	Adolescence or young adult Female predominance Largely unknown	Pervasive bodily concerns	Therapeutic alliance Stress management Psychotherapies Antidepressant medications	Unknown	Anorexia nervosa Psychosocial distress Avoidant or obsessive–compulsive personality disorder	Delusional disorder Depressive disorders Somatization disorder	Unconscious Self-esteem factors	Unconscious psychological factors
Pain disorder	Pain syndrome simulated	Female predominance 2:1 Older: 4th or 5th decade Familial Up to 40% of pain populations	Simulation or intensity incompatible with known physiological mechanisms or anatomy	Therapeutic alliance Redefine goals of treatment Antidepressant medications	Guarded, variable	Depressive disorders Alcohol and other substance abuse Dependent or histrionic personality disorder	Depression Psychophysiological Physical disease Malingering and disability syndrome	Unconscious Acute stressor developmental Physical trauma may predispose	Unconscious psychological factors

Adapted from Folks DG, Ford CV, Houck CA. Somatoform disorders, factitious disorders, and malingering: In: Stoudemire A, ed. *Clinical Psychiatry for Medical Students*. Philadelphia: Lippincott, 1990;233.

   b. Genetic—positive family history; present in 10% to 20% of mothers and sisters of affected patients; twins—concordance rate of 29% in monozygotic and 10% in dizygotic twins.

  3. Laboratory and psychological tests. Minor neuropsychological abnormality in some patients (e.g., faulty assessment of somatosensory input).

  4. Pathophysiology. Prolonged use of medications such as painkillers or other treatments given in response to patients seeking medical attention may increase the risk of adverse effects of those medications. Some data indicate that abnormal regulation of cytokines—messengers affecting immune system—may be involved in nonspecific symptoms reported with the disease such as fatigue, anorexia, and other features.

  5. Diagnosis, signs, and symptoms

    a. Many somatic complaints with complicated medical histories.

    b. The most common complaints are pain, gastrointestinal symptoms, sexual complaints, and neurological signs (e.g., dizziness, amnesia).

    c. Suicidal ideation often present, but suicide is rare.

    d. Depression or anxiety related to complaints may be present; interpersonal problems are frequent. See Table 16–2.

Table 16–2
DSM-IV-TR **Diagnostic Criteria for Somatization Disorder**

A. A history of many physical complaints beginning before age 30 years that occur over a period of several years and result in treatment being sought or significant impairment in social, occupational, or other important areas of functioning.

B. Each of the following criteria must have been met, with individual symptoms occurring at any time during the course of the disturbance:

  1. *four pain symptoms:* a history of pain related to at least four different sites or functions (e.g., head, abdomen, back, joints, extremities, chest, rectum, during menstruation, during sexual intercourse, or during urination)

  2. *two gastrointestinal symptoms:* a history of at least two gastrointestinal symptoms other than pain (e.g., nausea, bloating, vomiting other than during pregnancy, diarrhea, or intolerance of several different foods)

  3. *one sexual symptom:* a history of at least one sexual or reproductive symptom other than pain (e.g., sexual indifference, erectile or ejaculatory dysfunction, irregular menses, excessive menstrual bleeding, vomiting throughout pregnancy)

  4. *one pseudoneurologic symptom:* a history of at least one symptom or deficit suggesting a neurologic condition not limited to pain (conversion symptoms such as impaired coordination or balance, paralysis or localized weakness, difficulty swallowing or lump in throat, aphonia, urinary retention, hallucinations, loss of touch or pain sensation, double vision, blindness, deafness, seizures; dissociative symptoms such as amnesia; or loss of consciousness other than fainting)

C. Either (1) or (2):

  1. after appropriate investigation, each of the symptoms in Criterion B cannot be fully explained by a known general medical condition or the direct effects of a substance (e.g., a drug of abuse, a medication)

  2. when there is a related general medical condition, the physical complaints or resulting social or occupational impairment are in excess of what would be expected from the history, physical examination, or laboratory findings

D. The symptoms are not intentionally feigned or produced (as in factitious disorder or malingering).

From American Psychiatric Association. *Diagnostic and Statistical Manual of Mental Disorders,* 4th ed. Text rev. Washington, DC: American Psychiatric Association; 2000, with permission.

6. **Differential diagnosis.** Distinguishing features of actual medical conditions that might help exclude their consideration in these patients include:
   a. **Multiple sclerosis:** muscular weakness throughout body.
   b. **Chronic fatigue syndrome:** Epstein-Barr virus may be present.
   c. **Porphyria:** abdominal pain, red urine.
   d. **Schizophrenia:** thought disorder, hallucinations. Somatic delusions may be present.
   e. **Panic attacks:** intermittent, episodic. Symptoms of anxiety or panic.
   f. **Conversion disorder:** characterized by few symptoms with clearer symbolic meaning.
   g. **Factitious disorder:** conscious faking of symptoms to achieve role of patient; usually eager to be in hospital.
   h. **Pain disorder:** pain is usually the only complaint.
7. **Course and prognosis.** Chronic course with few remissions; however, severity of complaints can fluctuate. Complications include unnecessary surgery, repeated medical workups, substance dependence, and adverse effects of unnecessary prescribed drugs. Depression is frequent.
8. **Treatment**
   a. **Pharmacological:** avoid psychotropics, except during period of acute anxiety or depression, because patients tend to become psychologically dependent. Antidepressants are useful in secondary depression.
   b. **Psychological:** long-term insight or supportive psychotherapy is required to provide understanding of dynamics, support through distressing life events, or both; important to follow patient to prevent substance abuse, doctor shopping, unnecessary procedures, and diagnostic tests.
B. **Conversion disorder**
   1. **Definition.** Characterized by involuntary alteration or limitation of voluntary motor or sensory functioning that results from psychological conflict or need (previously known as hysteria).
   2. **Epidemiology**
      a. Incidence and prevalence: 10% of hospital inpatients and 5% to 15% of all psychiatric outpatients.
      b. Age: early adulthood, but can occur in middle or old age.
      c. Occurs in twice as many women as in men.
      d. Family history: more frequent in family members.
      e. More common in persons of low socioeconomic status and less well-educated persons.
   3. **Etiology**
      a. **Biological**
         (1) Symptoms depend on activation of inhibitory brain mechanisms.
         (2) Excessive cortical arousal triggers inhibitory central nervous system (CNS) mechanisms at synapses, brainstem, and reticular activating system that may account for sensory deficits.
         (3) Increased susceptibility in patients with frontal lobe trauma or other neurological deficits.

b. Psychological

(1) Expression of unconscious psychological conflict that is repressed.

(2) Premorbid personality disorder—avoidant, histrionic.

(3) Impulse (e.g., sex or aggression) is unacceptable to ego and is disguised through symptoms.

(4) Identification with family member who has same symptoms caused by real disease; learned in childhood.

c. Psychodynamics

(1) *La belle indifférence* is a lack of concern about illness or obvious impairment and is present in some patients.

(2) *Primary gain* refers to the reduction of anxiety by repression of an unacceptable impulse. Symbolization of impulse onto symptom thus occurs (e.g., paralysis of arm prevents expression of aggressive impulse).

(3) *Secondary gain* refers to benefits of illness (e.g., compensation from lawsuit [compensation neurosis], avoidance of work, dependence on family). Patient usually lacks insight about this dynamic.

(4) Other defense mechanisms as source of symptoms: reaction formation, denial, displacement.

4. Laboratory and psychological tests

a. Evoked potentials show disturbed somatosensory perception; diminished or absent on side of defect.

b. Mild cognitive impairment, attentional deficits, and visuoperceptual changes on Halstead-Reitan Battery.

c. Minnesota Multiphasic Personality Inventory-2 (MMPI-2) and Rorschach test show increased instinctual drives, sexual repression, and inhibited aggression.

d. Drug-assisted interview—intravenous amobarbital (Amytal) (100 to 500 mg) in slow infusion often causes conversion symptoms to abate. For example, patient with hysterical aphonia will begin to talk. Test can be used to aid in diagnosis but is not always reliable.

5. Pathophysiology. No changes; some brain imaging studies show hypometabolism in the dominant hemisphere and hypermetabolism in the nondominant hemisphere.

6. Diagnosis, signs, and symptoms. See Table 16–3.

a. Motor abnormalities—paralysis, ataxia, dysphagia, vomiting, aphonia.

b. Seizure symptoms—pseudoseizures, unconsciousness.

c. Sensory disturbances—blindness, deafness, anosmia, anesthesia, analgesia, diplopia, glove-and-stocking anesthesia (does not follow known sensory pathways).

d. Close temporal relationship between symptom and stress or intense emotion.

e. Left-sided symptoms more common than right-sided symptoms.

f. The person is not conscious of intentionally producing the symptoms.

Table 16–3
DSM-IV-TR **Diagnostic Criteria for Conversion Disorder**

A. One or more symptoms or deficits affecting voluntary motor or sensory function that suggest a neurological or other general medical condition.

B. Psychological factors are judged to be associated with the symptom or deficit because the initiation or exacerbation of the symptom or deficit is preceded by conflicts or other stressors.

C. The symptom or deficit is not intentionally produced or feigned (as in factitious disorder or malingering).

D. The symptom or deficit cannot, after appropriate investigation, be fully explained by a general medical condition, or by the direct effects of a substance, or as a culturally sanctioned behavior or experience.

E. The symptom or deficit causes clinically significant distress or impairment in social, occupational, or other important areas of functioning or warrants medical evaluation.

F. The symptom or deficit is not limited to pain or sexual dysfunction, does not occur exclusively during the course of somatization disorder, and is not better accounted for by another mental disorder.

Specify type of symptom or deficit:

With motor symptom or deficit
With sensory symptom or deficit
With seizures or convulsions
With mixed presentation

From American Psychiatric Association. *Diagnostic and Statistical Manual of Mental Disorders,* 4th ed. Text rev. Washington, DC: American Psychiatric Association; 2000, with permission.

7. **Differential diagnosis.** Major task is to distinguish from organically based disorder. Eventually, a medical disorder is diagnosed in 25% to 50% of patients; therefore, a thorough medical and neurological workup is always indicated.

   a. **Paralysis:** in conversion disorder, paralysis is inconsistent; it does not follow motor pathways. No pathological reflexes (e.g., Babinski's sign) are present. Spastic paralysis, clonus, and cogwheel rigidity are absent in conversion disorder.

   b. **Ataxia:** bizarre movements in conversion disorder. In organic lesions, the leg may be dragged and circumduction not possible. *Astasia–abasia* is an inconsistency patterned, unsteady gait that does not cause the patient with conversion disorder to fall or sustain injury.

   c. **Blindness:** no pupillary response is seen in true neurological blindness (except note that occipital lobe lesions can produce cortical blindness with intact pupillary response). Tracking movements are also absent in true blindness. Monocular diplopia, triplopia, and tunnel vision can be conversion complaints. Ophthalmologists use tests with distorting prisms and colored lenses to detect hysterical blindness.

   d. **Deafness:** loud noise will awaken sleeping patient with conversion disorder but not patient with organic deafness. Audiometric tests reveal varying responses in conversion.

   e. **Sensory:** on examination, reported sensory loss does not follow anatomic distribution of dermatomes, that is, hemisensory loss, which stops at midline, or glove-and-stocking anesthesia in conversion disorder.

    f. Hysterical: pain most often relates to head, face, back, and abdomen. No organic cause for pain in evidence.

    g. Pseudoseizures: incontinence, loss of motor control, and tongue biting are rare in pseudoseizures; an aura usually is present in organic epilepsy. Look for abnormal electroencephalogram (EEG); however, EEG results are abnormal in 10% of the normal adult population. Babinski's sign occurs in organic seizure and postictal state but not in conversion seizures.

    h. Schizophrenia: thought disorder is present.

    i. Mood disorder: depression or mania from examination or history.

    j. Malingering and factitious disorder with physical symptoms: difficult to distinguish from conversion, but malingerers are aware that they are faking symptoms and have insight into what they are doing; patients with factitious disorder also are aware that they are faking, but they do so because they want to be patients and be in a hospital.

8. **Course and prognosis.** Tends to be recurrent. Episodes are separated by asymptomatic periods. Major concern is not to miss an early neurological symptom that subsequently progresses into a full-blown syndrome (e.g., multiple sclerosis may begin with spontaneously remitting diplopia or hemiparesis). Table 16–4 lists factors associated with good and bad prognoses.

9. **Treatment**

    a. Pharmacological. Benzodiazepines for anxiety and muscular tension; antidepressants or serotonergic agents for obsessive rumination about symptoms.

    b. Psychological

      (1) Insight-oriented therapy is useful in helping the patient to understand the dynamic principles and conflicts behind symptoms. Patient learns to accept sexual or aggressive impulses and not to use conversion disorder as a defense.

      (2) Behavior therapy is used to induce relaxation.

      (3) Hypnosis and reeducation are useful in uncomplicated situations.

Table 16–4
Factors Associated with Good and Poor Prognoses in Conversion Disorder

Good prognosis
  Sudden onset
  Clearly identifiable stress at onset
  Short time between onset and treatment
  Above-average IQ
  Symptoms of paralysis, aphonia, blindness
Poor prognosis
  Comorbid mental disorders
  Ongoing litigation
  Symptoms of tremor, seizures

      (4) Do not accuse the patient of trying to get attention or of not wanting to get better.

      (5) Narcoanalysis sometimes removes symptoms.

C. Pain disorder

1. **Definition.** Pain disorder is a preoccupation with pain in the absence of physical disease to account for its intensity. It does not follow a neuroanatomic distribution. Stress and conflict may closely correlate with the initiation or exacerbation of the pain.

2. **Epidemiology.** Onset can be at any age, but especially in the 30s and 40s. More common in women than in men. Some evidence of first-degree biological relatives having a high incidence of pain, depression, and alcoholism.

3. **Etiology**

    a. Behavioral: pain behaviors are reinforced when rewarded (e.g., pain symptoms may become intense when followed by attentive behavior from others or avoidance of disliked activity).

    b. Interpersonal: pain is a way to manipulate and gain advantage in a relationship (e.g., to stabilize a fragile marriage).

    c. Biological: some patients may have pain disorder, rather than another mental disorder, because of sensory and limbic structural or chemical abnormalities that predispose them to pain.

    d. Psychodynamics: patients may be symbolically expressing an intrapsychic conflict through the body. Persons may unconsciously regard emotional pain as weak and displace it to the body. Pain can be a method to obtain love or can be used as a punishment. Defense mechanisms involved in the disorder include displacement, substitution, and repression.

4. **Diagnosis**

    a. Clinically significant amount of pain complaints that result in emotional distress and social or occupational impairment.

    b. Psychological factors play a major role in onset and severity of symptoms. See Table 16–5.

5. **Differential diagnosis**

    a. Physical pain due to a medical condition: difficult to distinguish because physical pain is also sensitive to emotional and situational factors. Pain that does not vary, wax, or wane or is not relieved by analgesics is more often psychogenic. Absence of a medical or surgical condition to account for pain is an important factor.

    b. Hypochondriasis: tend to have more symptoms than patients with pain disorder.

    c. Conversion disorder: usually have more motor and sensory disturbances than pain disorder.

6. **Course and prognosis**

    a. Variable course but tends to be chronic.

    b. Patients with comorbid depression have poor prognosis, as do patients with secondary gain (e.g., litigation).

Table 16–5
***DSM-IV-TR* Diagnostic Criteria for Pain Disorder**

A. Pain in one or more anatomic sites is the predominant focus of the clinical presentation and is of sufficient severity to warrant clinical attention.

B. The pain causes clinically significant distress or impairment in social, occupational, or other important areas of functioning.

C. Psychological factors are judged to have an important role in the onset, severity, exacerbation, or maintenance of the pain.

D. The symptom or deficit is not intentionally produced or feigned (as in factitious disorder or malingering).

E. The pain is not better accounted for by a mood, anxiety, or psychotic disorder and does not meet criteria for dyspareunia.

Code as follows:

Pain disorder associated with psychological factors: psychological factors are judged to have the major role in the onset, severity, exacerbation, or maintenance of the pain. (If a general medical condition is present, it does not have a major role in the onset, severity, exacerbation, or maintenance of the pain.) This type of pain disorder is not diagnosed if criteria are also met for somatization disorder.

Specify if:

Acute: duration of less than 6 months
Chronic: duration of 6 months or longer

Pain disorder associated with both psychological factors and a general medical condition: both psychological factors and a general medical condition are judged to have important roles in the onset, severity, exacerbation, or maintenance of the pain. The associated general medical condition or anatomic site of the pain is coded on Axis III.

Specify if:

Acute: duration of less than 6 months
Chronic: duration of 6 months or longer

From American Psychiatric Association. *Diagnostic and Statistical Manual of Mental Disorders*, 4th ed. Text rev. Washington, DC: American Psychiatric Association; 2000, with permission.

7. Treatment

a. Pharmacotherapy

(1) Antidepressants, particularly selective serotonin reuptake inhibitors (SSRIs), are useful.

(2) Augmentation with small doses of amphetamine may benefit some patients, but dosages must be monitored carefully.

(3) Avoid opioids for analgesia because of risk of abuse.

b. Psychotherapy

(1) Psychodynamic therapy is of use in motivated patients.

(2) Cognitive therapy has proved beneficial in altering negative life attitudes.

(3) Other approaches include hypnosis, biofeedback acupuncture, and massage.

 CLINICAL HINT:
Do not confront patients with comments such as "This is all in your head." For the patient, the pain is real. An entry point is to examine how the pain affects the patient's life, not whether the pain is imaginary.

D. Hypochondriasis

1. **Definition.** Morbid fear or belief that one has a serious disease even though none exists.

2. **Epidemiology**
   a. Prevalence: 10% of all medical patients.
   b. Men and women are affected equally.
   c. Occurs at all ages; peaks in 30s for men and 40s for women.
   d. Seen in monozygotic twins and first-degree relatives.
3. **Etiology**
   a. **Biological.** Some patients may have congenital hypersensitivity to bodily functions and sensations and low threshold for pain or physical discomfort.
   b. **Psychogenic.** Repression of anger toward others; displacement of anger toward the self with development of physical complaints; pain and suffering used as punishment for unacceptable guilty impulses. Specific disease feared may have important symbolic meaning.
4. **Laboratory and psychological tests**
   a. Results of repeated physical examinations to rule out medical illness are negative.

 CLINICAL HINT:

Hypochondriacs will usually be reassured when they are informed that a test result about a disease they feared is negative. If the patient is not reassured under any circumstances, the clinician should suspect a delusional disorder of the somatic type.

---

   b. MMPI-2 shows elevated hysterical scale.
   c. Many color responses on Rorschach test indicate emotional lability.
5. **Diagnosis, signs, and symptoms.** See Table 16–6.
   a. Any organ or functional system can be involved; gastrointestinal and cardiovascular systems most commonly affected.

 Table 16–6
DSM-IV-TR Diagnostic Criteria for Hypochondriasis

A. Preoccupation with fears of having, or the idea that one has, a serious disease based on the person's misinterpretation of bodily symptoms.
B. The preoccupation persists despite appropriate medical evaluation and reassurance.
C. The belief in Criterion A is not of delusional intensity (as in delusional disorder, somatic type) and is not restricted to a circumscribed concern about appearance (as in body dysmorphic disorder).
D. The preoccupation causes clinically significant distress or impairment in social, occupational, or other important areas of functioning.
E. The duration of the disturbance is at least 6 months.
F. The preoccupation is not better accounted for by generalized anxiety disorder, obsessive–compulsive disorder, panic disorder, a major depressive episode, separation anxiety, or another somatoform disorder.
Specify if:
   With poor insight: if, for most of the time during the current episode, the person does not recognize that the concern about having a serious illness is excessive or unreasonable

From American Psychiatric Association. *Diagnostic and Statistical Manual of Mental Disorders*, 4th ed. Text rev. Washington, DC: American Psychiatric Association; 2000, with permission.

b. Patient believes that disease or malfunction is present.

c. Negative physical examination or laboratory test results reassure patient, but only briefly; symptoms then return. (In somatic delusion, patient cannot be reassured.)

d. Disturbance lasts at least 6 months.

e. The belief is not of delusional intensity.

6. **Differential diagnosis.** Diagnosis is made by inclusion, *not* by exclusion. Physical disorders must be ruled out; however, 15% to 30% of patients with hypochondriacal disorder have physical problems, but they are often overinvested with meaning or consequence. Workup for medical disease may aggravate the condition by placing too much emphasis on the physical complaint.

   a. Depression: patient may have a somatic complaint, or somatic complaint can be part of a depressive syndrome. Look for signs of depression (e.g., apathy, anhedonia, feelings of worthlessness).

   b. Anxiety disorder: manifested by marked anxiety or obsessive–compulsive signs or symptoms; *la belle indifférence* is not present.

   c. Somatization disorder: multiple organ systems involved; vague complaints.

   d. Pain disorder: pain is major and usually sole complaint.

   e. Malingering and factitious disorders: history is associated with frequent hospitalizations, marked secondary gain; symptoms lack symbolic value and are under conscious control. *La belle indifférence* is not present.

   f. Sexual dysfunction: if sex is complaint, diagnose as sexual disorder.

7. **Course and prognosis.** Chronic course with remissions. Exacerbations are usually associated with identifiable life stress. Good prognosis is associated with minimal premorbid personality, poor prognosis with antecedent, or superimposed physical disorder.

8. **Treatment**

   a. Pharmacological. Pharmacological targeting of symptoms; antianxiety drugs and antidepressant drugs for anxiety and depression. Serotonergic drugs useful for depression and obsessive–compulsive disorder. Drug-assisted interview can induce catharsis and potential removal of symptoms; however, such relief usually is only temporary.

   b. Psychotherapy.

   (1) Insight-oriented dynamic psychotherapy uncovers symbolic meaning of symptom and is useful. Long-term relationship with physician or psychiatrist is valuable, with reassurance that no physical disease is present.

   (2) Hypnosis and behavior therapy are useful to induce relaxation. Prolonged inactivity can produce physical deterioration (e.g., muscle atrophy or contractures, osteoporosis), so attention to these issues is necessary.

CLINICAL HINT:
Regularly scheduled physical examinations are useful to reassure patients that they are not ill and that their complaints are being taken seriously. However, invasive diagnostic and therapeutic measures should be avoided.

E. Body dysmorphic disorder

1. **Definition.** Imagined belief (not of delusional proportions) that a defect in the appearance of all or a part of the body is present.

2. **Epidemiology.** Onset from adolescence through early adulthood. Men and women are affected equally.

3. **Etiology**

   a. **Biological:** responsiveness to serotonergic agents suggests involvement of serotonin or relation to another mental disorder.

   b. **Psychological:** unconscious conflict relating to a distorted body part may be present.

   c. **Psychodynamics:** defense mechanisms involved include repression (of unconscious conflict), distortion and symbolization (of body part), and projection (belief that other persons also see imagined deformity).

4. **Laboratory and psychological tests.** Draw-a-Person test shows exaggeration, diminution, or absence of affected body part.

5. **Pathophysiology.** No known pathological abnormalities. Minor body deficits may actually exist upon which imagined belief develops.

6. **Diagnosis, signs, and symptoms.** Patient complains of defect (e.g., wrinkles, hair loss, small breasts or penis, age spots, stature). Complaint is out of proportion to objective abnormality. If a slight physical anomaly is present, the person's concern is grossly excessive; however, the belief is not of delusional intensity. The person can acknowledge the possibility that he or she may be exaggerating the extent of the defect or that there may be no defect at all. In delusional disorder, the belief is fixed and not subject to reality testing. See Table 16–7.

7. **Differential diagnosis.** Distorted body image can also occur in schizophrenia, mood disorders, medical disorders, anorexia nervosa, bulimia nervosa, obsessive–compulsive disorder, gender identity disorder, and so-called specific "culture-bound syndromes" (e.g., *koro,* worry that penis is shrinking into abdomen).

 Table 16–7
***DSM-IV-TR* Diagnostic Criteria for Body Dysmorphic Disorder**

A. Preoccupation with an imagined defect in appearance. If a slight physical anomaly is present, the person's concern is markedly excessive.

B. The preoccupation causes clinically significant distress or impairment in social, occupational, or other important area of functioning.

C. The preoccupation is not better accounted for by another mental disorder (e.g., dissatisfaction with body shape and size in anorexia nervosa).

From American Psychiatric Association. *Diagnostic and Statistical Manual of Mental Disorders,* 4th ed. Text rev. Washington, DC: American Psychiatric Association; 2000, with permission.

Table 16–8
DSM-IV-TR **Diagnostic Criteria for Undifferentiated Somatoform Disorder**

A. One or more physical complaints (e.g., fatigue, loss of appetite, gastrointestinal or urinary complaints).
B. Either (1) or (2):
    1. after appropriate investigation, the symptoms cannot be fully explained by a known general medical condition or the direct effects of a substance (e.g., a drug of abuse, a medication)
    2. when there is a related general medical condition, the physical complaints or resulting social or occupational impairment is in excess of what would be expected from the history, physical examination, or laboratory findings
C. The symptoms cause clinically significant distress or impairment in social, occupational, or other important areas of functioning.
D. The duration of the disturbance is at least 6 months.
E. The disturbance is not better accounted for by another mental disorder (e.g., another somatoform disorder, sexual dysfunction, mood disorder, anxiety disorder, sleep disorder, or psychotic disorder).
F. The symptom is not intentionally produced or feigned as in factitious disorder or malingering.

From American Psychiatric Association. *Diagnostic and Statistical Manual of Mental Disorders*, 4th ed. Text rev. Washington, DC: American Psychiatric Association; 2000, with permission.

---

    8. Course and prognosis. Chronic course with repeated visits to doctors, plastic surgeons, or dermatologists. Secondary depression may occur. In some cases, imagined body distortion progresses to delusional belief.

    9. Treatment

        a. Pharmacological: serotonergic drugs (e.g., fluoxetine [Prozac], clomipramine [Anafranil]) effectively reduce symptoms in at least 50% of patients. Treatment with surgical, dermatologic, and dental procedures is rarely successful.

        b. Psychological: psychotherapy is useful; uncovers conflicts relating to symptoms, feelings of inadequacy.

  F. Undifferentiated somatoform disorder. Undifferentiated somatoform disorder consists of unexplained physical signs and symptoms that do not meet any of the criteria listed above for somatization disorder, that last for at least 6 months, and that cannot be explained by a known medical condition. See Table 16–8. Complaints relate to the autonomic nervous system with cardiovascular, gastrointestinal, and respiratory symptoms predominating. Fatigue is also common, and chronic fatigue syndrome must be considered. The differential diagnosis also includes anxiety and depressive disorder.

  G. Somatoform disorder not otherwise specified (NOS). Somatoform disorder NOS is a residual category for other conditions that cannot be classified in any of the above listed categories. Pseudocyesis (false pregnancy) is an example. See Table 16–9.

III. Factitious Disorders

  A. Definition. Intentional report and misrepresentation of symptoms, or self-infliction of physical signs of symptoms, of medical or mental disorders. The only apparent objective is to assume the role of a patient without an external incentive. Hospitalization is often a primary objective and a way of life. The disorders have a compulsive quality, but the behaviors are deliberate and

Table 16–9
DSM-IV-TR Diagnostic Criteria for Somatoform Disorder Not Otherwise Specified

This category includes disorders with somatoform symptoms that do not meet the criteria for any specific somatoform disorder. Examples include:
1. Pseudocyesis: a false belief of being pregnant that is associated with objective signs of pregnancy, which may include abdominal enlargement although the umbilicus does not become everted, reduced menstrual flow, amenorrhea, subjective sensation of fetal movement, nausea, breast engorgement and secretions, and labor pains at the expected date of delivery. Endocrine changes may be present, but the syndrome cannot be explained by a general medical condition that causes endocrine changes (e.g., a hormone-secreting tumor).
2. A disorder involving nonpsychotic hypochondriacal symptoms of less than 6 months' duration.
3. A disorder involving unexplained physical complaints (e.g., fatigue or body weakness) of less than 6 months' duration that are not due to another mental disorder.

From American Psychiatric Association. *Diagnostic and Statistical Manual of Mental Disorders*, 4th ed. Text rev. Washington, DC: American Psychiatric Association; 2000, with permission.

voluntary, even if they cannot be controlled. Also known as *Munchausen syndrome*.

B. **Epidemiology.** Unknown. More common in men than in women. Usually adult onset. Factitious illness, especially feigned fever, accounts for 5% to 10% of all hospital admissions. More common in health care workers.

C. **Etiology.** Early real illness coupled with parental abuse or rejection is typical. Patient recreates illness as an adult to gain loving attention from doctors. Can also express masochistic gratification for some patients who want to undergo surgical procedures. Others identify with an important past figure who had psychological or physical illness. No genetic or biological etiological factors have been identified.

D. **Psychodynamics.** Mechanisms of repression, identification with the aggressor, regression, and symbolization may be present.

E. **Diagnosis, signs, and symptoms**

1. **With predominantly physical signs and symptoms.** Intentional production of physical symptoms—nausea, vomiting, pain, or seizures. Patients may intentionally put blood in feces or urine, artificially raise body temperature, or take insulin to lower blood sugar. Gridiron abdomen sign is the result of scars from multiple surgical operations.

2. **With predominantly psychological signs and symptoms.** Intentional production of psychiatric symptoms—hallucinations, delusions, depression, or bizarre behavior. Patients may make up a story that they suffered major life stress to account for symptoms. *Pseudologia fantastica* consists of making up extravagant lies that the patient believes. Substance abuse, especially of opioids, is common in both types.

3. **With combined physical and psychological signs and symptoms.** Intentional production of both physical and psychological symptoms.

4. **Factitious disorder not otherwise specified.** Includes disorders that do not meet criteria for factitious disorder (e.g., factitious disorder by proxy—intentionally feigning symptoms in another person who is under the person's care so as to assume the sick role indirectly). *Factitious*

disorder by proxy is most common in mothers who feign an illness in their child, but accounts for fewer than 1,000 of the almost 3 million cases of child abuse reported annually.

F. Differential diagnosis

1. **Physical illness.** Physical examination and laboratory workup should be performed; results will be negative. The nursing staff should observe carefully for deliberate elevation of temperature or alteration of body fluids.

2. **Somatoform disorder.** Symptoms are voluntary in factitious disorder and not caused by unconscious or symbolic factors. *La belle indifférence* is not present in factitious disorder. Hypochondriacs do not want to undergo extensive tests or surgery.

3. **Malingering.** Most difficult differential diagnosis to make. Malingerers have specific goals (e.g., insurance payments, avoidance of jail term). Evidence of an intrapsychic need to maintain the sick role (e.g., to satisfy dependency needs) is more characteristic of factitious disorder.

4. **Ganser's syndrome.** Found in prisoners who give approximate answers to questions and talk past the point. Classified as a dissociative disorder not otherwise specified.

5. **Personality disorder.** Antisocial personalities are manipulative but do not usually feign illness or agree to invasive procedures or hospitalization. Borderline personalities usually have more chaotic lifestyles, parasuicidal behavior, and more disturbed interpersonal relationships.

G. Course and prognosis. Course is usually chronic. Begins in adulthood, but onset may be earlier. Frequent consultation with doctors and history of hospitalizations as patient seeks repeated care. High risk for substance abuse over time. Prognosis improves if associated depression or anxiety is present that responds to pharmacotherapy. Risk for death if patient undergoes multiple life-threatening surgical procedures.

H. Treatment

1. Avoid unnecessary laboratory tests or medical procedures. Confront patient with diagnosis of factitious disorder and feigned symptoms. Patients rarely enter psychotherapy because of poor motivation; however, working alliance with doctor is possible over time, and patient may gain insight into behavior. Good management, however, is more likely than a cure. A databank of patients with repeated hospitalizations for factitious illness is available in some areas of the United States.

2. Psychopharmacological therapy is useful for associated anxiety or depression. Substance abuse should be treated if present.

3. Contact child welfare services if a child is at risk (e.g., with factitious disorder by proxy).

IV. Malingering

A. Definition. Voluntary production of physical or psychological symptoms to accomplish specific, tangible goal (e.g., to receive insurance payments, avoid jail term or punishment).

B. Epidemiology. Unknown. Malingering occurs most frequently in settings with a preponderance of men—the military, prisons, factories, and other industrial settings—although the condition also occurs in women.

C. Etiology. Unknown. May be associated with antisocial personality disorder.

D. Diagnosis, signs, and symptoms. Patients have many vague or poorly localized complaints that are presented in great detail; they are easily irritated if a doctor is skeptical of the history. Psychosocial history reveals a need to avoid some situation or obtain money or the presence of legal problems. Look for defined goal (secondary gain).

E. Differential diagnosis

1. **Factitious disorders.** No obvious secondary gain. Assumption of the sick role for more chronic psychological needs is more typical of this disorder.

2. **Somatoform disorder.** Symbolic or unconscious component to symptom. Symptoms are not voluntarily and willfully produced.

F. Treatment. Result of physical and laboratory workups often are negative. Patient should be monitored as if a real disease is present, but no treatment should be offered. At some time, identify areas of secondary gain and encourage patient to ventilate. Help provide ways of managing stress. Patient may then be willing to give up symptoms.

 CLINICAL HINT:
Some patients may have to be confronted directly and forcefully by the clinician when he or she thinks the patient is malingering. That may be the only way to get the patient to admit to lying about signs and symptoms.

For more detailed discussion of this topic, see Somatoform Disorders, Ch 15, p. 1927; Factitious Disorders, Ch 16, p. 1949; and Malingering, Sec 26.1, p. 2479, in CTP/IX.

17

Dissociative Disorders

I. General Introduction

The *Diagnostic and Statistical Manual of Mental Disorders,* fourth edition, text revision (*DSM-IV-TR*) states that the essential feature of dissociative disorders is a disruption of the normally integrated functions of consciousness, environmental perception, memory, and identity. Such disturbances may be transient or chronic, and are either a sudden occurrence or something that happens gradually. Dissociation usually happens in response to a traumatic event. There are four specific dissociative disorders recognized by the *DSM-IV-TR*: dissociative amnesia, dissociative fugue, dissociative identity disorder, and depersonalization disorder, as well as dissociative disorder not otherwise specified (NOS).

II. Dissociative Amnesia

A. Definition. Dissociative phenomenon is specifically amnesic in that the patient is unable to recall an important memory, which is usually traumatic or stressful, but retains the capacity to learn new material. There is no medical explanation for the occurrence, nor is the condition caused by a drug.

B. Diagnosis. The diagnostic criteria for dissociative amnesia emphasizes that the forgotten information is usually of traumatic or stressful nature. The forgotten memories are usually related to day-to-day information that is a routine part of conscious awareness (i.e., who a person is). Patients are capable of learning and remembering new information, and their general cognitive functioning and language capacity are usually intact. Onset of dissociative amnesia is often abrupt, and history usually shows a precipitating emotional trauma charged with painful emotions and psychological conflict. Patients are aware that they have lost their memories, and while some may be upset at the loss, others appear to be unconcerned or indifferent. Patients are usually alert before and after amnesia; however, some report a slight clouding of consciousness during the period immediately surrounding onset of amnesia. Depression and anxiety are common predisposing factors. Amnesia may provide a primary or a secondary gain (i.e., a woman who is amnestic about the birth of a dead infant). Dissociative amnesia may take one of several forms: localized amnesia (loss of memory for the events over a short time), generalized amnesia (loss of memory for a whole lifetime of experiences), and selective or systematized amnesia (inability to recall some but not all events over a short time). The amnesia is not the result of a general medical condition or the ingestion of a substance. See Table 17–1.

C. Epidemiology

1. Most common dissociative disorder.

2. Occurs more often in women than in men.

Table 17–1
DSM-IV-TR Diagnostic Criteria for Dissociative Amnesia

A. The predominant disturbance is one or more episodes of inability to recall important personal information, usually of a traumatic or stressful nature, that is too extensive to be explained by ordinary forgetfulness.
B. The disturbance does not occur exclusively during the course of dissociative identity disorder, dissociative fugue, posttraumatic stress disorder, acute stress disorder, or somatization disorder and is not due to the direct physiologic effects of a substance (e.g., a drug of abuse, a medication) or a neurologic or other general medical condition (e.g., amnestic disorder due to head trauma).
C. The symptoms cause clinically significant distress or impairment in social, occupational, or other important areas of functioning.

From American Psychiatric Association. *Diagnostic and Statistical Manual of Mental Disorders*, 4th ed. Text rev. Washington, DC: American Psychiatric Association, 2000, with permission.

    3. Occurs more often in adolescents and young adults than in older adults.
    4. Incidence increases during times of war and natural disasters.
  D. Etiology
    1. Precipitating emotional trauma.
    2. Rule out medical causes.
  E. Psychodynamics
    1. Defenses include repression, denial, and dissociation.
    2. Memory loss is secondary to painful psychological conflict.
  F. Differential diagnosis. See Table 17–2.
    1. Dementia or delirium. Amnesia is associated with many cognitive symptoms.
    2. Epilepsy. Sudden memory impairment associated with motor or electroencephalogram (EEG) abnormalities.

Table 17–2
Differential Diagnostic Considerations in Dissociative Amnesia

Dementia
Delirium
Amnestic disorder due to a general medical condition
    Anoxic amnesia
    Cerebral infections (e.g., herpes simplex affecting temporal lobes)
    Cerebral neoplasms (especially limbic and frontal)
    Epilepsy
    Metabolic disorders (e.g., uremia, hypoglycemia, hypertensive encephalopathy, porphyria)
    Postconcussion (posttraumatic) amnesia
    Postoperative amnesia
Electroconvulsive therapy (or other strong electric shock)
Substance-induced (e.g., ethanol, sedative–hypnotics, anticholinergics, steroids, lithium, β-adrenergic receptor antagonists, pentazocine, phencyclidine, hypoglycemic agents, cannabis, hallucinogens, methyldopa)
Transient global amnesia
Wernicke–Korsakoff's syndrome
Sleep-related amnesia (e.g., sleepwalking disorder)
Other dissociative disorders
Posttraumatic stress disorder
Acute stress disorder
Somatoform disorders (somatization disorder, conversion disorder)
Malingering (especially when associated with criminal activity)

3. **Transient global amnesia.** Associated with anterograde amnesia during episode; patients tend to be more upset and concerned about the symptoms and are able to retain personal identity; memory loss is generalized, and remote events are recalled better than recent events. Patients usually have cardiovascular disorders.

G. **Course and prognosis.** The symptoms of dissociative amnesia terminate abruptly. Recovery is complete with few recurrences. The condition may last a long time in some patients, especially in cases involving secondary gain. Patient's lost memories should be restored as soon as possible, or the repressed memory may form a nucleus in the unconscious mind where future amnestic episodes may develop. Recovery generally is spontaneous but is accelerated with treatment.

H. **Treatment**
   1. **Psychotherapy.** Psychotherapy helps patients to incorporate the memories into their conscious state. Hypnosis is used primarily as a means to relax the patient sufficiently to recall forgotten information.
   2. **Pharmacotherapy.** Drug-assisted interviews with short-acting barbiturates, such as sodium amobarbital (Amytal) given intravenously, and benzodiazepines may be used to help patients recover their forgotten memories.

III. **Dissociative Fugue**
   A. **Definition.** Dissociative fugue is characterized by sudden, unexpected travel away from home, with the inability to recall some or all of one's past. This is accompanied by confusion about identity and, often, the assumption of an entirely new identity.
   B. **Diagnosis.** Memory loss is sudden and is associated with purposeful, unconfused travel, often for extended periods of time. Patients lose part or complete memory of their past life and are often unaware of the memory loss. They assume an apparently normal, nonbizarre new identity. However, perplexity and disorientation may occur. Once they suddenly return to their former selves, they recall the time antedating the fugue, but they are amnestic for the period of the fugue itself. See Table 17–3.

Table 17–3
DSM-IV-TR Diagnostic Criteria for Dissociative Fugue

A. The predominant disturbance is sudden, unexpected travel away from home or one's customary place of work, with inability to recall one's past.
B. Confusion about personal identity or assumption of a new identity (partial or complete).
C. The disturbance does not occur exclusively during the course of dissociative identity disorder and is not due to the direct physiologic effects of a substance (e.g., a drug of abuse, a medication) or a general medical condition (e.g., temporal lobe epilepsy).
D. The symptoms cause clinically significant distress or impairment in social, occupational, or other important areas of functioning.

From American Psychiatric Association. *Diagnostic and Statistical Manual of Mental Disorders*, 4th ed. Text rev. Washington, DC: American Psychiatric Association, 2000, with permission.

C. **Epidemiology**
   1. Rare, with a prevalence rate of 0.2% in the general population.
   2. Occurs most often during times of war, during natural disasters, and as a result of personal crises with intense internal conflict.
   3. Sex ratio and age of onset are variable.

D. **Etiology**
   1. Precipitating emotional trauma.
   2. Psychosocial factors include marital, financial, occupational, and wartime stressors.
   3. Predisposing factors include borderline, histrionic, schizoid personality disorders; alcohol abuse; mood disorders; organic disorders (especially epilepsy); and a history of head trauma.
   4. Rule out medical causes.

E. **Differential diagnosis**
   1. **Cognitive disorder.** Wandering is not as purposeful or complex.
   2. **Temporal lobe epilepsy.** Generally no new identity is assumed.
   3. **Dissociative amnesia.** No purposeful travel or new identity.
   4. **Malingering.** Difficult to distinguish. Clear secondary gain should raise suspicion.
   5. **Dissociative identity disorder.** Patients have multiple forms of complex amnesia and multiple identities.
   6. **Bipolar disorder.** Patients are able to recall behavior during depressed or manic state.
   7. **Schizophrenia.** Memory loss of events during wandering episodes is due to psychosis.

F. **Course and prognosis.** Fugues appear to be brief, lasting from hours to days. Most individuals recover, although refractory dissociative amnesia may persist in rare cases. Recovery is spontaneous and rapid. Recurrences are possible.

G. **Treatment.** Psychiatric interviews, drug-assisted interviews, and hypnosis help reveal to the clinician and the patient the psychological stressors that precipitated the fugue episode. Psychotherapy helps patients incorporate the precipitating stressors into their psyches in a healthy and integrated manner.

IV. **Dissociative Identity Disorder**
   A. **Definition.** Formerly known as multiple personality disorder, dissociative identity disorder is usually the result of a traumatic event, often physical or sexual abuse in childhood. This disorder involves the manifestation of two or more distinct personalities, which, when present, will dominate the person's behaviors and attitudes as if no other personality existed.
   B. **Diagnosis.** Diagnosis requires the presence of two distinct personality states. Original personality is generally amnestic for and unaware of other personalities. The median number of personalities ranges from 5 to 10, although *DSM-IV-TR* finds an average of 8 personalities for men and 15 for women. Usually two or three identities are evident at diagnosis, and others are recognized during the course of treatment. See Table 17–4.

Table 17–4
DSM-IV-TR Diagnostic Criteria for Dissociative Identity Disorder

A. The presence of two or more distinct identities or personality states (each with its own relatively enduring pattern of perceiving, relating to, and thinking about the environment and self).
B. At least two of these identities or personality states recurrently take control of the person's behavior.
C. Inability to recall important personal information that is too extensive to be explained by ordinary forgetfulness.
D. The disturbance is not due to the direct physiologic effects of a substance (e.g., blackouts or chaotic behavior during alcohol intoxication) or a general medical condition (e.g., complex partial seizures). **Note:** in children, the symptoms are not attributable to imaginary playmates or other fantasy play.

From American Psychiatric Association. *Diagnostic and Statistical Manual of Mental Disorders*, 4th ed. Text rev. Washington, DC: American Psychiatric Association, 2000, with permission.

Transition from one personality to another tends to be abrupt. During a personality state, patients are amnestic about other states and events that took place when another personality was dominant. Some personalities may be aware of aspects of other personalities; each personality may have its own set of memories and associations, and each generally has its own name or description. Different personalities may have different physiological characteristics (e.g., different eyeglass prescriptions) and different responses to psychometric testing (e.g., different IQ scores). Personalities may be of different sexes, ages, or races. One or more of the personalities may exhibit signs of a coexisting psychiatric disorder (e.g., mood disorder, personality disorder). Signs of dissociative identity disorder are listed in Table 17–5.

C. **Epidemiology**
   1. Occurs in 5% of psychiatric patients.
   2. More common in females than in males.
   3. Most common in late adolescence and young adulthood, although symptoms may be present for 5 to 10 years before diagnosis.

Table 17–5
Signs of Dissociative Identity Disorder

1. Reports of time distortions, lapses, and discontinuities.
2. Being told of behavioral episodes by others that are not remembered by the patient.
3. Being recognized by others or called by another name by people whom the patient does not recognize.
4. Notable changes in the patient's behavior reported by a reliable observer: the patient may call himself or herself by a different name or refer to himself or herself in the third person.
5. Other personalities are elicited under hypnosis or during amobarbital interviews.
6. Use of the word "we" in the course of an interview.
7. Discovery of writings, drawings, or other productions or objects (e.g., identification cards, clothing) among the patient's personal belongings that are not recognized or cannot be accounted for.
8. Headaches.
9. Hearing voices originating from within and not identified as separate.
10. History of severe emotional or physical trauma as a child (usually before the age of 5 years).

From Cummings JL. Dissociative states, depersonalization, multiple personality, episodic memory lapses. In: Cummings JL, ed. *Clinical Neuropsychiatry.* Orlando, FL: Grune & Stratton, 1985:122, with permission.

4. More common in first-degree biological relatives with the disorder.

5. As many as two thirds of patients attempt suicide.

D. Etiology

1. Severe sexual and psychological abuse in childhood.

2. Lack of support from significant others.

3. Epilepsy may be involved.

4. Rule out medical causes.

E. Psychodynamics. Severe psychological and physical abuse leads to a profound need to distance oneself from horror and pain. Each personality expresses some necessary emotion or state (e.g., rage, sexuality, flamboyance, competence) that the original personality dares not express. During abuse, the child attempts to protect himself or herself from trauma by dissociating from the terrifying acts, becoming in essence another person or persons who are not experiencing abuse and who could not be subjected to abuse. The dissociated selves become a long-term, ingrained method of self-protection from perceived emotional threats.

F. Differential diagnosis

1. **Schizophrenia.** Different identities are of delusional belief and patients have formal thought disorder and social deterioration.

2. **Malingering.** The most difficult differential diagnosis; clear secondary gain must raise suspicion. Drug-assisted interview may help.

3. **Borderline personality disorder.** Erratic mood, behavior, and interpersonal instability may mimic dissociative identity.

4. **Bipolar disorder with rapid cycling.** Discrete personalities are absent.

5. **Neurological disorders.** The symptoms of complex partial epilepsy are the most likely to mimic those of dissociative identity disorder.

 CLINICAL HINT:

Do not confuse imaginary companions, which begin in childhood and may persist through adulthood, with a multiple. The companion is recognized as a separate being that may or may not communicate with the patient; the companion is always known and never takes over the patient's personality.

G. Course and prognosis. The earlier the onset of dissociative identity disorder, the worse the prognosis. It is the most chronic and severe of the dissociative disorders. Levels of impairment range from moderate to severe depending on the number, type, and chronicity of the various personalities. Recovery is generally incomplete. Individual personalities may have their own separate mental disorders, mood disorders, and personality disorders, with other dissociative disorders being the most common.

H. Treatment

1. **Psychotherapy.** Insight-oriented psychotherapy, often with hypnotherapy or drug-assisted interviewing, is the most efficacious approach. Hypnotherapy is useful in obtaining additional history, identifying

previously unrecognized identities, and fostering abreaction. Psychotherapeutic treatment begins by confirming the diagnosis and by identifying and characterizing the various personalities. Goals of therapy include reconciliation of disparate, split-off affects by helping the patient understand that the original reasons for the dissociation (overwhelming rage, fear, and confusion secondary to abuse) no longer exist, and that the affects can be expressed by one whole personality without the self being destroyed. Hospitalization may be necessary in some cases.

2. **Pharmacotherapy.** Drug-assisted interviewing is helpful in obtaining additional history and identifying unrecognized identities. Antidepressant and antianxiety medications can be useful as adjuvants to psychotherapy. In selected patients, anticonvulsant medications, such as carbamazepine (Tegretol), have been helpful.

V. Depersonalization Disorder

A. Definition. According to the *DSM-IV-TR*, persistently feeling detached or estranged from oneself is the essential feature of depersonalization. The patient may report feeling as though they are watching themselves in a movie or feeling as if they are dreaming, and feels as if they are not in control of their actions.

B. Diagnosis. The *DSM-IV-TR* diagnostic criteria for depersonalization disorder include persistent or recurrent episodes of depersonalization resulting in significant distress to patients or in impairment in their social, occupational, or interpersonal relationships. Reality testing is intact. Patient's inner mental processes and external events remain unchanged, yet they no longer appear to have any relation or significance to the person. The central characteristic of this disorder is a sense of unreality and estrangement. Distortions in sense of time and space, a feeling that extremities are too large or too small, and derealization (sense of strangeness about external world) are common. See Table 17–6.

C. Epidemiology

1. Occasional isolated depersonalization episodes are common and occur in 70% of a given population. Pathological depersonalization is rare.

Table 17–6
DSM-IV-TR Diagnostic Criteria for Depersonalization Disorder

A. Persistent or recurrent experiences of feeling detached from, and as if one is an outside observer of, one's mental processes or body (e.g., feeling like one is in a dream).
B. During the personalization experience, reality testing remains intact.
C. The depersonalization causes clinically significant distress or impairment in social, occupational, or other important areas of functioning.
D. The depersonalization experience does not occur exclusively during the course of another mental disorder, such as schizophrenia, panic disorder, acute stress disorder, or another dissociative disorder, and is not due to the direct physiologic effects of a substance (e.g., a drug of abuse, a medication) or a general medical condition (e.g., temporal lobe epilepsy).

From American Psychiatric Association. *Diagnostic and Statistical Manual of Mental Disorders*, 4th ed. Text rev. Washington, DC: American Psychiatric Association, 2000, with permission.

    2. Occurs more often in women than in men.

    3. Mean age of occurrence is 16 years. Rarely found in persons over the age of 40 years.

D. Etiology

    1. Predisposing factors include anxiety, depression, and severe stress.

    2. May be caused by a psychological, neurological, or systemic disease.

    3. Associated with an array of substances including alcohol, barbiturates, benzodiazepines, scopolamine, β-adrenergic antagonists, marijuana, and virtually any phencyclidine (PCP)-like or hallucinogenic substance.

    4. Frequently associated with anxiety disorders, depressive disorders, and schizophrenia.

E. Differential diagnosis. As a symptom, depersonalization can occur in many syndromes, both psychiatric and medical. Mood disorders, anxiety disorders, schizophrenia, dissociative identity disorder, substance use, adverse effects of medication, brain tumors or injury, and seizure disorders (e.g., temporal lobe epilepsy) must be ruled out. Depersonalization disorder describes the condition in which depersonalization is predominant. Depersonalization is differentiated from psychotic disorders in that reality testing is intact. See Table 17–7.

F. Course and prognosis

    1. Symptoms appear suddenly, most often between 15 and 30 years of age.

    2. In more than 50% of cases, the disorder is long-lasting.

G. Treatment. Usually responds to anxiolytics and to both supportive and insight-oriented therapy. As anxiety is reduced, episodes of depersonalization decrease.

Table 17–7
Causes of Depersonalization

Neurological disorders	Idiopathic mental disorders
Epilepsy	Schizophrenia
Migraine	Depressive disorders
Brain tumors	Manic episodes
Cerebrovascular disease	Conversion disorder
Cerebral trauma	Anxiety disorders
Encephalitis	Obsessive–compulsive disorder
General paresis	Personality disorders
Dementia of the Alzheimer's type	Phobic–anxiety depersonalization syndrome
Huntington's disease	**In normal persons**
Spinocerebellar degeneration	Exhaustion
Toxic and metabolic disorders	Boredom; sensory deprivation
Hypoglycemia	Emotional shock
Hypoparathyroidism	**In hemidepersonalization**
Carbon monoxide poisoning	Lateralized (usually right parietal) focal brain lesion
Mescaline intoxication	
Botulism	
Hyperventilation	
Hypothyroidism	

Adapted from Cummings JL. Dissociative states, depersonalization, multiple personality, episodic memory lapses. In: Cummings JL, ed. *Clinical Neuropsychiatry.* Orlando, FL: Grune & Stratton 1985:123, with permission.

Table 17–8
Summary of Dissociative Disorders

	Dissociative Amnesia	Dissociative Fugue	Dissociative Identity Disorder	Depersonalization Disorder
Signs and symptoms	Loss of memory, usually with abrupt onset Patient aware of loss Alert before and after loss	Purposeful wandering, often long distances Amnesia for past life Often unaware of loss of memory Often assumes new identity Normal behavior during fugue	More than one distinct personality within one person, each of which dominates person's behavior and thinking when it is present Sudden transition from one personality to another Generally amnesia for other personalities	Persistent sense of unreality about one's body and self Intact reality testing Ego-dynamic
Epidemiology	Most common dissociative disorder More common following disasters or during war Female > male Adolescence young adulthood	Rare More common following disasters or during war Variable sex ratio and age of onset	Not nearly as rare as once thought Affects as many as 5% of psychiatric patients Adolescence–young adulthood (although may begin much earlier) Female > male Increased in first-degree relatives	Although pure disorder rare, intermittent episodes of depersonalization common Rare over age 40 May be more common in women
Etiology	Precipitating emotional trauma (e.g., domestic violence) Rule out medical causes	Precipitating emotional trauma Heavy alcohol abuse may predispose Borderline, histrionic, schizoid personality disorders predispose Rule out medical causes	Severe sexual and psychological abuse in childhood Lack of support from significant others Epilepsy may be involved Rule out medical causes	Severe stress, anxiety, depression predispose Rule out medical causes
Course and prognosis	Abrupt termination Few recurrences	Usually brief, hours or days Can last months and involve extensive travel Recovery generally spontaneous and rapid Recurrences rare	Most severe and chronic of dissociative disorders Incomplete recovery	Onset usually sudden Tends to be chronic

VI. Dissociative Disorder NOS

A. Definition. Dissociative disorders NOS are disorders in which the predominant feature is a dissociative symptom, such as a disruption in consciousness or memory, but that does not meet the criteria for specific dissociative disorder. In order for a patient to be diagnosed with dissociative disorder NOS, the patient must fail to meet the criteria for acute stress disorder, PTSD, or somatization disorder, all of which include dissociative symptoms.

B. Examples

1. **Ganser's syndrome**—giving approximate answers to questions (e.g., 2 + 2 = 5) or talking past the point; commonly associated with other symptoms (e.g., amnesia, disorientation, perceptual disturbances, fugue, conversion symptoms).

2. **Dissociative trance disorder**—disturbances in consciousness, identity, or memory that are indigenous to particular locations and cultures (e.g., *amok* [rage reaction], *pibloktog* [self-injurious behavior]). Trance states are altered states of consciousness with markedly diminished or selectively focused responsiveness to environmental stimuli. In children, such states may follow physical abuse or trauma.

3. **Recovered memory syndrome**—the recovery of a memory of a painful experience or conflict during hypnosis or psychotherapy (e.g., sexual or physical abuse). The patient not only recalls the experience, but may also relive it with the appropriate affective response (a process called *abreaction*).

4. Dissociated states in persons who have been subjected to periods of prolonged and intense coercive persuasion (e.g., brainwashing or indoctrination while the captive of terrorists or cultists).

   See Table 17–8 for an overview of all the dissociative disorders.

For more detailed discussion of this topic, see Dissociative Disorders, Ch 17, p. 1965, in CTP IX.

18

Sexual Dysfunctions, Paraphilias, and Gender Identity Disorders

I. Sexual Dysfunctions

A. Definition. Sexual function is affected by a complex interaction of factors. A person's sexuality is enmeshed with other personality factors, with one's biological makeup and with a general sense of self. A problem in one or more of these areas can result in sexual dysfunction. The final common pathway to dysfunction is performance anxiety, which inhibits sexual response and tends to perpetuate the sexual problem. The dysfunctions can be a **lifelong type** or an **acquired type** (i.e., developing after a period of normal functioning); a **generalized type** or **situational type** (i.e., limited to a certain partner or a specific situation); and the consequence of **physiological factors, psychological factors,** or **combined factors.**

In *Diagnostic and Statistical Manual of Mental Disorders,* fourth edition, text revision *(DSM-IV-TR)* a *sexual dysfunction* is defined as a disturbance in the sexual response cycle or as pain with sexual intercourse. Seven major categories of sexual dysfunction are listed in *DSM-IV-TR*: sexual desire disorders, sexual arousal disorders, orgasm disorders, sexual pain disorders, sexual dysfunction caused by a general medical condition, substance-induced sexual dysfunction, and sexual dysfunction not otherwise specified. Table 18–1 lists each *DSM-IV-TR* phase of the sexual response cycle and the sexual dysfunctions usually associated with it.

B. Sexual desire disorders. Sexual desire disorders are divided into two classes: hypoactive sexual desire disorder, characterized by a deficiency or absence of sexual fantasies and the desire for sexual activity, and sexual aversion disorder, characterized by an aversion to and avoidance of genital sexual contact with a sexual partner or an avoidance of masturbation.

Patients with desire problems may use inhibition of desire defensively to protect against unconscious fears about sex. A lack of desire can also accompany chronic anxiety or depression, or the use of various psychotropic drugs and other drugs that depress the central nervous system (CNS). In sex therapy clinic populations, lack of desire is one of the most common complaints among married couples, with women more affected than men.

C. Sexual arousal disorders. The sexual arousal disorders are divided by *DSM-IV-TR* into female sexual arousal disorder, characterized by the persistent or recurrent partial or complete failure to attain or maintain the lubrication-swelling response of sexual excitement until the completion of the sexual act, and male erectile disorder, characterized by the recurrent and persistent partial or complete failure to attain or maintain an erection until completion of the sex act.

Table 18–1
DSM-IV-TR Phases of the Sexual Response Cycle and Associated Sexual Dysfunctions[a]

Phases	Characteristics	Dysfunction
1. Desire	Distinct from any identified solely through physiology and reflects the patient's motivations, drives, and personality; characterized by sexual fantasies and the desire to have sex.	Hypoactive sexual desire disorder; sexual aversion disorder; hypoactive sexual desire disorder due to a general medical condition (male or female); substance-induced sexual dysfunction with impaired desire.
2. Excitement	Subjective sense of sexual pleasure and accompanying physiological changes; all physiological responses noted in Masters and Johnson's excitement and plateau phases are combined in this phase.	Female sexual arousal disorder; male erectile disorder (may also occur in stages 3 and 4); male erectile disorder due to a general medical condition; dyspareunia due to a general medical condition (male or female); substance-induced sexual dysfunction with impaired arousal.
3. Orgasm	Peaking of sexual pleasure, with release of sexual tension and rhythmic contraction of the perineal muscles and pelvic reproductive organs.	Female orgasmic disorder; male orgasmic disorder; premature ejaculation; other sexual dysfunction due to a general medical condition (male or female); substance-induced sexual dysfunction with impaired orgasm.
4. Resolution	A sense of general relaxation, well-being, and muscle relaxation; men are refractory to orgasm for a period of time that increases with age, whereas women can have multiple orgasms without a refractory period.	Postcoital dysphoria; postcoital headache.

[a]*DSM-IV-TR* consolidates Masters and Johnson's excitement and plateau phases into a single excitement phase, which is preceded by the desire (appetitive) phase. The orgasm and resolution phases remain the same as originally described by Masters and Johnson.

1. **Women.** The prevalence of female sexual arousal disorder is generally underestimated. In one study of subjectively happily married couples, 33% of women described arousal problems. Difficulty in maintaining excitement can reflect psychological conflicts (e.g., anxiety, guilt, and fear) or physiological changes. Alterations in levels of testosterone, estrogen, prolactin, serotonin, dopamine, and thyroxin have been implicated in arousal disorders, as have antihistamine medications. See Table 18–2.

2. **Men.** The prevalence of erectile disorder, or impotence, in young men is estimated at 8%. This disorder may first appear later in life. A number of procedures, from benign to invasive, are used to differentiate organically (i.e., physiologically) caused impotence from functional (i.e., psychological) impotence. The most commonly used procedure is monitoring of nocturnal penile tumescence (erections that occur during sleep), normally associated with rapid eye movement (REM) sleep. See Table 18–3.

   A good history is invaluable in determining the cause. A history of spontaneous erections, morning erections, or good erections with masturbation or with partners other than the usual one indicates functional

Table 18–2
DSM-IV-TR Diagnostic Criteria for Female Sexual Arousal Disorder

A. Persistent or recurrent inability to attain, or to maintain until completion of the sexual activity, an adequate lubrication-swelling response of sexual excitement.
B. The disturbance causes marked distress or interpersonal difficulty.
C. The sexual dysfunction is not better accounted for by another Axis I disorder (except another sexual dysfunction) and is not due exclusively to the direct physiologic effects of a substance (e.g., a drug of abuse, a medication) or a general medical condition.
Specify type:
  Lifelong type
  Acquired type
Specify type:
  Generalized type
  Situational type
Specify:
  Due to psychological factors
  Due to combined factors

From American Psychiatric Association. *Diagnostic and Statistical Manual of Mental Disorders*, 4th ed. Text rev. Washington, DC: American Psychiatric Association; 2000, with permission.

impotence. Psychological causes of erectile dysfunction include a punitive conscience or superego, an inability to trust, or feelings of inadequacy. Erectile dysfunction also may reflect relationship difficulties between partners.

D. Orgasmic disorders

 1. Female. See Table 18–4. Female orgasmic disorder (anorgasmia) is a recurrent or persistent delay in or absence of orgasm following a normal sexual excitement phase. The estimated proportion of married women over age 35 who never have achieved orgasm is 5%. The proportion is higher in unmarried women and younger women. The overall prevalence

Table 18–3
DSM-IV-TR Diagnostic Criteria for Male Erectile Disorder

A. Persistent or recurrent inability to attain, or to maintain until completion of the sexual activity, an adequate erection.
B. The disturbance causes marked distress or interpersonal difficulty.
C. The erectile dysfunction is not better accounted for by another Axis I disorder (other than a sexual dysfunction) and is not due exclusively to the direct physiologic effects of a substance (e.g., a drug of abuse, a medication) or a general medical condition.
Specify type:
  Lifelong type
  Acquired type
Specify type:
  Generalized type
  Situational type
Specify:
  Due to psychological factors
  Due to combined factors

From American Psychiatric Association. *Diagnostic and Statistical Manual of Mental Disorders*, 4th ed. Text rev. Washington, DC: American Psychiatric Association; 2000, with permission.

Table 18–4
***DSM-IV-TR* Diagnostic Criteria for Female Orgasmic Disorder**

A. Persistent or recurrent delay in, or absence of, orgasm following a normal sexual excitement phase. Women exhibit wide variability in the type or intensity of stimulation that triggers orgasm. The diagnosis of female orgasmic disorder should be based on the clinician's judgment that the woman's orgasmic capacity is less than would be reasonable for her age, sexual experience, and the adequacy of sexual stimulation she receives.
B. The disturbance causes marked distress or interpersonal difficulty.
C. The orgasmic dysfunction is not better accounted for by another Axis I disorder (except another sexual dysfunction) and is not due exclusively to the direct physiologic effects of a substance (e.g., a drug of abuse, a medication) or a general medical condition.
Specify type:
  Lifelong type
  Acquired type
Specify type:
  Generalized type
  Situational type
Specify:
  Due to psychological factors
  Due to combined factors

From American Psychiatric Association. *Diagnostic and Statistical Manual of Mental Disorders*, 4th ed. Text rev. Washington, DC: American Psychiatric Association; 2000, with permission.

of inhibited female orgasm is 30%. Psychological factors associated with inhibited orgasm include fears of impregnation or rejection by the sex partner, hostility toward men, feelings of guilt about sexual impulses, or marital conflicts.

2. **Male.** In male orgasmic disorder (inhibited male orgasm), the man achieves ejaculation during coitus with great difficulty, if at all. Lifelong inhibited male orgasm usually indicates more severe psychopathology. Acquired ejaculatory inhibition frequently reflects interpersonal difficulties. The most common biological reason for this condition is treatment with selective serotonin reuptake inhibitors (SSRIs), which cause delayed orgasm.

3. **Premature ejaculation.** Premature ejaculation is the chief complaint of 35% to 40% of men treated for sexual disorders. The man persistently or recurrently achieves orgasm and ejaculates before he wishes to. It is more prevalent among young men, men with a new partner, and college-educated men than among men with less education; the problem with the latter group is thought to be related to concern for partner satisfaction.

Difficulty in ejaculatory control may be associated with anxiety regarding the sex act and with unconscious fears about the vagina. It may also be the result of conditioning if the man's early sexual experiences occurred in situations in which discovery would have been embarrassing. A stressful marriage exacerbates the disorder.

This dysfunction is the one most amenable to cure when behavioral techniques are used in treatment. However, a subgroup of premature ejaculators may be biologically predisposed; they are more vulnerable to sympathetic stimulation or they have a shorter bulbocavernosus reflex nerve latency time, and they should be treated pharmacologically with SSRIs or other antidepressants. A side effect of these drugs is the inhibition of ejaculation.

E. **Sexual pain disorders**
1. **Vaginismus.** Vaginismus is an involuntary muscle constriction of the outer third of the vagina that interferes with penile insertion and intercourse. This dysfunction most frequently afflicts women in higher socioeconomic groups. A sexual trauma, such as rape or childhood sexual abuse, can be the cause. Women with psychosexual conflicts may perceive the penis as a weapon. A strict religious upbringing that associates sex with sin or problems in the dyadic relationship are also noted in these cases.
2. **Dyspareunia.** Dyspareunia is recurrent or persistent genital pain occurring before, during, or after intercourse. Medical causes (endometriosis, vaginitis, cervicitis, and other pelvic disorders) must be ruled out in patients with this complaint.

   Chronic pelvic pain is a common complaint in women with a history of rape or childhood sexual abuse. Painful coitus may result from tension and anxiety. Dyspareunia is uncommon in men and is usually associated with a medical condition (e.g., Peyronie's disease).
F. **Sexual dysfunction due to a general medical condition**
1. **Male erectile disorder.** Statistics indicate that erectile disorder is medically based in 50% of affected men. Medical causes of male erectile dysfunction are listed in Table 18–5.
2. **Dyspareunia.** Pelvic disease is found in 30% to 40% of women with this complaint who are seen in sex therapy clinics. An estimated 30% of surgical procedures on the female pelvic or genital area also result in temporary dyspareunia. In most cases, however, dynamic factors are considered causative.

   Medical conditions leading to dyspareunia include irritated or infected hymenal remnants, episiotomy scars, infection of a Bartholin's gland, various forms of vaginitis and cervicitis, endometriosis, and postmenopausal vaginal atrophy.
3. **Hypoactive sexual desire disorder.** Desire commonly decreases after major illness or surgery, particularly when the body image is affected after such procedures as mastectomy, ileostomy, hysterectomy, and prostatectomy. Drugs that depress the CNS, decrease testosterone or dopamine concentrations, or increase serotonin or prolactin concentrations can decrease desire.
4. **Other male sexual dysfunctions.** Male orgasmic dysfunction may have physiological causes and can occur after surgery on the genitourinary tract. It may also be associated with Parkinson's disease and other neurological disorders involving the lumbar or sacral sections of the spinal cord. Certain drugs (e.g., guanethidine monosulfate [Ismelin]) have been implicated in retarded ejaculation (Table 18–6).
5. **Other female sexual dysfunctions.** Some medical conditions—specifically, such endocrine diseases as hypothyroidism, diabetes mellitus, and primary hyperprolactinemia—can affect a woman's ability to have orgasms.
G. **Substance-induced sexual dysfunction.** In general, sexual function is negatively affected by serotonergic agents, dopamine antagonists, drugs that

Table 18–5
Medical Conditions Implicated in Erectile Dysfunction

Infectious and parasitic diseases	**Neurological disorders**
Elephantiasis	Multiple sclerosis
Mumps	Transverse myelitis
Cardiovascular disease	Parkinson's disease
Atherosclerotic disease	Temporal lobe epilepsy
Aortic aneurysm	Traumatic and neoplastic spinal cord diseases
Leriche's syndrome	Central nervous system tumor
Cardiac failure	Amyotrophic lateral sclerosis
Renal and urological disorders	Peripheral neuropathy
Peyronie's disease	General paresis
Chronic renal failure	Tabes dorsalis
Hydrocele and varicocele	**Pharmacological contributants**
Hepatic disorders	Alcohol and other dependence-inducing
Cirrhosis (usually associated with alcohol	substances (heroin, methadone, morphine,
dependence)	cocaine, amphetamines, and barbiturates)
Pulmonary disorders	Prescribed drugs (psychotropic drugs,
Respiratory failure	antihypertensive drugs, estrogens, and
Genetic disorders	antiandrogens)
Klinefelter's syndrome	**Poisoning**
Congenital penile vascular and structural	Lead (plumbism)
abnormalities	Herbicides
Nutritional disorders	**Surgical procedures**
Malnutrition	Perineal prostatectomy
Vitamin deficiencies	Abdominal–perineal colon resection
Endocrine disorders	Sympathectomy (frequently interferes with
Diabetes mellitus	ejaculation)
Dysfunction of the pituitary–adrenal–testis	Aortoiliac surgery
axis	Radical cystectomy
Acromegaly	Retroperitoneal lymphadenectomy
Addison's disease	**Miscellaneous**
Chromophobe adenoma	Radiation therapy
Adrenal neoplasia	Pelvic fracture
Myxedema	Any severe systemic disease or debilitating
Hyperthyroidism	condition

increase prolactin, and drugs that affect the autonomic nervous system. With commonly abused substances, dysfunction occurs within a month of significant substance intoxication or withdrawal. In small doses, some substances (e.g., amphetamines) may enhance sexual performance, but abuse impairs erectile, orgasmic, and ejaculatory capacities.

The interrelation between female sexual dysfunction and pharmacological agents has been less extensively evaluated than have male reactions. Oral contraceptives are reported to decrease libido in some women, and some drugs with anticholinergic side effects may impair arousal as well as orgasm. Benzodiazepines have been reported to decrease libido, but in some patients, the diminution of anxiety caused by those drugs enhances sexual function. Both increase and decrease in libido have been reported with psychoactive agents. It is difficult to separate those effects from the underlying condition or from improvement of the condition. Sexual dysfunction associated with the use of a drug disappears when the drug is discontinued. Table 18–7 lists psychiatric medications that may inhibit female orgasm.

Table 18–6
Pharmacological Agents Implicated in Male Sexual Dysfunctions

Drug	Impairs Erection	Impairs Ejaculation
Psychiatric drugs		
Selective serotonin reuptake inhibitors[a]		
Citalopram (Celexa)	–	+
Fluoxetine (Prozac)	–	+
Paroxetine (Paxil)	–	+
Sertraline (Zoloft)	–	+
Cyclic drugs		
Imipramine (Tofranil)	+	+
Protriptyline (Vivactil)	+	+
Desipramine (Pertofrane)	+	+
Clomipramine (Anafranil)	+	+
Amitriptyline (Elavil)	+	+
Monoamine oxidase inhibitors		
Tranylcypromine (Parnate)	+	
Phenelzine (Nardil)	+	+
Pargyline (Eutonyl)	–	+
Isocarboxazid (Marplan)	–	+
Other mood-active drugs		
Lithium (Eskalith)	+	
Amphetamines	+	+
Trazodone (Desyrel)[b]	–	–
Venlafaxine (Effexor)	–	+
Antipsychotics[c]		
Fluphenazine (Prolixin)	+	
Thioridazine (Mellaril)	+	+
Chlorprothixene (Taractan)	–	+
Mesoridazine (Serentil)	–	+
Perphenazine (Trilafon)	–	+
Trifluoperazine (Stelazine)	–	+
Reserpine (Serpasil)	–	+
Haloperidol (Haldol)	–	+
Antianxiety agent[d]		
Chlordiazepoxide (Librium)	–	+
Antihypertensive drugs		
Clonidine (Catapres)	+	
Methyldopa (Aldomet)	+	+
Spironolactone (Aldactone)	+	–
Hydrochlorothiazide (Hydrodiuril)	+	–
Guanethidine (Ismelin)	+	+
Commonly abused substances		
Alcohol	+	+
Barbiturates	+	+
Cannabis	+	–
Cocaine	+	+
Heroin	+	+
Methadone	+	–
Morphine	+	+
Miscellaneous drugs		
Antiparkinsonian agents	+	+
Clofibrate (Atromid-S)	+	–
Digoxin (Lanoxin)	+	–
Glutethimide (Doriden)	+	+
Indomethacin (Indocin)	+	–
Phentolamine (Regitine)	–	+
Propranolol (Inderal)	+	–

[a]SSRIs also impair desire.

[b]Trazodone has been causative in some cases of priapism.

[c]Impairment of sexual function is less likely with atypical antipsychotics. Priapism has occasionally occurred in association with the use of antipsychotics.

[d]Benzodiazepines have been reported to decrease libido, but in some patients, the diminution of anxiety caused by those drugs enhances sexual function.

Table 18–7
Some Psychiatric Drugs That Inhibit Female Orgasm

Tricyclic antidepressants	**Dopamine receptor antagonists**
Imipramine (Tofranil)	Thioridazine (Mellaril)
Clomipramine (Anafranil)	Trifluoperazine (Stelazine)
Nortriptyline (Aventyl)	**Selective serotonin reuptake inhibitors**
Monoamine oxidase inhibitors	Fluoxetine (Prozac)
Tranylcypromine (Parnate)	Paroxetine (Paxil)
Phenelzine (Nardil)	Sertraline (Zoloft)
Isocarboxazid (Marplan)	Fluvoxamine (Luvox)
	Citalopram (Celexa)

H. Sexual dysfunction not otherwise specified. Includes sexual dysfunctions
that do not meet the criteria for any specific dysfunction. Examples include
orgasmic anhedonia (i.e., not experiencing pleasure during orgasm) and compulsive sexual behavior.

I. Treatment. Methods that have proved effective singly or in combination
include (1) training in behavioral–sexual skills, (2) systematic desensitization, (3) directive marital therapy, (4) psychodynamic approaches, (5) group
therapy, (6) pharmacotherapy, (7) surgery, and (8) hypnotherapy. Evaluation and treatment must address the possibility of accompanying personality
disorders and physical conditions.

    1. Analytically oriented sex therapy. One of the most effective treatment
modalities is the integration of sex therapy (training in behavioral–sexual
skills) with psychodynamic and psychoanalytically oriented psychotherapy. Psychodynamic conceptualizations are added to behavioral techniques for the treatment of patients with sexual disorders associated with
other psychopathology.

    2. Behavioral techniques. The aim of these techniques is to establish or
reestablish verbal and sexual communication between partners. Specific
exercises are prescribed to help the person or couple with their particular
problem. All exercises are carried out in privacy, never in the presence of
the therapist.

        Beginning exercises focus on verbal interchange and then on height-
ening sensory awareness to sight, touch, and smell. Initially, intercourse is
prohibited and partners caress each other, with stimulation of the genitalia
excluded. Performance anxiety is reduced because responses of genital
excitement and orgasm are unnecessary for the completion of the initial
exercises.

        During these sensate focus exercises, patients receive encouragement
and reinforcement to reduce their anxiety. They are urged to use fantasies
to distract them from obsessive concerns about performance (spectator-
ing). The expression of mutual needs is encouraged. Resistances, such
as claims of fatigue or not enough time to complete the exercises, are
common and must be dealt with by the therapist. Genital stimulation is
eventually added to general body stimulation. Finally, intromission and
intercourse are permitted. Therapy sessions follow each new exercise

period, and problems and satisfactions, both sexual and related to other areas of the patients' lives, are discussed.

a. Dysfunction-specific techniques and exercises. Different techniques are used for specific dysfunctions.

  (1) **Vaginismus**—the woman is advised to dilate her vaginal opening with her fingers or with dilators.

  (2) **Premature ejaculation**—the squeeze technique is used to raise the threshold of penile excitability. The patient or his partner forcibly squeezes the coronal ridge of the glans at the first sensation of impending ejaculation. The erection is diminished and ejaculation inhibited. A variation is the stop–start technique. Stimulation is stopped as excitement increases, but no squeeze is used.

  (3) **Male erectile disorder**—the man is sometimes told to masturbate to demonstrate that full erection and ejaculation are possible.

  (4) **Female orgasmic disorder (primary anorgasmia)**—the woman is instructed to masturbate, sometimes with the use of a vibrator. The use of fantasy is encouraged.

  (5) **Retarded ejaculation**—managed by extravaginal ejaculation initially and gradual vaginal entry after stimulation to the point of near ejaculation.

b. Behavioral techniques. Reported to be successful 40% to 85% of the time. Individual psychotherapy is required in 10% of refractory cases. Approximately one third of dysfunctional couples who are refractory to behavioral techniques alone require some combination of marital and sex therapy.

3. Biological

a. Pharmacotherapy. Most pharmacological treatments are for male sexual dysfunctions. Studies are being conducted to test the use of drugs to treat women. Pharmacotherapy may be used to treat sexual disorders of physiological, psychological, or mixed causes. In the latter two cases, pharmacological treatment is usually used in addition to a form of psychotherapy.

  (1) **Treatment of erectile disorder and premature ejaculation.** Sildenafil (Viagra), a nitric oxide enhancer, facilitates the inflow of blood to the penis necessary for an erection for about 4 hours. The medication does not work in the absence of sexual stimulation. Its use is contraindicated for people taking organic nitrates. New nitric oxide enhancers are vardenafil (Levitra) and tadalafil (Cialis). Tadalafil is effective for up to 36 hours.

 CLINICAL HINT:
When prescribing any of these drugs, be sure to explain to the patient that the pill does not produce an erection spontaneously. Sexual stimulation is necessary if an erection is to occur.

Other medications act as vasodilators in the penis. They include oral prostaglandin (Vasomax); alprostadil (Caverject), an injectable phentolamine; and a transurethral alprostadil suppository (MUSE).

α-Adrenergic agents such as methylphenidate (Ritalin), dextroamphetamine (Dexedrine), and yohimbine (Yocon) are also used to treat erectile disorder.

SSRIs and heterocyclic antidepressants alleviate premature ejaculation because of their side effect of inhibiting orgasm.

(2) **Treatment of sexual aversion disorder.** Cyclic antidepressants and SSRIs are used if people with this dysfunction are considered phobic of the genitalia.

b. **Surgery.** Penile implants, revascularization.

II. Gender Identity Disorders

A. **Definition.** A group of disorders that have as their main symptom a persistent preference for the role of the opposite sex and the feeling that one was born into the wrong sex. The feeling of discontent with one's biological sex is labeled *gender dysphoria.*

People with disordered gender identity try to live as or pass as members of the opposite sex. *Transsexuals* want biological treatment (surgery, hormones) to change their biological sex and acquire the anatomic characteristics of the opposite sex. The disorders may coexist with other pathology or be circumscribed, with patients functioning ably in many areas of their lives.

B. **Diagnosis, signs, and symptoms.** See Table 18–8.

C. **Epidemiology**

1. Unknown, but rare.
2. Male-to-female ratio is 4:1.
   a. Almost all gender-disordered females have a homosexual orientation.
   b. Fifty percent of gender-disordered males have a homosexual orientation, and 50% have a heterosexual, bisexual, or asexual orientation.
3. The prevalence rate for transsexualism is 1 per 10,000 males and 1 per 30,000 females.

D. **Etiology**

1. **Biological.** Testosterone affects brain neurons that contribute to masculinization of the brain in such areas as the hypothalamus. Whether testosterone contributes to so-called masculine or feminine behavioral patterns in gender identity disorders remains controversial. Sex steroids influence the expression of sexual behavior in mature men and women (i.e., testosterone can increase libido and aggressiveness in women, and estrogen or progesterone can decrease libido and aggressiveness in men).

2. **Psychosocial.** The absence of same-sex role models and explicit or implicit encouragement from caregivers to behave like the other sex contributes to gender identity disorder in childhood. Mothers may be

Table 18–8
DSM-IV-TR Diagnostic Criteria for **Gender Identity Disorder**

A. A strong and persistent cross-gender identification (not merely a desire for any perceived cultural advantages of being the other sex).

In children, the disturbance is manifested by four (or more) of the following:
1. repeatedly stated desire to be, or insistence that he or she is, the other sex
2. in boys, preference for cross-dressing or simulating female attire; in girls, insistence on wearing only stereotypical masculine clothing
3. strong and persistent preferences for cross-sex roles in make-believe play or persistent fantasies of being the other sex
4. intense desire to participate in the stereotypical games and pastimes of the other sex
5. strong preference for playmates of the other sex

In adolescents and adults, the disturbance is manifested by symptoms such as a stated desire to be the other sex, frequent passing as the other sex, desire to live or be treated as the other sex, or the conviction that he or she has the typical feelings and reactions of the other sex.

B. Persistent discomfort with his or her sex or sense of inappropriateness in the gender role of that sex.

In children, the disturbance is manifested by any of the following: in boys, assertion that his penis or testes are disgusting or will disappear, assertion that it would be better not to have a penis, or aversion toward rough-and-tumble play and rejection of male stereotypical toys, games, and activities; in girls, rejection of urinating in a sitting position, assertion that she has or will grow a penis, assertion that she does not want to grow breasts or menstruate, or marked aversion toward normative feminine clothing.

In adolescents and adults, the disturbance is manifested by symptoms such as preoccupation with getting rid of primary and secondary sex characteristics (e.g., request for hormones, surgery, or other procedures to physically alter sexual characteristics to stimulate the other sex) or belief that he or she was born the wrong sex.

C. The disturbance is not concurrent with a physical intersex condition.

D. The disturbance causes clinically significant distress or impairment in social, occupational, or other important areas of functioning.

Code based on current age:
   Gender identity disorder in children
   Gender identity disorder in adolescents or adults
Specify it (tor sexually mature individuals):
   Sexually attracted to males
   Sexually attracted to females
   Sexually attracted to both
   Sexually attracted to neither

From American Psychiatric Association. *Diagnostic and Statistical Manual of Mental Disorders*, 4th ed. Text rev. Washington, DC: American Psychiatric Association; 2000, with permission.

depressed or withdrawn. Inborn temperamental traits sometimes result in sensitive, delicate boys and energetic, aggressive girls.

E. Differential diagnosis

1. **Transvestic fetishism.** Cross-dressing for purpose of sexual excitement; can coexist (dual diagnosis).

2. **Intersex conditions.** See Table 18–9.

3. **Schizophrenia.** Rarely, true delusions of being other sex.

F. Course and prognosis

1. **Children.** Course varies. Symptoms may diminish spontaneously or with treatment. Prognosis depends on age of onset and intensity of symptoms. The disorder begins in boys before the age of 4 years, and peer conflict develops at about the age of 7 or 8 years. Tomboyism is generally better tolerated. The age of onset is also early for girls, but most give up

Table 18–9
Classification of Intersexual Disorders[a]

Syndrome	Description
Virilizing adrenal hyperplasia (adrenogenital syndrome)	Results from excess androgens in fetus with XX genotype; most common female intersex disorder; associated with enlarged clitoris, fused labia, hirsutism in adolescence.
Turner's syndrome	Results from absence of second female sex chromosome (XO); associated with web neck, dwarfism, cubitus valgus; no sex hormones produced; infertile; usually assigned as females because of female-looking genitals.
Klinefelter's syndrome	Genotype is XXY; male habitus present with small penis and rudimentary testes because of low androgen production; weak libido; usually assigned as male.
Androgen insensitivity syndrome (testicular-feminizing syndrome)	Congenital X-linked recessive disorder that results in inability of tissues to respond to androgens; external genitals look female and cryptorchid testes present; assigned as females, even though they have XY genotype; in extreme form patient has breasts, normal external genitals, short blind vagina, and absence of pubic and axillary hair.
Enzymatic defects in XY genotype (e.g., 5-α reductase deficiency, 17-hydroxysteroid deficiency)	Congenital interruption in production of testosterone that produces ambiguous genitals and female habitus; usually assigned as female because of female-looking genitalia.
Hermaphroditism	True hermaphrodite is rare and characterized by both testes and ovaries in same person (may be 46 XX or 46 XY).
Pseudohermaphroditism	Usually the result of endocrine or enzymatic defect (e.g., adrenal hyperplasia) in persons with normal chromosomes; female pseudohermaphrodites have masculine-looking genitals but are XX; male pseudohermaphrodites have rudimentary testes and external genitals and are XY; assigned as males or females, depending on morphology of genitals.

[a]Intersexual disorders include a variety of syndromes that produce persons with gross anatomical or physiological aspects of the opposite sex.

masculine behavior by adolescence. Fewer than 10% of children go on to transsexualism.

   2. Adults. Course tends to be chronic.

      a. Transsexualism—after puberty, distress with one's biological sex and a desire to eliminate one's primary and secondary sex characteristics and acquire those of the other sex. Most transsexuals have had gender identity disorder in childhood; cross-dressing is common; associated mental disorder is common, especially borderline personality disorder or depressive disorder; suicide is a risk, but persons may mutilate their sex organs to coerce surgeons to perform sex reassignment surgery.

G. Treatment

   1. Children. Improve existing role models or, in their absence, provide one from the family or elsewhere (e.g., big brother or sister). Caregivers are helped to encourage sex-appropriate behavior and attitudes. Any associated mental disorder is addressed.

   2. Adolescents. Difficult to treat because of the coexistence of normal identity crises and gender identity confusion. Acting out is common, and

Table 18–10
Paraphilias

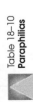

Disorder	Definition	General Considerations	Treatment
Exhibitionism	Exposing genitals in public; rare in females.	Person wants to shock female—her reaction is affirmation to patient that penis is intact.	Insight-oriented psychotherapy, aversive conditioning. Female should try to ignore exhibitionistic male, who is offensive but not dangerous, or call police.
Fetishism	Sexual arousal with inanimate objects (e.g., shoes, hair, clothing).	Almost always in men. Behavior often followed by guilt.	Insight-oriented psychotherapy; aversive conditioning; implosion, that is, patient masturbates with fetish until it loses its arousal effect (masturbatory satiation).
Frotteurism	Rubbing genitals against female to achieve arousal and orgasm.	Occurs in crowded places, such as subways usually by passive, nonassertive men.	Insight-oriented psychotherapy, aversive conditioning, group therapy, antiandrogenic medication.
Pedophilia	Sexual activity with children under age 13; most common paraphilia.	95% heterosexual, 5% homosexual. High risk of repeated behavior. Fear of adult sexuality in patient; low self-esteem. 10%–20% of children have been molested by age 18.	Place patient in treatment unit, group therapy, insight-oriented psychotherapy, antiandrogen medication to diminish sexual urge.
Sexual masochism	Sexual pleasure derived from being abused physically or mentally or from being humiliated (moral masochism).	Defense against guilt feelings related to sex—punishment turned inwards.	Insight-oriented psychotherapy; group therapy.
Sexual sadism	Sexual arousal resulting from causing mental or physical suffering to another person.	Mostly seen in men. Named after Marquis de Sade. Can progress to rape in some cases.	Insight-oriented psychotherapy; aversive conditioning.
Transvestic fetishism	Cross-dressing.	Most often used in heterosexual arousal. Most common is male-to-female cross-dressing. Do not confuse with transsexualism—wanting to be opposite sex.	Insight-oriented psychotherapy.
Voyeurism	Sexual arousal by watching sexual acts (e.g., coitus or naked person). Can occur in women but more common in men. Variant is listening to erotic conversations (e.g., telephone sex).	Masturbation usually occurs during voyeuristic activity. Usually arrested for loitering or peeping tomism.	Insight-oriented psychotherapy; aversive conditioning.
Other paraphilias Excretory paraphilias	Defecating (coprophilia) or urinating (urophilia) on a partner or vice versa	Fixation at anal stage of development; klismaphilia (enemas).	Insight-oriented psychotherapy.
Zoophilia	Sex with animals.	More common in rural areas; may be opportunistic.	Behavior modification; insight-oriented psychotherapy.

adolescents rarely have a strong motivation to alter their stereotypic cross-gender roles.

3. **Adults**

   a. **Psychotherapy**—set the goal of helping patients become comfortable with the gender identity they desire; the goal is not to create a person with a conventional sexual identity. Therapy also explores sex-reassignment surgery and the indications and contraindications for such procedures, which severely distressed and anxious patients often decide to undergo impulsively.

   b. **Sex-reassignment surgery**—definitive and irreversible. Patients must go through a 3- to 12-month trial of cross-dressing and receive hormone treatment. Seventy percent to 80% of patients are satisfied by the results. Dissatisfaction correlates with severity of preexisting psychopathology. A reported 2% commit suicide.

   c. **Hormonal treatments**—many patients are treated with hormones in lieu of surgery.

III. Paraphilias

These are disorders characterized by sexual impulses, fantasies, or practices that are unusual, deviant, or bizarre. More common in men than in women. Cause is unknown. A biological predisposition (abnormal electroencephalogram, hormone levels) may be reinforced by psychological factors, such as childhood abuse. Psychoanalytic theory holds that paraphilia results from fixation at one of the psychosexual phases of development or is an effort to ward off castration anxiety. Learning theory holds that association of the act with sexual arousal during childhood leads to conditioned learning.

Paraphiliac activity often is compulsive. Patients repeatedly engage in deviant behavior and are unable to control the impulse. When stressed, anxious, or depressed, the patient is more likely to engage in the deviant behavior. The patient may make numerous resolutions to stop the behavior but is generally unable to abstain for long, and acting out is followed by strong feelings of guilt. Treatment techniques, which result in only moderate success rates, include insight-oriented psychotherapy, behavior therapy, and pharmacotherapy alone or in combination. Table 18–10 lists the common paraphilias.

For more detailed discussion of this topic, see Normal Human Sexuality and Sexual and Gender Identity Disorder, Ch 18, p. 2027, in CTP/IX.

19

Eating Disorders

I. Anorexia Nervosa

Anorexia nervosa is a syndrome characterized by three essential criteria: (1) a self-induced starvation to a significant degree, (2) a relentless drive for thinness or a morbid fear of fatness, and (3) the presence of medical signs and symptoms resulting from starvation. It is often associated with disturbances of body image—the perception that one is distressingly large despite obvious thinness.

A. Epidemiology. The most common age of onset is between 14 and 18 years. Anorexia nervosa is estimated to occur in about 0.5% to 1% of adolescent girls. It occurs 10 to 20 times more often in females than in males. The prevalence of young women with some symptoms of anorexia nervosa who do not meet the diagnostic criteria is estimated to be close to 5%. It seems to be most frequent in developed countries, and it may be seen with greatest frequency among young women in professions that require thinness, such as modeling and ballet.

B. Etiology. Biological, social, and psychological factors are implicated in the causes of anorexia nervosa. Some evidence points to higher concordance rates in monozygotic twins than in dizygotic twins. Major mood disorders are more common in family members than in the general population.

1. **Biological factors.** Starvation results in many biochemical changes, some of which are also present in depression, such as hypercortisolemia and nonsuppression by dexamethasone. An increase in familial depression, alcohol dependence, or eating disorders has been noted. Some evidence of increased anorexia nervosa in sisters has also been noted. Neurobiologically, a reduction in 3-methoxy-4-hydroxyphenylglycol (MHPG) in urine and cerebrospinal fluid (CSF) suggests lessened norepinephrine turnover and activity. Endogenous opioid activity appears lessened as a consequence of starvation. In one positron emission tomography (PET) study, caudate nucleus metabolism was higher during the anorectic state than after weight gain. Magnetic resonance imaging (MRI) may show volume deficits of gray matter during illness, which may persist during recovery. A genetic predisposition may be a factor.

2. **Social factors.** Patients with anorexia nervosa find support for their practices in society's emphasis on thinness and exercise. Families of children who present with eating disorders, especially binge-eating or purging subtypes, may exhibit high levels of hostility, chaos, and isolation and low levels of nurturance and empathy. Vocational and avocational interests interact with other vulnerability factors to increase the probability of developing eating disorders (i.e., ballet in young women and wrestling in high school boys).

Table 19–1
DSM-IV-TR Diagnostic Criteria for Anorexia Nervosa

A. Refusal to maintain body weight at or above a minimally normal weight for age and height (e.g., weight loss leading to maintenance of body weight less than 85% of that expected; or failure to make expected weight gain during period of growth, leading to body weight less than 85% of that expected).
B. Intense fear of gaining weight or becoming fat, even though underweight.
C. Disturbance in the way in which one's body weight or shape is experienced, undue influence of body weight or shape on self-evaluation, or denial of the seriousness of the current low body weight.
D. In postmenarchal females, amenorrhea, i.e., the absence of at least three consecutive menstrual cycles. (A woman is considered to have amenorrhea if her periods occur only following hormone, e.g., estrogen, administration.)

Specify type:
Restricting type: during the current episode of anorexia nervosa, the person has not regularly engaged in binge-eating or purging behavior (i.e., self-induced vomiting or the misuse of laxatives, diuretics, or enemas)
Binge-eating/purging type: during the current episode of anorexia nervosa, the person has regularly engaged in binge-eating or purging behavior (i.e., self-induced vomiting or the misuse of laxatives, diuretics, or enemas)

From American Psychiatric Association. *Diagnostic and Statistical Manual of Mental Disorders*, 4th ed. Text rev. Washington, DC: American Psychiatric Association; 2000, with permission.

3. **Psychological and psychodynamic factors.** Patients with the disorder substitute their preoccupations, which are similar to obsessions, with eating and weight gain for other, normal adolescent pursuits. These patients typically lack a sense of autonomy and self-hood.
C. **Diagnosis and clinical features.** The onset of anorexia nervosa usually occurs between the ages of 10 and 30 years. It is present when (1) an individual voluntarily reduces and maintains an unhealthy degree of weight loss or fails to gain weight proportional to growth; (2) an individual experiences an intense fear of becoming fat, has a relentless drive for thinness despite obvious medical starvation, or both; (3) an individual experiences significant starvation-related medical symptomatology, often, but not exclusively, abnormal reproductive hormone functioning, but also hypothermia, bradycardia, orthostasis, and severely reduced body fat stores; and (4) the behaviors and psychopathology are present for at least 3 months (Table 19–1). Obsessive–compulsive behavior, depression, and anxiety are other psychiatric symptoms of anorexia nervosa most frequently noted in the literature. Poor sexual adjustment is frequently described in patients with the disorder.
D. **Subtypes**
1. **Restricting type (no binge eating).** Present in approximately 50% of cases. Food intake is highly restricted (usually with attempts to consume fewer than 300 to 500 calories per day and no fat grams), and the patient may be relentlessly and compulsively overactive, with overuse athletic injuries. Persons with restricting anorexia nervosa often have obsessive–compulsive traits with respect to food and other matters.
2. **Binge-eating/purging type.** Patients alternate attempts at rigorous dieting with intermittent binge or purge episodes, with the binges, if present, being either subjective (more than the patient intended, or because of

social pressure, but not enormous) or objective. Purging represents a secondary compensation for the unwanted calories, most often accomplished by self-induced vomiting, frequently by laxative abuse, less frequently by diuretics, and occasionally with emetics. The suicide rate is higher than in those with the restricting type.

E. Pathology and laboratory examination. A complete blood count often reveals leukopenia with a relative lymphocytosis in emaciated patients with anorexia nervosa. If binge eating and purging are present, serum electrolyte determination reveals hypokalemic alkalosis. Fasting serum glucose concentrations are often low during the emaciated phase, and serum salivary amylase concentrations are often elevated if the patient is vomiting. The ECG may show ST-segment and T-wave changes, which are usually secondary to electrolyte disturbances; emaciated patients have hypotension and bradycardia.

F. Differential diagnosis

1. **Medical conditions and substance use disorders.** Medical illness (e.g., cancer, brain tumor, gastrointestinal disorders, drug abuse) that can account for weight loss.

2. **Depressive disorder.** Depressive disorders and anorexia nervosa have several features in common, such as depressed feelings, crying spells, sleep disturbance, obsessive ruminations, and occasional suicidal thoughts. However, generally a patient with a depressive disorder has decreased appetite, whereas a patient with anorexia nervosa claims to have normal appetite and feels hungry; only in the severe stages of anorexia nervosa do patients actually have a decreased appetite. Also, in contrast to depressive agitation, the hyperactivity seen in anorexia nervosa is planned and ritualistic. The preoccupation with recipes, the caloric content of foods, and the preparation of gourmet feasts is typical with anorexia nervosa not with depressive disorder. In depressive disorders, patients have no intense fear of obesity or disturbance of body image. Comorbid major depression or dysthymia has been found in 50% of patients with anorexia.

3. **Somatization disorder.** Weight loss not as severe; no morbid fear of becoming overweight; amenorrhea unusual.

4. **Schizophrenia.** Delusions about food (e.g., patients believe the food to be poisoned). Patients rarely fear becoming obese and are not as hyperactive.

5. **Bulimia nervosa.** Patient's weight loss is seldom more than 15%. Bulimia nervosa develops in 30% to 50% of patients with anorexia nervosa within 2 years of the onset of anorexia.

 CLINICAL HINT:
Anorexia nervosa patients often give a history of few or no sexual experiences and generally have low libido, whereas bulimia patients are often sexually active with a normal or high libido.

G. Course and prognosis. The course of anorexia nervosa varies greatly—spontaneous recovery without treatment, recovery after a variety of treatments, a fluctuating course of weight gains followed by relapses, and a gradually deteriorating course resulting in death caused by complications of starvation. The short-term response of patients to almost all hospital treatment programs is good. Those who have regained sufficient weight, however, often continue their preoccupation with food and body weight, have poor social relationships, and exhibit depression. In general, the prognosis is not good. Studies have shown a range of mortality rates from 5% to 18%. About half of patients with anorexia nervosa eventually have the symptoms of bulimia, usually within the first year after the onset of anorexia nervosa.

H. Treatment

1. **Hospitalization.** The first consideration in the treatment of anorexia nervosa is to restore patients' nutritional state. Patients with anorexia nervosa who are 20% below the expected weight for their height are recommended for inpatient programs, and patients who are 30% below their expected weight require psychiatric hospitalization for 2 to 6 months. Inpatient psychiatric programs for patients with anorexia nervosa generally use a combination of a behavioral management approach, individual psychotherapy, family education and therapy, and, in some cases, psychotropic medications. Patients must become willing participants for treatment to succeed in the long run. After patients are discharged from the hospital, clinicians usually find it necessary to continue outpatient supervision of the problems identified in the patients and their families.

2. **Psychotherapy**

   a. **Cognitive–behavioral therapy (CBT).** Cognitive and behavioral therapy principles can be applied in both inpatient and outpatient settings.

   > Behavior therapy has been found effective for inducing weight gain; no large, controlled studies of cognitive therapy with behavior therapy in patients with anorexia nervosa have been reported. Patients are taught to monitor their food intake, their feelings and emotions, their binging and purging behaviors, and their problems in interpersonal relationships. Patients are taught cognitive restructuring to identify automatic thoughts and to challenge their core beliefs. Problem solving is a specific method whereby patients learn how to think through and devise strategies to cope with their food-related and interpersonal problems. Patients' vulnerability to rely on anorectic behavior as a means of coping can be addressed if they can learn to use these techniques effectively.

   b. **Dynamic Psychotherapy.** Patients' resistance may make the process difficult and painstaking. Because patients view their symptoms as constituting the core of their specialness, therapists must avoid excessive investment in trying to change their eating behavior.

   > The opening phase of the psychotherapy process must be geared to building a therapeutic alliance. Patients may experience early interpretations as though someone else were telling them what they really feel and thereby minimizing and invalidating their own experiences. Therapists who empathize with patients' points of view and take an active interest in what their patients think and feel, however, convey to patients that their autonomy is respected. Above all, psychotherapists must be flexible, persistent, and durable in the face of patients' tendencies to defeat any efforts to help them.

    c. Family Therapy. A family analysis should be done for all patients with anorexia nervosa who are living with their families, as a basis for a clinical judgment on what type of family therapy or counseling is advisable. In some cases, family therapy is not possible; however, issues of family relationships can then be addressed in individual therapy. Sometimes, brief counseling sessions with immediate family members is the extent of family therapy required.

3. Pharmacotherapy. Some reports support the use of cyproheptadine (Periactin), a drug with antihistaminic and antiserotonergic properties, for patients with the restricting type of anorexia nervosa. Amitriptyline (Elavil) has also been reported to have some benefit. Concern exists about the use of tricyclic drugs in low-weight, depressed patients with anorexia nervosa, who may be vulnerable to hypotension, cardiac arrhythmia, and dehydration. Once an adequate nutritional status has been attained, the risk of serious adverse effects from the tricyclic drugs may decrease; in some patients, the depression improves with weight gain and normalized nutritional status.

    Other medications that have been tried by patients with anorexia nervosa with variable results include clomipramine (Anafranil), pimozide (Orap), and chlorpromazine (Thorazine). Trials of fluoxetine (Prozac) have resulted in some reports of weight gain, and serotonergic agents may yield positive responses. In patients with anorexia nervosa and coexisting depressive disorders, the depressive condition should be treated.

II. Bulimia Nervosa

Bulimia nervosa is defined as binge eating combined with inappropriate ways of stopping weight gain. Social interruption or physical discomfort—that is, abdominal pain or nausea—terminates the binge eating, which is often followed by feelings of guilt, depression, or self-disgust. Unlike patients with anorexia nervosa, those with bulimia nervosa may maintain a normal body weight.

A. Epidemiology. Bulimia nervosa is more prevalent than anorexia nervosa. Estimates of bulimia nervosa range from 2% to 4% of young women. As with anorexia nervosa, bulimia nervosa is significantly more common in women than in men, but its onset is often later in adolescence than that of anorexia nervosa. The onset may even occur in early adulthood. Approximately 20% of college women experience transient bulimic symptoms at some point during their college years. Although bulimia nervosa is often present in normal-weight young women, they sometimes have a history of obesity. In industrialized countries, the prevalence is about 1% of the general population.

B. Etiology

    1. Biological factors. Serotonin and norepinephrine have been implicated. Because plasma endorphin levels are raised in some bulimia nervosa patients who vomit, the feeling of well-being after vomiting that some of these patients experience may be mediated by raised endorphin levels. Increased frequency of bulimia nervosa is found in first-degree relatives of persons with the disorder.

2. **Social factors.** Patients with bulimia nervosa, as with those with anorexia nervosa, tend to be high achievers and to respond to societal pressures to be slender. As with anorexia nervosa patients, many patients with bulimia nervosa are depressed and have increased familial depression, but the families of patients with bulimia nervosa are generally less close and more conflictual than the families of those with anorexia nervosa. Patients with bulimia nervosa describe their parents as neglectful and rejecting.

3. **Psychological factors.** Patients with bulimia nervosa have difficulties with adolescent demands, but are more outgoing, angry, and impulsive than patients with anorexia nervosa. Alcohol dependence, shoplifting, and emotional lability (including suicide attempts) are associated with bulimia nervosa. These patients generally experience their uncontrolled eating as more ego-dystonic and seek help more readily.

C. **Diagnosis and clinical features.** Bulimia nervosa is present when (1) episodes of binge eating occur relatively frequently (twice a week or more) for at least 3 months; (2) compensatory behaviors are practiced after binge eating to prevent weight gain—primarily self-induced vomiting, laxative abuse, use of diuretics, or abuse of emetics (80% of cases), and, less commonly, severe dieting and strenuous exercise (20% of cases); (3) weight is not severely lowered as in anorexia nervosa; and (4) the patient has a morbid fear of fatness, a relentless drive for thinness, or both and a disproportionate amount of self-evaluation depends on body weight and shape (Table 19–2). When making a diagnosis of bulimia nervosa, clinicians should explore the possibility that the patient has experienced a brief or prolonged prior bout

Table 19–2
DSM-IV-TR Diagnostic Criteria for Bulimia Nervosa

A. Recurrent episodes of binge eating. An episode of binge eating is characterized by both of the following:
  1. eating, in a discrete period of time (e.g., within any 2-hour period), an amount of food that is definitely larger than most people would eat during a similar period of time and under similar circumstances
  2. a sense of lack of control over eating during the episode (e.g., a feeling that one cannot stop eating or control what or how much one is eating)
B. Recurrent inappropriate compensatory behavior in order to prevent weight gain, such as self-induced vomiting; misuse of laxatives, diuretics, enemas, or other medications; fasting; or excessive exercise.
C. The binge eating and inappropriate compensatory behaviors both occur, on average, at least twice a week for 3 months.
D. Self-evaluation is unduly influenced by body shape and weight.
E. The disturbance does not occur exclusively during episodes of anorexia nervosa.
Specify type:
  Purging type: during the current episode of bulimia nervosa, the person has regularly engaged in self-induced vomiting or the misuse of laxatives, diuretics, or enemas
  Nonpurging type: during the current episode of bulimia nervosa, the person has used other inappropriate compensatory behaviors, such as fasting or excessive exercise, but has not regularly engaged in self-induced vomiting or the misuse of laxatives, diuretics, or enemas

From American Psychiatric Association. *Diagnostic and Statistical Manual of Mental Disorders*, 4th ed. Text rev. Washington, DC: American Psychiatric Association; 2000, with permission.

of anorexia nervosa, which is present in approximately half of those with bulimia nervosa. Binging usually precedes vomiting by about 1 year. Depression, sometimes called *postbinge anguish*, often follows the episode. During binges, patients eat food that is sweet, high in calories, and generally soft or smooth textured, such as cakes and pastry. The food is eaten secretly and rapidly and is sometimes not even chewed. Most patients are sexually active. Pica and struggles during meals are sometimes revealed in the histories of patients with bulimia nervosa.

D. Subtypes
1. **Purging type.** Patients regularly engage in self-induced vomiting or the use of laxatives or diuretics. May be at risk for certain medical complications, such as hypokalemia from vomiting or laxative abuse and hypochloremic alkalosis. Those who vomit repeatedly are at risk for gastric and esophageal tears, although these complications are rare.
2. **Nonpurging type (binge eaters).** Patients use strict dieting, fasting, or vigorous exercise, but do not regularly engage in purging. Patients tend to be obese.

E. Pathology and laboratory examinations. Bulimia nervosa can result in electrolyte abnormalities and various degrees of starvation. In general, thyroid function remains intact in bulimia nervosa, but patients may show nonsuppression on the dexamethasone suppression test. Dehydration and electrolyte disturbances are likely to occur in patients with bulimia nervosa who purge regularly. These patients commonly exhibit hypomagnesemia and hyperamylasemia. Although not a core diagnostic feature, many patients with bulimia nervosa have menstrual disturbances. Hypotension and bradycardia occur in some patients.

F. Differential diagnosis
1. **Anorexia nervosa.** The diagnosis of bulimia nervosa cannot be made if the binge-eating and purging behaviors occur exclusively during episodes of anorexia nervosa. In such cases, the diagnosis is anorexia nervosa, binge-eating/purging type.
2. **Neurological disease.** Clinicians must ascertain that patients have no neurological disease, such as epileptic-equivalent seizures, central nervous system tumors, Klüver–Bucy syndrome, or Kleine–Levin syndrome.
3. **Seasonal affective disorder.** Patients with bulimia nervosa who have concurrent seasonal affective disorder and patterns of atypical depression (with overeating and oversleeping in low-light months) may manifest seasonal worsening of both bulimia nervosa and depressive features. In these cases, binges are typically much more severe during winter months.
4. **Borderline personality disorder.** Patients sometimes binge eat, but the eating is associated with other signs of the disorder.
5. **Major depressive disorder.** Patients rarely have peculiar attitudes or idiosyncratic practices regarding food.

G. Course and prognosis. Bulimia nervosa is characterized by higher rates of partial and full recovery compared with anorexia nervosa. Those treated have a fair chance at recovery, much better than those who are untreated do. Untreated patients tend to remain chronic or may show small but generally unimpressive degrees of improvement with time. A history of substance use problems and a longer duration of the disorder at presentation predicted worse outcome.

H. Treatment

1. **Hospitalization.** Most patients with uncomplicated bulimia nervosa do not require hospitalization. In some cases—when eating binges are out of control, outpatient treatment does not work, or a patient exhibits such additional psychiatric symptoms as suicidality and substance abuse— hospitalization may become necessary. In addition, electrolyte and metabolic disturbances resulting from severe purging may necessitate hospitalization.

 CLINICAL HINT:
Bulimia patients should have careful dental checkups, as the acid content of vomit often erodes tooth enamel.

---

2. **Psychotherapy**
   a. **Cognitive–behavioral therapy.** CBT should be considered the bench- mark, first-line treatment for bulimia nervosa. CBT implements a number of cognitive and behavioral procedures to (1) interrupt the self-maintaining behavioral cycle of binging and dieting and (2) alter the individual's dysfunctional cognitions; beliefs about food, weight, body image; and overall self-concept.
   b. **Dynamic psychotherapy.** Psychodynamic treatment of patients with bulimia nervosa has revealed a tendency to concretize introjective and projective defense mechanisms. In a manner analogous to split- ting, patients divide food into two categories: items that are nutritious and those that are unhealthy. Food that is designated nutritious may be ingested and retained because it unconsciously symbolizes good introjects. But, junk food is unconsciously associated with bad intro- jects and, therefore, is expelled by vomiting, with the unconscious fantasy that all destructiveness, hate, and badness are being evacu- ated. Patients can temporarily feel good after vomiting because of the fantasized evacuation, but the associated feeling of "being all good" is short lived because it is based on an unstable combination of splitting and projection.
3. **Pharmacotherapy.** Antidepressant medications have been shown to be helpful in treating bulimia. This includes the selective serotonin reuptake inhibitors (SSRIs), such as fluoxetine. Imipramine (Tofranil), desipramine (Norpramin), trazodone (Desyrel), and monoamine oxidase inhibitors (MAOIs) have been helpful. In general, most of the antidepressants have

Table 19–3
DSM-IV-TR Diagnostic Criteria for Eating Disorder Not Otherwise Specified

The eating disorder not otherwise specified category is for disorders of eating that do not meet the criteria for any specific eating disorder. Examples include
1. For females, all of the criteria for anorexia nervosa are met except that the individual has regular menses.
2. All of the criteria for anorexia nervosa are met except that, despite significant weight loss, the individual's current weight is in the normal range.
3. All of the criteria for bulimia nervosa are met except that the binge eating and inappropriate compensatory mechanisms occur at a frequency of less than twice a week or for a duration of less than 3 months.
4. The regular use of inappropriate compensatory behavior by an individual of normal body weight after eating small amounts of food (e.g., self-induced vomiting after the consumption of two cookies).
5. Repeatedly chewing and spitting out, but not swallowing, large amounts of food.
6. Binge-eating disorder: recurrent episodes of binge eating in the absence of the regular use of inappropriate compensatory behaviors characteristic of bulimia nervosa.

From American Psychiatric Association. *Diagnostic and Statistical Manual of Mental Disorders*, 4th ed. Text rev. Washington, DC: American Psychiatric Association; 2000, with permission.

been effective at doses usually given in the treatment of depressive disorders. Carbamazepine (Tegretol) and lithium (Eskalith) have not shown impressive results as treatments for binge eating, but they have been used in the treatment of patients with bulimia nervosa with comorbid mood disorders, such as bipolar I disorder.

Table 19–4
DSM-IV-TR Research Criteria for Binge-Eating Disorder

A. Recurrent episodes of binge eating. An episode of binge eating is characterized by both of the following:
   1. eating, in a discrete period of time (e.g., within any 2-hour period), an amount of food that is definitely larger than what most people would eat in a similar period of time under similar circumstances
   2. a sense of lack of control over eating during the episode (e.g., a feeling that one cannot stop eating or control what or how much one is eating)
B. The binge-eating episodes are associated with three (or more) of the following:
   1. eating much more rapidly than normal
   2. eating until feeling uncomfortably full
   3. eating large amounts of food when not feeling physically hungry
   4. eating alone because of being embarrassed by how much one is eating
   5. feeling disgusted with oneself, depressed, or very guilty after overeating
C. Marked distress regarding binge eating is present.
D. The binge eating occurs, on average, at least 2 days a week for 6 months.
   Note: The method of determining frequency differs from that used for bulimia nervosa; future research should address whether the preferred method of setting a frequency threshold is counting the number of days on which binges occur or counting the number of episodes of binge eating.
E. The binge eating is not associated with the regular use of inappropriate compensatory behaviors (e.g., purging, fasting, excessive exercise) and does not occur exclusively during the course of anorexia nervosa or bulimia nervosa.

From American Psychiatric Association. *Diagnostic and Statistical Manual of Mental Disorders*, 4th ed. Text rev. Washington, DC: American Psychiatric Association; 2000, with permission.

III. Eating Disorder Not Otherwise Specified

The text revision of the fourth edition of the *Diagnostic Statistical Manual of Mental Disorders* (*DSM-IV-TR*) diagnostic classification eating disorder not otherwise specified is a residual category used for eating disorders that do not meet the criteria for a specific eating disorder (Table 19–3). Binge-eating disorder—that is, recurrent episodes of binge eating in the absence of the inappropriate compensatory behaviors characteristic of bulimia nervosa (Table 19–4)—falls into this category. Such patients are not fixated on body shape and weight.

For more detailed discussion of this topic, see Eating Disorders, Ch 19, p. 2128 in CTP/IX.

Obesity and the Metabolic Syndrome

I. Introduction

In industrialized nations, the prevalence of obesity has reached epidemic proportions. It is associated with increased morbidity and mortality and is the leading cause of preventable death in the United States.

II. Definition

Obesity refers to an excess of body fat.

A. In healthy individuals, body fat accounts for approximately 25% of body weight in women and 18% in men.

B. Overweight refers to weight above some reference norm, typically standards derived from actuarial or epidemiological data. In most cases, increasing weight reflects increasing obesity.

C. Body mass index (BMI) is calculated by dividing weight in kilograms by height in meters squared. Although there is debate about the ideal BMI, it is generally thought that a BMI of 20 to 25 kg^2 represents healthy weight, a BMI of 25 to 27 kg^2 is associated with somewhat elevated risk, a BMI above 27 kg/m^2 represents clearly increased risk, and a BMI above 30 kg/m^2 carries greatly increased risk.

III. Epidemiology

A. In the United States, over 50% of the population is overweight (defined as a BMI of 25.0 to 29.9 kg/m^2), whereas 30% are obese (defined as a BMI >30 kg/m^2). Extreme obesity (BMI ≥ 40 kg/m^2) is found in about 3% of men and 7% of women.

B. The prevalence of obesity is highest in minority populations, particularly among non-Hispanic black women.

C. More than one half of these individuals 40 years of age or older are obese and more than 80% are overweight.

D. The prevalence of overweight and obesity in children and adolescents in the United States has also increased substantially. About 18% of adolescents and about 10% of 2- to 5-year-olds are overweight.

IV. Etiology

Persons accumulate fat by eating more calories than are expended as energy, thus intake of energy exceeds its dissipation. If fat is to be removed from the body, fewer calories must be put in or more calories must be taken out than are put in. An error of no more than 10% in either intake or output would lead to a 30-pound change in body weight in 1 year's time.

A. Satiety. The feeling that results when hunger is satisfied is satiety. A metabolic signal derived from food receptor cells, probably in the hypothalamus, produce satiety. Studies have shown evidence for dysfunction in serotonin, dopamine, and norepinephrine involvement in regulating eating behavior through the hypothalamus. Other hormonal factors that may be involved include corticotrophin releasing factor, neuropeptide Y, gonadotropin-releasing hormone, and thyroid-stimulating hormone. A new substance, obestatin, made in the stomach, is a hormone that, in animal experiments, produces satiety and may have potential use as a weight-loss agent in humans.

Eating is also affected by cannabinoid receptors, which, when stimulated, increases appetite. Marijuana acts on that receptor, which accounts for the "munchies" associated with marijuana use. The drug rimonabant is an inverse agonist to the cannabidiol receptor, meaning that it blocks appetite. It may have clinical use.

B. Olfactory system. The olfactory system may play a role in satiety. Experiments have shown that strong stimulation of the olfactory bulbs in the nose with food odors by use of an inhaler saturated with a particular smell produces satiety for that food. This may have implications for therapy of obesity.

V. Factors that Contribute to Obesity

A. Genetic factors. About 80% of patients who are obese have a family history of obesity, although no specific genetic marker of obesity has been found. Studies show that identical twins raised apart can both be obese, an observation that suggests a hereditary role.

B. Developmental factors

1. Obesity that begins early in life is characterized by adipose tissue with an increased number of adipocytes (fat cells) of increased size. Obesity that begins in adult life, on the other hand, results solely from an increase in the size of the adipocytes. In both instances, weight reduction produces a decrease in cell size.

2. The distribution and amount of fat vary in individuals, and fat in different body areas has different characteristics. Fat cells around the waist, flanks, and abdomen (the so-called potbelly) are more active metabolically than those in the thighs and buttocks.

3. A hormone called leptin, made by fat cells, acts as a fat thermostat. When the blood level of leptin is low, more fat is consumed; when it is high, less fat is consumed.

C. Physical activity factors. The marked decrease in physical activity in affluent societies seems to be the major factor in the rise of obesity as a public health problem. Physical inactivity restricts energy expenditure and may contribute to increased food intake. Although food intake increases with increasing energy expenditure over a wide range of energy demands, intake does not decrease proportionately when physical activity falls below a certain minimum level.

D. Brain-damage factors. Destruction of the ventromedial hypothalamus can produce obesity in animals, but this is probably a very rare cause of obesity in humans. There is evidence that the central nervous system, particularly in the lateral and ventromedial hypothalamic areas, adjusts to food intake in response to changing energy requirements so as to maintain fat stores at a baseline determined by a specific set point. This set point varies from one person to another and depends on height and body build.

E. Health factors

1. In only a small number of cases of obesity, the consequence is identifiable illness. Such cases include a variety of rare genetic disorders, such as Prader-Willi syndrome, as well as neuroendocrine abnormalities. Hypothalamic obesity results from damage to the ventromedial region of the hypothalamus (VMH), which has been studied extensively in laboratory animals and is a known center of appetite and weight regulation. In humans, damage to the VMH may result from trauma, surgery, malignancy, or inflammatory disease.

2. Some forms of depression, particularly seasonal affective disorder, are associated with weight gain. Most persons who live in seasonal climates report increases in appetite and weight during the fall and winter months, with decreases in the spring and summer. Depressed patients usually lose weight, but some gain weight (e.g., atypical depression).

F. Other factors

1. **Clinical disorders.** A variety of clinical disorders are associated with obesity. Cushing's disease is associated with a characteristic fat distribution and moonlike face. Myxedema is associated with weight gain, although not invariably. Other neuroendocrine disorders include adiposogenital dystrophy (Fröhlich's syndrome), which is characterized by obesity and sexual and skeletal abnormalities.

2. **Psychotropic drugs.** Long-term use of steroid medications is associated with significant weight gain, as is the use of several psychotropic agents. Patients treated for major depression, psychotic disturbances, and bipolar disorder typically gain 3 to 10 kg, with even larger gains with chronic use. This can produce the so-called metabolic syndrome discussed later.

3. **Psychological factors.** Although psychological factors are evidently crucial to the development of obesity, how such psychological factors result in obesity is not known. The food-regulating mechanism is susceptible to environmental influence, and cultural, family, and psychodynamic factors have all been shown to contribute to the development of obesity. Although many investigators have proposed that specific family histories, precipitating factors, personality structures, or unconscious conflicts cause obesity, overweight persons may suffer from any conceivable psychiatric disorder and come from a variety of disturbed backgrounds. Many obese patients are emotionally disturbed persons who, because of the availability of the overeating mechanism in their environments, have learned to use hyperphagia as a means of coping with psychological problems. Some patients may

show signs of serious mental disorder when they attain normal weight because they no longer have that coping mechanism.

VI. Diagnosis and Clinical Features

The diagnosis of obesity, if done in a sophisticated way, involves the assessment of body fat. Because this is rarely practical, the use of height and weight to calculate BMI is recommended.

In most cases of obesity, it is not possible to identify the precise etiology, given the multitude of possible causes and their interactions. Instances of secondary obesity are rare but should not be overlooked.

The habitual eating patterns of many obese persons often seem similar to patterns found in experimental obesity. Impaired satiety is a particularly important problem. Obese persons seem inordinately susceptible to food cues in their environment, to the palatability of foods, and to the inability to stop eating if food is available. Obese persons are usually susceptible to all kinds of external stimuli to eating, but they remain relatively unresponsive to the usual internal signals of hunger. Some are unable to distinguish between hunger and other kinds of dysphoria.

VII. Differential Diagnosis

A. The night-eating syndrome, in which persons eat excessively after they have had their evening meal, seems to be precipitated by stressful life circumstances and, once present, tends to recur daily until the stress is alleviated. Night eating may also occur as a result of using sedatives to sleep that may produce sleep-walking and eating. This has been reported with the use of zolpidem (Ambien) in patients.

B. The binge-eating syndrome (bulimia) is characterized by the sudden, compulsive ingestion of very large amounts of food in a short time, usually with great subsequent agitation and self-condemnation. Binge eating also appears to represent a reaction to stress. In contrast to the night-eating syndrome, however, these bouts of overeating are not periodic, and they are far more often linked to specific precipitating circumstances. (See Section 19.2 for a complete discussion of bulimia.) The Pickwickian syndrome is said to exist when a person is 100% over desirable weight and has associated respiratory and cardiovascular pathology.

C. Body dysmorphic disorder (dysmorphophobia). Some obese persons feel that their bodies are grotesque and loathsome and that others view them with hostility and contempt. This feeling is closely associated with self-consciousness and impaired social functioning. Emotionally healthy obese persons have no body image disturbances, and only a minority of neurotic obese persons has such disturbances. The disorder is confined mainly to persons who have been obese since childhood; even among them, less than half suffer from it. (Body dysmorphic disorder is discussed further in Chapter 16 on Somatoform Disorders.)

Table 20–1
Metabolic Syndrome: T or More Risk Factors Required for NCEP Definition

Risk Factor	Defining Level
Abdominal obesity	**Waist circumference (at umbilicus)**
Men	>102 cm (>40 in)
Women	>88 cm (>35 in)
Triglycerides	≥150 mg/dL
Men	<40 mg/dL
Women	<50 mg/dL
Blood pressure	≥130/≥85 mm Hg
Fasting glucose	≥100 mg/dL

NCEP, National Cholesterol Education Program.

VIII. Metabolic Syndrome

The metabolic syndrome consists of a cluster of metabolic abnormalities associated with obesity and that contribute to an increased risk of cardiovascular disease and type II diabetes. The syndrome is diagnosed when a patient has three or more of the following five risk factors: (1) abdominal obesity, (2) high triglyceride level, (3) low high-density lipoprotein (HDL) cholesterol level, (4) hypertension, and (5) an elevated fasting blood glucose level. (See Table 20–1.) The syndrome is believed to occur in about 30% of the U.S. population, but it is also well known in other industrialized countries around the world.

The cause of the syndrome is unknown, but obesity, insulin resistance, and a genetic vulnerability are involved. Treatment involves weight loss, exercise, and the use of statins and antihypertensives as needed to lower lipid levels and blood pressure. Because of the increased risk of mortality, it is important that the syndrome be recognized early and treated.

Second-generation (atypical) antipsychotic medication has been implicated as a cause of metabolic syndrome. In patients with schizophrenia, treatment with these medications can cause a rapid increase in body weight in the first few months of therapy that may continue for more than 1 year. In addition, insulin resistance leading to type II diabetes has been associated with an atherogenic lipid profile.

Clozapine and olanzapine (Zyprexa) are the two drugs most implicated, but other atypical antipsychotics may also be involved. Patients who are prescribed second-generation antipsychotic medication should be monitored periodically with fasting blood glucose levels at the beginning of treatment and during its course. Lipid profiles should also be obtained. Children, adolescents, and young adults are the most likely groups to gain weight from these drugs.

Psychological reactions to the metabolic syndrome depend on the signs and symptoms experienced by the patient. Those who suffer primarily from obesity must deal with self-esteem issues from being overweight as well as the stress of participating in weight loss programs. In many cases of obesity, eating is a way of satisfying deep-seated dependency needs. As weight is lost, some patients become depressed or anxious. Cases of psychosis have been reported in a few markedly obese patients during or after the process of losing a vast amount of weight. Other metabolic discrepancies, particularly variations in blood sugar, may be accompanied by irritability or other mood changes. Finally, fatigue is a common occurrence in patients with this syndrome. As the condition improves, especially if exercise is part of the regimen, fatigue eventually diminishes, but patients may be misdiagnosed as having a dysthymic disorder or chronic fatigue syndrome if metabolic causes of fatigue are not considered.

IX. Course and Prognosis

A. Effects on health

1. Obesity has adverse effects on health and is associated with a broad range of illnesses. There is a strong correlation between obesity and cardiovascular disorders. Hypertension (blood pressure >160/95 mm Hg) is three times higher for persons who are overweight, and hypercholesterolemia (blood cholesterol >250 mg/dL) is twice as common.

2. Studies show that blood pressure and cholesterol levels can be reduced by weight reduction. Diabetes, which has clear genetic determinations, can often be modified with weight reduction, especially type II diabetes (mature-onset or noninsulin-dependent diabetes mellitus).

3. Obese men, regardless of smoking habits, have a higher mortality from colon, rectal, and prostate cancer than men of normal weight. Obese women have a higher mortality from cancer of the gallbladder, biliary passages, breast (postmenopause), uterus (including cervix and endometrium), and ovaries than women of normal weight.

B. Longevity

1. The more overweight a person is, the higher that person's risk for death is. A person who reduces weight to acceptable levels has a mortality decline to normal rates.

2. Weight reduction may be lifesaving for patients with extreme obesity, defined as weight that is twice the desirable weight. Such patients may have cardiorespiratory failure, especially when asleep (sleep apnea).

3. A number of studies have demonstrated that decreasing caloric intake by 30% or more in young or middle-aged laboratory animals prevents or retards age-related chronic diseases and significantly prolongs maximal life span.

C. Prognosis

1. The prognosis for weight reduction is poor, and the course of obesity tends toward inexorable progression. Of patients who lose significant amounts of weight, 90% regain it eventually. The prognosis is particularly poor for those who become obese in childhood.

2. Juvenile-onset obesity tends to be more severe, more resistant to treatment, and more likely to be associated with emotional disturbance than is adult obesity.

X. Treatment

A. Diet

1. The basis of weight reduction is simple—establish a caloric deficit by bringing intake below output. The simplest way to reduce caloric intake is by means of a low-calorie diet. The best long-term effects are achieved with a balanced diet that contains readily available foods. For most persons, the most satisfactory reducing diet consists of their usual foods in amounts determined with the aid of tables of food values that are available in standard books on dieting. Such a diet gives the best chance of long-term maintenance of weight loss.

2. Total unmodified fasts are used for short-term weight loss, but they have associated morbidity including orthostatic hypotension, sodium diuresis, and impaired nitrogen balance.

3. Ketogenic diets are high-protein, high-fat diets used to promote weight loss. They have a high cholesterol content and produce ketosis, which is associated with nausea, hypotension, and lethargy.

4. In general, the best method of weight loss is a balanced diet of 1,100 to 1,200 calories. Such a diet can be followed for long periods but should be supplemented with vitamins, particularly iron, folic acid, zinc, and vitamin B_6.

B. Exercise

1. Increased physical activity is an important part of a weight-reduction regimen. Because caloric expenditure in most forms of physical activity is directly proportional to body weight, obese persons expend more calories than persons of normal weight with the same amount of activity.

2. Increased physical activity may actually decrease food intake by formerly sedentary persons. This combination of increased caloric expenditure and decreased food intake makes an increase in physical activity a highly desirable feature of any weight-reduction program.

3. Exercise also helps maintain weight loss.

C. Pharmacotherapy

1. Drug treatment is effective because it suppresses appetite, but tolerance to this effect may develop after several weeks of use. An initial trial period of 4 weeks with a specific drug can be used; then, if the patient responds with weight loss, the drug can be continued to see whether tolerance develops.

2. One weight-loss medication approved by the Food and Drug Administration (FDA) for long-term use (in 1999) is orlistat (Xenical), which is a selective gastric and pancreatic lipase inhibitor that reduces the absorption of dietary fat (which is then excreted in stool). In clinical trials, orlistat (120 mg, three times a day), in combination with a low-calorie diet, induced losses of approximately 10% of initial weight in the first 6 months, which were generally well maintained for periods up to 24 months.

3. Another medication, Sibutramine (Meridia) is a β-phenylethylamine that inhibits the reuptake of serotonin and norepinephrine (and dopamine to a limited extent). It was approved by the FDA in 1997 for weight loss and the maintenance of weight loss (i.e., long-term use).

4. **Rimonabant**

   a. Rimonabant has a unique mechanism of action: It is a selective cannabinoid-1 receptor blocker. Rimonabant has been shown to reduce body weight and improve cardiovascular risk factors in obese patients.

   b. It appears to help suppress metabolic abnormalities that lead to type II diabetes, obesity, and atherosclerosis. The use of Rimonabant to mitigate psychopharmacological metabolic disturbances may be justified in some patients.

D. Surgery

1. Surgical methods that cause malabsorption of food or reduce gastric volume have been used in persons who are markedly obese.

2. *Gastric bypass* is a procedure in which the stomach is made smaller by transecting or stapling one of the stomach curvatures.

3. In *gastroplasty,* the size of the stomach stoma is reduced so that the passage of food slows. Results are successful, although vomiting, electrolyte imbalance, and obstruction may occur.

> A syndrome called dumping, which consists of palpitations, weakness, and sweating, may follow surgical procedures in some patients if they ingest large amounts of carbohydrates in a single meal. The surgical removal of fat (lipectomy) has no effect on weight loss in the long run nor does liposuction, which has value only for cosmetic reasons. Bariatric surgery is now recommended in individuals who have serious obesity-related health complications and a BMI of greater than 35 kg/m² (or a BMI >40 kg/m² in the absence of major health complications). Before surgery, candidates should have tried to lose weight using the safer, more traditional options of diet, exercise, and weight loss medication.

E. Psychotherapy. Some patients may respond to insight-oriented psychodynamic therapy with weight loss, but this treatment has not had much success. Uncovering the unconscious causes of overeating may not alter the behavior of persons who overeat in response to stress, although it may serve to augment other treatment methods. Years after successful psychotherapy, many persons who overeat under stress continue to do so. Obese persons seem particularly vulnerable to overdependency on a therapist, and the inordinate regression that may occur during the uncovering psychotherapies should be carefully monitored.

Behavior modification has been the most successful of the therapeutic approaches for obesity and is considered the method of choice. Patients are taught to recognize external cues that are associated with eating and to keep diaries of foods consumed in particular circumstances, such as at the movies or while watching television, or during certain emotional states, such as anxiety or depression. Patients are also taught to develop new eating patterns, such as eating slowly, chewing food well, not reading while eating, and not eating between meals or when not seated. Operant conditioning therapies that use rewards such as praise or new clothes to reinforce weight loss have also been successful. Group therapy helps to maintain motivation, to promote identification among members who have lost weight, and to provide education about nutrition.

For further reading on this subject please refer to Obesity, Section 24.4, p. 2273, CTP IX.

21
Sleep Disorders

I. General Introduction

Sleep is a universal behavior that has been demonstrated in every animal species studied, from insects to mammals. It is one of the most significant of human behaviors, occupying roughly one third of human life. Approximately 30% of adults in the United States experience a sleep disorder during their lifetime, and over half do not seek treatment. Lack of sleep can lead to the inability to concentrate, memory complaints, deficits in neuropsychological testing, and decreased libido. Additionally, sleep disorders can have serious consequences, including fatal accidents related to sleepiness. Disturbed sleep can be a primary diagnosis itself or a component of another medical or psychiatric disorder (Table 21–1). Careful diagnosis and specific treatment are essential. Female sex, advanced age, medical and mental disorders, and substance abuse are associated with an increased prevalence of sleep disorders.

In the text revision of the fourth edition of the *Diagnostic Statistical Manual of Mental Disorders* (*DSM-IV-TR*), sleep disorders are classified on the basis of clinical diagnostic criteria and presumed etiology. The three major categories are (1) primary sleep disorders, (2) sleep disorders related to another mental disorder, and (3) other sleep disorders (due to a general medical condition and substance induced).

A. Sleep stages. Sleep is comprised of two physiological states: rapid eye movement (REM) sleep and nonrapid eye movement (NREM) sleep. NREM sleep consists of four sleep stages, named stage I through stage IV. Dreaming occurs mostly in REM sleep, but additionally, some dreaming occurs in stages III and IV sleep. Sleep is measured with a polysomnograph, which simultaneously measures brain activity (electroencephalogram [EEG]), eye movement (electrooculogram), and muscle tone (electromyogram). Other physiological tests can be applied during sleep and measured along with the above. EEG findings are used to describe sleep stages (Table 21–2).

It takes the average person 15 to 20 minutes to fall asleep; this is the sleep latency. During the next 45 minutes, one descends from stages I and II of sleep to stages III and IV. Stages III and IV comprise the deepest sleep; that is, the largest stimulus is needed to arouse one in these stages of sleep. Approximately 45 minutes after stage IV begins, the first REM period is reached. Therefore, the average REM latency (the time from sleep onset to REM onset) is 90 minutes. Throughout the night, one cycles through the four stages of sleep followed by REM sleep. As the night progresses, each REM period becomes longer, and stages III and IV disappear. Hence, further into the night, persons sleep more lightly and dream (mostly REM sleep) more. The sleep stages in an adult are approximately 25% REM sleep and 75% NREM sleep, consisting of 5% in stage I, 45% in stage II, 12% in stage III, and 13% in stage IV.

Table 21-1
Common Causes of Insomnia

Symptom	Insomnia Secondary to Medical Conditions	Insomnia Secondary to Psychiatric or Environmental Conditions
Difficulty in falling asleep	Any painful or uncomfortable condition CNS lesions Conditions listed below, at times	Anxiety Tension anxiety, muscular Environmental changes Circadian rhythm sleep disorder
Difficulty in remaining asleep	Sleep apnea syndromes Nocturnal myoclonus and restless legs syndrome Dietary factors (probably) Episodic events (parasomnias) Direct substance effects (including alcohol) Substance withdrawal effects (including alcohol) Substance interactions Endocrine or metabolic diseases Infectious, neoplastic, or other diseases Painful or uncomfortable conditions Brainstem or hypothalamic lesions or diseases Aging	Depression, especially primary depression Environmental changes Circadian rhythm sleep disorder Posttraumatic stress disorder Schizophrenia

Courtesy of Ernest L. Hartmann, M.D.

B. Characteristics of REM sleep (also called paradoxical sleep)

1. Autonomic instability
   a. Increased heart rate (HR), blood pressure (BP), and respiratory rate (RR).
   b. Increased variability in HR, BP, and RR from minute to minute.
   c. Appears similar to an awake person on EEG.
2. Tonic inhibition of skeletal muscle tone leading to paralysis.
3. Rapid eye movements.
4. Dreaming.
5. Reduced hypercapnic respiratory drive, no increase in tidal volume as partial pressure of carbon dioxide decreases.

Table 21-2
Sleep Stages

Awake:	Low voltage, random, very fast
Drowsy:	Alpha waves (8–12 CPS), random and fast
Stage I:	Theta waves (3–7 CPS), slight slowing
Stage II:	Further slowing, K complex (triphasic complexes), sleep spindles, true sleep onset
Stage III:	Delta waves (0.5–2 CPS), high amplitude slow waves.
Stage IV:	At least 50% delta waves. Stages III and IV comprise delta sleep.
REM:	Sawtooth waves, similar to drowsy sleep on EEG

CPS, cycles per second.

6. Relative poikilothermia (cold-bloodedness).

7. Penile tumescence or vaginal lubrication.

8. Reduced sensitivity to sounds.

II. Primary Sleep Disorders

The *DSM-IV-TR* defines primary sleep disorders as those not caused by another mental disorder, a physical condition, or a substance but, rather, are caused by an abnormal sleep–wake mechanism and often by conditioning. The two main primary sleep disorders are dyssomnias and parasomnias.

A. Dyssomnias. A heterogeneous group of sleep disorders characterized by abnormalities in the quality, amount, or timing of sleep.

1. Primary insomnia. Diagnosed when the chief complaint is difficulty in initiating or maintaining sleep or nonrestorative sleep for at least 1 month.

a. Insomnia is the most common type of sleep disorder.

b. Causes are listed in Table 21–1.

c. Treatment includes deconditioning techniques, transcendental meditation, relaxation tapes, sedative–hypnotic drugs, and nonspecific measures, such as sleep hygiene, described in Table 21–3.

2. Primary hypersomnia. Diagnosed when there is no other cause found for greater than 1 month of excessive somnolence (daytime sleepiness) or excessive amounts of daytime sleep. Usually begins in childhood. Treatment consists of stimulant drugs.

3. Narcolepsy

a. Narcolepsy consists of the following characteristics:

(1) Excessive daytime somnolence (sleep attacks) is the primary symptom of narcolepsy.

(a) Distinguished from fatigue by irresistible sleep attacks of short duration (less than 15 minutes).

(b) Sleep attacks may be precipitated by monotonous or sedentary activity.

(c) Naps are highly refreshing and effects usually last 30 to 120 minutes.

Table 21–3
Nonspecific Measures to Induce Sleep (Sleep Hygiene)

1. Arise at the same time daily.
2. Limit daily in-bed time to the usual amount before the sleep disturbance.
3. Discontinue CNS-acting drugs (caffeine, nicotine, alcohol, stimulants).
4. Avoid daytime naps (except when sleep chart shows they induce better night sleep).
5. Establish physical fitness by means of a graded program of vigorous exercise early in the day.
6. Avoid evening stimulation; substitute radio or relaxed reading for television.
7. Try very hot, 20-minute, body temperature–raising bath soaks near bedtime.
8. Eat at regular times daily; avoid large meals near bedtime.
9. Practice evening relaxation routines, such as progressive muscle relaxation or meditation.
10. Maintain comfortable sleeping conditions.

From Regestein QR. Sleep disorders. In: Stoudemire A, ed. *Clinical Psychiatry for Medical Students.* Philadelphia: Lippincott, 1990:578.

   (2) Cataplexy

      (a) Reported by over 50% of narcoleptic patients.

      (b) Brief (seconds to minutes) episodes of muscle weakness or paralysis.

      (c) No loss of consciousness if episode is brief.

      (d) When attack is over, the patient is completely normal.

      (e) May manifest as partial loss of muscle tone (weakness, slurred speech, buckled knees, dropped jaw).

      (f) Often triggered by laughter (common), anger (common), athletic activity, excitement or elation, sexual intercourse, fear, or embarrassment.

      (g) Flat affect or lack of expressiveness develops in some patients as an attempt to control emotions.

      (h) A diagnosis of cataplexy automatically results in a diagnosis of narcolepsy. If cataplexy does not occur, multiple other characteristics are necessary for the diagnosis of narcolepsy.

   (3) Sleep paralysis

      (a) Temporary partial or complete paralysis in sleep–wake transitions.

      (b) Conscious but unable to move or open eyes.

      (c) Most commonly occurs on awakening.

      (d) Generally described as an anxiety-provoking, "scary" event.

      (e) Generally lasts less than 1 minute.

      (f) Reported by 25% to 50% of the general population, though for a much shorter duration.

   (4) Hypnagogic and hypnopompic hallucinations

      (a) Dreamlike experience during transition from wakefulness to sleep and vice versa.

      (b) Vivid auditory or visual hallucinations or illusions.

   (5) Sleep-onset REM periods (SOREMPs)

      (a) Defined as appearance of REM within 15 minutes of sleep onset (normally approximately 90 minutes).

      (b) Narcolepsy can be distinguished from other disorders of excessive daytime sleepiness by SOREMPs seen on polysomnographic recording.

      (c) A multiple sleep latency test (MSLT) measures excessive sleepiness. An MSLT consists of at least four recorded naps at 2-hour intervals. More than two SOREMPs is considered diagnostic of narcolepsy (seen in 70% of patients with narcolepsy, in fewer than 10% of patients with other hypersomnias).

b. Increased incidence of other clinical findings in narcolepsy:

   (1) Periodic leg movement.

   (2) Sleep apnea—predominantly central.

   (3) Short sleep latency.

   (4) Frequent nighttime arousals; from REM sleep to stage I or wakefulness, the patient usually is unaware of the awakenings.

(5) Memory problems.

(6) Ocular symptoms—blurring, diplopia, flickering.

(7) Depression.

(8) Automatic behaviors can occur for which people have no memory.

c. Onset and clinical course.

(1) Typically, full syndrome emerges in late adolescence or early 20s.

(2) Once established, condition is chronic without major remissions.

(3) A long delay may occur between the earliest symptoms (excessive somnolence) and the late appearance of cataplexy.

d. Causes.

(1) Plausibly caused by an abnormality of REM-inhibiting mechanisms.

(2) Human leukocyte antigen (HLA)-DR2 and narcolepsy.

(a) Strong (greater than 70%) association between narcolepsy and HLA-DR2, a type of human lymphocyte antigen.

(b) HLA-DR2 is also found in up to 30% of unaffected persons.

(3) Recent research involving hypocretin, a neurotransmitter, suggests that hypocretin is significantly reduced in narcolepsy patients.

e. Treatment.

(1) Regular bedtime.

(2) Daytime naps scheduled at a regular time of day.

(3) Safety considerations, such as caution while driving and avoiding furniture with sharp edges.

(4) Stimulants (e.g., modafinil [Provigil]) for daytime sleepiness. High-dose propranolol (Inderal) may be effective.

(5) Tricyclics and selective serotonin reuptake inhibitors (SSRIs) for REM-related symptoms, especially cataplexy. Other treatments are listed in Table 21–4.

4. **Breathing-related sleep disorder.** Characterized by sleep disruption that is caused by a sleep-related breathing disturbance, leading to excessive sleepiness, insomnia, or hypersomnia. Breathing disturbances include apneas, hypoapneas, and oxygen desaturations.

a. **Apnea.** The three types of sleep apnea are (1) obstructive, (2) central, and (3) mixed. Greater than 40% of patients evaluated for somnolence using polysomnography are found to have sleep apnea. Sleep apnea may account for a number of unexplained deaths.

(1) **Obstructive sleep apnea**

(a) Caused by cessation of air flow through the nose or mouth in the presence of continuing thoracic breathing movements, resulting in decreases in arterial oxygen saturation and a transient arousal, after which respiration resumes normally.

(b) Typically occurs in middle-aged, overweight men (Pickwickian syndrome).

(c) Also occurs more frequently in patients with smaller jaws or micrognathia, acromegaly, and hypothyroidism.

Table 21–4
Narcolepsy Drugs Currently Available

Drug	Maximal Daily Dosage (mg) (All Drugs Administered Orally)
Treatment of excessive daytime somnolence (EDS)	
Stimulants	
Methylphenidate	≤60
Pemoline	≤150
Modafinil	≤400
Amphetamine–dextroamphetamine	≤60
Dextroamphetamine	≤60
Adjunct-effect drugs (i.e., improve EDS if associated with stimulant)	
Protriptyline	≤10
Treatment of cataplexy, sleep paralysis, and hypnagogic hallucinations	
Tricyclic antidepressants (with atropinelike side effects)	
Protriptyline	≤20
Imipramine	≤200
Clomipramine	≤200
Desipramine	≤200
Antidepressants (without major atropinelike side effects)	
Bupropion	≤300
SSRIs	
Sertraline	≤200
Citalopram	≤40

Adapted from Guilleminault C. Narcolepsy syndrome. In: Kryger MH, Roth T, Dement WC, eds. *Principles and Practice of Sleep Medicine.* Philadelphia: Saunders, 1989:344, with permission.

(d) Main symptoms are loud snoring with intervals of apnea.

(e) Additional symptoms include extreme daytime sleepiness with long and unrefreshing daytime sleep attacks.

(f) Other symptoms include severe morning headaches, morning confusion, depression, and anxiety.

(g) Medical consequences include cardiac arrhythmias, systemic and pulmonary hypertension, and decreased sexual drive or function with progressive worsening without treatment.

(h) Apneic events occur in both REM (more severe) and NREM (more frequent) sleep.

(i) Each event lasts 10 to 20 seconds. There are usually 5 to 10 events per hour of sleep.

(j) In severe cases, patients may have more than 300 episodes of apnea per night.

(k) Patients are unaware of episodes of apnea.

(l) Treatment consists of nasal continuous positive airway pressure (CPAP), uvulopharyngopalatoplasty, weight loss, buspirone (BuSpar), and SSRIs and tricyclic drugs (to reduce REM periods, the stage during which obstructive apnea is usually more frequent). If a specific abnormality of the upper airway is found, surgical intervention is indicated.

(m) Sedatives and alcohol should be avoided because they can considerably exacerbate the condition, which may then become life threatening.

(2) **Central sleep apnea**

(a) Cessation of air flow secondary to lack of respiratory effort.

(b) Rare, usually in elderly.

(c) Treatment consists of mechanical ventilation or nasal CPAP.

(3) **Mixed type.** Elements of both obstructive and central sleep apnea.

b. **Central alveolar hypoventilation.** Central apnea followed by an obstructive phase.

(1) Impaired ventilation that appears or greatly worsens only during sleep and in which significant apneic episodes are absent.

(2) The ventilatory dysfunction is characterized by inadequate tidal volume or respiratory rate during sleep.

(3) Death may occur during sleep (Ondine's curse).

(4) Central alveolar hypoventilation is treated with mechanical ventilation (e.g., nasal ventilation).

5. **Circadian rhythm sleep disorders.** Includes a wide range of conditions involving a misalignment between desired and actual sleep periods.

a. Disturbance types include (1) delayed sleep phase, (2) jet lag, (3) shift work, and (4) unspecified (e.g., advanced sleep phase, non–24-hour, and irregular or disorganized sleep–wake pattern).

b. Quality of sleep is basically normal.

c. Self-limited. Resolves as body readjusts to new sleep–wake schedule.

d. Adjusting to an advance of sleep time is more difficult than adjusting to a delay.

e. Most effective treatment of sleep–wake schedule disorders is a regular schedule of bright light therapy to entrain the sleep cycle. More useful for transient than for persistent disturbances. Melatonin, a natural hormone that induces sleep, which is produced by the pineal gland, has been used orally to alter sleep–wake cycles, but its effect is uncertain.

6. **Dyssomnia not otherwise specified**

a. **Periodic leg movement disorder** (formerly called *nocturnal myoclonus*).

(1) Stereotypic, periodic leg movements (every 20 to 60 seconds) during NREM sleep (at least five leg movements per hour).

(2) No seizure activity.

(3) Most prevalent in patients over age 55.

(4) Frequent awakenings.

(5) Unrefreshing sleep.

(6) Daytime sleepiness a major symptom.

(7) Patient unaware of the myoclonic events.

(8) Associated with renal disease, iron deficiency, and vitamin B_{12} deficiency. May also be associated with attention-deficit/hyperactivity disorder (ADHD).

(9) Various drugs have been reported to help. These include clonazepam (Klonopin), opioids, quinine, and levodopa (Larodopa).

(10) Other treatments include stress management and anxiety-relieving programs.

b. Restless leg syndrome (Ekbom syndrome)

(1) Uncomfortable sensations in legs at rest.

(2) Peaks in middle age; occurs in 5% of the population.

(3) Can interfere with falling asleep, though symptoms not limited to sleep.

(4) Relieved by movement.

(5) Patient may have associated sleep-related myoclonus.

(6) Associated with pregnancy, renal disease, iron deficiency, and vitamin B_{12} deficiency.

(7) Treatment includes benzodiazepines, levodopa, quinine, opioids, propranolol, valproate, carbamazepine, and carbidopa. A relatively new drug, ropinirole (Requip), has been reported to be effective.

c. Kleine–Levin syndrome

(1) Periodic disorder of episodic hypersomnolence.

(2) Usually affects young men, ages 10 to 21.

(3) May sleep excessively for several weeks and awaken only to eat (voraciously).

(4) Associated with hypersexuality, extreme hostility, irritability, and occasionally hallucinations during episode.

(5) Amnesia follows attacks.

(6) May resolve spontaneously after several years.

(7) Patients are normal between episodes.

(8) Treatment consists of stimulants (amphetamines, methylphenidate [Ritalin], and pemoline [Cylert]) for hypersomnia and preventive measures for other symptoms. Lithium also has been used successfully.

d. Menstruation-associated syndrome. Some women experience intermittent marked hypersomnia, altered behavior patterns, and voracious eating at or shortly before the onset of menses.

e. Insufficient sleep. Characterized by complaints of daytime sleepiness, irritability, inability to concentrate, and impaired judgment by a person who persistently fails to sleep enough to support alert wakefulness.

f. Sleep drunkenness

(1) Inability to become fully alert for sustained period after awakening.

(2) Most commonly seen in persons with sleep apnea or after sustained sleep deprivation.

(3) Can occur as an isolated disorder.

(4) No specific treatment. Stimulants may be of limited value.

    g. **Altitude insomnia**

      (1) Insomnia secondary to change in sleep onset ventilatory set point and resulting breathing problems.

      (2) More severe at higher altitudes as oxygen level declines.

      (3) Patients may awaken with apnea.

      (4) Acetazolamide (Diamox) can increase ventilatory drive and decrease hypoxemia.

B. Parasomnias. Characterized by unusual or undesirable phenomena during sleep or on the threshold of wakefulness.

  1. Nightmare disorder

    a. Nightmares are vivid dreams in which one awakens frightened.

    b. About 50% of the adult population may report occasional nightmares.

    c. Almost always occur during REM sleep.

    d. Can occur at any time of night, but usually after a long REM period late in the night.

    e. Good recall (quite detailed).

    f. Less anxiety, vocalization, motility, and autonomic discharge than in sleep terrors.

    g. No harm results from awakening a person who is having a nightmare.

    h. Benzodiazepines, tricyclics, and SSRIs may be of help. Minipress (Prazosin), 1 to 3 mg at night may be tried for relief.

  2. Sleep terror disorder

    a. Sudden awakening, usually sitting up, with intense anxiety.

    b. Autonomic overstimulation, movement, crying out, increased heart rate, and diaphoresis.

    c. Especially common in children (about 1% to 6%), more common in boys, and tends to run in families.

    d. Patient does not remember the event in the morning.

    e. Occurs during deep, NREM sleep, usually stage III or IV sleep.

    f. Often occurs within the first few hours of sleep.

    g. Occurrence starting in adolescence or later may be the first symptom of temporal lobe epilepsy.

    h. Treatment rarely needed in childhood.

    i. Awakening child before night terror for several days may eliminate terrors for extended periods.

    j. In rare cases, when medication is required, diazepam in small doses at bedtime may be beneficial.

  3. Sleepwalking disorder (*somnambulism*)

    a. Complex activity—with brief episodes of leaving bed and walking about without full consciousness.

    b. Usually begins between the ages of 4 and 8, with peak prevalence at about 12 years old; generally disappears spontaneously with age.

    c. About 15% of children have an occasional episode and is more common in boys.

    d. Patients often have familial history of other parasomnias.

   e. Amnesia for the event—patient does not remember the episode.
   f. Occurs during deep NREM sleep (stages III and IV sleep).
   g. Initiated during first third of the night.
   h. Can usually be guided back to bed.
   i. Can sometimes be initiated by placing a child who is in stage IV sleep in the standing position.
   j. In adults and elderly persons, may reflect psychopathology—rule out central nervous system (CNS) pathology.
   k. Potentially dangerous. Precautions include window guards and other measures to prevent injury.
   l. Treatment includes education and reassurance.
   m. Drugs that suppress stage IV sleep, such as benzodiazepines, can be used to treat somnambulism.

4. **Parasomnia not otherwise specified**
   a. **Sleep bruxism (tooth grinding)**
      (1) Occurs throughout the night, though primarily occurs in stages I and II sleep or during partial arousals or transitions.
      (2) Occurs in greater than 5% of the population.
      (3) Treatment consists of bite plates to prevent dental damage.
   b. **REM sleep behavior disorder**
      (1) Loss of atonia during REM sleep, with emergence of complex, often violent behaviors (acting out dreams).
      (2) Chronic and progressive, chiefly in elderly men.
      (3) Potential for serious injury.
      (4) Neurological cause in many cases such as small stroke or early Parkinson's disease.
      (5) May occur as rebound to sleep deprivation.
      (6) May develop in patients treated with stimulants and SSRIs.
      (7) Treat with 0.5 to 2.0 mg of clonazepam daily, or 100 mg of carbamazepine (Tegretol) three times daily.
   c. **Sleep talking (somniloquy)**
      (1) Common in children and adults.
      (2) Sometimes accompanies night terrors and sleepwalking.
      (3) Found in all stages of sleep.
      (4) Requires no treatment.
   d. **Rhythmic movement disorder *(jactatio capitis nocturna)***
      (1) Rhythmic head or body rocking just before or during sleep; may extend into light sleep.
      (2) Usually limited to childhood.
      (3) No treatment required in most infants and young children. Crib padding or helmets may be used. Behavior modification, benzodiazepines, and tricyclic drugs may be effective.
   e. **Sleep paralysis (not associated with narcolepsy)**
      (1) Isolated symptom.
      (2) Episode terminates with touch, noise (some external stimulus), or voluntary repetitive eye movements.

    f. Other. Confusional arousals, sleep starts, nocturnal leg cramps, impaired or painful sleep-related penile erections, REM sleep-related sinus arrest, sleep enuresis, nocturnal paroxysmal dystonia, sleep-related abnormal swallowing syndrome, and primary snoring.

III. Sleep Disorders Related to Another Mental Disorder

Characterized by insomnia that is related to a psychiatric disorder (e.g., major depressive disorder, panic disorder, schizophrenia) and that lasts for at least 1 month.

    A. Insomnia related to axis I or axis II disorder. One who complains of insomnia for greater than 1 year is 40 times more likely than the general population to have a diagnosable psychiatric disorder. In 35% of patients who present to sleep disorder centers with a complaint of insomnia, the underlying cause is a psychiatric disorder. Half of these patients have major depression. Roughly, 80% of patients with major depression complain of insomnia. In patients with major depression, sleep involves relatively normal onset, but then repeated awakenings in the second half of the night, premature morning awakening, decreased stages III and IV sleep, a short REM latency, and a long first REM period. Treatment for insomnia in a depressed patient may include use of a sedating antidepressant, for example, treating with amitriptyline (Elavil). Posttraumatic stress disorder patients typically describe insomnia and nightmares.

    B. Hypersomnia related to axis I or axis II disorder. Hypersomnia related to a mental disorder is usually found in a variety of conditions, such as the early stages of mild depressive disorder, grief, personality disorders, dissociative disorders, and somatoform disorders. Treatment of the primary disorder should resolve the hypersomnia.

IV. Other Sleep Disorders

    A. Sleep disorder resulting from a general medical condition

        1. Insomnia, hypersomnia, parasomnia, or a combination can be caused by a general medical condition, such as:

            a. Sleep-related epileptic seizures. Seizures occur almost exclusively during sleep (sleep epilepsy).

            b. Sleep-related cluster headaches. Sleep-related cluster headaches are severe and unilateral, appear often during sleep, and are marked by an on–off pattern of attacks.

            c. Chronic paroxysmal hemicrania. Chronic paroxysmal hemicrania is a unilateral headache that occurs frequently and has a sudden onset (only occurs during REM).

            d. Sleep-related abnormal swallowing syndrome. A condition during sleep in which inadequate swallowing results in aspiration of saliva, coughing, and choking. It is intermittently associated with brief arousals or awakenings.

            e. Sleep-related asthma. Asthma that is exacerbated by sleep. In some people, it may result in significant sleep disturbances.

  f. Sleep-related cardiovascular symptoms. Associated with disorders of cardiac rhythm, congestive heart failure, valvular disease, and blood pressure variability that may be induced or exacerbated by alterations in cardiovascular physiology during sleep.

  g. Sleep-related gastroesophageal reflux. Patient awakes from sleep with burning substernal pain, a feeling of tightness or pain in the chest, or a sour taste in the mouth. Often associated with hiatal hernia. Gastroesophageal reflux disorder (GERD) can also lead to sleep-related asthma due to reflux into the lungs.

  h. Sleep-related hemolysis (paroxysmal nocturnal hemoglobinuria). Rare, acquired, chronic hemolytic anemia. The hemolysis and consequent hemoglobinuria are accelerated during sleep so that the morning urine appears brownish red.

  i. Painful conditions, such as arthritis, may lead to insomnia.

 2. Treatment, whenever possible, should be of the underlying medical condition.

B. Substance-induced sleep disorder. Insomnia, hypersomnia, parasomnia, or a combination caused by the use a medication or by intoxication or withdrawal from a drug of abuse.

 1. Somnolence can be related to tolerance or withdrawal from a CNS stimulant or to sustained use of CNS depressants.

 2. Insomnia is associated with tolerance to or withdrawal from sedative–hypnotic drugs, with CNS stimulants, and with long-term alcohol consumption.

 3. Sleep problems may occur as a side effect of many drugs (e.g., antimetabolites, thyroid preparations, anticonvulsant agents, antidepressants).

V. Sleep and Aging
A. Subjective reports by elderly
 1. Time in bed increases.
 2. Number of nocturnal awakenings increases.
 3. Total sleep time at night decreases.
 4. Sleep latency increases.
 5. Dissatisfaction with sleep.
 6. Tired and sleepy in the daytime.
 7. More frequent napping.

B. Objective evidence of age-related changes in sleep cycle
 1. Reduced total REM sleep.
 2. Reduced stages III and IV.
 3. Frequent awakenings.
 4. Reduced duration of nocturnal sleep.
 5. Need for daytime naps.
 6. Propensity for phase advance.

C. Certain sleep disorders are more common in the elderly
 1. Nocturnal myoclonus.
 2. Restless legs syndrome.

   3. REM sleep behavior disturbance.
   4. Sleep apnea.
   5. Sundowning (confusion from sedation).
D. Medications and medical disorders also contribute to the problem.

For more detailed discussion of this topic, see Sleep Disorders, Ch 20, p. 2150, CTP/IX.

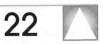

Impulse-Control and Adjustment Disorders

I. Impulse-Control Disorders

A. Introduction. Persons with impulse control disorders are unable to resist an intense drive or temptation to perform a particular act that is obviously harmful to themselves, others, or both. Before the event, the individual usually experiences mounting tension and arousal, sometimes—but not consistently—mingled with conscious anticipatory pleasure. Completing the action brings gratification and relief. Within a variable time afterward, the individual experiences a conflation of remorse, guilt, self-reproach, and dread. These feelings may stem from obscure unconscious conflicts or awareness of the deed's impact on others (including the possibility of serious legal consequences in syndromes such as kleptomania). Shameful secretiveness about the repeated impulsive activity frequently expands to pervade the individual's entire life, often significantly delaying treatment. Listed below are the six types of impulsive control disorders described in the text revision of the fourth edition of the *Diagnostic Statistical Manual of Mental Disorders* (*DSM-IV-TR*):

1. **Intermittent explosive disorder**—episodes of aggression resulting in harm to others (Table 22–1).
2. **Kleptomania**—repeated shoplifting or stealing (Table 22–2).
3. **Pyromania**—deliberately setting fires (Table 22–3).
4. **Pathological gambling**—repeated episodes of gambling that result in socioeconomic disruption, indebtedness, and illegal activities (Table 22–4).
5. **Trichotillomania**—compulsive hair pulling that produces bald spots (alopecia areata) (Table 22–5).
6. **Impulse-control disorder not otherwise specified**—residual category. Examples: compulsive buying, Internet addiction, compulsive sexual behavior (also known as sex addiction).

B. Epidemiology

1. Intermittent explosive disorder, pathological gambling, pyromania—men are affected more than women.
2. Kleptomania, trichotillomania—women affected more than men. The female-to-male ratio is 3:1 in clinical samples.
3. Pathological gambling—affects up to 3% of adult population in the United States. The disorder is more common in men than in women, and the rate is higher in locations where gambling is legal.

C. Etiology. Usually unknown. Some disorders (e.g., intermittent explosive disorder) may be associated with abnormal electroencephalogram (EEG) results, mixed cerebral dominance, or soft neurological signs. Alcohol or drugs (e.g., marijuana) reduce the patient's ability to control impulses (disinhibition).

Table 22–1
DSM-IV-TR Diagnostic Criteria for Intermittent Explosive Disorder

A. Several discrete episodes of failure to resist aggressive impulses that result in serious assaultive acts or destruction of property.
B. The degree of aggressiveness expressed during the episodes is grossly out of proportion to any precipitating psychosocial stressors.
C. The aggressive episodes are not better accounted for by another mental disorder (e.g., antisocial personality disorder, borderline personality disorder, a psychotic disorder, a manic episode, conduct disorder, or attention-deficit/hyperactivity disorder) and are not due to the direct physiologic effects of a substance (e.g., a drug of abuse, a medication) or a general medical condition (e.g., head trauma, Alzheimer's disease).

From American Psychiatric Association. *Diagnostic and Statistical Manual of Mental Disorders*, 4th ed. Text rev. Washington, DC: American Psychiatric Association; 2000, with permission.

D. Psychodynamics. Acting out of impulses relates to the need to express sexual or aggressive drive. Gambling is often associated with underlying depression and represents an unconscious need to lose and experience punishment.

E. Differential diagnosis. See Table 22–6.

1. **Temporal lobe epilepsy.** Characteristic foci of EEG abnormalities in the temporal lobe account for aggressive outbursts, kleptomania, or pyromania.

2. **Head trauma.** Brain imaging techniques may show residual signs of trauma.

3. **Bipolar I disorder.** Gambling may be an associated feature of manic episodes.

4. **Substance-related disorder.** History of drug or alcohol use or a positive test result on a drug screen may suggest that the behavior is drug- or alcohol-related.

5. **Medical condition.** Rule out brain tumor, degenerative brain disease, and endocrine disorder (e.g., hyperthyroidism) on the basis of characteristic findings for each.

6. **Schizophrenia.** Delusions or hallucinations account for impulsive behavior.

F. Course and prognosis. Course usually is chronic for all impulse-control disorders. See Table 22–6.

Table 22–2
DSM-IV-TR Diagnostic Criteria for Kleptomania

A. Recurrent failure to resist impulses to steal objects that are not needed for personal use or for their monetary value.
B. Increasing sense of tension immediately before committing the theft.
C. Pleasure, gratification, or relief at the time of committing the theft.
D. The stealing is not committed to express anger or vengeance and is not in response to a delusion or a hallucination.
E. The stealing is not better accounted for by conduct disorder, a manic episode, or antisocial personality disorder.

From American Psychiatric Association. *Diagnostic and Statistical Manual of Mental Disorders*, 4th ed. Text rev. Washington, DC: American Psychiatric Association; 2000, with permission.

Table 22–3
DSM-IV-TR Diagnostic Criteria for Pyromania

A. Deliberate and purposeful fire setting on more than one occasion.
B. Tension or affective arousal before the act.
C. Fascination with, interest in, curiosity about, or attraction to fire and its situational contexts (e.g., paraphernalia, uses, consequences).
D. Pleasure, gratification, or relief when setting fires, or when witnessing or participating in their aftermath.
E. The fire setting is not done for monetary gain, as an expression of sociopolitical ideology, to conceal criminal activity, to express anger or vengeance, to improve one's living circumstances, in response to a delusion or hallucination, or as a result of impaired judgment (e.g., in dementia, mental retardation, substance intoxication).
F. The fire setting is not better accounted for by conduct disorder, a manic episode, or antisocial personality disorder.

From American Psychiatric Association. *Diagnostic and Statistical Manual of Mental Disorders*, 4th ed. Text rev. Washington, DC: American Psychiatric Association; 2000, with permission.

G. Treatment

1. **Intermittent explosive disorder.** Combined pharmacotherapy and psychotherapy is most effective. May have to try different medications (e.g., β-adrenergic receptor antagonists, anticonvulsants [carbamazepine (Tegretol), lithium (Eskalith)]) before result is achieved. Serotonergic drugs such as buspirone (BuSpar), trazodone (Desyrel), and selective serotonin reuptake inhibitors (SSRIs) (e.g., fluoxetine [Prozac]) may be helpful. Benzodiazepines can aggravate the condition through disinhibition. Other measures include supportive psychotherapy, behavior therapy with limit setting, and family therapy. Group therapy must be used cautiously if the patient is liable to be aggressive toward other group members.

Table 22–4
DSM-IV-TR Diagnostic Criteria for Pathological Gambling

A. Persistent and recurrent maladaptive gambling behavior as indicated by five (or more) of the following:
   1. is preoccupied with gambling (e.g., preoccupied with reliving past gambling experiences, handicapping or planning the next venture, or thinking of ways to get money with which to gamble)
   2. needs to gamble with increasing amounts of money in order to achieve the desired excitement
   3. has repeated unsuccessful efforts to control, cut back, or stop gambling
   4. is restless or irritable when attempting to cut down or stop gambling
   5. gambles as a way of escaping from problems or of relieving a dysphoric mood (e.g., feelings of helplessness, guilt, anxiety, depression)
   6. after losing money gambling, often returns another day to get even ("chasing" one's losses)
   7. lies to family members, therapist, or others to conceal the extent of involvement with gambling
   8. has committed illegal acts such as forgery, fraud, theft, or embezzlement to finance gambling
   9. has jeopardized or lost a significant relationship, job, or educational or career opportunity because of gambling
   10. relies on others to provide money to relieve a desperate financial situation caused by gambling
B. The gambling behavior is not better accounted for by a manic episode.

From American Psychiatric Association. *Diagnostic and Statistical Manual of Mental Disorders*, 4th ed. Text rev. Washington, DC: American Psychiatric Association; 2000, with permission.

Table 22–5
DSM-IV-TR Diagnostic Criteria for Trichotillomania

A. Recurrent pulling out of one's hair resulting in noticeable hair loss.
B. An increasing sense of tension immediately before pulling out the hair or when attempting to resist the behavior.
C. Pleasure, gratification, or relief when pulling out the hair.
D. The disturbance is not better accounted for by another mental disorder and is not due to a general medical condition (e.g., a dermatologic condition).
E. The disturbance causes clinically significant distress or impairment in social, occupational, or other important areas of functioning.

From American Psychiatric Association. *Diagnostic and Statistical Manual of Mental Disorders*, 4th ed. Text rev. Washington, DC: American Psychiatric Association; 2000, with permission.

Table 22–6
Differential Diagnosis, Course, and Prognosis for Impulse-control Disorders

Disorder	Differential Diagnosis	Course and Prognosis
Intermittent explosive disorder	Delirium, dementia Personality change due to a general medical condition, aggressive type Substance intoxication or withdrawal Oppositional defiant disorder, conduct disorder, antisocial disorder, manic episode, schizophrenia Purposeful behavior, malingering Temporal lobe epilepsy	May increase in severity with time
Kleptomania	Ordinary theft Malingering Antisocial personality disorder, conduct disorder Manic episode Delusions, hallucinations (e.g., schizophrenia) Dementia Temporal lobe epilepsy	Frequently arrested for shoplifting
Pyromania	Arson: profit, sabotage, revenge, political statement Childhood experimentation Conduct disorder Manic episode Antisocial personality disorder Delusions, hallucinations (e.g., schizophrenia) Dementia Mental retardation Substance intoxication Temporal lobe epilepsy	Often produces increasingly larger fires over time
Pathological gambling	Social or professional gambling Manic episode Antisocial personality disorder	Progressive, with increasing financial losses, writing bad checks, total deterioration
Trichotillomania	Alopecia areata, male pattern baldness, chronic discoid lupus erythematosus, lichen planopilaris, or other cause of alopecia Obsessive–compulsive disorder Stereotypic movement disorder Delusion, hallucination Factitious disorder	Remissions and exacerbations

CLINICAL HINT:
The successful use of SDAs (quetiapine [Seroquel]) to control acting out of impulses has been reported.

2. **Kleptomania.** Insight-oriented psychotherapy is helpful in understanding motivation (e.g., guilt, need for punishment) and to control impulse. Behavior therapy can be effective to learn new patterns of behavior. SSRIs, tricyclics, trazodone, lithium, and valproate (Depakote) may be effective in some patients.

3. **Pathological gambling.** Total abstinence is the goal. Insight-oriented psychotherapy coupled with peer support groups is recommended, especially Gamblers Anonymous; however, the dropout rate is high. Treat associated depression, mania, or substance abuse. Family therapy may be helpful.

4. **Pyromania.** Insight-oriented therapy and behavior therapy are used for the treatment of pyromania. Patients require close supervision because of repeated fire-setting behavior and consequent danger to others. May require inpatient facility, night hospital, or other structured setting. Fire setting by children must be treated in a timely manner. Treatment should include family therapy and close supervision.

5. **Trichotillomania.** Treatment usually involves psychiatrists and dermatologists in a joint endeavor. Supportive and insight-oriented psychotherapies are of value, but medications may also be required: benzodiazepines for patients with high level of anxiety; or antidepressant drugs, especially serotonergic agents (e.g., SSRIs, clomipramine [Anafranil]), for patients with or without depressed mood. Hypnosis and biofeedback may be of use.

6. **Other impulse control disorders:**
   a. **Compulsive shopping.** Treatment is difficult with best results from self-help groups such as Debtors Anonymous. Dynamic psychotherapy of cognitive therapy, individually or in groups is useful. Drug therapy trials with antidepressants, mood stabilizers, anxiolytics, and antipsychotics to treat co-morbid psychiatric disorders should be used.
   b. **Mobile phone compulsion.** Understanding of psychodynamic fear of being alone, excessive dependency and needs, and phobic tendencies may be of help in changing behavior. Cognitive therapy and behavioral modification techniques are useful.
   c. **Compulsive sexual behavior.** Abstinence is goal achieved through self-help groups such as sex-addicts anonymous. In severe cases, antiandrogen medication may be used in men. Underlying psychiatric conditions, most commonly depression, should be treated.

II. Adjustment Disorders
A. **Definition.** Defined as clinically significant emotional or behavioral symptoms that develop in response to an identifiable psychosocial stressor or stressors.

Table 22–7
DSM-IV-TR Diagnostic Criteria for Adjustment Disorders

A. The development of emotional or behavioral symptoms in response to an identifiable stressor(s) occurring within 3 months of the onset of the stressor(s).
B. These symptoms or behaviors are clinically significant as evidenced by either of the following: 1. marked distress that is in excess of what would be expected from exposure to the stressor   2. significant impairment in social or occupational (academic) functioning
C. The stress-related disturbance does not meet the criteria for another specific Axis I disorder and is not merely an exacerbation of a preexisting Axis I or Axis II disorder.
D. The symptoms do not represent bereavement.
E. Once the stressor (or its consequences) has terminated, the symptoms do not persist for more than an additional 6 months.
Specify if: Acute: If the disturbance lasts less than 6 months.   Chronic: If the disturbance lasts for 6 months or longer.   Adjustment disorders are coded based on the subtype, which is selected to the predominant symptoms. The specific stressor(s) can be specified on Axis IV.   With depressed mood.   With anxiety.   With mixed anxiety and depressed mood.   With disturbance of conduct.   With mixed disturbance of emotions and conduct.   Unspecified.

From American Psychiatric Association. *Diagnostic and Statistical Manual of Mental Disorders*, 4th ed. Text rev. Washington, DC: American Psychiatric Association; 2000, with permission.

B. Diagnosis. Marked distress in reaction to a stressor. The reaction is disproportionate to the nature of the stressor, and social or occupational functioning is significantly impaired. Stressors are within the range of normal experience (e.g., birth of a baby, going away to school, marriage, loss of job, divorce, illness). See Table 22–7.

C. Epidemiology. Most frequent in adolescence, but can occur at any age. Estimated to be present in 2% to 8% of the general population.

D. Etiology

1. **Genetic.** High-anxiety temperament more prone to overreacting to a stressful event and experiencing subsequent adjustment disorder.

2. **Biologic.** Greater vulnerability with history of serious medical illness or disability.

3. **Psychosocial.** Greater vulnerability in persons who lost a parent during infancy or who had poor mothering experiences. Ability to tolerate frustration in adult life correlates with gratification of basic needs in infant life.

E. Differential diagnosis

1. **Acute and posttraumatic stress disorders.** Psychosocial stressor determines diagnosis. Stressor is outside the range of normal human experience (e.g., war, rape, mass catastrophe, floods, being taken hostage).

2. **Brief psychotic disorder.** Characterized by hallucinations, delusions, and disorganized behavior.

3. **Uncomplicated bereavement.** Occurs before, immediately, or shortly after death of a loved one; occupational or social functioning is impaired within expected bounds and remits spontaneously.

4. **Anxiety and mood disorders.** Symptoms not directly related to stressor and occur frequently.

F. **Course and prognosis.** Most patients return to their previous level of functioning within 3 months. Some persons (particularly adolescents) who have adjustment disorder later have mood disorders or substance-related disorders. Adolescents usually require a longer time to recover than adults do.

G. **Treatment**

    1. **Psychological**

        a. **Psychotherapy**—the treatment of choice. Explore meaning of stressor to the patient, provide support, encourage alternative ways of coping, and offer empathy. Biofeedback, relaxation techniques, and hypnosis for anxious mood are examples of possible treatment methods for adjustment disorders.

        b. **Crisis intervention**—aimed at helping the person resolve the situation quickly through supportive techniques, suggestion, reassurance, environmental modifications, and hospitalization, if necessary.

    2. **Pharmacological.** Patients can be treated with anxiolytic or antidepressant agents depending on the type of adjustment disorder (e.g., with anxiety, with depressed mood), but be careful to avoid drug dependency, especially if benzodiazepines are used.

For more detailed discussion of these topics, see Impulse-Control Disorders Not Elsewhere Classified, Ch 21, p. 2178, and Adjustment Disorders, Ch 22, p. 2187, in CTP/IX.

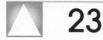

23
Psychosomatic Medicine

I. Psychosomatic Disorders

A. Definition. Psychosomatic (psychophysiological) medicine has been a specific area of study within the field of psychiatry for more than 75 years. It is informed by two basic assumptions: There is a unity of mind and body (reflected in term mind–body medicine); and psychological factors must be taken into account when considering all disease states. Although most physical disorders are influenced by stress, conflict, or generalized anxiety, some disorders are more affected than others.

B. Classification. In the text revision of the fourth edition of the *Diagnostic Statistical Manual of Mental Disorders (DSM-IV-TR)*, psychosomatic disorders are classified under the heading *psychological factors affecting medical condition,* which covers physical disorders caused by emotional or psychological factors and mental or emotional disorders caused or aggravated by physical illness (Table 23–1).

C. Diagnosis. To meet the diagnostic criteria for psychological factors affecting a medical condition, the following two criteria must be met: (1) a medical condition is present and (2) psychological factors affect it adversely (e.g., the psychologically meaningful environmental stimulus is temporally related to the initiation or exacerbation of the specific physical condition or disorder). The physical condition must demonstrate either organic disease (e.g., rheumatoid arthritis) or a known pathophysiological process (e.g., migraine headache). A number of physical disorders meet these criteria and are listed in Table 23–2.

D. Etiology

1. **Stress factors.** This etiologic theory states that any prolonged stress can cause physiological changes that result in a physical disorder. Each person has a shock organ that is genetically vulnerable to stress: Some patients are cardiac reactors, others are gastric reactors, and others are skin reactors. Persons who are chronically anxious or depressed are more vulnerable to physical or psychosomatic disease. Table 23–3 lists life stressors that may herald a psychosomatic disorder.

2. **Neurotransmitter response.** Stress activates noradrenergic system release of catecholamines and serotonin, which are increased. Dopamine is increased via mesoprefrontal pathways.

3. **Endocrine response.** Corticotropin-releasing factor (CRF) is secreted from the hypothalamus, which releases cortisol. Glucocorticoids promote energy use in the short term. Increased thyroid hormone turnover also occurs during stress states.

4. **Immune response.** Release of humoral immune factors (called cytokines) such as interleukin-1 and -2 occurs. Cytokines can increase

Table 23–1
DSM-IV-TR Diagnostic Criteria for Psychological Factors Affecting Medical Condition

A. A general medical condition (coded on Axis III) is present.
B. Psychological factors adversely affect the general medical condition in one of the following ways:
    1. The factors have influenced the course of the general medical condition as shown by a close temporal association between the psychological factors and the development or exacerbation of, or delayed recovery from, the general medical condition.
    2. The factors interfere with the treatment of the general medical condition.
    3. The factors constitute additional health risks for the individual.
    4. Stress-related physiologic responses precipitate or exacerbate symptoms of a general medical condition.
Choose name based on the nature of the psychological factors; if more than one factor is present indicate the most prominent:
    Mental disorder affecting medical condition (e.g., an Axis I disorder such as major depressive disorder delaying recovery from a myocardial infarction).
    Psychological symptoms affecting medical condition (e.g., depressive symptoms delaying recovery from surgery, anxiety, exacerbating asthma).
    Personality traits or coping style affecting medical condition (e.g., pathological denial of the need for surgery in a patient with cancer, hostile, pressured behavior contributing to cardiovascular disease).
    Maladaptive health behaviors affecting medical condition (e.g., lack of exercise, unsafe sex, overeating)
    Stress-related physiologic response affecting general medical condition (e.g., stress-related exacerbation of ulcer hypertension, arrhythmia, or tension headache).
    Other or unspecified psychological factors affecting medical condition (e.g., interpersonal, cultural, or religious factors).

From American Psychiatric Association. *Diagnostic and Statistical Manual of Mental Disorders*, 4th ed. Text rev. Washington, DC: American Psychiatric Association; 2000, with permission.

Table 23–2
Physical Conditions Affected by Psychological Factors

Disorder	Observations/Comments/Theory/Approach
Angina, arrhythmias, coronary spasms	Type A person is aggressive, irritable, easily frustrated, and prone to coronary artery disease. Arrhythmias common in anxiety states. Sudden death from ventricular arrhythmia in some patients who experience massive psychological shock or catastrophe. Lifestyle changes: cease smoking, curb alcohol intake, lose weight, lower cholesterol to limit risk factors. Propranolol (Inderal) prescribed for patients who develop tachycardia as part of social phobia—protects against arrhythmia and decreased coronary blood flow.
Asthma	Attacks precipitated by stress, respiratory infection, allergy. Examine family dynamics, especially when child is the patient. Look for overprotectiveness and try to encourage appropriate independent activities. Propranolol and beta blockers contraindicated in asthma patients for anxiety. Psychological theories: strong dependency and separation anxiety; asthma wheeze is suppressed cry for love and protection.
Connective tissue diseases: systemic lupus erythematosus, rheumatoid arthritis	Disease can be heralded by major life stress, especially death of loved one. Worsens with chronic stress, anger, or depression. Important to keep patient as active as possible to minimize joint deformities. Treat depression with antidepressant medications or psychostimulants, and treat muscle spasm and tension with benzodiazepines.

(continued)

Table 23–2—*continued*
Physical Conditions Affected by Psychological Factors

Disorder	Observations/Comments/Theory/Approach
Headaches	Tension headache results from contraction of strap muscles in neck, constricting blood flow. Associated with anxiety, situational stress. Relaxation therapy, antianxiety medication useful. Migraine headaches are unilateral and can be triggered by stress, exercise, foods high in tyramine. Manage with ergotamine (Cafergot). Propranolol prophylaxis can produce associated depression. Sumatriptan (Imitrex) can be used to treat nonhemiplegic and nonbasilar migraine attacks.
Hypertension	Acute stress produces catecholamines (epinephrine), which raise systolic blood pressure. Chronic stress associated with essential hypertension. Look at lifestyle. Prescribe exercise, relaxation therapy, biofeedback. Benzodiazepines of use in acute stress if blood pressure rises as shock organ. Psychological theories: inhibited rage, guilt over hostile impulses, need to gain approval from authority.
Hyperventilation syndrome	Accompanies panic disorder, generalized anxiety disorder with associated hyperventilation, tachycardia, vasoconstriction. May be hazardous in patients with coronary insufficiency. Antianxiety agents of use: Some patients respond to monoamine oxidase inhibitors, tricyclic antidepressants, or serotonergic agents.
Inflammatory bowel diseases: Crohn's disease, irritable bowel syndrome, ulcerative colitis	Depressed mood associated with illness; stress exacerbates symptoms. Onset after major life stress. Patients respond to stable doctor–patient relationship and supportive psychotherapy in addition to bowel medication. Psychological theories: passive personality, childhood intimidation, obsessive traits, fear of punishment, masked hostility.
Metabolic and endocrine disorders	Thyrotoxicosis following sudden severe stress. Glycosuria in chronic fear and anxiety. Depression alters hormone metabolism, especially adrenocorticotropic hormone (ACTH).
Neurodermatitis	Eczema in patients with multiple psychosocial stressors—especially death of loved one, conflicts over sexuality, repressed anger. Some respond to hypnosis in symptom management.
Obesity	Hyperphagia reduces anxiety. Night-eating syndrome associated with insomnia. Failure to perceive appetite, hunger, and satiation. Psychological theories: conflicts about orality and pathological dependency. Behavioral techniques, support groups, nutritional counseling, and supportive psychotherapy useful. Treat underlying depression.
Osteoarthritis	Lifestyle management includes weight reduction, isometric exercises to strengthen joint musculature, maintenance of physical activity, pain control. Treat associated anxiety or depression with supportive psychotherapy.
Peptic ulcer disease	Idiopathic type not related to specific bacterium or physical stimulus. Increased gastric acid and pepsin relative to mucosal resistance: both sensitive to anxiety, stress, coffee, alcohol. Lifestyle changes. Relaxation therapy. Psychological theories: strong frustrated dependency needs, cannot express anger, superficial self-sufficiency.
Raynaud's disease	Peripheral vasoconstriction associated with smoking, stress, lifestyle changes: cessation of smoking, moderate exercise. Biofeedback can raise hand temperature by increased vasodilation.
Syncope, hypotension	Vasovagal reflex with acute anxiety or fear produces hypotension and fainting. More common in patients with hyperreactive autonomic nervous system. Aggravated by anemia, antidepressant medications (produce hypotension as side effect).
Urticaria, angioedema	Idiopathic type not related to specific allergens or physical stimulus. May be associated with stress, chronic anxiety, depression. Pruritus worse with anxiety; self-excoriation associated with repressed hostility. Some phenothiazines have antipruritic effect. Psychological theories: conflict between dependence–independence, unconscious guilt feelings, itching as sexual displacement.

Table 23–3
Ranking of 10 Life-change Stressors

1. Death of spouse
2. Divorce
3. Death of close family member
4. Marital separation
5. Serious personal injury or illness
6. Fired from work
7. Jail term
8. Death of a close friend
9. Pregnancy
10. Business readjustment

Adapted from Richard H. Rahe, M.D., and Thomas Holmes.

glucocorticoids. Some persons develop severe organ damage from over-load of cytokine release under stress.

5. Physiological factors

    a. Hans Selye described the *general adaption syndrome*, which is the sum of all the nonspecific systemic reactions of the body that follow pro-longed stress. The hypothalamic–pituitary–adrenal axis is affected, with excess secretion of cortisol-producing structural damage to various organ systems.

    b. George Engel postulated that in the stressed state, all neuroregulatory mechanisms undergo functional changes that depress the body's home-ostatic mechanisms, so that the body is left vulnerable to infection and other disorders. Neurophysiological pathways thought to mediate stress reactions include the cerebral cortex, limbic system, hypothala-mus, adrenal medulla, and sympathetic and parasympathetic nervous systems. Neuromessengers include hormones such as cortisol and thy-roxine (Table 23–4).

    c. Walter Cannon demonstrated that under stress the autonomic ner-vous system is activated to ready the organism to the "fight-or-flight" response. When there is no option for either, psychosomatic disorders may result.

E. Differential diagnosis. A host of medical and neurological disorders (Table 23–5) may present with psychiatric symptoms, which must be differentiated

Table 23–4
Functional Responses to Stress

Neurotransmitter response
  Increased synthesis of brain norepinephrine.
  Increased serotonin turnover may result in eventual depletion of serotonin.
  Increased dopaminergic transmission.
Endocrine response
  Increased adrenocorticotropic hormone (ACTH) stimulates adrenal cortisol.
  Testosterone decrease with prolonged stress.
  Decrease in thyroid hormone.
Immune response
  Immune activation occurs with release of hormonal immune factors (cytokines) in acute stress.
  Number and activity of natural killer cells decreased in chronic stress.

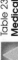

Table 23-5
Medical Problems That Present with Psychiatric Symptoms

Disease	Sex and Age Prevalence	Common Medical Symptoms	Psychiatric Symptoms and Complaints	Impaired Performance and Behavior	Diagnostic Problems
AIDS	Males > females: IV drug abusers, homosexuals, female sex partners of bisexual men	Lymphadenopathy, fatigue, opportunistic infections, Kaposi's sarcoma	Depression, anxiety, disorientation	Dementia with global impairment	Seropositive HIV virus is diagnostic when clinical signs present
Hyperthyroidism (thyrotoxicosis)	Females 3:1; 20 to 50 years	Tremor, sweating, loss of weight and strength, heat intolerance	Anxiety, depression	Occasional hyperactive or grandiose behavior	Long lead time; rapid onset resembles anxiety attack
Hypothyroidism (myxedema)	Females 5:1; 30 to 50 years	Puffy face, dry skin, cold intolerance	Lethargy, anxiety with irritability, thought disorder, somatic delusions, hallucinations	Myxedema madness; delusional, paranoid, belligerent behavior	Madness may mimic schizophrenia; mental status is clear, even during most disturbed behavior
Hyperparathyroidism	Females 3:1, 40 to 60 years	Weakness, anorexia, fractures, colliculi, peptic ulcers			Anorexia and fatigue of slow-growing adenoma resembles involutional depression
Hypoparathyroidism	Females, 40 to 60 years	Hyperreflexia, spasms, tetany	Either state may cause anxiety, hyperactivity, and irritability or depression, apathy, and withdrawal	Either state may proceed to a toxic psychosis: confusion, disorientation, and clouded sensorium	None; rare condition except after surgery
Hyperadrenalism (Cushing's disease)	Adults, both sexes	Weight gain, fat alteration, easy fatigability	Varied; depression, anxiety, thought disorder with somatic delusions	Rarely produces aberrant behavior	Bizarre somatic delusions caused by bodily changes; resemble those of schizophrenia
Adrenal cortical insufficiency (Addison's disease)	Adults, both sexes	Weight loss, hypotension, skin pigmentation	Depression—negativism, apathy; thought disorder—suspiciousness	Toxic psychosis with confusion and agitation	Long lead time; weight loss, apathy, despondency resemble involutional depression
Porphyria—acute intermittent type	Females, 20 to 40 years	Abdominal crises, paresthesias, weakness	Anxiety—sudden onset, severe; mood swings	Extremes of excitement or withdrawal; emotional or angry outbursts	Patients often have truly neurotic lifestyles; crises resemble conversion reactions or anxiety attacks

Pernicious anemia	Females, 40 to 60 years	Weight loss, weakness, glossitis, extremity neuritis	Depression—feelings of guilt and worthlessness	Eventual brain damage with confusion and memory loss	Long lead time, sometimes many months; easily mistaken for involutional depression; normal early blood studies may give false reassurance
Hepatolenticular degeneration (Wilson's disease)	Males 2:1; adolescence	Liver and extrapyramidal symptoms	Mood swings—sudden and changeable; anger—explosive	Eventual brain damage with memory and IQ loss; combativeness	In late teens, may resemble adolescent storm, incorrigibility, or schizophrenia
Hypoglycemia (islet cell adenoma)	Adults, both sexes	Tremor, sweating, hunger, fatigue, dizziness	Anxiety—fear and dread, depression with fatigue	Agitation, confusion; eventual brain damage	Can mimic anxiety attack or acute alcoholism; bizarre behavior may draw attention away from somatic symptoms
Intracranial tumors	Adults, both sexes	None early; headache, vomiting, papilledema later	Varied; depression, anxiety, personality changes	Loss of memory, judgment; self-criticism; clouding of consciousness	Tumor location may not determine early symptoms
Pancreatic carcinoma	Males 3:1, 50 to 70 years	Weight loss, abdominal pain, weakness, jaundice	Depression, sense of imminent doom but without severe guilt	Loss of drive and motivation	Long lead time; exact age and symptoms of involutional depression
Pheochromocytoma	Adults, both sexes	Headache, sweating during elevated blood pressure	Anxiety, panic, fear, apprehension, trembling	Inability to function during an attack	Classic symptoms of anxiety attack; intermittently normal blood pressures may discourage further studies
Multiple sclerosis	Females, 20 to 40 years	Motor and sensory losses, scanning speech, nystagmus	Varied; personality changes, mood swings, depression; bland euphoria uncommon	Inappropriate behavior resulting from personality changes	Long lead time; early neurological symptoms mimic hysteria or conversion disorders
Systemic lupus erythematosus	Females 8:1; 20 to 40 years	Multiple symptoms of cardiovascular, genitourinary, gastrointestinal, other systems	Varied; thought disorder, depression, confusion	Toxic psychosis unrelated to steroid treatment	Long lead time, perhaps many years; psychiatric picture variable over time; thought disorder resembles schizophrenia, steroid psychosis

Adapted from Maurice J. Martin, M.D.

Table 23–6
Conditions Mimicking Psychosomatic Disorders

Diagnosis	Definition and Example
Conversion disorder	There is an alteration of physical function that suggests a physical disorder but is an expression of psychological conflict (e.g., psychogenic aphonia). The symptoms are falsely neuroanatomic in distribution, are symbolic in nature, and allow much secondary gain.
Body dysmorphic disorder	Preoccupation with an imagined physical defect in appearance in a normal-appearing person (e.g., preoccupation with facial hair).
Hypochondriasis	Imagined overconcern about physical disease when objective examination reveals none to exist (e.g., angina pectoris with normal heart functioning).
Somatization disorder	Recurrent somatic and physical complaints with no demonstrable physical disorder despite repeated physical examinations and no organic basis.
Pain disorder	Preoccupation with pain with no physical disease to account for intensity. It does not follow a neuroanatomic distribution. There may be a close correlation between stress and conflict and the initiation or exacerbation of pain.
Physical complaints associated with classic psychological disorders	Somatic accompaniment of depression (e.g., weakness, asthenia).
Physical complaints with substance abuse disorder	Bronchitis and cough associated with nicotine and tobacco dependence.

from psychiatric disorders. Some psychiatric disorders have associated physical symptoms. In most cases, there is no demonstrable organic pathological lesion to account for the symptoms (e.g., aphonia in conversion disorder). See Table 23–6.

F. Treatment

1. **Collaborative approach.** Collaborate with internist or surgeon who manages the physical disorder and with psychiatrist attending to psychiatric aspects.

2. **Psychotherapy**

   a. **Supportive psychotherapy.** When patients have a therapeutic alliance, they are able to ventilate fears of illness, especially death fantasies, with the psychiatrist. Many patients have strong dependency needs, which are partially gratified in treatment.

   b. **Dynamic insight-oriented psychotherapy.** Explore unconscious conflicts regarding sex and aggression. Anxiety associated with life stresses is examined and mature defenses are established. More patients will benefit from supportive psychotherapy than insight-oriented therapy when they have psychosomatic disorders.

   c. **Group therapy.** Group therapy is of use for patients who have similar physical conditions (e.g., patients with colitis, those undergoing hemodialysis). They share experiences and learn from one another.

   d. **Family therapy.** Family relationships and processes are explored, with emphasis placed on how the patient's illness affects other family members.

   e. Cognitive–behavioral therapy
     (1) Cognitive. Patients learn how stress and conflict translate into somatic illness. Negative thoughts about disease are examined and altered.
     (2) Behavioral. Relaxation and biofeedback techniques affect the autonomic nervous system positively. Of use in asthma, allergies, hypertension, and headache.
   f. Hypnosis. Effective in smoking cessation and dietary change augmentation.

Table 23–7
Common Consultation–Liaison Problems

Reason for Consultation	Comments
Suicide attempt or threat	High-risk factors are men over 45, no social support, alcohol dependence, previous attempt, incapacitating medical illness with pain, and suicidal ideation. If risk is present, transfer to psychiatric unit or start 24-hour nursing care.
Depression	Suicidal risks must be assessed in every depressed patient (see above); presence of cognitive defects in depression may cause diagnostic dilemma with dementia; check for history of substance abuse or depressant drugs (e.g., reserpine, propranolol); use antidepressants cautiously in cardiac patients because of conduction side effects, orthostatic hypotension.
Agitation	Often related to cognitive disorder, withdrawal from drugs (e.g., opioids, alcohol, sedative–hypnotics); haloperidol most useful drug for excessive agitation; use physical restraints with great caution; examine for command hallucinations or paranoid ideation to which patient is responding in agitated manner; rule out toxic reaction to medication.
Hallucinations	Most common cause in hospital is delirium tremens; onset 3 to 4 days after hospitalization. In intensive care units, check for sensory isolation; rule out brief psychotic disorder, schizophrenia, cognitive disorder. Treat with antipsychotic medication.
Sleep disorder	Common cause is pain; early morning awakening associated with depression; difficulty in falling asleep associated with anxiety. Use antianxiety or antidepressant agent, depending on cause. Those drugs have no analgesic effect, so prescribe adequate painkillers. Rule out early substance withdrawal.
No organic basis for symptoms	Rule out conversion disorder, somatization disorder, factitious disorder, and malingering; glove and stocking anesthesia with autonomic nervous system symptoms seen in conversion disorder; multiple body complaints seen in somatization disorder; wish to be hospitalized seen in factitious disorder; obvious secondary gain in malingering (e.g., compensation case).
Disorientation	Delirium versus dementia; review metabolic status, neurological findings, substance history. Prescribe small dose of antipsychotics for major agitation; benzodiazepines may worsen condition and cause sundown syndrome (ataxia, confusion); modify environment so patient does not experience sensory deprivation.
Noncompliance or refusal to consent to procedure	Explore relationship of patient and treating doctor; negative transference is most common cause of noncompliance; fears of medication or of procedure require education and reassurance. Refusal to give consent is issue of judgment; if impaired, patient can be declared incompetent, but only by a judge; cognitive disorder is main cause of impaired judgment in hospitalized patients.

g. **Biofeedback.** Control of certain autonomic nervous system functions by training. Used for tension, migraine headaches, and hypertension.

h. **Acupressure and acupuncture.** Alternative therapy used with variable results in almost all psychosomatic disorders.

i. **Relaxation exercises**

(1) **Muscle relaxation.** Patients are taught to relax muscle groups, such as those involved in "tension headaches." When they

Table 23–8
Transplantation and Surgical Problems

Organ	Biological Factors	Psychological Factors
Kidney	50%–90% success rate; may not be done if patient is over age 55; increasing use of cadaver kidneys rather than those from living donors	Living donors must be emotionally stable; parents are best donors, siblings may be ambivalent; donors are subject to depression. Patients who panic before surgery may have poor prognoses; altered body image with fear of organ rejection is common. Group therapy for patients is helpful.
Bone marrow	Used in aplastic anemias and immune system disease	Patients are usually ill and must deal with death and dying; compliance is important. The procedure is commonly done in children who present problems of prolonged dependence; siblings are often donors and may be angry or ambivalent about procedure.
Heart	End-stage coronary artery disease and cardiomyopathy	Donor is legally dead; relatives of the deceased may refuse permission or be ambivalent. No fallback is available if the organ is rejected; kidney rejection patient can go on hemodialysis. Some patients seek transplantation hoping to die. Postcardiotomy delirium is seen in 25% of patients.
Breast	Radical mastectomy versus lumpectomy	Reconstruction of breast at time of surgery leads to postoperative adaptation; veteran patients are used to counsel new patients; lumpectomy patients are more open about surgery and sex than are mastectomy patients; group support is helpful.
Uterus	Hysterectomy performed on 10% of women over 20	Fear of loss of sexual attractiveness with sexual dysfunction may occur in a small percentage of women; loss of childbearing capacity is upsetting.
Brain	Anatomic location of lesion determines behavioral change	Environmental dependence syndrome in frontal lobe tumors is characterized by inability to show initiative; memory disturbances are involved in periventricular surgery; hallucinations are involved in parieto-occipital area.
Prostate	Cancer surgery has more negative psycho-biological effects and is more technically difficult than surgery for benign hypertrophy	Sexual dysfunction is common except in transurethral prostatectomy. Perineal prostatectomy produces the absence of emission, ejaculation, and erection; penile implant may be of use.
Colon and rectum	Colostomy and ostomy are common outcomes, especially for cancer	One third of patients with colostomies feel worse about themselves than before bowel surgery; shame and self-consciousness about the stoma can be alleviated by self-help groups that deal with those issues.
Limbs	Amputation performed for massive injury, diabetes, or cancer	Phantom-limb phenomenon occurs in 98% of cases; the experience may last for years; sometimes the sensation is painful, and neuroma at the stump should be ruled out; the condition has no known cause or treatment; it may stop spontaneously.

encountered and were aware of situations that caused tension in their muscles, the patients were trained to focus on the muscles involved.

j. Time management. Time-management methods are designed to help individuals restore a sense of balance to their lives. To accomplish this goal, individuals might be asked to keep a record of how they spend their time each day, noting the amount of time spent in important categories such as work, family, exercise, or leisure activities. With awareness comes increased motivation to make changes.

3. Pharmacotherapy

a. Always take nonpsychiatric symptoms seriously and use appropriate medication (e.g., laxatives for simple constipation). Consult with referring physician.

b. Use antipsychotic drugs when associated psychosis is present. Be aware of side effects and their impact on the disorder.

c. Antianxiety drugs diminish harmful anxiety during period of acute stress. Limit use so as to avoid dependency, but do not hesitate to prescribe in a timely manner.

d. Antidepressants can be used with depression resulting from a medical condition. Selective serotonin reuptake inhibitors (SSRIs) can help when the patient obsesses or ruminates about his or her illness.

II. Consultation–Liaison Psychiatry

Psychiatrists serve as consultants to medical colleagues (either another psychiatrist or, more commonly, a nonpsychiatric physician) or to other mental health professionals (psychologist, social worker, or psychiatric nurse). In addition, consultation–liaison psychiatrists provide consultation regarding patients in medical or surgical settings and provide follow-up psychiatric treatment as needed. Consultation–liaison psychiatry is associated with all the diagnostic, therapeutic, research, and teaching services that psychiatrists perform in the general hospital and serves as a bridge between psychiatry and other specialties.

Because more than 50% of medical inpatients have psychiatric problems that may require treatment, the consultation–liaison psychiatrist is important in the hospital setting. Table 23–7 lists the most common consultation–liaison problems encountered in general hospitals.

III. Special Medical Settings

Other than the usual medical wards in a hospital, special settings produce uncommon, distinctive forms of stress.

A. ICU. ICUs contain seriously ill patients who have life-threatening illnesses (e.g., coronary care units). Among the defensive reactions encountered are fear, anxiety, acting out, signing out against medical advice, hostility, dependency, depression, grief, and delirium.

B. Hemodialysis. Patients on hemodialysis have a lifelong dependency on machines and health care providers. They have problems with prolonged dependency, regression to childhood states, hostility, and negativism in

Table 23–9
Phytomedicinals with Psychoactive Effects*

Name	Ingredients	Use	Adverse Effects	Interactions	Dosage	Comments
Echinacea L. *Echinacea purpurea*	Flavonoids, polysaccharides, caffeic acid derivatives, alkamides	Stimulates immune system; for lethargy, malaise, respiratory and lower urinary tract infections	Allergic reaction, fever, nausea, vomiting	Undetermined.	1–3 g/day	Use in HIV and AIDS patients is controversial.
Ephedra, Ma-huang L. *Ephedra sinica*	Ephedrine, pseudoephedrine	Stimulant; for lethargy, malaise, diseases of respiratory tract	Sympathomimetic overload: arrhythmias, increased blood pressure, headache, irritability, nausea, vomiting	Synergistic with sympathomimetics, serotoninergic agents. Avoid with MAOIs.	1–2 g/day	Administer for short periods as tachyphylaxis and dependence can occur.
Ginkgo L. *Ginkgo biloba*	Flavonoids,[†] ginkgolide	Symptomatic relief of delirium, dementia; improves concentration and memory deficits; possible antidote to SSRI-induced sexual dysfunction	Allergic skin reactions, gastrointestinal upset, muscle spasms, headache	Anticoagulant: Use with caution because of its inhibitory effect on platelet-activating factor; increased bleeding possible.	120–240 mg/day	Studies indicate improved cognition in Alzheimer's patients after 4 to 5 weeks of use, possibly because of increased blood flow.
Ginseng L. *Panax ginseng*	Triterpenes, ginsenosides	Stimulant; for fatigue, elevation of mood immune system	Insomnia, hypertonia, and edema (called *ginseng abuse syndrome*)	Not to be used with sedatives, hypnotic agents, MAOIs, antidiabetic agents, or steroids.	1–2 g/day	Several varieties exist: Korean (most highly valued), Chinese, Japanese, American (*Panax quinquefolius*).
Kava kava L. *Piperis methysticum rhizoma*	Kava lactones, kava pyrone	Sedative-hypnotic, antispasmodic	Lethargy, impaired cognition, dermatitis with long-term unreported use	Synergistic with anxiolytics, alcohol; avoid with levodopa and dopaminergic agents.	600–800 mg/day	May be GABAergic. Contraindicated in patients with endogenous depression; may increase the danger of suicide.

Herb	Active constituents	Uses/Actions	Adverse effects	Interactions/Cautions	Dosage	Comments
St. John's wort L. *Hypericum Perforatum*	Hypericin, flavonoids, xanthones	Antidepressant, sedative, anxiolytic	Headaches, photosensitivity (may be severe), constipation	Report of manic reaction when used with sertraline (Zoloft). Do not combine with SSRIs or MAOIs; possible serotonin syndrome. Do not use with alcohol opioids.	100–950 mg/day	Under investigation by National Institutes of Health. May act as MAOI or SSRI. Allow a 4- to 6-week trial for mild depressive moods; if no apparent improvement, another therapy should be tried.
Valerian L. *Valeriana officinalis*	Valepotriates, valerenic acid, caffeic acid	Sedative, muscle relaxant, hypnotic	Cognitive and motor impairment, gastrointestinal upset, hepatotoxicity; with long-term use: contact allergy, headache, restlessness, insomnia, mydriasis, cardiac dysfunction	Avoid concomitant use with alcohol or CNS depressants.	1–2 g/day	May be chemically unstable.

*No reliable, consistent, or valid data on dosages or adverse effects are available for most phytomedicinals.
† Flavonoids are common to many herbs. They are plant by-products that act as antioxidants (i.e., agents that prevent the deterioration of material such as DNA via oxidation).

MAOI, monoamine oxidase inhibitor; GABA, γ–aminobutyric acid; SSRI, selective serotonin reuptake inhibitor.

following doctors' directions. It is advisable that all patients for whom dialysis is being considered undergo a psychological evaluation.

Dialysis dementia is a disorder characterized by a loss of cognitive functions, dystonias, and seizures. It usually ends in death. It tends to occur in patients who have been on dialysis for long periods of time.

C. **Surgery.** Patients who have undergone severe surgical procedures have a variety of psychological reactions, depending on their premorbid personality and the nature of the surgery. These reactions are summarized in Table 23–8.

IV. Alternative (or Complementary) Medicine

The use of alternative medicine is increasing. One in three persons uses such therapies at some point for such common ailments as depression, anxiety, chronic pain, low back pain, headaches, and digestive problems. Some commonly taken herbal preparations with psychoactive properties are listed in Table 23–9.

For a more detailed discussion of this topic, see Psychosomatic Medicine, Ch 24, p. 2241, in CTP/IX.

24
Personality Disorders

I. General Introduction
A. Definition. The term *personality* is universally used to describe the characteristic behavior responses of an individual, based of his or her internal or external experiences; it is predictable and stable. A personality disorder is diagnosed when an individual's behavior deviates from the normal range of variation found in the majority of people, resulting in significant impairment of adaptive functioning and/or personal distress.

B. Classification. The text revision of the fourth edition of the *Diagnostic Statistical Manual of Mental Disorders* (*DSM-IV-TR*) groups the personality disorders into three clusters.

1. **Cluster A.** The *odd and eccentric cluster* consists of the paranoid, schizoid, and schizotypal personality disorder. These disorders involve the use of fantasy and projection and are associated with a tendency toward psychotic thinking. Patients may have a biological vulnerability toward cognitive disorganization when stressed.

2. **Cluster B.** The *dramatic, emotional, and erratic cluster* includes the histrionic, narcissistic, antisocial, and borderline personality disorders. These disorders involve the use of dissociation, denial, splitting, and acting out. Mood disorders may be common.

3. **Cluster C.** The *anxious or fearful cluster* includes the avoidant, dependent, and obsessive–compulsive personality disorders. These disorders involve the use of isolation, passive aggression, and hypochondriasis.

4. Some personality disorders are included in an appendix to *DSM-IV-TR* (depressive and passive–aggressive personality disorders). Personality disorder not otherwise specified is also listed. When a patient meets the criteria for more than one personality disorder, clinicians should diagnose each; this circumstance is not uncommon.

II. Odd and Eccentric Cluster
A. Paranoid personality disorder
1. **Definition.** Characterized by their intense distrust and suspiciousness of others, patients with paranoid personality disorder are often hostile, irritable, hypersensitive, envious, or angry and will not take responsibility for their own actions, often projecting such responsibility onto others. They may be bigots, injustice collectors, pathologically jealous spouses, or litigious cranks.

2. **Epidemiology**
   a. The prevalence is 0.5% to 2.5% in the general population; 10% to 30% for inpatients; and 2% to 10% for outpatients.
   b. The prevalence is higher among minorities, immigrants, and the deaf.

    c. The incidence is increased in relatives of patients with schizophrenia and delusional disorders.

    d. The disorder is more common in men than in women.

3. Etiology

    a. A genetic component is established.

    b. Nonspecific early family difficulties are often present. Histories of childhood abuse are common.

4. Psychodynamics

    a. The classic defenses are projection, denial, and rationalization.

    b. Shame is a prominent feature.

    c. The superego is projected onto authority.

    d. Unresolved separation and autonomy issues are a factor.

5. Diagnosis. The critical feature of such patients is a pervasive and unwarranted tendency to perceive the actions of others as deliberately demeaning or threatening. This tendency begins by early adulthood. Patients expect to be exploited or harmed by others and frequently dispute the loyalty and trustworthiness of family, friends, or associates without justification. These patients tend to be reluctant to confide. They have a formal manner, can exhibit considerable muscle tension, and may scan the environment. They are often humorless and serious. Although the premises of their arguments may be false at times, their speech is goal directed and logical. Projection is employed, and they can be quite prejudiced. Some are involved in extremist groups. In marriage and sexual relationships, they are often pathologically jealous and question the fidelity of their partners. They tend to internalize their own emotions and use the defense of projection. They attribute to others the impulses and thoughts that they are unable to accept in themselves. Ideas of reference and logically defended false beliefs are common. See Table 24–1.

Table 24–1
***DSM-IV-TR* Diagnostic Criteria for Paranoid Personality Disorder**

A. A pervasive distrust and suspiciousness of others such that their motives are interpreted as malevolent, beginning by early adulthood and present in a variety of contexts, as indicated by four (or more) of the following:
1. suspects, without sufficient basis, that others are exploiting, harming, or deceiving him or her
2. is preoccupied with unjustified doubts about the loyalty or trustworthiness of friends or associates
3. is reluctant to confide in others because of unwarranted fear that the information will be used maliciously against him or her
4. reads hidden demeaning or threatening meanings into benign remarks or events
5. persistently bears grudges, that is, is unforgiving of insults, injuries, or slights
6. perceives attacks on his or her character or reputation that are not apparent to others and is quick to react angrily or to counterattack
7. has recurrent suspicions, without justification, regarding fidelity of spouse or sexual partner
B. Does not occur exclusively during the course of schizophrenia, a mood disorder with psychotic features, or another psychotic disorder, and is not due to the direct physiologic effects of a general medical condition.
Note: If criteria are met prior to the onset of schizophrenia, add "premorbid," for example, "paranoid personality disorder (premorbid)."

From American Psychiatric Association. *Diagnostic and Statistical Manual of Mental Disorders,* 4th ed. Text rev. Washington, DC: American Psychiatric Association; 2000, with permission.

6. **Differential diagnosis**
   a. **Delusional disorder**—the patient has fixed delusions.
   b. **Paranoid schizophrenia**—the patient has hallucinations and a formal thought disorder.
   c. **Schizoid, borderline, and antisocial personality disorders**—the patient does not show similar active involvement with others and is less stable.
   d. Substance abuse (e.g., stimulants) can produce paranoid features.
7. **Course and prognosis.** Whereas the disorder is lifelong in some patients, it is a harbinger of schizophrenia in others. Generally, patients with paranoid personality disorder have problems working and living with others. Occupational and marital problems are common.
8. **Treatment**
   a. **Psychotherapy.** Psychotherapy is the treatment of choice. Therapists should be straightforward and remember that trust and toleration of intimacy are difficult areas for such patients. Group therapy is not a method of choice with these patients, although it can be useful in improving social skills and diminishing suspiciousness.
   b. **Pharmacotherapy.** Pharmacotherapy is useful in dealing with agitation and anxiety. In most cases, an antianxiety agent such as diazepam (Valium) or clonazepam (Klonopin) is sufficient. It may sometimes be necessary to use an antipsychotic, such as olanzapine (Zyprexa) or haloperidol (Haldol), in small dosages and for brief periods to manage agitation and quasi-delusional thinking. The antipsychotic drug pimozide (Orap) has been successfully used to reduce paranoid ideation in some patients.

B. **Schizoid personality disorder**
1. **Definition.** Often perceived as eccentric and introverted, patients with schizoid personality disorder are characterized by their isolated lifestyles and their lack of interest in social interaction.
2. **Epidemiology**
   a. This disorder may affect 7.5% of the general population.
   b. The incidence is increased among family members of schizophrenic and schizotypal personality disorder probands.
   c. The incidence is greater among men than among women, with a possible ratio of 2:1.
3. **Etiology**
   a. Genetic factors are likely.
   b. A history of disturbed early family relationships often is elicited.
4. **Psychodynamics**
   a. Social inhibition is pervasive.
   b. Social needs are repressed to ward off aggression.
5. **Diagnosis.** These patients are ill at ease with others and may show poor eye contact. Their affect is often constricted, aloof, or inappropriately serious. Humor may be adolescent or off the mark. They may give short answers, avoid spontaneous speech, and use occasional odd metaphors. They may be

Table 24–2
DSM-IV-TR Diagnostic Criteria for Schizoid Personality Disorder

A. A pervasive pattern of detachment from social relationships and a restricted range of suppression of emotions in interpersonal settings, beginning by early adulthood and present in a variety of contexts, as indicated by four (or more) of the following:
1. neither desires nor enjoys close relationships, including being part of a family
2. almost always chooses solitary activities
3. has little, if any, interest in having sexual experiences with another person
4. takes pleasure in few, if any, activities
5. lacks close friends or confidants other than first-degree relatives
6. appears indifferent to the praise or criticism of others
7. shows emotional coldness, detachment, or flattened affectivity
B. Does not occur exclusively during the course of schizophrenia, a mood disorder with psychotic features, another psychotic disorder, or a pervasive developmental disorder and is not due to the direct physiologic effects of a general medical condition.
Note: If criteria are met prior to the onset of schizophrenia, add "premorbid," for example, "schizoid personality disorder (premorbid)."

From American Psychiatric Association. *Diagnostic and Statistical Manual of Mental Disorders*, 4th ed. Text rev. Washington, DC: American Psychiatric Association; 2000, with permission.

fascinated with inanimate objects or metaphysical constructs, or interested in mathematics, astronomy, or philosophical movements. Their sensorium is intact, their memory functions well, and their proverb interpretations are appropriately abstract. See Table 24–2.

6. **Differential diagnosis**
   a. **Paranoid personality disorder**—the patient is involved with others, has a history of aggressive behavior, and projects his or her feelings onto others.
   b. **Schizotypal personality disorder**—the patient exhibits oddities and eccentricities of manners, has schizophrenic relatives, and may not have a successful work history.
   c. **Avoidant personality disorder**—the patient is isolated but wants to be involved with others.
   d. **Schizophrenia**—the patient exhibits thought disorder and delusional thinking.

7. **Course and prognosis.** The onset of this disorder usually occurs in early childhood. The course is long-lasting, but not necessarily lifelong. Complications of delusional disorder, schizophrenia, other psychoses, or depression may develop.

8. **Treatment**
   a. **Psychotherapy.** Unlike paranoid personality disorder, schizoid patients are often introspective, and they may become devoted, if distant, psychotherapy patients. As trust builds, the patient may reveal a plethora of fantasies, imaginary friends, and fears of unbearable dependence—even of merging with the therapist. In group therapy, schizoid patients may be silent for long periods of time, but they do not completely lack involvement. The other group members become important to the patient as time goes by and may become the patient's only social contacts.

  b. **Pharmacotherapy.** Small dosages of antipsychotics, antidepressants, and psychostimulants have been effective in some patients. Serotonergic agents may make patients less sensitive to rejection. Benzodiazepines may be of use to diminish interpersonal anxiety.

C. **Schizotypal personality disorder**

  1. **Definition.** Persons with schizotypal personality disorder are characterized by magical thinking, peculiar notations, ideas of reference, illusions, and derealization. Such individuals are perceived as strikingly odd or strange, even to laypersons.

  2. **Epidemiology**

     a. The prevalence of this disorder is 3%.

     b. The prevalence is increased in families of schizophrenic probands. A higher concordance in monozygotic twins has been shown.

     c. The sex ratio is unknown; however, it is frequently diagnosed in women with fragile X syndrome.

  3. **Etiology.** Etiologic models of schizophrenia may apply. See Chapter 12.

  4. **Psychodynamics.** Dynamics of magical thinking, splitting, isolation of affect.

  5. **Diagnosis.** Schizotypal personality disorder is diagnosed on the basis of the patient's oddities of thinking, behavior, and appearance. Taking the history of such patients may be difficult due to their bizarre way of communicating. These patients may be superstitious or claim powers of clairvoyance and may believe that they have other special powers of thought and insight. They may be isolated and have few friends due to their inability to maintain interpersonal relationships and their inappropriate actions. While under stress, patients may decompensate and show psychotic symptoms. See Table 24–3.

  6. **Differential diagnosis**

     a. **Paranoid personality disorder**—the patient is suspicious and guarded, but lacks odd behavior.

     b. **Schizoid personality disorder**—the patient has no particular eccentricities.

     c. **Borderline personality disorder**—the patient shows emotional instability, intensity, and impulsiveness.

     d. **Schizophrenia**—the patient's reality testing is lost.

  7. **Course and prognosis.** Up to 10% of patients commit suicide. Schizophrenia can develop in some patients. Prognosis is guarded.

  8. **Treatment**

     a. **Psychotherapy.** Treatment of patients with schizotypal personality disorder is similar to that of schizoid patients. Patients have eccentric patterns of thinking and some may be involved in cults, strange religious practices, and the occult. Clinicians must not appear skeptical nor ridicule or judge schizotypal patients for these beliefs.

     b. **Pharmacotherapy.** In dealing with ideas of reference, illusions, and other symptoms, antipsychotic agents may be useful and can be

Table 24–3
DSM-IV-TR Diagnostic Criteria for Schizotypal Personality Disorder

A. A pervasive pattern of social and interpersonal deficits marked by acute discomfort with and reduced capacity for close relationships as well as by cognitive or perceptual distortions and eccentricities of behavior, beginning by early adulthood and present in a variety of contexts, as indicated by five (or more) of the following:
  1. ideas of reference (excluding delusions of reference)
  2. odd beliefs or magical thinking that influences behavior and is inconsistent with subcultural norms (e.g., superstitiousness, belief in clairvoyance, telepathy, or "sixth sense"; in children and adolescents, bizarre fantasies or preoccupations)
  3. unusual perceptual experiences, including bodily illusions
  4. odd thinking and speech (e.g., vague, circumstantial, metaphoric, overelaborate, or stereotyped)
  5. suspiciousness or paranoid ideation
  6. inappropriate or constricted affect
  7. behavior of appearance that is odd, eccentric, or peculiar
  8. lack of close friends or confidants other than first-degree relatives
  9. excessive social anxiety that does not diminish with familiarity and tends to be associated with paranoid fears rather than negative judgments about self
B. Does not occur exclusively during the course of schizophrenia, a mood disorder with psychotic features, another psychotic disorder, or a pervasive developmental disorder.
Note: If criteria are met prior to the onset of schizophrenia, add "premorbid," for example, "schizotypal personality disorder (premorbid)."

From American Psychiatric Association. *Diagnostic and Statistical Manual of Mental Disorders*, 4th ed. Text rev. Washington, DC: American Psychiatric Association; 2000, with permission.

combined with psychotherapy. Antidepressants may be used when depression is present.

III. Dramatic, Emotional, and Erratic Cluster
A. Antisocial personality disorder
1. **Definition.** Persons with antisocial personality disorder are characterized by their inability to conform to the social norms that govern individual behavior. Such persons are impulsive, egocentric, irresponsible, and cannot tolerate frustration. Patients with antisocial personality disorder reject discipline and authority and have an underdeveloped conscience. It should be noted that though this disorder is associated with criminality, it is not synonyms with it.
2. **Epidemiology**
   a. The prevalence is 3% in men (it may be as high as 7%) and 1% in women in the general population. In prison populations, it may be as high as 75%.
   b. Antisocial personality disorder, somatization disorder, and alcoholism cluster in some families. The disorder is five times more common among first-degree relatives of men than among controls.
   c. The disorder is more common in lower socioeconomic groups.
   d. Predisposing conditions include attention-deficit/hyperactivity disorder (ADHD) and conduct disorder.
3. **Etiology**
   a. Adoptive studies demonstrate that genetic factors are involved in this disorder.

    b. Brain damage or dysfunction is a feature of this disorder, which can be secondary to such conditions as perinatal brain injury, head trauma, and encephalitis.

    c. Histories of parental abandonment or abuse are very common. Repeated, arbitrary, or harsh punishment by parents is thought to be a factor.

4. Psychodynamics

    a. Patients with this disorder are impulse-ridden, with associated ego deficits in planning and judgment.

    b. Superego deficits or lacunae are present; conscience is primitive or poorly developed.

    c. Object relational difficulties are significant, with a failure in empathy, love, and basic trust.

    d. Aggressive features are prominent.

    e. Associated features are sadomasochism, narcissism, and depression.

5. Diagnosis. Patients with antisocial personality disorder can fool the most experienced clinician. They may appear composed and credible, but beneath the façade lies tension, hostility, irritability, and rage. A stress interview, one where patients are vigorously confronted with inconsistencies in their histories, may be needed to reveal the pathology. A diagnostic workup should include a thorough neurological examination. Patients often show abnormal electroencephalogram (EEG) results and soft neurological signs suggestive of minimal brain damage in childhood. Typical experiences beginning in childhood include lying, truancy, running away from home, thefts, fights, substance abuse, and illegal activities. Promiscuity, spouse abuse, child abuse, and drunk driving are common. Patients lack remorse for their actions and appear to lack a conscience. See Table 24–4.

Table 24–4
_D3M-IV TR_ Diagnostic Criteria for Antisocial Personality Disorder

A. There is a pervasive pattern of disregard for and violation of the rights of others occurring since age 15 years as indicated by three (or more) of the following:
  1. failure to conform to social norms with respect to lawful behaviors as indicated by repeatedly performing acts that are grounds for arrest
  2. deceitfulness, as indicated by repeated lying, use of all cases, or conning others for personal profit or pleasure
  3. impulsivity or failure to plan ahead
  4. irritability and aggressiveness, as indicated by repeated physical fights or assaults
  5. reckless disregard for safety of self or others
  6. consistent irresponsibility as indicated by repeated failure to sustain consistent work behavior or honor financial obligations
  7. lack of remorse, as indicated by being indifferent to or rationalizing having hurt, mistreated, or stolen from another
B. The individual is at least age 18 years.
C. There is evidence of conduct disorder with onset before age 15 years.
D. The occurrence of antisocial behavior is not exclusively during the course of schizophrenia or a manic episode.

From American Psychiatric Association. *Diagnostic and Statistical Manual of Mental Disorders*, 4th ed. Text rev. Washington, DC: American Psychiatric Association; 2000, with permission.

6. **Differential diagnosis**
   a. **Adult antisocial behavior**—the patient does not meet all the criteria in Table 24–4.
   b. **Substance use disorders**—the patient may exhibit antisocial behavior as a consequence of substance abuse and dependence.
   c. **Mental retardation**—the patient may demonstrate antisocial behavior as a consequence of impaired intellect and judgment.
   d. **Psychoses**—the patient may engage in antisocial behavior as a consequence of psychotic delusions.
   e. **Borderline personality disorder**—the patient often attempts suicide and exhibits self-loathing and intense, ambivalent attachments.
   f. **Narcissistic personality disorder**—the patient is law-abiding.
   g. **Personality change secondary to a general medical condition**—the patient has had a different premorbid personality or shows features of an organic disorder.
   h. **ADHD**—cognitive difficulties and impulse dyscontrol are present.

7. **Course and prognosis.** The prognosis of antisocial personality disorder varies. The condition often significantly improves after early or middle adulthood. Complications include death by violence, substance abuse, suicide, physical injury, legal and financial difficulties, and depressive disorders.

8. **Treatment**
   a. **Psychotherapy.** Psychotherapy is often difficult if not impossible. It improves if the patient is institutionalized so that they cannot act out. Self-help groups, especially with other antisocial personalities, are often useful. Firm limits are crucial before treatment can begin. Clinicians must deal with patients' self-destructive behavior. They must frustrate the patient's desire to run from honest human encounters and overcome the patient's fear of intimacy. In doing so, therapists face the challenge of separating control from punishment and of separating the need to be confrontational from the patient's unconscious fear of rejection.
   b. **Pharmacotherapy.** Pharmacotherapy is used to deal with symptoms such as anxiety, anger, and depression, but drugs must be used judiciously due to the risk of substance abuse. If the patient exhibits evidence of ADHD, psychostimulants such as methylphenidate (Ritalin) may be useful. There have been attempts to alter catecholamine metabolism with drugs and to control impulsive behavior with antiepileptic drugs such as carbamazepine (Tegretol) or valproate (Depakote), especially in cases of abnormal waveforms on an EEG. β-Adrenergics have been used to reduce aggression.

B. **Borderline personality disorder**
   1. **Definition.** Patients with borderline personality disorder are literally on the border between neurosis and psychosis. They are characterized by extraordinarily unstable mood, affect, behavior, object relations, and self-image. Suicide attempts and acts of self-mutilation are common

occurrences among borderline patients. These individuals are very impulsive, and suffer from identity problems as well as feelings of emptiness and boredom. Borderline personality disorder has also been called *ambulatory schizophrenia, as-if personality, pseudoneurotic schizophrenia,* and *psychotic character disorder.*

2. **Epidemiology**
   a. The prevalence of borderline personality disorder is about 2% of the general population, 10% of outpatients, 20% of inpatients, and 30% to 60% of patients with personality disorders.
   b. It is more common in women than in men.
   c. Of these patients, 90% have one other psychiatric diagnosis, and 40% have two.
   d. The prevalence of mood and substance-related disorders and antisocial personality disorder in families is increased.
   e. The disorder is five times more common among relatives of probands with the disorder. The prevalence of borderline personality disorder is increased in the mothers of borderline patients.

3. **Etiology**
   a. Brain damage may be present and represent perinatal brain injury, encephalitis, head injury, and other brain disorders.
   b. Histories of physical and sexual abuse, abandonment, or overinvolvement are the rule.

4. **Psychodynamics**
   a. Splitting—the patient divides persons into those who like and those who hate the patient, and into those who are all "good" and all "bad." These feelings are changeable and can become a problem for a treatment team managing a patient. Also known as primitive idealization.
   b. Projective identification—the patient attributes idealized positive or negative features to another, then seeks to engage the other in various interactions that confirm the patient's belief. The patient tries, unconsciously, to induce the therapist to play the projected role.
   c. The patient has both intense aggressive needs and intense object hunger, often alternating.
   d. The patient has a marked fear of abandonment.
   e. The rapprochement subphase of separation–individuation (theory of M. Mahler) is unresolved; object constancy is impaired. This results in a failure of internal structuralization and control.
   f. Turning against the self—self-hate, self-loathing—is prominent.
   g. Generalized ego dysfunction results in identity disturbance.

5. **Diagnosis.** Patients with borderline personality disorder are marked by their pervasive and excessive instability of affects, self-image, and interpersonal relationships and their distinct impulsivity. They tend to have micropsychotic episodes, often with paranoia or transient dissociative symptoms. Self-destructive, self-mutilating, or suicidal gestures, threats, or acts occur frequently. They are impulsive in regard to money and sex and engage in substance abuse, reckless driving, or binge eating. They

Table 24–5
DSM-IV-TR Diagnostic Criteria for Borderline Personality Disorder

A pervasive pattern of instability of interpersonal relationships, self-image, and affects, and marked impulsivity beginning by early adulthood and present in a variety of contexts, as indicated by five (or more) of the following:
1. frantic efforts to avoid real or imagined abandonment (**Note:** Do not include suicidal or self-mutilating behavior, covered in Criterion 5)
2. a pattern of unstable and intense interpersonal relationships characterized by alternating between extremes of idealization and devaluation
3. identity disturbance: markedly and persistently unstable self-image or sense of self
4. impulsivity in at least two areas that are potentially self-damaging (e.g., spending, sex, substance abuse, reckless driving, binge eating) (**Note:** Do not include suicidal or self-mutilating behavior covered in Criterion 5)
5. recurrent suicidal behavior, gestures, or threats, or self-mutilating behavior
6. affective instability due to a marked reactivity of mood (e.g., intense episodic dysphoria, irritability, or anxiety usually lasting a few hours and only rarely more than a few days)
7. chronic feelings of emptiness
8. inappropriate, intense anger or difficulty controlling anger (e.g., frequent displays of temper, constant anger, recurrent physical fights)
9. transient, stress-related paranoid ideation or severe dissociative symptoms

From American Psychiatric Association. *Diagnostic and Statistical Manual of Mental Disorders*, 4th ed. Text rev. Washington, DC: American Psychiatric Association; 2000, with permission.

---

may show shortened rapid eye movement (REM) latency and sleep continuity disturbances, abnormal dexamethasone suppression test (DST) results, and abnormal thyrotropin-releasing hormone (TRH) test results. Pananxiety and chaotic sexuality are also common features. Patients with borderline personality disorder always appear to be in a state of crisis. Mood swings are common. See Table 24–5.

6. **Differential diagnosis**
   a. **Psychotic disorder**—impaired reality testing persists.
   b. **Mood disorders**—the mood disturbance is usually nonreactive. Major depressive disorder with atypical features is often a difficult differential diagnosis. At times, only a treatment trial will tell. However, atypical patients often have sustained episodes of depression.
   c. **Personality change secondary to a general medical condition**—results of testing for medical illness are positive.
   d. **Schizotypal personality disorder**—the affective features are less severe.
   e. **Antisocial personality disorder**—the defects in conscience and attachment ability are more severe.
   f. **Histrionic personality disorder**—suicide and self-mutilation are less common. The patient tends to have more stable interpersonal relationships.
   g. **Narcissistic personality disorder**—identity formation is more stable.
   h. **Dependent personality disorder**—attachments are stable.
   i. **Paranoid personality disorder**—suspiciousness is more extreme and consistent.

7. Course and prognosis. Prognosis is variable; some improvement may occur in later years. Suicide, self-injury, mood disorders, somatoform disorders, psychoses, substance abuse, and sexual disorders are possible complications.

8. Treatment. Patients with borderline personality disorder can be problematic. The patient may have "affect storms" and require considerable attention.

    a. Psychotherapy. Psychotherapy is the treatment of choice, although it is difficult for both the therapist and the patient. Patients easily regress, act out their impulses, and show labile or fixed negative or positive transferences, which are difficult to analyze. Projective identification and splitting may also make treatment problematic; therefore, a reality-oriented approach is preferred to exploration of the unconscious. Behavior therapy may be useful to control impulses and angry outbursts and to reduce sensitivity to criticism and rejection. Social skills training is useful to improve their interpersonal behavior. Dialectical behavior therapy may be used in cases of parasuicidal behavior, such as frequent cutting. Intensive psychotherapy in the hospital setting is useful on both an individual basis and a group basis.

    b. Pharmacotherapy. Antipsychotics are useful in controlling anger, hostility, and brief psychotic episodes. Antidepressants are useful in improving depressed mood. Monoamine oxidase inhibitors (MAOIs) may be effective in modulating impulse behavior. Benzodiazepines, particularly alprazolam (Xanax), can be helpful with anxiety and depression, but some patients show a disinhibition with these drugs. Anticonvulsants such as carbamazepine (Tegretol) may improve global functioning. Serotonergic agents such as fluoxetine (Prozac) have proved to be useful.

C. Histrionic personality disorder

    1. Definition. Characterized by their flamboyant, dramatic, excitable, and overreactive behavior, persons with histrionic personality disorder are intent on gaining attention. They tend to be immature, dependent, and are often seductive. These individuals have difficulty maintaining long-lasting relationships.

    2. Epidemiology

        a. The prevalence of histrionic personality disorder is 2% to 3%. Of the patients in treatment, 10% to 15% are reported to have this disorder.

        b. The prevalence is greater in women than in men, but the disorder is probably underdiagnosed in men.

        c. This disorder may be associated with somatization disorder, mood disorders, and alcohol use.

    3. Etiology

        a. Early interpersonal difficulties may have been resolved by dramatic behavior.

        b. Distant or stern father with a seductive mother may be a pattern.

4. **Psychodynamics**

   a. Fantasy in "playing a role," with emotionality and a dramatic style, is typical.

   b. Common defenses include repression, regression, identification, somatization, conversion, dissociation, denial, and externalization.

   c. A faulty identification with the same-sex parent and an ambivalent and seductive relationship with the opposite-sex parent are often noted.

   d. Fixation at the early genital level.

   e. Prominent oral traits.

   f. Fear of sexuality, despite overt seductiveness.

5. **Diagnosis.** Patients with histrionic personality disorder are often cooperative and eager to be helped. Gestures and dramatic punctuation in their conversation are common and their language is colorful. Cognitive test results are usually normal; however, a lack of perseverance may be shown on arithmetic or concentration tasks. Emotionality may also be shallow or insincere and patients may be forgetful of affect-laden material. They tend to exaggerate thoughts and feelings to get attention, and they display temper tantrums, tears, and accusations when they do not get the attention they crave. They constantly need reassurance and their relationships tend to be superficial. See Table 24–6.

6. **Differential diagnosis**

   a. **Borderline personality disorder**—more overt despair and suicidal and self-mutilating features; the disorders can coexist.

   b. **Somatization disorder**—physical complaints predominate.

   c. **Conversion disorder**—physical symptoms are prominent.

   d. **Dependent personality disorder**—the emotional flamboyance is lacking.

7. **Course and prognosis.** The course is variable. Patients often show fewer symptoms with age; however, because they lack the energy of earlier years, the decrease in symptoms may be more apparent than real. Possible complications are somatization disorders, conversion disorders, dissociative disorders, sexual disorders, mood disorders, and substance abuse.

Table 24–6
DSM-IV-TR Diagnostic Criteria for Histrionic Personality Disorder

A pervasive pattern of excessive emotionality and attention seeking, beginning by early adulthood and present in a variety of contexts, as indicated by five (or more) of the following:
1. is uncomfortable in situations in which he or she is not the center of attention
2. interaction with others is often characterized by inappropriate sexually seductive or provocative behavior
3. displays rapidly shifting and shallow expression of emotions
4. consistently uses physical appearance to draw attention to self
5. has a style of speech that is excessively impressionistic and lacking in detail
6. shows self-dramatization, theatricality, and exaggerated expression of emotion
7. is suggestible, that is, easily influenced by others or circumstances
8. considers relationships to be more intimate than they actually are

From American Psychiatric Association. *Diagnostic and Statistical Manual of Mental Disorders*, 4th ed. Text rev. Washington, DC: American Psychiatric Association; 2000, with permission.

8. **Treatment**
   a. **Psychotherapy.** Histrionic patients are often unaware of their real feelings, so clarification of their feelings is essential to the therapeutic process. Treatment is usually individual psychotherapy, insight-oriented, or supportive, depending on ego strength. The focus is on the patient's deeper feelings and use of superficial drama as a defense against them.
   b. **Pharmacotherapy.** Pharmacotherapy can be adjunctive when symptoms are targeted. Antidepressants can be used for depression and somatic complaints. Antianxiety agents are useful for anxiety. Antipsychotics can be used for derealization and illusions.

D. **Narcissistic personality disorder**
   1. **Definition.** Persistent pattern of grandiosity, a heightened sense of self-importance, preoccupation with fantasies of ultimate success, exaggerated responses to criticism, an overconcern with self-esteem and self-image, and disturbance in interpersonal relationships.
   2. **Epidemiology**
      a. The established prevalence is less than 1% in the general population.
      b. The prevalence is 2% to 16% in the clinical population.
      c. More common in men than in women.
      d. A familial transmission is suspected.
   3. **Etiology.** A commonly cited factor is a failure in maternal empathy, with early rejection or loss.
   4. **Psychodynamics.** Grandiosity and empathic failure defend against primitive aggression. The grandiosity is commonly viewed as a compensation for a sense of inferiority.
   5. **Diagnosis.** Patients with narcissistic personality disorder have a grandiose sense of self-importance, whether in fantasy or in behavior. They have a great need for admiration, lack empathy, and often have chronic, intense envy. They handle criticism or defeat poorly; they become either enraged or depressed. Fragile self-esteem and interpersonal relationships are evident. Common stresses produced by their behavior are interpersonal difficulties, occupational problems, rejection, and loss. See Table 24–7.
   6. **Differential diagnosis**
      a. **Antisocial personality disorder**—the patient overtly disregards the law and the rights of others.
      b. **Paranoid schizophrenia**—the patient has overt delusions.
      c. **Borderline personality disorder**—the patient shows greater emotionality and greater instability.
      d. **Histrionic personality disorder**—the patient displays more emotion.
   7. **Course and prognosis.** The disorder can be chronic and difficult to treat. Aging is handled poorly because it is a narcissistic injury; therefore, they are more vulnerable to midlife crises. Possible complications include mood disorders, transient psychoses, somatoform disorders, and substance use disorders. The overall prognosis is guarded.

Table 24–7
DSM-IV-TR Diagnostic Criteria for Narcissistic Personality Disorder

A pervasive pattern of grandiosity (in fantasy or behavior), need for admiration, and lack of empathy, beginning by early adulthood and present in a variety of contexts, as indicated by five (or more) of the following:

1. has a grandiose sense of self-importance (e.g., exaggerates achievements and talents, expects to be recognized as superior without commensurate achievements)
2. is preoccupied with fantasies of unlimited success, power, brilliance, beauty, or ideal love
3. believes that he or she is "special" and unique and can only be understood by, or should associate with, other special or high-status people (or institutions)
4. requires excessive admiration
5. has a sense of entitlement, that is, unreasonable expectations of especially favorable treatment or automatic compliance with his or her expectations
6. is interpersonality exploitative, that is, takes advantage of others to achieve his or her own ends
7. lacks empathy: is unwilling to recognize or identify with the feelings and needs of others
8. is often envious of others or believes that others are envious of him or her
9. shows arrogant, naughty behavior or attitudes

From American Psychiatric Association. *Diagnostic and Statistical Manual of Mental Disorders*, 4th ed. Text rev. Washington, DC: American Psychiatric Association; 2000, with permission.

8. **Treatment**
   a. **Psychotherapy.** Patients must renounce narcissism to make progress, making treatment rather difficult. Some clinicians suggest psychoanalytic approaches to effect change, but more research is needed. Group therapy has proved useful in helping patients share with others and develop an empathic response to others.
   b. **Pharmacotherapy.** Lithium (Eskalith) is useful in patients with mood swings. Antidepressants, especially serotonergic agents, are useful with depression.

IV. **Anxious or Fearful Cluster**
   A. **Obsessive–compulsive personality disorder**
      1. **Definition.** Characterized by perfectionism, orderliness, inflexibility, stubbornness, emotional constriction, and indecisiveness. Also called *anancastic personality disorder*.
      2. **Epidemiology**
         a. The prevalence is 1% in the general population and 3% to 10% in outpatients.
         b. The prevalence is greater in men than in women.
         c. Familial transmission is likely.
         d. The concordance is increased in monozygotic twins.
         e. The disorder is diagnosed most often in oldest children.
      3. **Etiology.** Patients may have backgrounds characterized by harsh discipline.
      4. **Psychodynamics**
         a. Isolation, reaction formation, undoing, intellectualization, and rationalization are the classic defenses.
         b. Emotions are distrusted.

Table 24–8
DSM-IV-TR Diagnostic Criteria for Obsessive–Compulsive Personality Disorder

A pervasive pattern of preoccupation with orderliness, perfectionism, and mental and interpersonal control, at the expense of flexibility, openness, and efficiency, beginning by early adulthood and present in a variety of contexts, as indicated by four (or more) of the following:
1. is preoccupied with details, rules, lists, order, organization, or schedules to the extent that the major point of the activity is lost
2. shows perfectionism that interferes with task completion (e.g., is unable to complete a project because his or her own overly strict standards are not met)
3. is excessively devoted to work and productivity to the exclusion of leisure activities and friendships (not accounted for by obvious economic necessity)
4. is overconscientious, scrupulous, and inflexible about matters of morality, ethics, or values (not accounted for by cultural or religious identification)
5. is unable to discard worn-out or worthless objects even when they have no sentimental value
6. is reluctant to delegate tasks or work with others unless they submit to exactly his or her way of doing things
7. adopts a miserly spending style toward both self and others; money is viewed as something to be hoarded for future catastrophes
8. shows rigidity and stubbornness

From American Psychiatric Association. *Diagnostic and Statistical Manual of Mental Disorders,* 4th ed. Text rev. Washington, DC: American Psychiatric Association; 2000, with permission.

    c. Issues of defiance and submission are psychologically important.

    d. Fixation at the anal period.

5. Diagnosis. Patients with obsessive–compulsive personality disorder have a stiff, formal, and rigid demeanor. They lack spontaneity and their mood is usually serious. In an interview, patients may be anxious about not being in control and their answers to questions are unusually detailed. Patients with obsessive–compulsive personality disorder are preoccupied with rules, regulations, orderliness, neatness, and details. Patients lack interpersonal skills; they often lack a sense of humor, alienate people, and are unable to compromise. However, they are eager to please powerful figures and carry out these people's wishes in an authoritarian manner. See Table 24–8.

6. Differential diagnosis. The patient with obsessive–compulsive disorder has true obsessions or compulsions, whereas the patient with obsessive–compulsive personality disorder does not.

7. Course and prognosis. The course of this disorder is variable and unpredictable. The patient may flourish in arrangements in which methodical or detailed work is required. The patient's personal life is likely to remain barren. Complications of anxiety disorders, depressive disorders, and somatoform disorders may develop.

8. Treatment

    a. Psychotherapy. Patients with obsessive–compulsive personality disorder are aware of their suffering and often seek treatment on their own. Treatment is often long and complex, and counter transference problems are common. Patients value free association and nondirective therapy.

b. **Pharmacotherapy.** Clonazepam (Klonopin) is useful in reducing symptoms. Clomipramine (Anafranil) and serotonergic agents such as fluoxetine, with dosages of 60 to 80 mg/day may be useful if obsessive–compulsive signs and symptoms break through. Atypical antipsychotics such as quetiapine (Seroquel) may be of use in severe cases.

B. Avoidant personality disorder

1. **Definition.** Patients have a shy or timid personality and show an intense sensitivity to rejection. They are not asocial and show a great desire for companionship; however, they have a strong need for reassurance and a guarantee of uncritical acceptance. They are sometimes described as having an inferiority complex.

2. **Epidemiology**

   a. The prevalence is 0.05% to 1% of the general population and 10% of outpatients.

   b. Possible predisposing factors include avoidant disorder of childhood or adolescence or a deforming physical illness.

3. **Etiology.** Overt parental deprecation, overprotection, or phobic features in the parents themselves are possible etiologic factors.

4. **Psychodynamics**

   a. The avoidance and inhibition are defensive.

   b. The overt fears of rejection cover underlying aggression, either oedipal or preoedipal.

5. **Diagnosis.** In clinical interviews, patients are often anxious about talking to the interviewer. Their nervous and tense manner appears to wax and wane with their perception of whether the interviewer likes them. Patients may be vulnerable to the interviewer's comments and suggestions and may perceive a clarification or an interpretation as criticism. See Table 24–9.

6. **Differential diagnosis**

   a. **Schizoid personality disorder**—the patient has no overt desire for involvement with others.

Table 24–9
DSM-IV-TR Diagnostic Criteria for Avoidant Personality Disorder

A pervasive pattern of social inhibition, feeling of inadequacy, and hypersensitivity to negative evaluation, beginning by early adulthood and present in a variety of contexts, as indicated by four (or more) of the following:

1. avoids occupational activities that involve significant interpersonal contact, because of fears of criticism, disapproval, or rejection
2. is unwilling to get involved with people unless certain of being liked
3. shows restraint within intimate relationships because of the fear of being shamed or ridiculed
4. is preoccupied with being criticized or rejected in social situations
5. is inhibited in new interpersonal situations because of feelings of inadequacy
6. views self as socially inept, personally unappealing, or inferior to others
7. is unusually reluctant to take personal risks or to engage in any new activities because they may prove embarrassing

From American Psychiatric Association. *Diagnostic and Statistical Manual of Mental Disorders*, 4th ed. Text rev. Washington, DC: American Psychiatric Association; 2000, with permission.

    b. Social phobia—specific social situations, rather than personal relationships, are avoided. The disorders may coexist.

    c. Dependent personality disorder—the patient does not avoid attachments and has a greater fear of abandonment. Disorders may coexist.

    d. Borderline and histrionic personality disorders—the patient is demanding, irritable, and unpredictable.

7. Course and prognosis. Patients function best in a protected environment. Possible complications are social phobia and mood disorders.

8. Treatment

    a. Psychotherapy. Psychotherapeutic treatment depends on solidifying an alliance with patients. As trust develops, it is crucial that a clinician conveys an accepting attitude toward the patient's fears, especially that of rejection. Clinicians should be cautious about giving assignments to exercise the patient's new social skills outside of therapy, because failure may reinforce patients' poor self-esteem. Group therapy is helpful in gaining an understanding of the effects that sensitivity to rejection has on themselves and others. Assertive training in behavior therapy may help teach patients to openly express their needs and to enhance their self-esteem.

    b. Pharmacotherapy. Pharmacotherapy is useful in managing anxiety and depression. β-Adrenergic receptor antagonists, such as atenolol (Tenormin), is helpful in managing hyperactivity in the autonomic nervous system, which is especially high when approaching feared situations. Serotonergic agents are helpful with rejection sensitivity. Dopaminergic agents may cause more novelty-seeking behavior in these patients, but the patient needs to be psychologically prepared for any new experiences that may occur as a result.

C. Dependent personality disorder

1. Definition. Patients are predominantly dependent and submissive. They lack self-confidence and get others to assume responsibility for major areas of their lives.

2. Epidemiology

    a. The disorder is more prevalent in women than in men; however, it may be underdiagnosed in men.

    b. The disorder is common, possibly accounting for 2.5% of all personality disorders.

    c. More common in young children than in older ones.

3. Etiology. Chronic physical illness, separation anxiety, or parental loss in childhood may predispose.

4. Psychodynamics

    a. Unresolved separation issues are present.

    b. The dependent stance is a defense against aggression.

5. Diagnosis. Persons with dependent personality disorder have an intense need to be taken care of, which leads to clinging behavior, submissiveness, fear of separation, and interpersonal dependency. In interviews, they appear rather compliant; they try to cooperate, welcome specific questions,

Table 24–10
DSM-IV-TR Diagnostic Criteria for Dependent Personality Disorder

A pervasive and excessive need to be taken care of that leads to submissive and clinging behavior and fears of separation, beginning by early adulthood and present in a variety of contexts, as indicated by five (or more) of the following:
1. has difficulty making everyday decisions without an excessive amount of advice and reassurance from others
2. needs others to assume responsibility for most major areas of his or her life
3. has difficulty expressing disagreement with others because of fear of loss of support or approval (**Note:** Do not include realistic fears of retribution)
4. has difficulty initiating projects or doing things on his or her own (because of a lack of self-confidence in judgment or abilities rather than a lack of motivation or energy)
5. goes to excessive lengths to obtain nurturance and support from others, to the point of volunteering to do things that are unpleasant
6. feels uncomfortable or helpless when alone because of exaggerated fears of being unable to care for himself or herself
7. urgently seeks another relationship as a source of care and support when a close relationship ends
8. is unrealistically preoccupied with fears of being left to take care of himself or herself

From American Psychiatric Association. *Diagnostic and Statistical Manual of Mental Disorders,* 4th ed. Text rev. Washington, DC: American Psychiatric Association; 2000, with permission.

and look for guidance. They are passive and have difficulty expressing disagreement. Patients are pessimistic, indecisive, and fear expressing sexual or aggressive feelings. In *folie à deux* (shared psychotic disorder), one member of the pair usually suffers from this disorder; the submissive partner takes on the delusional system of the more aggressive, assertive partner on whom he or she is dependent. See Table 24–10.

6. **Differential diagnosis**
   a. **Agoraphobia**—the patient is afraid of leaving or being away from home.
   b. **Histrionic and borderline personality disorders**—the patient has a series of dependent relationships and is overly manipulative.
7. **Course and prognosis.** The course of dependent personality disorder is variable. Depressive complications are possible if a relationship is lost. The prognosis can be favorable with treatment. The patient may not be able to tolerate the "healthy" step of leaving an abusive relationship.
8. **Treatment**
   a. **Psychotherapy.** Insight-oriented therapies are helpful in enabling patients to understand the antecedents of their behavior, thereby enabling them to become more independent, assertive, and self-reliant. Behavior therapy, assertiveness training, family therapy, and group therapy have also been successful. Clinicians must respect patients' feelings of attachment in pathological relationships.
   b. **Pharmacotherapy.** Pharmacotherapy has been used in managing specific symptoms such as anxiety or depression. Alprazolam (Xanax) has been useful in patients who experience panic attacks. If a patient's depression or withdrawal symptoms respond to psychostimulants, they may be used. Benzodiazepines and serotonergic agents have also been used successfully.

V. Other Personality Disorders

A. Passive–aggressive personality disorder

1. Definition. Patients with this disorder show aggression in passive ways characterized by obstructionism, procrastination, stubbornness, and inefficiency. It is also called *negativistic personality disorder*.

2. Epidemiology. Unknown.

3. Etiology

a. May involve learned behavior and parental modeling.

b. Early difficulties with authority common.

4. Psychodynamics

a. Conflicts regarding authority, autonomy, and dependence.

b. Uses passive modes to express defiance and aggression.

5. Diagnosis. Patients with passive–aggressive personality disorder are passive, sullen, and argumentative. They resist demands for adequate performance in social and occupational tasks and unreasonably criticize and scorn authority. They complain of being misunderstood and unappreciated and exaggerate personal misfortune. They are both envious and resentful of those whom they deem more fortunate. They tend to alternate between hostile defiance and guilt. See Table 24–11.

6. Differential diagnosis

a. Histrionic and borderline personality disorders—the patient's behavior is more flamboyant, dramatic, and openly aggressive.

b. Antisocial personality disorder—the patient's defiance is overt.

c. Obsessive–compulsive personality disorder—the patient is overtly perfectionistic and submissive.

7. Course and prognosis. Association with depressive disorders and alcohol abuse in approximately 50% of patients. Prognosis is guarded without treatment.

8. Treatment

a. Psychotherapy. Psychotherapy can be successful with these patients but requires that clinicians point out the consequences of passive–aggressive

Table 24–11
DSM-IV-TR Research Criteria for Passive–Aggressive Personality Disorder

A. A pervasive pattern of negativistic attitudes and passive resistance to demands for adequate performance, beginning by early adulthood and present in a variety of contexts, as indicated by four (or more) of the following:
  1. passively resists fulfilling routine social and occupational tasks
  2. complains of being misunderstood and unappreciated by others
  3. is sullen and argumentative
  4. unreasonably criticizes and scorns authority
  5. expresses envy and resentment toward those apparently more fortunate
  6. voices exaggerated and persistent complaints of personal misfortune
  7. alternates between hostile defiance and contrition
B. Does not occur exclusively during major depressive episodes and is not better accounted for by dysthymic disorder.

From American Psychiatric Association. *Diagnostic and Statistical Manual of Mental Disorders*, 4th ed. Text rev. Washington, DC: American Psychiatric Association; 2000, with permission.

behaviors as they occur. Such confrontations may be more helpful than a correct interpretation in changing patients' behavior. Clinicians must treat suicide gestures as a covert expression of anger rather than as object loss in major depressive disorder.

b. Pharmacotherapy. Antidepressants are used when clinical indications of depression and suicidal ideation exist. Some patients respond to benzodiazepines and psychostimulants, depending on the clinical features.

B. Depressive personality disorder

1. **Definition.** Patients are characterized by depressive traits that have been prevalent throughout their lives, such as pessimism, self-doubt, and chronic unhappiness. They are introverted passive and duty bound.

2. **Epidemiology**
   a. The disorder is thought to be common, but no data are available.
   b. Probably occurs equally in men and women.
   c. Probably occurs in families with depression.

3. **Etiology.** Chronic physical illness, separation anxiety, or parental loss in childhood may predispose.

4. **Psychodynamics**
   a. Unresolved separation issues are present.
   b. The dependent stance is a defense against aggression.

5. **Diagnosis.** Patients with depressive personality disorder often complain of chronic feelings of unhappiness. They admit to low self-esteem and have difficulty finding anything joyful, hopeful, or optimistic in their lives. They are self-critical and derogatory and are likely to denigrate their work, themselves, and their relationships with others. Their physiognomy often reflects their mood—poor posture, depressed faces, soft voice, and psychomotor retardation. See Table 24–12.

6. **Differential diagnosis**
   a. Dysthymic disorder—fluctuations in mood are greater than in depressive personality disorder.
   b. Avoidant personality disorder—the patient tends to be more anxious than depressed.

Table 24–12
DSM-IV-TR Research Criteria for Depressive Personality Disorder

A. A pervasive pattern of depressive cognitions and behaviors beginning by early adulthood and present in a variety of contexts, as indicated by five (or more) of the following:
  1. usual mood is dominated by dejection, gloominess, cheerlessness, joylessness, unhappiness
  2. self-concept centers around beliefs of inadequacy, worthlessness, and low self-esteem
  3. is critical, blaming, and derogatory toward self
  4. is brooding and given to worry
  5. is negativistic, critical, and judgmental toward others
  6. is pessimistic
  7. is prone to feeling guilty or remorseful
B. Does not occur exclusively during major depressive episodes and is not better accounted for by dysthymic disorder.

From American Psychiatric Association. *Diagnostic and Statistical Manual of Mental Disorders*, 4th ed. Text rev. Washington, DC: American Psychiatric Association; 2000, with permission.

7. **Course and prognosis.** A risk for dysthymic disorder, major depressive disorder, and current or lifetime mood disorder is thought to be likely.

8. **Treatment**

   a. **Psychotherapy.** Insight-oriented psychotherapy enables patients to gain insight into the psychodynamics of their illness and to appreciate the effect it has on their interpersonal relationships. Cognitive therapy corrects the cognitive manifestation of their low self-esteem and pessimism. Group therapy, interpersonal therapy, and self-help measures are also useful.

   b. **Pharmacotherapy.** Pharmacotherapy for depressive personality disorder patients includes the use of antidepressant medications. Serotonergic agents are especially useful. Small dosages of psychostimulants, such as amphetamine at 5 to 15 mg/day, have been helpful for some patients. These approaches should be combined with psychotherapy for best results.

C. **Sadomasochistic personality disorder.** Not an official diagnostic category in *DSM-IV-TR*, but one of major interest to physicians clinically and historically. It is characterized by elements of sadism, the desire to cause others pain sexually, physically, or psychologically, and masochism, inflicting pain on oneself either sexually or morally. Treatment with insight-oriented psychotherapy, including psychoanalysis, can be effective.

D. **Sadistic personality disorder.** Patients show a pervasive pattern of cruel, demeaning, and aggressive behavior toward others. Physical cruelty and violence is used to inflict pain on others with no actual goal. Such patients are usually fascinated with weapons, violence, injury, and torture. It is often related to parental abuse.

E. **Self-defeating personality disorder.** Patients are classified by their avoidance of pleasurable situations and their appeal toward situations or relationships in which they will suffer. They reject help or good outcomes and have a dysphoric response to success.

F. **Personality disorder due to a general medical condition.** Patients are characterized by a marked change in personality style and traits from their previous level of functioning. There must be evidence of a causative organic factor antedating the onset of the personality change. Management usually involves treatment of the underlying organic condition when possible. Psychopharmacological treatment of specific symptoms may be needed. Alcohol should be avoided, and social engagements should be curtailed when patients have tendencies to act in a grossly offensive manner.

G. **Personality disorder not otherwise specified.** This diagnosis is made if the patient has a personality disorder with mixed features of other personality disorders.

For more detailed discussion of this topic, see Personality Disorders, Ch 23, p. 2197, in CTP/IX.

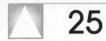 **25**

Suicide, Violence, and Other Psychiatric Emergencies

I. Suicide
A. Definition
1. The word *suicide* is derived from Latin, meaning "self-murder." If successful, it is a fatal act that fulfills the person's wish to die. Various terms used to describe parasuicidal thoughts or behaviors (i.e., suicidality, ideation) should be used with clear meaning and purpose. See Table 25–1 for definitions of terms related to suicide.
2. Identification of the potentially suicidal patient is among the most critical tasks in psychiatry.

B. Incidence and prevalence
1. About 35,000 persons commit suicide per year in the United States.
2. The rate is 12.5 persons per 100,000.
3. About 250,000 persons attempt suicide per year.
4. The United States is at the midpoint worldwide in numbers of suicides (e.g., 25 persons per 100,000 in Scandinavian countries). The rate is lowest in Spain and Italy.

C. Associated risk factors. Table 25–2 lists high- and low-risk factors in the evaluation of suicide risk.
1. **Gender.** Men commit suicide three times more often than women. Women attempt suicide four times more often than men.
2. **Method.** Men's higher rate of successful suicide is related to the methods they use (e.g., firearms, hanging), while women more commonly take an overdose of psychoactive substances or a poison.
3. **Age.** Rates increase with age.
   a. Among men, the suicide rate peaks after age 45; among women, it peaks after age 65.
   b. Older persons attempt suicide less often but are more successful.
   c. After age 75, the rate rises in both sexes.
   d. Currently, the most rapid rise is among male 15- to 24-year-olds.
4. **Race.** In the United States, white males commit two of every three suicides. The risk is lower in nonwhites. Suicide rates are higher than average in Native Americans and Inuits.
5. **Religion.** Rate highest in Protestants; lowest in Catholics, Jews, and Muslims.
6. **Marital status.** Rate is twice as high in single persons than in married persons. Divorced, separated, or widowed persons have rates four to five times higher than married persons. Divorced men register 69 suicides per 100,000, compared with 18 per 100,000 for divorced women. Death of spouse increases risk. For women, having young children at home is

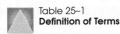

Table 25–1
Definition of Terms

- Suicide—self-inflicted death with evidence (either explicit or implicit) that the person intended to die.
- Suicide attempt—self-injurious behavior with a nonfatal outcome accompanied by evidence (either explicit or implicit) that the person intended to die.
- Aborted suicide attempt—potentially self-injurious behavior with evidence (either explicit or implicit) that the person intended to die but stopped the attempt before physical damage occurred.
- Parasuicidal—patients who injure themselves by self-mutilation (e.g., cutting the skin) but usually do not wish to die.
- Suicidal ideation—thoughts of wanting to die; may vary in seriousness depending on the specificity of suicide plans and the degree of suicidal intent.
- Suicidal intent—subjective expectation and desire to end one's life.
- Lethality of suicidal behavior—objective danger to life associated with a suicide method or action (e.g., jumping from heights is highly lethal, while cutting wrist is less lethal).

From Assessment and Treatment of Patients with Suicidal Behaviors. *The American Psychiatric Association's Practice Guidelines*, 2004.

Table 25–2
Evaluation of Suicide Risk

Variable	High Risk	Low Risk
Demographic and social profile		
Age	Over 45 years	Below 45 years
Sex	Male	Female
Marital status	Divorced or widowed	Married
Employment	Unemployed	Employed
Interpersonal relationship	Conflictual	Stable
Family background	Chaotic or conflictual	Stable
Health		
Physical	Chronic illness	Good health
	Hypochondriac	Feels healthy
	Excessive substance intake	Low substance use
Mental	Severe depression	Mild depression
	Psychosis	Neurosis
	Severe personality disorder	Normal personality
	Substance abuse	Social drinker
	Hopelessness	Optimism
Suicidal activity		
Suicidal ideation	Frequent, intense, prolonged	Infrequent, low intensity, transient
Suicide attempt	Multiple attempts	First attempt
	Planned	Impulsive
	Rescue unlikely	Rescue inevitable
	Unambiguous wish to die	Primary wish for change
	Communication internalized (self-blame)	Communication externalized (anger)
	Method lethal and available	Method of low lethality or not readily available
Resources		
Personal	Poor achievement	Good achievement
	Poor insight	Insightful
	Affect unavailable or poorly controlled	Affect available and appropriately controlled
Social	Poor rapport	Good rapport
	Socially isolated	Socially integrated
	Unresponsive family	Concerned family

From Adam K. Attempted suicide. *Psychiatric Clin North Am* 1985;8:183, with permission.

Table 25–3
Medical and Mental Disorders Associated with Increased Suicide Risk

- AIDS
- Amnesia
- Attention-deficit/hyperactivity disorder (ADHD)
- Bipolar disorder
- Borderline personality disorder
- Delirium
- Dementia
- Dysthymic disorder
- Eating disorders
- Impulse-control disorders
- Learning disability
- Major depression
- Panic disorder
- Posttraumatic stress disorder
- Schizoaffective disorder
- Schizophrenia
- Substance use disorders

protective against suicide. Homosexual persons are at higher risk than heterosexuals.

7. **Physical health.** Medical or surgical illness is a high-risk factor, especially if associated with pain or chronic or terminal illness (Table 25–3).

8. **Mental illness**

a. **Depressive disorders.** Mood disorders are the diagnoses most commonly associated with suicide. Fifty percent of all persons who commit suicide are depressed. Fifteen percent of depressed patients kill themselves. Patients with mood disorder accompanied by panic or anxiety attacks are at highest risk.

b. **Schizophrenia.** The onset of schizophrenia is typically in adolescence or early childhood, and most of these patients who commit suicide do so during the first few years of their illness. In the United States, an estimated 4,000 schizophrenic patients commit suicide each year. Ten percent of persons who commit suicide are schizophrenic with prominent delusions. Patients who have command hallucinations telling them to harm themselves are at increased risk.

c. **Alcohol and other substance dependence.** Alcohol dependence increases risk of suicide, especially if the person is also depressed. Studies show that many alcohol-dependent patients who eventually commit suicide are rated depressed during hospitalization, and that up to two-thirds are assessed as having mood disorder symptoms during the period in which they commit suicide. The suicide rate for persons who are heroin dependent or dependent on other drugs is approximately 20 times the rate for the general population.

d. **Personality disorders.** Borderline personality disorder is associated with a high rate of parasuicidal behavior. An estimated 5% of patients with antisocial personality disorder commit suicide, especially those in prisons. Prisoners have the highest suicide rate of any group.

    e. **Dementia and delirium.** Increased risk in patients with dementia and delirium, especially secondary to alcohol abuse or with psychotic symptoms.

    f. **Anxiety disorder.** Unsuccessful suicide attempts are made by almost 20% of patients with a panic disorder and social phobia. If depression is an associated feature, the risk of suicide rises. Panic disorder has been diagnosed in 1% of persons who successfully kill themselves.

9. Other risk factors

    a. Unambiguous wish to die.

    b. Unemployment.

    c. Sense of hopelessness.

    d. Rescue unlikely.

    e. Hoarding pills.

    f. Access to lethal agents or to firearms.

    g. Family history of suicide or depression.

    h. Fantasies of reunion with deceased loved ones.

    i. Occupation: dentist, physician, nurse, scientist, police officer, or farmer.

    j. Previous suicide attempt.

    k. History of childhood physical or sexual abuse.

    l. History of impulsive or aggressive behavior.

    m. **Social context.** Key features of the epidemiology of suicide, however, can vary among different countries or ethnic groups. For example, in China, women commit suicide more than men. Rates vary from some South American countries reporting rates of 3/100,000 to rates in the Russian Federation of 60/100,000.

D. Management of the suicidal patient. A general strategy for evaluating and managing suicidal patients is presented in Table 25–4.

    1. Do not leave a suicidal patient alone; remove any potentially dangerous objects from the room.

    2. Assess whether the attempt was planned or impulsive. Determine the lethality of the method, the chances of discovery (whether the patient was alone or notified someone), and the reaction to being saved (whether the patient is disappointed or relieved). Also, determine whether the factors that led to the attempt have changed.

    3. Patients with severe depression may be treated on an outpatient basis if their families can supervise them closely and if treatment can be initiated rapidly. Otherwise, hospitalization is necessary.

    4. The suicidal ideation of alcoholic patients generally remits with abstinence in a few days. If depression persists after the physiological signs of alcohol withdrawal have resolved, a high suspicion of major depression is warranted. All suicidal patients who are intoxicated by alcohol or drugs must be reassessed when they are sober.

    5. Suicidal ideas in schizophrenic patients must be taken seriously because they tend to use violent, highly lethal, and sometimes bizarre methods.

Table 25–4
General Strategy in Evaluating Patients

I. Protect yourself
   A. Know as much as possible about the patients before meeting them.
   B. Leave physical restraint procedures to those who are trained to handle them.
   C. Be alert to risks for impending violence.
   D. Attend to the safety of the physical surroundings (e.g., door access, room objects).
   E. Have others present during the assessment, if needed.
   F. Have others in the vicinity.
   G. Attend to developing an alliance with the patient (e.g., do not confront or threaten patients with paranoid psychoses).
II. Prevent harm
   A. Prevent self-injury and suicide. Use whatever methods are necessary to prevent patients from hurting themselves during the evaluation.
   B. Prevent violence toward others. During the evaluation, briefly assess the patient for the risk of violence. If the risk is deemed significant, consider the following options:
       1. Inform the patient that violence is not acceptable.
       2. Approach the patient in a nonthreatening manner.
       3. Reassure and calm the patient or assist in reality testing.
       4. Offer medication.
       5. Inform the patient that restraint or seclusion will be used if necessary.
       6. Have teams ready to restrain the patient.
       7. When patients are restrained, always closely observe them and frequently check their vital signs. Isolate restrained patients from agitating stimuli. Immediately plan a further approach—medication, reassurance, medical evaluation.
III. Rule out cognitive disorders
IV. Rule out impending psychosis

6. Patients with personality disorders benefit mostly from empathic confrontation and assistance in solving the problem that precipitated the suicide attempt and to which they have usually contributed.

7. Long-term hospitalization is recommended for conditions that contribute to self-mutilation; brief hospitalization does not usually affect such habitual behavior. Parasuicidal patients may benefit from long-term rehabilitation, and brief hospitalization may be necessary from time to time, but short-term treatment cannot be expected to alter their course significantly.

CLINICAL HINTS: SUICIDE

- *Ask about suicidal ideas, especially plans to harm oneself. Asking about suicide does not plant the idea.*
- *Do not hesitate to ask patients if they "want to die." A straightforward approach is the most effective.*
- *Conduct the interview in a safe place. Patients have been known to throw themselves out of a window.*
- *Do not offer false reassurance (e.g., "Most people think about killing themselves at some time").*
- *Always ask about past suicide attempts, which can be related to future attempts.*
- *Always ask about access to firearms; access to weapons increases the risk in a suicidal patient.*

- *Do not release patients from the emergency department if you are not certain that they will not harm themselves.*
- *Never assume that family or friends will be able to watch a patient 24 hours a day. If that is required, admit the patient to the hospital.*
- *Never worry alone—If you are unsure about the level of risk or course of action, involve others.*

E. Legal issues
1. Successful suicide is a major cause of lawsuits against psychiatrists.
2. Courts recognize that not all suicides can be prevented, but they do require thorough evaluation of suicide risk and careful treatment plan.
3. Careful documentation of suicidal patients is necessary, including record of decision-making process (e.g., discharge of patient from hospital to home, provision for follow-up care).

II. Violence
A. Definition
1. Intentional act of doing bodily harm to another person.
2. Includes assault, rape, robbery, and homicide.
3. Physical and sexual abuse of adults, children, and the elderly are included in violent acts.
B. Incidence and prevalence
1. About 8 million violent acts are committed each year in the United States.
2. Lifetime risk of becoming a homicide victim is about 1 in 85 for men and 1 in 280 for women. Men are the victims of violence more often than women.
C. Disorders associated with violence. The psychiatric conditions most commonly associated with violence include such psychotic disorders as schizophrenia and mania (particularly if the patient is paranoid or is experiencing command hallucinations), intoxication with alcohol and drugs, withdrawal from alcohol and sedative–hypnotics, catatonic excitement, agitated depression, personality disorders characterized by rage and poor impulse control (e.g., borderline and antisocial personality disorders), and cognitive disorders (especially those associated with frontal and temporal lobe involvement).
D. Predicting violent behavior. See Table 25–5. Best predictors are past acts of violence. Predictors, however, are often very nonspecific among psychiatric populations. Some evidence suggests that a fluctuating course or altered pattern of symptoms in a psychiatric illness, rather than the cumulative specific symptoms per se, might be predictive of greater violence risk.
1. Several symptom scales such as the Modified Overt Aggression Scale (MOAS) or the Broset Violence Checklist have been studied with respect to the prediction of violence, although mostly in terms of immediate risk in inpatient treatment settings. One key value of such scales may be to fix more concerted attention and management of staff to patients as well as track clinical course.

Table 25-5
Assessing and Predicting Violent Behavior

Signs of impending violence

Recent acts of violence, including property violence.

Verbal or physical threats (menacing).

Carrying weapons or other objects that may be used as weapons (e.g., forks, ashtrays).

Progressive psychomotor agitation.

Alcohol or other substance intoxication.

Paranoid features in a psychotic patient.

Command violent auditory hallucinations—some but not all patients are at high risk.

Brain diseases, global or with frontal lobe findings; less commonly with temporal lobe findings (controversial).

Catatonic excitement.

Certain manic episodes.

Certain agitated depressive episodes.

Personality disorders (rage, violence, or impulse dyscontrol).

Assess the risk for violence

Consider violent ideation, wish, intention, plan, availability of means, implementation of plan, wish for help.

Consider demographics—sex (male), age (15–24), socioeconomic status (low), social supports (few).

Consider the patient's history: violence, nonviolent antisocial acts, impulse dyscontrol (e.g., gambling, substance abuse, suicide or self-injury, psychosis).

Consider overt stressors (e.g., marital conflict, real or symbolic loss).

E. Evaluation and management

1. **Protect yourself.** Assume that violence is always a possibility, and be on guard for a sudden violent act. Never interview an armed patient. The patient should always surrender a weapon or potential weapon to secure personnel. Know as much as possible about the patient before the interview. Never interview a potentially violent patient alone or in an office with the door closed. Consider removing neckties, necklaces, and other articles of clothing or jewelry you are wearing that the patient can grab or pull. Stay within sight of other staff members. Leave physical restraint to staff members who are trained in that. Do not give the patient access to areas where weapons may be available (e.g., a crash cart or a treatment room). Do not sit close to a paranoid patient, who may feel threatened. Keep yourself at least an arm's length away from any potentially violent patient. Do not challenge or confront a psychotic patient. Be alert to the signs of impending violence. Always leave yourself a route of rapid escape in case the patient attacks you. Never turn your back on the patient.

2. Signs of impending violence include recent violent acts against people or property, clenched teeth and fists, verbal threats (menacing), possession of weapons or objects potentially usable as weapons, psychomotor agitation (considered to be an important indicator), alcohol or drug intoxication, paranoid delusions, and command hallucinations.

3. Physical restraint should be applied only by persons with appropriate training. Patients with suspected phencyclidine intoxication should not be physically restrained (limb restraints especially should be avoided) because they may injure themselves. Usually, a benzodiazepine or an

antipsychotic is given immediately after physical restraints have been applied to provide a chemical restraint, but the choice of drug depends on the diagnosis. Provide a nonstimulating environment.

4. Perform a definitive diagnostic evaluation. The patient's vital signs should be assessed, a physical examination performed, and a psychiatric history obtained. Evaluate the patient's risk for suicide and create a treatment plan that provides for the management of potential subsequent violence. Elevated vital signs may suggest withdrawal from alcohol or sedative–hypnotics.

5. Explore possible psychosocial interventions to reduce the risk for violence. If violence is related to a specific situation or person, try to separate the patient from that situation or person. Try family interventions and other modifications of the environment. Would the patient still be potentially violent while living with other relatives?

6. Hospitalization may be necessary to detain the patient and prevent violence. Constant observation may be necessary, even on a locked inpatient psychiatric ward.

7. If psychiatric treatment is not appropriate, you may involve the police and the legal system.

8. Intended victims must be warned of the continued possibility of danger (e.g., if the patient is not hospitalized).

 CLINICAL HINT: VIOLENT PATIENTS

- *If the patient is brought to the emergency department by police with restraining devices (e.g., handcuffs), do not immediately remove them.*
- *Conduct the interview in a safe environment with attendants on call in case the patient becomes agitated.*
- *Position yourself so that you cannot be blocked by the patient from exiting the examination room.*
- *Do not interview a patient if sharp or potentially dangerous objects are in the interview room (e.g., a letter opener on a desk).*
- *Trust your feelings. If you feel apprehensive or fearful, terminate the interview.*
- *Ask about past attempts at violence (including cruelty to animals). They are predictors for future violent events.*
- *Admit a patient for observation if there is any question of his or her being a danger to others.*
  Never worry alone—If you are unsure about the level of risk or course of action, involve others.

F. **History and diagnosis.** Risk factors for violence include a statement of intent, formulation of a specific plan, available means, male sex, young age (15 to 24 years), low socioeconomic status, poor social support system, past history of violence, other antisocial acts, poor impulse control, history of

Table 25–6
Risk Factors for Violence

Current mental status findings
  Hostile, irritable, menacing, threatening
  Agitation
  Victim(s) apparently picked out
  Weapons available
  Acute Intoxication
  Paranoia
  Delusions or hallucinations, especially command-type or that are used by patients to explain or justify their behavior
  Impaired empathy
Disorders
  Mania (when characterized by prominent irritability), as in bipolar disorder or schizoaffective disorder, bipolar type
  Paranoid schizophrenia
  Anabolic steroid abuse
  Personality change (with disinhibition, e.g., frontal lobe syndrome)
  Dementia
  Delirium
  Mental retardation
  Paranoid personality disorder
  Antisocial personality disorder
  Borderline personality disorder
  Alcohol intoxication
  Stimulant intoxication (cocaine, amphetamines)
  Intermittent explosive disorder
  Delusional disorder
Personal history
  History of violent behavior, impulsivity, in similar circumstances
  Recent act(s) of violence/destruction of property
  History of being physically abused in childhood
  Growing up in a family where parents were violent toward each other
  Childhood history of enuresis, cruelty to animals, and fire setting (the "triad")
Demographic
  Male > female
  Young (late teens or early 20s) > older

suicide attempts, and recent stressors. A history of violence is the best predictor of violence. Additional important factors include a history of childhood victimization; a childhood history of the triad of bed-wetting, fire setting, and cruelty to animals; a criminal record; military or police service; reckless driving; and a family history of violence. See Table 25–6 for commonly attributed risk factors.

G. Drug treatment

  1. Drug treatment depends on the specific diagnosis.

  2. Benzodiazepines and antipsychotics are used most often to tranquilize a patient. Haloperidol (Haldol) given at a dose of 5 mg by mouth or intramuscularly, 2 mg of risperidone (Risperdal) by mouth, or 2 mg of lorazepam (Ativan) by mouth or intramuscularly may be tried initially. An intramuscular form of olanzapine is also commonly used.

Text continues on page 347.

Table 25–7
Common Psychiatric Emergencies

Syndrome or Presenting Symptom	Emergency Problem	Emergency Treatment Issues
Abuse of child or adult	Is there another explanation? Protect from further injury.	Management of medical problems: psychiatric evaluation, notification of protective services.
AIDS	Unrealistic or obsessive concern about having contracted the illness; changes in behavior secondary to organic effects; symptoms of depression or anxiety in someone who has the illness; grief over the loss of a friend or lover from AIDS.	Explore the patient's primary concern; if there is a realistic possibility of the patient having contracted the virus, arrange for counseling and HIV titer; rule out an organic component in the HIV-positive patient, facilitate grieving for the patient who has suffered a loss by identifying the depression and referring for brief psychotherapy treatment or AIDS-support group.
Adjustment disorder	Agitation, sleep disorder, or depression; substance abuse; anxiety.	Explore briefly the meaning of the stress that has precipitated the adjustment reaction; refer for brief focused therapy; do not prescribe medications for the symptoms of adjustment disorder in the emergency department because many of the symptoms abate once the patient is aware of their origins and has a chance to deal with the associated feelings.
Adolescent crisis	Suicidal ideation or attempts, running-away behaviors, drug use, pregnancy, psychosis, assaultive behavior toward family members, and eating disorders.	Family crisis intervention is ideal if that can be accomplished; for the adolescent who is completely estranged from the family, inquire about an interested adult relative or friend who can be involved; evaluate for sexual or other physical abuse; evaluate for suicidal ideation; refer to adolescent crisis services if those are available; consider hospitalization if necessary.
Agoraphobia	Determination of the reason for the patient's emergency department visit.	Agoraphobia is a long-standing problem; refer the patient for psychiatric treatment; do not prescribe medications in the emergency department unless there will be continuity of care in follow up.
Akathisia	Is this a new onset? Is the patient on maintenance antipsychotics?	Determine the causative agent; diphenhydramine (Benadryl) orally or intravenously, or benztropine (Cogentin) orally or intramuscularly. Explain to patient and family the cause of the symptom.
Alcohol-related emergencies	Confusion; psychosis; assaultive behavior, suicidal ideation or behavior; hallucinations.	Determine blood alcohol concentration; concentrations above 300 mg/dL suggest fairly long-standing alcohol abuse; assess the need for emergency intervention; antipsychotic agents as needed for psychotic symptoms; confront the patient about the degree of alcohol abuse and hold in emergency department until level decreases sufficiently for an appropriate assessment of suicidality and judgment; refer to an alcohol treatment program.

(continued)

Table 25–7—*continued*
Common Psychiatric Emergencies

Syndrome or Presenting Symptom	Emergency Problem	Emergency Treatment Issues
Alcohol idiosyncratic intoxication	Marked aggressive or assaultive behavior; "the patient just isn't himself (or herself)!"	Rule out organic cause; benzodiazepines as needed to calm the patient; decrease external stimulation and restrain the patient, if necessary; after a determination is made that the patient can be safely discharged, warn the patient about the likelihood that the idiosyncratic reaction will recur with further drinking.
Alcohol withdrawal	Irritability, shakiness; confusion and disorientation; abnormal vital signs, including tachycardia, hyperthermia, and hypertension.	Benzodiazepines as needed to reduce symptoms; observe patient closely and monitor vital signs over several hours to detect onset of delirium tremens; when the patient is ready for discharge, inform the patient firmly about the diagnosis of alcohol dependence and refer for treatment.
Korsakoff's syndrome, Wernicke's encephalopathy	Confusion, amnesia; multiple organic symptoms, including ataxia, confusion, and disturbances of eye muscles.	Determine onset if possible; institute treatment with thiamine, determine capacity for patient to care for self; hospitalize, if necessary; inform the patient firmly about the diagnosis of alcoholism.
Amnesia	Identification; differential diagnosis, particularly of an organic component.	Explore circumstances in which patient came to the emergency department; consider an amobarbital (Amytal) interview; evaluate patient to rule out organic cause.
Amphetamine, cocaine, or amphetaminelike intoxication	Psychosis; agitation or assaultive behavior; paranoia.	Decrease stimulation, consider restraints and antipsychotics to control behavior, consider hospitalization as amphetamine-induced psychotic disorder may persist for weeks to months; cocaine withdrawal may produce suicidal feelings.
Anxiety, acute	Differential diagnosis, particularly of medical or substance-induced cause; management of the acute symptomatology.	Explore patient's capacity for insight regarding the precipitant; refer for outpatient psychiatric treatment; avoid prescribing medications from the emergency department because the principal agents that are effective are also commonly abused.
Borderline personality disorder	Determination of the immediate need for the emergency department visit; determination of the patient's agenda.	Evaluate for acute suicidal ideation; consider hospitalization if clinician is uncomfortable; state limits as clearly as able to enforce; state clear follow-up plan.
Catatonia	Differential diagnosis of an organic cause; management of the acute symptoms.	Rule out organic causes; consider rapid tranquilization if the emergency department has the capacity to monitor the patient over several hours.
Delirium, dementia	Fluctuating sensorium; determine acuity; differential diagnosis; need for physical restraint while the patient is evaluated.	Evaluate patient for organic cause; remember that prescribed medications are very common causes for acute cognitive disorders.

(continued)

Table 25–7—*continued*
Common Psychiatric Emergencies

Syndrome or Presenting Symptom	Emergency Problem	Emergency Treatment Issues
Delusions	Degree to which delusional beliefs interfere with the patient's ability to negotiate activities of daily living; degree to which the patient's response to these delusional beliefs is likely to cause problems for the patient.	Explore the time of onset, the pervasiveness of the delusions, and the degree to which the delusional beliefs interfere with the patient's daily functioning, particularly if there is anything to suggest that the patient might try to harm self or others because of these delusions; rule out organic causes; refer for ongoing treatment, or hospitalize if there is an immediate life threat or need for further organic evaluation.
Depression	Recognition of the diagnosis; onset; risk of suicide; assessment of the need to protect the patient.	Explore onset of symptoms; evaluate for suicidal ideation; evaluate nonpsychiatric causes; drug-related depression; consider hospitalization if the patient does not respond to the interpersonal interaction of the emergency evaluation or seems hopeless or helpless even after the evaluation; tell the patient the presumptive diagnosis and refer for treatment; initiation of pharmacological treatment for depression should not take place from an emergency department unless there will be continuity of care for the patient in the some system.
Dystonia, acute	Patient's psychological and physical discomfort; identification of causative agent.	Determine the causative agent; treat with diphenhydramine or benztropine and contact the agency or therapist that prescribed the medication for follow-up care; refer the patient back to treating agency after explaining the cause of the symptoms.
Family crises, marital cases	Determination of danger to members of the family; resolution of the crisis sufficiently to get the couple or family out of the emergency department.	Offer an opportunity for the family unit to meet briefly to explore the issue that brought them to the emergency department; do not make any recommendations that seem self-evident, because there is always more than meets the eye when a crisis propels a family to use an emergency department as an intervention; rule out issues of domestic violence, child abuse, or substance abuse; refer as appropriate.
Geriatric crises	Identification of contributory medical or pharmacological problems; identification of family agenda.	Determine acuity; try to uncover the family agenda; rule out organicity, especially as it relates to the reason for the emergency department visit now; rule out elder abuse; refer as appropriate.

(continued)

Table 25–7—*continued*
Common Psychiatric Emergencies

Syndrome or Presenting Symptom	Emergency Problem	Emergency Treatment Issues
Grief and bereavement	Identification of an excessive or pathological reaction, determination of the need for professional referral; facilitation of the grieving process in the emergency department.	Explore any extreme or pathological reactions to the loss, especially undue use of medications, drugs, or alcohol; rule out major depressive disorder; acknowledge the validity of the feelings, and refer for appropriate treatment or to support groups as necessary; avoid prescribing any medications from the emergency department unless there is the capacity for continuity of care and follow-up.
Hallucinations	Onset; differential diagnosis, particularly for a medical or substance-related cause.	Evaluate for possible organic cause, especially for visual, tactile, or olfactory hallucinations; assess for suicidal or homicidal content and consider hospitalization or referral for immediate care, if indicated.
High fever	Potential life threat; determine cause; potential offenders include lithium, anticholinergics, agranulocytosis induced by clozapine (Clozaril) or phenothiazines; neuroleptic malignant syndrome.	Emergency treatment for high fever; stop offending medication and treat underlying cause.
Homicidal and assaultive behavior	Danger to staff and other patients; determination of risk for suicide; cause of the behavior.	Determine whether there is an acute psychiatric condition determining the homicidal or assaultive behavior; use sufficient personnel and restraints to ensure the safety of staff and other patients; rule out medical or substance-related components.
Homosexual panic	Circumstances precipitating the behavior; emergency department capacity to accommodate patient's immediate need.	Allow the patient an opportunity to talk; medication, including benzodiazepines or antipsychotics, may be needed to calm the patient; be particularly cautious about any physical assessment of the patient.
Hyperventilation	Physical symptoms; patient's anxiety with respect to the symptoms.	Explain briefly to the patient how the symptoms are caused by hyperventilation; instruct the patient to breathe into a paper bag for several minutes; it may be useful to encourage the patient to hyperventilate again in the clinician's presence to confirm the cause of the symptoms.
Insomnia	Determination of an acute precipitant; identification of the patient's primary concern.	Determine the cause of the symptoms, rule out depression or incipient psychosis; refer as appropriate; do not prescribe medications from the emergency department for the condition.
Lithium (Eskalith) toxicity	Medical instability; contributing medical conditions.	Monitor for significant medical instability and consider hospitalization; stop lithium immediately; institute supportive measures as indicated.

(continued)

Table 25–7—*continued*
Common Psychiatric Emergencies

Syndrome or Presenting Symptom	Emergency Problem	Emergency Treatment Issues
Mania	Danger to self or others; need for restraints before behavior escalates out of control in the emergency department.	Reduce stimulation and consider the use of restraints; rule out organic cause if there is no history of a bipolar disorder or if the symptoms are significantly worse; consider hospitalization, especially if patient is unable to appreciate need for treatment.
Neuroleptic malignant syndrome	Medical instability; correct identification of the problem; need for rapid response.	Institute life support measures as indicated; the illness can progress rapidly; hospitalize; make clear to the receiving physicians the presumptive diagnosis.
Opioid intoxication or withdrawal	Correct identification of the problem.	Administer naloxone (Narcan) for overdose; opiate withdrawal is not life threatening, and patient may be treated symptomatically for relief of discomfort; refer to proper treatment program.
Panic reactions	Identification of an acute precipitant; response to the patient's need for immediate relief.	Talk the patient down; look for an organic cause, especially for a first episode; attempt to identify the acute precipitant, but it is a chronic problem that must be referred for adequate management; there is some evidence that encouraging the patient to face the precipitating stimulus again as soon as possible minimizes the long-term disability associated with panic reactions.
Paranoia	Underlying psychosis; possible organic cause.	Consider an underlying psychosis; stimulant abuse is the most common organic cause for paranoid symptoms; refer the patient as appropriate, or consider hospitalization if the paranoia poses a threat to the patient's life or to others'; suicidal behavior is not uncommon in acute paranoia.
Parkinsonism	Identification of the cause (i.e., idiopathic vs. side effects of medication).	Prescribe an antiparkinsonian agent and refer the patient to the original prescribing physician or to a neurologist or psychiatrist as indicated.
Phencyclidine intoxication	Identification of causative agent; danger to self or others.	Reduce stimulation; observe for significant physiological disturbances, such as temperature elevation; avoid antipsychotics; hospitalize, if necessary to protect the patient during intoxication, which may last for several days.
Phobias	Reason for current emergency department visit.	Assess onset of symptoms and the degree to which they are interfering with the patient immediately; refer for long-term management, probably to a behavioral treatment program.
Photosensitivity or rash	Confirm cause (phenothiazines).	Advise patient of necessary precautions (sunscreen, hat, avoidance of strong sunlight).

(continued)

Table 25–7—*continued*
Common Psychiatric Emergencies

Syndrome or Presenting Symptom	Emergency Problem	Emergency Treatment Issues
Posttraumatic stress disorder	Identification of the precipitant; identification of symptoms that are particularly disruptive to normal functioning, such as substance abuse, sleep disturbances, or isolation.	Assess onset of symptoms; try to identify the precipitant for the current visit; refer to a brief treatment program if a specific precipitant can be identified.
Priapism	Discomfort, anxiety; determine whether patient is on trazodone (Desyrel).	Discontinue trazodone; consult urologist if symptom persists.
Psychosis	Acuity; differential diagnosis; danger to self or others from suicidal ideation or psychotic ideation.	Evaluate for organic cause; explore possible precipitants; take whatever measures are indicated to protect the patient and others; consider rapid neuroleptization if medical or substance-related cause can be clearly ruled out.
Rape	Identification of any extreme features of the assault; need for support; medical components.	Be sure that all medical and forensic issues have been addressed, such as chain of evidence, prevention of pregnancy, and sexually transmitted disease; facilitate the patient's exploration of feelings about the assault; facilitate access to rape crisis counseling.
Repeaters	Reason for the return visit; emergency issues; danger to self or others; reason for failure of prior management or referral.	Once genuine reasons for a return visit have been ruled out, review how the emergency department may be encouraging the patient to use such a method of receiving care and attention rather than more traditional channels; consider substance abuse or medical condition as possible overlooked conditions.
Schizophrenia	Onset; reason for current emergency department visit; question whether there is a breakdown of long-term case management.	Determine reason for use of the emergency department rather than the patient's identified treatment program; contact program before making any decisions about treatment or hospitalization; consider suicide potential.
Sedative intoxication	Medical management; exploration of motivation (was it a suicidal act?) for intoxication.	Initiate treatment as indicated; consider suicidal intent even if patient denies it.
Seizures	Patient safety; determination of cause.	Observe for postictal confusion; discontinue or lower seizure-inducing medication; refer or hospitalize for comprehensive evaluation.
Substance abuse	Onset; reason for use of the emergency department; identification of agent; level of need for treatment (intoxication, withdrawal, or desire for abstinence).	Institute treatment as indicated for medically unstable patients; refer all others to formal treatment programs and do not institute treatment in the emergency department.

(continued)

Table 25–7—*continued*
Common Psychiatric Emergencies

Syndrome or Presenting Symptom	Emergency Problem	Emergency Treatment Issues
Suicidal behavior	Seriousness of intent; seriousness of attempt; need for medical intervention; need for hospitalization.	Consider hospitalization, particularly if patient has made prior attempts; has a family history of suicide; has had a significant recent loss, particularly by suicide; and does not seem to respond to the interpersonal interaction with the physician; hospitalize if uneasy.
Suicide thoughts or threats	Seriousness of intent; ability of patient to control thoughts; determination of usefulness of prior or current psychiatric treatment.	As above.
Tardive dyskinesia	Patient's discomfort; reason for emergency department visit; question whether there has been a breakdown of outpatient management.	This is a long-term problem, not an acute one; reduction of antipsychotic often increases the symptoms of tardive dyskinesia; refer the patient for appropriate psychiatric treatment.
Tremor	New onset? Determine cause, such as lithium toxicity, tardive dyskinesia, substance withdrawal, anxiety.	Treat according to cause.
Violence	Danger to others; determination of underlying psychiatric basis for behavior.	Use sufficient strength, in terms of numbers and competence of staff, and restraints to control the behavior quickly; delay or hesitation may escalate the violence; assess, and treat the patient as indicated according to the underlying cause; file charges if there has been any damage or injury because of the patient's behavior.

Table by Beverly J. Fauman, M.D.

3. If the patient is already taking an antipsychotic, give more of the same drug. If the patient's agitation has not decreased in 20 to 30 minutes, repeat the dose.
4. Avoid antipsychotics in patients who are at risk for seizures.
5. Benzodiazepines may be ineffective in patients who are tolerant, and they may cause disinhibition, which can potentially exacerbate violence.
6. For patients with epilepsy, first try an anticonvulsant (e.g., carbamazepine [Tegretol] or gabapentin [Neurontin]) and then a benzodiazepine (e.g., clonazepam [Klonopin]). Chronically violent patients sometimes respond to beta-blockers (e.g., propranolol [Inderal]).

III. Other Psychiatric Emergencies

A psychiatric emergency is a disturbance in thoughts, feelings, or actions that requires immediate treatment. It may be caused or accompanied by a medical or surgical condition that requires timely evaluation and treatment. Emergencies can occur in any location—home, office, street, and medical, surgical, and psychiatric units. Under ideal conditions, the patient will be brought to the psychiatric emergency unit, where physicians and psychiatrists who specialize in emergency medicine can evaluate the situation and institute treatment. Table 25–7 lists a broad range of conditions that fall into the category of psychiatric emergencies.

For a more detailed discussion of this topic, see Psychiatric Emergencies, Ch 29, p. 2717, in CTP/VIII.

Infant, Child, and Adolescent Disorders

I. Principles of Child and Adolescent Diagnostic Assessment

A comprehensive evaluation of a child includes interviews with the parents, the child, and the family; gathering of information regarding the child's current school functioning; and often, a standardized assessment of the child's intellectual level and academic achievement. In some cases, standardized measures of developmental level and neuropsychological assessments are useful. Psychiatric evaluations of children are rarely initiated by the child, so clinicians must obtain information from the family and the school to understand the reasons for the evaluation. In some cases, the court or a child protective service agency may initiate a psychiatric evaluation. Children often have difficulty with the chronology of symptoms and are sometimes reticent to report behaviors that got them into trouble. Very young children often cannot articulate their experiences verbally and are better at showing their feelings and preoccupations in a play situation.

The examiner should make sure that the following areas are covered:

A. Supplement data from patient interviews with information from family members, guardians, teachers, and outside agencies.

B. Understand normal development so as to understand fully what constitutes abnormality at a given age. Table 26–1 presents developmental milestones.

C. Be familiar with the current diagnostic criteria of disorders so as to guide anamnesis on the mental status examination.

D. Understand the family psychiatric history, which is necessary given the genetic predispositions and environmental influences associated with many disorders.

II. Child Development

Development results from the interplay of maturation of the central nervous system (CNS), neuromuscular apparatus, and endocrine system and various environmental influences (e.g., parents and teachers, who can either facilitate or thwart a child's attainment of his or her developmental potential). This potential is specific to each person's given genetic predisposition to (1) intellectual level and (2) mental disorders, temperament, and probably certain personality traits.

Development is continuous and lifelong but is most rapid in early life. The neonatal brain weighs 350 g, almost triples in weight by 18 months, and at 7 years is very close to the adult weight of 1,350 g. Whereas neurogenesis is virtually complete at birth, the arborization of axons and dendrites continues for many years. This and synaptogenesis appear to be influenced by the environment. Because of brain plasticity, some connections are strengthened

Table 26–1
Landmarks of Normal Behavioral Development

Age	Motor and Sensory Behavior	Adaptive Behavior	Personal and Social Behavior
Birth to 4 weeks	Hand to mouth reflex, grasping reflex Rooting reflex (puckering lips in response to perioral stimulation); Moro reflex (digital extension when startled); sucking reflex; Babinski reflex (toes spread when sole of foot touched) Differentiates sounds (orients to human voice) and sweet and sour tastes Visual tracking Fixed focal distance of 8 inches Makes alternating crawling movements Moves head laterally when placed in prone position	Anticipatory feeding-approach behavior of 4 days Responds to sound of rattle and bell Regards moving objects momentarily	Responsiveness to mother's face, eyes, and voice within first few hours of life Endogenous smile Independent play (until 2 years) Quiets when picked up Impassive face
4 weeks	Tonic neck reflex positions predominate Hands fisted Head sags but can hold head erect for a few seconds	Follows moving objects to the midline Shows no interest and drops objects immediately	Regards face and diminishes activity Responds to speech Smiles preferentially to mother
16 weeks	Visual fixation, stereoscopic vision (12 weeks) Symmetrical postures predominate Holds head balanced Head lifted 90 degrees when prone on forearm Visual accommodation	Follows a slowly moving object well Arms activate on sight of dangling object	Spontaneous social smile (exogenous) Aware of strange situations
28 weeks	Sits steadily, leaning forward on hands Bounces actively when placed in standing position	One-hand approach and grasp of toy Bangs and shakes rattle Transfers toys	Takes feet to mouth Pats mirror image Starts to imitate mother's sounds and actions
40 weeks	Sits alone with good coordination Creeps Pulls self to standing position Points with index finger	Matches two objects at midline Attempt to imitate scribble	Separation anxiety manifest when taken away from mother Responds to social play, such as pat-a-cake and peekaboo Feeds self cracker and holds own bottle
52 weeks	Walks with one hand held Stands alone briefly	Seeks novelty	Cooperates in dressing

Age	Motor	Social/Behavioral
15 months	Toddles Creeps up stairs	Points or vocalizes wants Throws objects in play or refusal
18 months	Coordinated walking, seldom falls Hurls ball Walks up stairs with one hand held	Feeds self in part, spills Pulls toy on string Carries or hugs a special toy, such as a doll Imitates some behavioral patterns with slight delay
2 years	Builds a tower of three or four cubes Scribbles spontaneously and imitates a writing stroke	Pulls on simple garment Domestic mimicry Refers to self by name Says "no" to mother
	Runs well, no falling Kicks large ball Goes up and down stairs alone Fine motor skills increase	Separation anxiety begins to diminish Organized demonstrations of love and protest Parallel play (plays side by side but does not interact with other children)
	Builds a tower of six or seven cubes Aligns cubes, imitating train Imitates vertical and circular strokes Develops original behaviors	
3 years	Rides tricycle Jumps from bottom steps Alternates feet going up stairs	Puts on shoes Unbuttons buttons Feeds self well Understands taking turns
	Builds tower of nine or ten cubes Imitates a three-cube bridge Copies a circle and a cross	
4 years	Walks down stairs one step to a tread Stands on one foot for 5–8 sec	Washes and dries own face Brushes teeth Associative or joint play (plays cooperatively with other children)
	Copies a cross Repeats four digits Counts three objects with correct pointing	
5 years	Skips, using feet alternately Usually has complete sphincter control Fine coordination improves	Dresses and undresses self Prints a few letters Plays competitive exercise games
	Copies a square Draws a recognizable human with a head, a body, limbs Counts 10 objects accurately	
6 years	Rides two-wheel bicycle	Ties shoelaces
	Prints name Copies triangle	

Adapted from Arnold Gesell, M.D., and Stella Chess, M.D.

and others are developed in response to environmental input. Myelinization continues for decades.

The most cited theorists in child development have been Sigmund Freud, Margaret Mahler, Erik Erikson, and Jean Piaget; their work is outlined in Table 26–2.

III. Learning Disorders

Learning disorder is diagnosed when reading, writing, and mathematical skills are significantly lower than expected. The text revision of the fourth edition of the *Diagnostic and Statistical Manual of Mental Disorders (DSM-IV-TR)* includes four diagnostic categories on learning disorders: reading disorder, mathematic disorder, disorder of written expression, and learning disorder not otherwise specified.

A. Reading disorder. Formally known as *dyslexia*, reading disorder is characterized by an impaired ability to recognize words, poor comprehension, and slow and inaccurate reading.

  1. Diagnosis. Reading ability is significantly below that expected of a child of the same age, education, and measured intelligence. It is usually identified by the age of 7 years (second grade); however, in some cases, particularly when the disorder is associated with high intelligence, it may not be apparent until the age of 9 years (fourth grade). Associated problems include language difficulties and difficulties in properly sequencing words. Younger children tend to feel shame and humiliation while older children tend to be angry and depressed and exhibit low self-esteem (Table 26–3).

  2. Epidemiology

   a. Occurs in 4% of school-aged children.

   b. Prevalence ranges from 2% to 8%.

   c. Equal rates among females and males.

  3. Etiology

   a. Possible link to chromosome 6 and chromosome 15.

   b. Occipital lobe lesions and hemispheric abnormality have been linked.

   c. Occurs in 35% to 40% of first-degree relatives.

  4. Differential diagnosis

   a. Mental retardation. Reading, along with other skills, is below the achievement expected for a child's chronologic age.

   b. Attention-deficit/hyperactivity disorder (ADHD). Difficulties with linguistic abilities are not consistent. Reading improves with medication.

   c. Hearing and visual impairments. Should be ruled out with screening tests.

  5. Course and prognosis. Most school-aged children do not need remediation past grade school, with only severe disorders requiring help into middle and high school level.

Text continues on page 358.

Table 26-2
A Synthesis of Developmental Theorists

Age (years)	Margaret Mahler	Sigmund Freud	Erik Erikson	Jean Piaget	Comments
0–1	Normal autistic phase (birth to 4 weeks) • State of half-sleep, half-wake • Major task of phase is to achieve homeostatic equilibrium with the environment Normal symbiotic phase (3–4 weeks to 4–5 months) • Dim awareness of caretaker, but infant still functions as if he or she and caretaker are in state of undifferentiation or fusion • Social smile characteristic (2–4 months) The subphases of separation–individuation proper First subphase: differentiation (5–10 months) • Process of hatching from autistic shell (i.e., developing more alert sensorium that reflects cognitive and neurologic maturation) • Beginning of comparative scanning (i.e., comparing what is and what is not mother) • Characteristic anxiety: stranger anxiety, which involves curiosity and fear (most prevalent around 8 months)	Oral phase (birth to 1 year) • Major site of tension and gratification is the mouth, lips, tongue—includes biting and sucking activities	Basic trust vs. basic mistrust (oral sensory) (birth to 1 year) • Social mistrust demonstrated via ease of feeding, depth of sleep, bowel relaxation • Depends on consistency and sameness of experience provided by caretaker • Second 6 months teething and biting move infant "from getting to taking" • Weaning leads to "nostalgia for lost paradise" • If basic trust is strong, child maintains hopeful attitude	Sensorimotor phase (birth to 2 years) • Intelligence rests mainly on actions and movements coordinated under schemata. (*Schemata* is a pattern of behavior in response to a particular environmental stimulus.) • Environment is mastered through *assimilation* and *accommodation* (*Assimilation* is the incorporation of new environmental stimuli; *accommodation* is the modification of behavior to adapt to new stimuli.) • *Object permanence* is achieved by age 2 years. Object still exists in mind if disappears from view: search for hidden object • *Reversibility* in action begins	In contrast to Mahler, other observers of mother-infant pairs are impressed with a mutuality and complementarity (not autism or fusion), which provides a groundwork for relatedness and language development, as if there were a prewiring for these abilities. Piaget and others emphasize the infant's active striving to manipulate the inanimate environment. This supplements Freud's work because the infant and young child's motivation for behavior is not simply to relieve drive tension and attain oral, anal, and phallic gratification.

(continued)

353

Table 26-2—continued
A Synthesis of Developmental Theorists

Age (years)	Margaret Mahler	Sigmund Freud	Erik Erikson	Jean Piaget	Comments

1–2	Second subphase: practicing (10–16 months)
	• Beginning of this phase marked by upright locomotion—child has new perspective and also mood of elation
	• Mother used as home base
	• Characteristic anxiety: separation anxiety
	
	Third subphase: rapprochement (16–24 months)
	• Infant now a toddler—more aware of physical separateness, which dampens mood of elation
	• Child tries to bridge gap between self and mother—concretely seen as bringing objects to mother
	• Mother's efforts to help toddler often not perceived as helpful, temper tantrums typical
	• Characteristic event: rapprochement crisis, wanting to be soothed by mother and yet not able to accept her help
	• Symbol of rapprochement: child standing on threshold of door not knowing which way to turn, helpless frustration
	• Resolution of crisis occurs as child's skills improve and child able to get gratification from doing things on own
		Anal phase (1–3 years)
		• Anus and surrounding area major source of interest
		• Acquisition of voluntary sphincter control (toilet training)
			Autonomy vs. shame and doubt (muscular–anal) (1–3 years)
			• Biologically includes learning to walk, feed self, talk
			• Muscular maturation sets stage for "holding on and letting go"
			• Need for outer control, firmness of caretaker before development of autonomy
			• *Shame* occurs when child is overtly self-conscious via negative exposure
			• *Self-doubt* can evolve if parents overly shame child (e.g., about elimination)
				Preoperational phase (2–7 years)
				• Appearance of *symbolic* functions, associated with language acquisition
				• *Egocentrism*: child understands everything exclusively from own perspective
				• Thinking is illogical and magical
				• Nonreversible thinking with absence of conversation
				  —*Animism*: belief that inanimate objects are alive (i.e., have feelings and intentions)
				  —"*Imminent justice*," belief that punishment for bad deeds is inevitable
					Supplementing the work of Freud and Mahler, theorists have postulated that severe problems in mother–infant/toddler interactions contribute to the formation of pathological character traits, gender identity disorder, or personality disorders. Angry, frustrating, narcissistic caretakers often produce angry, needy children and adults who cannot tolerate the normal frustrations and disappointments in relationships and whose character formation is grossly distorted.

Age				
2–3	Fourth subphase: consolidation and object constancy (24–36 months) • Child better able to cope with mother's absence and engage substitutes • Child can begin to feel comfortable with mother's absences by knowing she will return • Gradual internalization of image of mother as reliable and stable • Through increasing verbal skills and better sense of time, child can tolerate delay and endure separations			
3–4	Phalic-cedipal phase (3–5 years) • Genital focus of interest, stimulation, and excitement • Penis is organ of interest for both sexes • Genital masturbation common • Intense preoccupation with *castration anxiety* (fear of genital loss or injury) • *Penis envy* (discontent with one's own genitals and wish to possess genitals of male) seen in girls in this phase • *Oedipus complex* universal: child wishes to have sex with and marry parent of opposite sex and simultaneously be rid of parent of same sex	Initiative vs. guilt (locomotor genital) (3–5 years) • *Initiative* arises in relation to tasks for the sake of activity, both motor and intellectual • *Guilt* may arise over goals contemplated (especially aggressive) • Desire to mimic adult world; involvement in oedipal struggle leads to resolution via social role identification • Sibling rivalry frequent	Researchers have amended Freud's work. Children of both sexes explore and are aware of their own genitals during the second year of life and, with proper parental reinforcement, begin to correctly identify themselves as girls or boys. Penis envy is neither universal nor normative. Freud emphasized problems with oedipal resolution in psychopathogenesis. His theory accounts for only a part of psychopathology.
4–5				

(continued)

Table 26–2—continued
A Synthesis of Developmental Theorists

Age (years)	Margaret Mahler	Sigmund Freud	Erik Erikson	Jean Piaget	Comments
5–6		Latency phase (from 5–6 years to 11–12 years) • State of relative quiescence of sexual drive with resolution of oedipal complex • Sexual drives channeled into more socially appropriate aims (i.e., schoolwork and sports)			Contrary to Freud, the onset of latency (school age or middle childhood) is now considered primarily a consequence of changes in the CNS and less dependent on the nondemonstrable quiescence and sublimation of sexual drive. During the years 6–8, changes in the CNS are reflected in developmental progress of perceptual-sensory-motor functioning and thought processes. In Piaget's framework, it is the transition from the preoperational to the concrete (operational) phase. Compared with preschoolers, latency children are capable of greater learning, independent functioning, and socialization. Friendships develop with less dependence on parents (and less preoccupation with intrafamilial oedipal rivalries). Today, superego development is considered more prolonged and gradual and less related to oedipal resolution.
6–11		• Formation for superego, one of three psychic structures in mind responsible for moral and ethical development, including conscience • Other two psychic structures are ego, a group of functions mediating between drives and the external environment, and id, repository of sexual and aggressive drives • The id is present at birth, and the ego develops gradually from rudimentary structure present at birth	• Industry vs. inferiority (latency) (6–11 years) • Child is busy building, creating, and accomplishing • Receives systematic instruction as well as fundamentals of technology • Danger of sense of inadequacy and inferiority if child despairs of his or her tools/skills and status among peers • Socially decisive age	• Concrete (operational) phase (7–11 years) • Emergence of logical (cause–effect) thinking, including reversibility and ability to sequence and serialize • Understanding of part-whole relationships and classifications • Child able to take others' point of view • Conservation of number, length, weight, and volume	

11+

Genital phase (from 11–12 years and beyond) • Final stage of psychosexual development—begins with puberty and the biologic capacity for orgasm but involves the capacity for true intimacy	Identity vs. role diffusion (11 years through end of adolescence) • Struggle to develop *ego identity* (sense of inner sameness and continuity) • Preoccupation with appearance, hero worship, ideology • *Group identity* (peers) develops • Danger of *role confusion*, doubts about sexual and vocational identity • *Psychosocial moratorium*, stage between morality learned by the child and the ethics to be developed by the adult	Formal (abstract) phase (11 years through end of adolescence) • Hypothetical–deductive reasoning, not only on basis of objects but also on basis of hypotheses or propositions • Capable of thinking about one's thoughts • Combinative structures emerge, permitting flexible grouping of elements in a system • Ability to use two systems of reference simultaneously • Ability to grasp concept of probabilities	The interplay of child and caretaker is emphasized in the attachment theory of John Bowlby. Mary Ainsworth developed the "strange situation" protocol for examining infant–caretaker separations. "Goodness of fit" between child and caretaker is also stressed in the work on temperament by Chess and Thomas. Infants have inborn differences in certain behavioral dimensions, such as activity level, approach, or withdrawal, intensity of reaction. How parents respond to these behaviors influences development. Lawrence Kohlberg, who was influenced by Piaget, described three levels of moral development: preconventional, in which moral decisions are made to avoid punishment; conventional role conformity, with decisions made to maintain friendships; and in adolescence self-accepted moral principles, (i.e. voluntary compliance with ethical principles).

Adapted from Sylvia Karasu, M.D. and Richard Oberfield, M.D.

Table 26–3
DSM-IV-TR Diagnostic Criteria for Reading Disorder

A. Reading achievement, as measured by individually administered standardized tests of reading accuracy or comprehension, is substantially below that expected given the person's chronologic age, measured intelligence, and age-appropriate education.
B. The disturbance in Criterion A significantly interferes with academic achievement or activities of daily living that require reading skills.
C. If a sensory deficit is present, the reading difficulties are in excess of those usually associated with it.
Coding note: If a general medical (e.g., neurologic) condition or sensory deficit is present, code the breakcondition on Axis III.

From American Psychiatric Association. *Diagnostic and Statistical Manual of Mental Disorders*, 4th ed. Text rev. Washington, DC: American Psychiatric Association, 2000, with permission.

6. **Treatment**
   a. **Remediation.** Effective remediation programs begin with teaching the child to make accurate associations between letters and sounds. Once these skills have been mastered, remediation can target larger components of reading, such as syllables and words. Positive coping strategies include small, structured reading groups that offer individual attention.
   b. **Psychotherapy.** Coexisting emotional and behavioral problems are treated by appropriate psychotherapeutic means. Parental counseling may be helpful. Social skills improvement is an important component of psychotherapy.
   c. **Pharmacotherapy.** Used only for an associated psychiatric disorder, such as ADHD.
B. **Mathematics disorder.** Child has difficulty with learning and remembering numerals, remembering and applying basic facts about numbers, and is slow and inaccurate in computation.
   1. **Diagnosis.** Mathematical ability is significantly below what is expected when considering the child's age, education, and measured intelligence. Children have difficulty learning the names for numbers and signs for addition and subtraction, memorizing multiplication tables, applying computations to word problems, and doing calculations at a reasonable pace (Table 26–4).

Table 26–4
DSM-IV-TR Diagnostic Criteria for Mathematics Disorder

A. Mathematical ability, as measured by individually administered standardized tests, is substantially below that expected given the person's chronologic age, measured intelligence, and age-appropriate education.
B. The disturbance in Criterion A significantly interferes with academic achievement or activities of daily living that require mathematical ability.
C. If a sensory deficit is present, the difficulties in mathematical ability are in excess of those usually associated with it.
Coding note: If a general medical (e.g., neurologic) condition or sensory deficit is present, code the breakcondition on Axis III.

From American Psychiatric Association. *Diagnostic and Statistical Manual of Mental Disorders*, 4th ed. Text rev. Washington, DC: American Psychiatric Association, 2000, with permission.

2. **Epidemiology**
   a. Occurs in approximately 1% of school-aged children.
   b. May occur more often in females.
3. **Etiology**
   a. In part to genetic factors.
   b. Possible right hemisphere deficit, principally in occipital lobe areas.
4. **Differential diagnosis**
   a. **Mental retardation.** Arithmetic difficulties are accompanied by a generalized impairment in overall intellectual functioning.
   b. **ADHD or conduct disorder.** Should not be overlooked during diagnosis.
5. **Course and prognosis.** This disorder is usually identified by the age of 8 years (third grade); however, it can be seen as early as 6 years (first grade) or as late as 10 years (fifth grade). Children with moderate mathematics disorder who do not receive intervention may have complications such as continuing academic difficulties, shame, poor self-concept, frustration, and depression. Such complications can lead to reluctance to attend school, truancy, and hopelessness about academic success.
6. **Treatment**
   a. **Remediation.** Combines effective teaching of mathematical concepts along with continuous practice.
   b. **Psychoeducation.** Provides positive feedback for good performance in social areas.

C. **Disorders of written expression.** Characterized by frequent grammatical and punctuation errors and poor spelling and handwriting skills.
   1. **Diagnosis.** Child underperforms in composing written text when compared to similar-aged children and intellectual ability. The child has poor spelling, poor punctuation, poor handwriting, and poor organization of written stories. Features manifest in grade school. The child often becomes angry and frustrated because of feelings of inadequacy and failure in academic performance. In severe cases, depressive disorders may be present (Table 26–5).

Table 26–5
DSM-IV-TR Diagnostic Criteria for Disorder of Written Expression

A. Writing skills, as measured by individually administered standardized tests (or functional assessments of writing skills), are substantially below those expected given the person's chronologic age, measured intelligence, and age-appropriate education.
B. The disturbance in Criterion A significantly interferes with academic achievement or activities of daily living that require the composition of written texts (e.g., writing grammatically correct sentences and organized paragraphs).
C. If a sensory deficit is present, the difficulties in writing skills are in excess of those usually associated with it.
Coding note: If a general medical (e.g., neurologic) condition or sensory deficit is present, code the breakcondition on Axis III.

From American Psychiatric Association. *Diagnostic and Statistical Manual of Mental Disorders,* 4th ed. Text rev. Washington, DC: American Psychiatric Association, 2000, with permission.

2. **Epidemiology**
   a. Occurs in approximately 4% of school-aged children.
   b. Three times more likely in males.
3. **Etiology**
   a. Causes believed to be similar to those of reading disorder.
   b. Strong concordance between children and first-degree relatives with disorder of written expression.
4. **Differential diagnosis.** The confounding effects of ADHD and depressive disorder may interfere with the ability to concentrate. Therefore, treatment of the above disorders may improve the child's writing performance. Disorder of written expression may occur with other language and learning disorders such as reading disorder, mixed receptive–expressive language disorder, expressive language disorder, mathematics disorder, developmental coordination disorder, and disruptive behavior and attention-deficit disorders (ADDs).
5. **Course and prognosis.** In severe cases, symptoms appear by age 7 (second grade); in less severe cases, the disorder may appear by age 10 (fifth grade) or later. Patients with mild to moderate cases usually do well if they receive remedial education early in grade school. Severe cases require continual, extensive remedial treatment through high school and college. Prognosis relies on the severity of the disorder, the age or grade in which intervention is received, the length and continuity of treatment, and the presence or absence of associated or secondary emotional or behavioral problems.
6. **Treatment**
   a. **Remediation.** Treatment includes continuous practice of spelling and sentence writing and review of grammar. Intensive and individually tailored creative writing therapy may provide additional benefit.
   b. **Psychotherapy.** Psychological therapy including individual, group, or family therapy may be useful in cases of secondary behavioral and emotional problems.
D. **Learning disorder not otherwise specified.** A category in *DSM-IV-TR* for disorders that do not meet the criteria for any specific learning disorder, but cause impairment and reflects learning abilities below those expected for a child's intelligence, education, and age (Table 26–6). An example is a spelling skills deficit.

IV. **Motor Skills Disorder: Developmental Coordination Disorder**
   Characterized by poor performance in daily activities requiring coordination. This may present with delays in achieving such motor milestones as sitting, crawling, and walking. The disorder may also manifest by clumsy gross and fine motor skills, resulting in poor athletic performance and poor handwriting.
   A. **Diagnosis.** Disorder may manifest as early as infancy. Diagnosis is based on a history of delay in achieving early motor milestones. The diagnosis may be associated with below-normal scores on performance subtests of

Table 26–6
DSM-IV-TR Diagnostic Criteria for Learning Disorder Not Otherwise Specified

This category is for disorders in learning that do not meet criteria for any specific learning disorder. This category might include problems in all three areas (reading, mathematics, written expression) that together significantly interfere with academic achievement even though performance on tests measuring each individual skill is not substantially below that expected given the person's chronologic age, measured intelligence, and age-appropriate education.

From American Psychiatric Association. *Diagnostic and Statistical Manual of Mental Disorders*, 4th ed. Text rev. Washington, DC: American Psychiatric Association, 2000, with permission.

standardized intelligence tests and by normal or above-normal scores on verbal subtests (Table 26–7).

B. Epidemiology
1. Prevalence is approximately 5% of school-aged children.
2. Male-to-female ratio may range from 2:1 to 4:1; however, bias may exist.

C. Etiology
1. Unknown but probably multifactorial.
2. Risk factors may include prematurity, hypoxia, perinatal malnutrition, and low birth weight.
3. Frequently found in children with hyperactivity and learning disorders.

D. Differential diagnosis
1. **Neuromuscular disorders.** Patients exhibit more global muscle and neurologic impairment.
2. **Attention-deficit/hyperactivity disorder.** Rule out physical carelessness seen in individuals with ADHD.
3. **Mental retardation.** Coordination usually does not stand out as a significant deficit compared with other skills.

E. Course and prognosis. Few data available on outcome. Although clumsiness may continue, some children are able to compensate by developing interest in other skills. Clumsiness generally persists into adolescence and adult life.

Table 26–7
DSM-IV-TR Diagnostic Criteria for Developmental Coordination Disorder

A. Performance in daily activities that require motor coordination is substantially below that expected given the person's chronologic age and measured intelligence. This may be manifested by marked delays in achieving motor milestones (e.g., walking, crawling, sitting), dropping things, "clumsiness," poor performance in sports, or poor handwriting.
B. The disturbance in Criterion A significantly interferes with academic achievement or activities of daily living.
C. The disturbance is not due to a general medical condition (e.g., cerebral palsy, hemiplegia, or muscular dystrophy) and does not meet criteria for a pervasive developmental disorder.
D. If mental retardation is present, the motor difficulties are in excess of those usually associated with it.
Coding note: If a general medical (e.g., neurologic) condition or sensory deficit is present, code the condition on Axis III.

From American Psychiatric Association. *Diagnostic and Statistical Manual of Mental Disorders*, 4th ed. Text rev. Washington, DC: American Psychiatric Association, 2000, with permission.

F. **Treatment.** Usually includes versions of sensory integration programs and modified forms of physical education. Sensory integration programs consist of physical activities that increase awareness of motor and sensory function. Adaptive physical education programs incorporate certain sports actions, such as kicking or throwing a ball. Patients may benefit from social skills groups and other prosocial interventions. Secondary academic and emotional problems and coexisting communication disorders should be considered for individual treatments. Parental counseling may be beneficial in reducing parents' anxiety and guilt, increasing their awareness, and facilitating their confidence.

V. **Communication Disorders**

Communication disorders are characterized by impairment in understanding and expressing language and the production of speech. There are four major communication disorders: two language disorders (expressive and mixed receptive–expressive communication disorder) and two speech disorders (phonologic disorder and stuttering).

A. **Expressive language disorder.** Characterized by deficits in vocabulary, tenses, production of complex sentences, and recall of words.

1. **Diagnosis.** Patient presents selective deficits in language skills accompanied by normal function in nonverbal areas and receptive skills. Diagnosis should be confirmed by standardized tests of expressive language and nonverbal intelligence. Severity of the disorder can be determined by the child's verbal and sign language in various places (i.e., the schoolyard, classroom, home, and playroom) and interaction with other children. In severe cases, the disorder presents by approximately 18 months (Table 26–8).

2. **Epidemiology**
   a. Occurs in 3% to 5% of school-aged children.
   b. Two to three times more common in males.
   c. History of relatives with other communication disorders.

Table 26–8
***DSM-IV-TR* Diagnostic Criteria for Expressive Language Disorder**

A. The scores obtained from standardized individually administered measures of expressive language development are substantially below those obtained from standardized measures of both nonverbal intellectual capacity and receptive language development. The disturbance may be manifest clinically by symptoms that include having a markedly limited vocabulary, making errors in tense, or having difficulty recalling words or producing sentences with developmentally appropriate length or complexity.
B. The difficulties with expressive language interfere with academic or occupational achievement or with social communication.
C. Criteria are not met for mixed receptive–expressive language disorder or a pervasive developmental disorder.
D. If mental retardation, a speech-motor or sensory deficit, or environmental deprivation is present, the language difficulties are in excess of those usually associated with these problems.

From American Psychiatric Association. *Diagnostic and Statistical Manual of Mental Disorders*, 4th ed. Text rev. Washington, DC: American Psychiatric Association, 2000, with permission.

3. **Etiology**
   a. Subtle cerebral damage and maturational lags in cerebral development may be a cause.
   b. Associated with left-handedness and ambilaterality.
   c. Concordance for monozygotic twins.
   d. Genetic, environmental, and educational factors appear to play a role.
4. **Differential diagnosis**
   a. **Mental retardation.** Child has an overall impairment in intellectual functioning, and nonverbal intellectual capacity is not within normal limits.
   b. **Mixed receptive–expressive language disorder.** Comprehension of language (decoding) is below the expected age-appropriate level.
   c. **Pervasive developmental disorder.** Child has no inner language or appropriate use of gestures and shows little or no frustration with the inability to communicate verbally.
   d. **Aphasia or dysphasia.** Child has a history of early normal language development; onset of the disordered language is after a head trauma or other neurologic disorder (i.e., seizure disorder).
   e. **Selective mutism.** Child has a history of normal language development.
5. **Course and prognosis.** The rapidity and degree of recovery depends on the severity of the disorder, the child's motivation to participate in therapies, and the timely institution of speech and other therapeutic interventions. As many as 50% of children with mild cases recover spontaneously, while severe cases continue to display some features of language impairment.
6. **Treatment**
   a. **Remedial.** Language therapy is aimed at using words to improve communication strategies and social interactions.
   b. **Psychotherapy.** Can be used as a positive model for more effective communication and broadening social skills in patients where language impairment has affected self-esteem. Supportive parental counseling may be useful in some cases.
B. **Mixed receptive–expressive language disorder.** Children are impaired in both understanding and expressing language. Scores on standardized tests in both receptive (comprehension) and expressive language fall substantially below those obtained from standardized measurements of nonverbal intellectual capacity. According to *DSM-IV-TR,* it is not advised to diagnose receptive language disorder in the absence of expressive language disorder.
   1. **Diagnosis.** Measurements in both receptive and expressive language development are below measures of nonverbal intellectual capacity. On average, patients show symptoms before the age of 4 years, with severe cases apparent by the age of 2 years and mild cases by age 7 years (second grade) or older (Table 26–9).

Table 26–9
DSM-IV-TR Diagnostic Criteria for Mixed Receptive–Expressive Language Disorder

A. The scores obtained from a battery of standardized individually administered measures of both receptive and expressive language development are substantially below those obtained from standardized measures of nonverbal intellectual capacity. Symptoms include those for expressive language disorder as well as difficulty understanding words, sentences, or specific types of words, such as spatial terms.
B. The difficulties with receptive and expressive language significantly interfere with academic or occupational achievement or with social communication.
C. Criteria are not met for a pervasive developmental disorder.
D. If mental retardation, a speech-motor or sensory deficit, or environmental deprivation is present, the language difficulties are in excess of those usually associated with these problems.

From American Psychiatric Association. *Diagnostic and Statistical Manual of Mental Disorders*, 4th ed. Text rev. Washington, DC: American Psychiatric Association, 2000, with permission.

2. **Epidemiology**
   a. Prevalence is 3% of school-aged children.
   b. Twice more common in males.
3. **Etiology**
   a. Evidence of familial aggregation of mixed receptive–expressive language disorder.
   b. Twin studies implicate a genetic contribution, but no mode of genetic transmission has been proven.
4. **Differential diagnosis**
   a. **Expressive language disorder.** Decoding remains within normal limits.
   b. **Phonological disorder or stuttering.** Have normal expressive and receptive language competence, despite speech impairments.
5. **Course and prognosis.** The prognosis is variable and depends on the nature and severity of the damage. Prognosis is less favorable than those with expressive language disorder alone. Some children achieve close-to-normal language functions. In young children, the disorder is usually severe, the short-term prognosis is poor, and it is likely that they may develop a learning disorder in the future.
6. **Treatment**
   a. **Remedial.** Most patients benefit from a small, special educational setting that allows more individualized learning.
   b. **Psychotherapy.** Beneficial in patients with associated emotional and behavioral problems. Family counseling in which parents and children can develop more effective, less frustrating means of communicating is beneficial.
C. **Phonologic disorder.** The child presents impairment in sound production by substituting one sound for another or omitting sounds that are part of words.
   1. **Diagnosis.** Delay or failure to produce developmentally expected speech sounds accompanied by normal language development. The child is unable to articulate certain phonemes correctly and may omit,

Table 26–10
DSM-IV-TR Diagnostic Criteria for Phonologic Disorder

A. Failure to use developmentally expected speech sounds that are appropriate for age and dialect (e.g., errors in sound production, use, representation, or organization such as, but not limited to, substitutions of one sound for another use of /t/ for target /k/ sound for omissions of sounds such as final consonants).
B. The difficulties in speech sound production interfere with academic or occupational achievement or with social communication.
C. If mental retardation, a speech-motor or sensory deficit, or environmental deprivation is present, the speech difficulties are in excess of those usually associated with these problems.

From American Psychiatric Association. *Diagnostic and Statistical Manual of Mental Disorders*, 4th ed. Text rev. Washington, DC: American Psychiatric Association, 2000, with permission.

substitute, or distort the affected phonemes. Most children usually outgrow the disorder by third grade; however, spontaneous recovery is unlikely after fourth grade (Table 26–10).

2. **Epidemiology**
   a. Variable prevalence of 0.5% by mid- to late adolescence.
   b. Two to three times more common in males.
   c. Common among first-degree relatives.

3. **Etiology**
   a. Likely to include perinatal problems, genetics, auditory processing problems, hearing impairment, and structural abnormalities related to speech.
   b. Genetic studies indicate a high concordance among monozygotic twins.

4. **Differential diagnosis**
   a. Physical abnormalities causing articulation errors must be ruled out.
   b. Dysarthria is less likely to spontaneously remit.
   c. Hearing impairment, mental retardation, and pervasive developmental disorders should be ruled out.

5. **Course and prognosis.** Spontaneous remission of symptoms is common in children whose misarticulations involve only a few phonemes. Articulation problems that persist after the age of 5 years may be comorbid with other speech and language impairments. Auditory perceptual problems are more likely in children with articulation problems after the age of 5 years. Spontaneous remission is rare after the age of 8 years (fourth grade).

6. **Treatment.** Speech therapy is the most successful form of treatment. It is indicated when the child's intelligibility is poor; the child is over the age of 8 years; the speech problem interferes with peer relations, learning, and self-image; the disorder is so severe that many consonants are misarticulated; and errors involve omissions and substitution of phonemes rather than distortions. Parental counseling and monitoring of child–peer relations and school behavior may be beneficial.

Table 26–11
***DSM-IV-TR* Diagnostic Criteria for Stutteing**

A. Disturbance in the normal fluency and time patterning of speech (inappropriate for the individual's age), characterized by frequent occurrences of one or more of the following:
1. sound and syllable repetitions
2. sound prolongations
3. interjections
4. broken words (e.g., pauses within a word)
5. available or silent blocking (filled or unfilled pauses in speech)
6. circumlocutions (word substitutions to avoid problematic words)
7. words produced with an excess of physical tension
8. monosyllabic whole-word repetitions (e.g., "I-I-I see him")
B. The disturbance in fluency interferes with academic or occupational achievement or with social communication.
C. If a speech–motor or sensory deficit is present, the speech difficulties are in excess of those usually associated with these problems.

From American Psychiatric Association. *Diagnostic and Statistical Manual of Mental Disorders,* 4th ed. Text rev. Washington, DC: American Psychiatric Association, 2000, with permission.

D. Stuttering. A condition characterized by involuntary disruptions in the flow of speech.

1. **Diagnosis.** Disturbance in normal fluency and time patterning of speech. Stuttering appears between the ages of 18 months and 9 years, with peaks at 2 to 3.5 years and 5 to 7 years. Symptoms gradually develop over weeks or months with a repetition of initial consonants (Table 26–11).

2. **Epidemiology**
   a. Prevalence is 3% to 4%.
   b. Affects three to four times more males.
   c. Typical onset is 2 to 7 years of age with a peak at 5 years of age.
   d. Spontaneous remission in about 80% of young children.

3. **Etiology.** Unknown; organic and learning models have been proposed.

4. **Differential diagnosis**
   a. **Normal speech dysfluency.** Patients are nonfluent with their speech but seem to be at ease.
   b. **Spastic dysphonia.** Patients have an abnormal breathing pattern.
   c. **Cluttering.** Patients are unaware of the disturbance in speech.

5. **Course and prognosis.** Course is usually long term with periods of remissions and exacerbations. Fifty percent to 80% of patients recover spontaneously, mostly with mild cases.

6. **Treatment**
   a. **Remediation.** Speech therapy, relaxation techniques, and breathing exercises have been employed. Other approaches using distraction include teaching the patient to talk in time to rhythmic movements of the arm, hand, or finger, but this only removes stuttering temporarily. Relaxation techniques are based on the premise that the relaxed state and stuttering are incompatible.

Table 26–12
DSM-IV-TR Diagnostic Criteria for Communication Disorder Not Otherwise Specified

This category is for disorders in communication that do not meet criteria for any specific communication disorder, for example, a voice disorder (i.e., an abnormality of vocal pitch, loudness, quality, tone, or resonance).
From American Psychiatric Association. *Diagnostic and Statistical Manual of Mental Disorders*, 4th ed. Text rev. Washington, DC: American Psychiatric Association, 2000, with permission.

   b. Psychotherapy. Classic psychoanalysis, insight-oriented psychotherapy, group therapy, and other psychotherapeutic techniques have not been successful in treating stuttering, but individual psychotherapy can be helpful in cases that include associated poor self-image, anxiety, or depression. Family therapy should be considered if there is evidence of family dysfunction, a family contribution to symptoms, or family stress caused by trying to cope with, or help, the stutter.

   c. Pharmacotherapy. Treatments such as haloperidol (Haldol) have been used in an attempt to increase relaxation; however, there are no data to assess its efficacy. Recent studies have suggested the use of serotonin–dopamine antagonists including olanzapine (Zyprexa) and risperidone (Risperdal) but data is inconclusive.

E. **Communication disorder not otherwise specified.** Disorders that do not meet the diagnostic criteria for any specific communication disorder. Examples include voice disorder, in which the patient has an abnormality in pitch, loudness, quality, tone, or resonance; or cluttering disorder, in which the disturbed rate and rhythm of speech impair intelligibility (Table 26–12).

VI. **Pervasive Developmental Disorders**

A group of disorders characterized by defects in understanding and expressing language and the production of speech. These disorders affect multiple areas of development (e.g., social skills, contact with reality), are manifested early in life, and cause persistent dysfunction. *DSM-IV-TR* includes five pervasive developmental disorders: autistic disorder, Rett's disorder, childhood disintegrative disorder, Asperger's disorder, and pervasive developmental disorder not otherwise specified.

A. **Autistic disorder.** Autistic disorder is characterized by qualitative deficits in reciprocal social interaction and communication skills and restricted patterns of behavior.

   1. **Diagnosis.** Among the principle criteria for diagnosing autism are deficits in language development and difficulty using language to communicate. At first glance, patients do not show physical signs of the disorder; however, they do have minor physical abnormalities such as ear malformations. Autistic children do not demonstrate special attention to important people in their lives and have impaired eye contact and attachment behavior to family members and notable deficits in

Table 26–13
DSM-IV-TR Diagnostic Criteria for Autistic Disorder

A. A total of six (or more) items from (1), (2), and (3), with at least two from (1) and one each from (2) and (3).
  1. Qualitative impairment in social interaction, as manifested by at least two of the following:
    a. marked impairment in the use of multiple nonverbal behaviors such as eye-to-eye gaze, facial expression, body postures, and gestures to regulate social interaction
    b. failure to develop peer relationships appropriate to developmental level
    c. a lack of spontaneous seeking to share enjoyment, interests, or achievements with other people (e.g., by showing, bringing, or pointing out objects of interest)
    d. lack of social or emotional reciprocity
  2. Qualitative impairments in communication as manifested by at least one of the following:
    a. delay in, or total lack of, the development of spoken language (not accompanied by an attempt to compensate through alternative modes of communication such as gesture or mime)
    b. in individuals with adequate speech, marked impairment in the ability to initiate or sustain a conversation with others
    c. stereotyped and repetitive use of language or idiosyncratic language
    d. lack of varied, spontaneous make-believe play or social imitative play appropriate to developmental level
  3. Restricted repetitive and stereotyped patterns of behavior, interests, and activities, as manifested by at least one of the following:
    a. encompassing preoccupation with one or more stereotyped and restricted patterns of interest that is abnormal either in intensity or focus
    b. apparently inflexible adherence to specific, nonfunctional routines or rituals
    c. stereotyped and repetitive motor mannerisms (e.g., hand or finger flapping or twisting, or complex whole-body movements)
    d. persistent preoccupation with parts of objects
B. Delays or abnormal functioning in at least one of the following areas, with onset prior to age 3 years: (1) social interaction, (2) language as used in social communication, or (3) symbolic at imaginative play.
C. The disturbance is not better accounted for by Rett's disorder or childhood disintegrative disorder.

From American Psychiatric Association. *Diagnostic and Statistical Manual of Mental Disorders*, 4th ed. Text rev. Washington, DC: American Psychiatric Association, 2000, with permission.

interacting with peers. One description of the cognitive style of children with autism is that they are unable to make attributions about the motivation or intentions of others; therefore, they cannot develop empathy. Activities and play are often rigid, repetitive, and monotonous. Common behavior problems include hyperkinesis, hypokinesis, aggression, head banging, biting, scratching, hair pulling, and resistance to change in routine. Prodigious cognitive or visuomotor capabilities may occur in a small subgroup (idiot or autistic savants). See Table 26–13.

2. **Epidemiology**
  a. Occurs in 0.05% of children.
  b. Four to five times more common in males; females with the disorder are more likely to have more severe mental retardation.
  c. Onset before age of 3 years.

3. **Etiology**
  a. Higher concordance rate in monozygotic than dizygotic twins; at least 2% to 4% of siblings are affected.
  b. Biologic factors implicated due to high rates of seizure disorder and mental retardation.

Table 26–14
Autistic Disorder Versus Schizophrenia with Childhood Onset

Criteria	Autistic Disorder	Schizophrenia (with Onset Before Puberty)
Age of onset	Before 38 months	Not under 5 years of age
Incidence	2–5 in 10,000	Unknown, possibly same or even rarer
Sex ratio (M:F)	3–4:1	1.67:1 (nearly equal, or slight preponderance of males)
Family history of schizophrenia	Not raised or probably not raised	Raised
Socioeconomic status (SES)	Overrepresentation of upper SES groups (artifact)	More common in lower SES groups
Prenatal and perinatal complications and cerebral dysfunction	More common in autistic disorder	Less common in schizophrenia
Behavioral characteristics	Failure to develop relatedness; absence of speech or echolalia; stereotyped phrases; language comprehension absent or poor; insistence on sameness and stereotypies	Hallucinations and delusions; thought disorder
Adaptive functioning	Usually always impaired	Deterioration in functioning
Level of intelligence	In majority of cases subnormal, frequently severely impaired (70% ≤70)	Usually within normal range, mostly dull normal (15% ≤70)
Pattern of IQ	Marked unevenness	More even
Grand mal seizures	4%–32%	Absent or lower incidence

Courtesy of Magda Campbell, M.D., and Wayne Green, M.D.

    c. Immunologic incompatibility and prenatal and perinatal insults might be contributory factors.

    d. Magnetic resonance imaging (MRI) studies have demonstrated increased brain volume in occipital, parietal, and temporal lobes.

    e. Subgroups have abnormal levels of dopamine and serotonin metabolites in cerebrospinal fluid (CSF).

    f. Psychosocial and family stressors are associated with exacerbation of symptoms.

4. Differential diagnosis

    a. Schizophrenia with childhood onset. Is rare in children under the age of 5 and is accompanied by hallucinations or delusions, with a lower incidence of seizures and mental retardation and a more even IQ (Table 26–14).

    b. Mental retardation with behavioral symptoms. Children usually relate to adults and other children in accordance with their mental age; they use the language they do have to communicate with others; and they have a relatively even profile of impairments without splinter functions.

    c. Acquired aphasia with convulsion. Child is normal for several years before losing both receptive and expressive language. Most have a few seizures and generalized electroencephalogram (EEG) abnormalities at onset that do not persist. A profound language comprehension disorder then follows, characterized by deviant speech pattern and speech impairment.

d. Congenital deafness or severe hearing impairment. Infants have a history of relatively normal babbling that tapers off gradually and may stop from 6 months to 1 year of age. Children respond only to loud sounds. Auditory or auditory-evoked potentials indicate significant hearing loss. Children usually relate to their parents, seek their affection, and enjoy being held as infants.

e. Psychosocial deprivation. Children improve rapidly when placed in a favorable and enriched psychosocial environment.

5. **Course and prognosis.** Autistic disorder is generally a lifelong disorder with a guarded prognosis. Two-thirds remain severely handicapped and dependent. Improved prognosis if IQ >70 and communication skills are seen by ages 5 to 7 years.

6. **Treatment**

a. **Remediation.** Structured classroom training in combination with behavioral methods is the most effective treatment method. Language and academic remediation are often required.

b. **Psychotherapy.** Parents are often distraught and need support and counseling.

c. **Pharmacotherapy.** The administration of antipsychotic medication reduces aggressive or self-injurious behavior. Serotoinin–dopamine antagonists (SDAs) such as risperidone (Risperdal), olanzapine (Zyprexa), quetiapine (Seroquel), clozapine (Clozaril), and ziprasidone (Geodon) have been used. Selective serotonin reuptake inhibitors (SSRIs), including fluoxetine (Prozac), and citalopram (Celexa) have been studied in autistic disorder, because of the association between the compulsive behaviors in OCD and stereotypic behaviors seen in autism. Atomoxetine (Strattera) has also shown improvement in children with pervasive developmental disorder (PDD).

B. **Rett's disorder.** Severe developmental deterioration following a normal developmental period of at least 6 months.

1. **Diagnosis.** Neurodegenerative disease that shows characteristic features after a period of at least 6 months of normal function and growth. Signs include microcephaly, lack of purposeful hand movements, stereotypic motions, poor receptive and expressive communication, apraxic gait, and poor coordination (Table 26–15).

2. **Epidemiology.** Prevalence is 6 to 7 per 100,000 of females.

3. **Etiology**

a. Progression is consistent with a metabolic disorder.

b. Complete concordance in monozygotic twins.

c. Males born with Rett's disorder are either still-born or die shortly after birth.

4. **Differential diagnosis.** Autistic disorder does not demonstrate deterioration of developmental milestones, head circumference, and overall growth.

Table 26–15
DSM-IV-TR Diagnostic Criteria for Rett's Disorder

A. All of the following: begin (3)
   1. apparently normal prenatal and perinatal development
   2. apparently normal psychomotor development through the first 5 months after birth
   3. normal head circumference at birth
B. Onset of all of the following after the period of normal development:
   1. deceleration of head growth between ages 5 and 48 months
   2. loss of previously acquired purposeful hand skills between ages 5 and 30 months with the subsequent development of stereotyped hand movements (e.g., hand wringing or hand washing)
   3. loss of social engagement early in the course (although often social interaction develops later)
   4. appearance of poorly coordinated gait or trunk movements
   5. severely impaired expressive and receptive language development with severe psychomotor retardation

From American Psychiatric Association. *Diagnostic and Statistical Manual of Mental Disorders*, 4th ed. Text rev. Washington, DC: American Psychiatric Association, 2000, with permission.

5. **Course and prognosis.** Course is progressive. Patients who live into adulthood remain at a cognitive and social level equivalent to that in the first year of life.

6. **Treatment.** Treatment is aimed at symptomatic intervention. Physiotherapy is beneficial for the muscular dysfunction, and anticonvulsant treatment is usually necessary to control the seizures. Behavior therapy and medication is helpful to control self-injurious behaviors and to regulate the breathing disorganization.

C. **Childhood disintegrative disorder.** Disintegration of intellectual, social, and language function after at least 2 years of normal development.

1. **Diagnosis.** Normal development for at least 2 years followed by abnormalities in reciprocal social interaction, communication skills, and stereotyped behavior. Core features include impaired ability in language, social behavior, adaptive behavior, bowel or bladder control, play, and motor skills. Majority of onset occurs at age 3 to 4 years (Table 26–16).

2. **Epidemiology**
   a. Occurs in 0.005% of children.
   b. Four to eight times more common in males.

3. **Etiology.** Unknown, but may be associated with other neurologic conditions such as seizure disorders, tuberous sclerosis, and various metabolic disorders.

4. **Differential diagnosis**
   a. **Autistic disorder.** Patient does not demonstrate deterioration of developmental milestones.
   b. **Rett's disorder.** Onset occurs earlier in life.

5. **Course and prognosis.** Course is variable, with a plateau reached in most cases. Most patients are left with some moderate mental retardation.

6. **Treatment.** Similar approach to treatment of autistic disorder; antipsychotic medication.

Table 26–16
DSM-IV-TR Diagnostic Criteria for Childhood Disintegrative Disorder

A. Apparently normal development for at least the first 2 years after birth or manifested by the presence of age-appropriate verbal and nonverbal communication, social relationships, play, and adaptive behavior.

B. Clinically significant loss of previously acquired skills (before age 10 years) in at least two of the following areas:
   1. expressive or receptive language
   2. social skills or adaptive behavior
   3. bowel or bladder control
   4. play
   5. motor skills

C. Abnormalities of functioning in at least two of the following areas:
   1. qualitative impairment in social interaction (e.g., impairment in nonverbal behaviors, failure to develop peer relationships, lack of social or emotional reciprocity)
   2. qualitative impairments in communication (e.g., delay or lack of spoken language, inability to initiate or sustain a conversation, stereotyped and repetitive use of language, lack of varied make-believe play)
   3. restrictive, repetitive, and stereotyped patterns of behavior, interests, and activities, including motor stereotypes and mannerisms

D. The disturbance is not better accounted for by another specific pervasive developmental disorder or by schizophrenia.

From American Psychiatric Association. *Diagnostic and Statistical Manual of Mental Disorders*, 4th ed. Text rev. Washington, DC: American Psychiatric Association, 2000, with permission.

D. Asperger's disorder. Patient shows impairment in social interaction and restricted repetitive patterns of behavior. There are no significant delays in language, cognitive development, or age-appropriate self-help skills.

1. **Diagnosis.** Features include at least two of the following: markedly abnormal nonverbal communicative gestures, failure to develop peer relationships, the lack of social or emotional reciprocity, and an impaired ability to express pleasure in other people's happiness. Restricted interests and patterns of behavior are always present (Table 26–17).

2. **Epidemiology.** Prevalence is greater than that of autistic disorder.

3. **Etiology.** The cause of Asperger's disorder is unknown. Family studies show a possible relation to autistic disorder, which supports the presence of genetic, metabolic, infectious, and perinatal contributing factors.

4. **Differential diagnosis.** Language delay is a core feature in autistic disorder.

5. **Course and prognosis.** Course and prognosis are variable. Good prognosis relies on normal IQ and high-level social skills.

6. **Treatment.** Treatment depends on the patient's level of adaptive functioning. Similar techniques (i.e., antipsychotic medication) used with autistic disorder for patients with severe social impairment.

E. Pervasive disorder not otherwise specified. Disorder with severe, pervasive impairment in social interaction or communication skills or the presence of stereotyped behavior, interests, and activities, but lacks the criteria for a specific pervasive developmental disorder, schizophrenia, schizotypal disorder, and avoidant personality disorder (Table 26–18).

Table 26–17
DSM-IV-TR Diagnostic Criteria for Asperger's Disorder

A. Quantitative impairment in social interaction, as manifested by at least two of the following:
  1. marked impairment in the use of multiple nonverbal behaviors such as eye-to-eye gaze, facial expression, body postures, and gestures to require social interaction
  2. failure to develop peer relationship appropriate to developmental level
  3. a lack of spontaneous seeking to share enjoyment, interests, or achievements with other people (e.g., by a lack of showing, bringing, or pointing out objects of interest to other people)
  4. lack of social or emotional reciprocity
B. Restricted repetitive and stereotyped patterns of behavior, interests, and activities, as manifested by at least one of the following:
  1. encompassing preoccupation with one or more stereotyped and restricted patterns of interest that is abnormal either in intensity or in focus
  2. apparently inflexible adherence to specific, nonfunctional routines or rituals
  3. stereotyped and repetitive motor mannerisms (e.g., hand or finger flapping or twisting, or complex whole-body movements)
  4. persistet preoccupation with parts of objects
C. The disturbance causes clinically significant impairment in social, occupational, or other important areas in functioning.
D. There is no clinically significant general delay in language (e.g., single words used by age 2 years, communicative phrases used by age 3 years).
E. There is no clinically significant delay in cognitive development or in the development of age-appropriate self-help skills, adaptive behavior (other than in social interaction), and curiosity about the environment in childhood.
F. Criteria are not met for another specific pervasive developmental disorder or schizophrenia.

From American Psychiatric Association. *Diagnostic and Statistical Manual of Mental Disorders*, 4th ed. Text rev. Washington, DC: American Psychiatric Association, 2000, with permission.

VII. Attention-Deficit Disorders

Disorders with a persistent and marked pattern of inattention and/or hyperactive and impulsive behavior. Includes attention-deficit/hyperactivity disorder and attention-deficit/hyperactivity disorder not otherwise specified.

A. Attention-deficit/hyperactivity disorder. Consists of a persistent pattern of inattention and/or hyperactivity and impulsive behavior that is more severe than expected of children of similar age and level of development. Symptoms must be present before the age of 7 years, must be present in at least two settings, and must interfere with the appropriate social, academic, and extracurricular functioning.

  1. Diagnosis. Principle signs are based on history of child's developmental patterns and direct observation in situations requiring

Table 26–18
DSM-IV-TR Diagnostic Criteria for Pervasive Developmental Disorder Not Otherwise Specified (Including Atypical Autism)

This category should be used when there is a severe and pervasive impairment in the development of reciprocal social interaction associated with impairment in either verbal or nonverbal communication skills or with the presence of stereotyped behavior, interests, and activities, but the criteria are not met for a specific pervasive developmental disorder, schizophrenia, schizotypal personality disorder, or avoidant personality disorder. For example, this category includes "atypical autism"—presentations that do not meet the criteria for autistic disorder because of late age at onset, atypical symptomatology, or subthreshold symptomatology, or all of these.

From American Psychiatric Association. *Diagnostic and Statistical Manual of Mental Disorders*, 4th ed. Text rev. Washington, DC: American Psychiatric Association, 2000, with permission.

Table 26–19
***DSM-IV-TR* Diagnostic Criteria for Attention-Deficit/Hyperactivity Disorder**

A. Either (1) or (2):
  1. Six (or more) of the following symptoms of inattention have persisted for at least 6 months to a degree that is maladaptive and inconsistent with developmental level:break
    a. often fails to give close attention to details or makes careless mistakes in schoolwork, work, or other activities
    b. often has difficulty sustaining attention in tasks or play activities
    c. often does not seem to listen when spoken to directly
    d. often does not follow through on instructions and fails to finish schoolwork, chores, or duties in the workplace (not oppositional behavior or failure to understand instructions)
    e. often has difficulty organizing tasks and activities
    f. often avoids, dislikes, or is reluctant to engage in tasks that require sustained mental effort (such as schoolwork or homework)
    g. often loses things necessary for tasks of activities (e.g., toys, school assignments, pencils, books, or tools)
    h. is often easily distracted by extraneous stimuli
    i. is often forgetful in daily activities
  2. Six (or more) of the following symptoms of **hyperactivity–impulsivity** have persisted for at least 6 months to a degree that is maladaptive and inconsistent with developmental level:
  Hyperactivity
    a. often fidgets with hands or feet or squirms in seat
    b. often leaves seat in classroom or in other situations in which remaining seated is expected
    c. often runs about or climbs excessively in situations in which it is inappropriate (in adolescents or adults, may be limited to subjective feelings of restlessness)
    d. often has difficulty playing or engaging in leisure activities quietly
    e. is often "on the go" or often acts as if "driven by a motor"
    f. often talks excessively
  Impulsivity
    g. often blurts out answers before questions have been completed
    h. often has difficulty awaiting turn
    i. often interrupts or intrudes on others (e.g., butts into conversations or games)
B. Some hyperactive–impulsive or inattentive symptoms that caused impairment were present before age 7 years.
C. Some impairment from the symptoms is present in two or more settings (e.g., of school (or work) and at home).
D. There must be clear evidence of clinically significant impairment in social, academic, or occupational functioning.
E. The symptoms do not occur exclusively during the course of a pervasive developmental disorder, schizophrenia or other psychotic disorder and are not better accounted for by another mental disorder (e.g., mood disorder, anxiety disorder, dissociative disorder, or a personality disorder).
Code based on type
Attention-deficit/hyperactivity disorder, combined type: if both Criteria A1 and A2 are met for the past 6 months
Attention-deficit/hyperactivity disorder, predominantly inattentive type: If Criterion A1 is met but Criterion A2 is not met for the past 6 months
Attention-deficit/hyperactivity disorder, predominantly hyperactive–impulsive type: If Criterion A2 is met but Criterion A1 is not met for the past 6 months
Coding note: For individuals (especially adolescents and adults) who currently have symptoms that no longer meet full criteria. "In partial remission" should be specified.

From American Psychiatric Association. *Diagnostic and Statistical Manual of Mental Disorders,* 4th ed. Text rev. Washington, DC: American Psychiatric Association, 2000, with permission.

attention. Typical signs include talking excessively, persevering, fidgeting, frequent interruptions, impatience, difficulty organizing and finishing tasks, distractibility, and forgetfulness (Table 26–19).
2. **Epidemiology**
  a. Occurs in 3% to 7% of grade-schoolers.

    b. Male-to-female ratio is 3:1 to 5:1.

    c. Symptoms often present by 3 years.

3. Etiology

    a. Possible causes include perinatal trauma and genetic and psychosocial factors.

    b. Evidence of noradrenergic and dopaminergic dysfunction in neurotransmitter systems.

    c. Frontal lobe hypoperfusion and lower frontal lobe metabolic rates have also been noted.

    d. Soft neurological signs are found in higher rates among children with ADHD.

4. Differential diagnosis

    a. Bipolar I disorder. There is more waxing and waning of symptoms.

    b. Mania. Irritability may be more common than euphoria.

    c. Learning disorders. Inability to do math or read is not because of inattention.

    d. Depressive disorder. Distinguished by hypoactivity and withdrawal.

    e. Anxiety disorder. May be manifested by overactivity and easy distractibility.

5. Course and prognosis. Course is variable. Most patients undergo partial remission. Inattention is frequently the last remitting symptom. Patients are vulnerable to antisocial behavior, substance use disorders, and mood disorders. Learning problems often continue throughout life.

6. Treatment

    a. Psychotherapy. Multimodality treatment is often necessary for child and family. These include social skills groups, behavioral intervention, individual psychotherapy, family therapy, and special education when indicated.

    b. Pharmacotherapy. Pharmacologic agents shown to have significant efficacy and excellent safety records are CNS stimulants such as methylphenidate (Ritalin, Ritalin SR, Concerta, Metadate CD, Metadate ER) and dextroamphetamine and amphetamine salt combinations (Adderall, Adderall XR). A prodrug of amphetamine, lisdexamfetamine (Vynase) was recently approved for once-daily dosing. The Daytrana patch (active ingredient methylphenidate) has been approved by the FDA in the treatment of ADHD in children age 6 to 12 years. Daytrana comes in patches that can deliver 15 mg, 20 mg, and 30 mg when worn for 9 hours per day. Second-line agents include antidepressants such as bupropion (Wellbutrin, Wellbutrin SR), venlafaxine (Effexor, Effexor XR), and α-adrenergic receptor agonists clonidine (Catapres) and guanfacine (Tenex). Atomoxetine (Strattera), a norepinephrine reuptake inhibitor, is also used.

B. Attention-deficit/hyperactivity disorder not otherwise specified. A residual category for disturbances with prominent symptoms of

Table 26–20
DSM-IV-TR Diagnostic Criteria for Attention-Deficit/Hyperactivity Disorder Not
Otherwise Specified

This category is for disorders with prominent symptoms of inattention or hyperactivity–impulsivity that
do not meet criteria for attention-deficit/hyperactivity disorder. Examples include:
1. Individuals whose symptoms and impairment meet the criteria for attention deficit/hyperactivity
   disorder, predominantly inattentive type but whose age at onset is 7 years or after
2. Individuals with clinically significant impairment who present with inattention and whose symptom
   pattern does not meet the full criteria for the disorder but have a behavioral pattern marked by
   sluggishness, daydreaming, and hypoactivity

From American Psychiatric Association. *Diagnostic and Statistical Manual of Mental Disorders*, 4th ed.
Text rev. Washington, DC: American Psychiatric Association, 2000, with permission.

inattention or hyperactivity that do not meet the criteria for ADHD. Treatment involves the use of amphetamines or methylphenidate (Table 26–20).

VIII. Disruptive Behavior Disorders

Includes two persistent constellations of disruptive symptoms categorized as
oppositional defiant disorder and conduct disorder, which result in impaired
social or academic function in a child.

A. Oppositional defiant disorder. Enduring pattern of negative, hostile
   behavior in absence of serious violation of societal norms or rules.

1. Diagnosis. A pattern of defiant, angry, and negative behavior enduring
   for at least 6 months. The child frequently loses his or her temper, is
   resentful and easily annoyed, and actively defies requests and rules in
   the presence of familiar adults and peers (Table 26–21).

2. Epidemiology
   a. Ranges from 2% to 16% in children.

Table 26–21
DSM-IV-TR Diagnostic Criteria for Oppositional Defiant Disorder

A. A pattern of negativistic, hostile, and defiant behavior lasting at least 6 months, during which four
   (or more) of the following are present:
   1. often loses temper
   2. often argues with adults
   3. often actively defies or refuses to comply with adults' requests or rules
   4. often deliberately annoys people
   5. often blames others for his or her mistakes or misbehavior
   6. is often touchy or easily annoyed by others
   7. is often angry and resentful
   8. is often spiteful or vindictive
   Note: Consider a criterion met only if the behavior occurs more frequently than is typically
   observed in individuals of comparable age and developmental level.
B. The disturbance in behavior causes clinically significant impairment in social, academic, or
   occupational functioning.
C. The behaviors do not occur exclusively during the course of a psychotic or mood disorder.
D. Criteria are not met for conduct disorder, and if the individual is age 18 years or older, criteria are
   not met for antisocial personality disorder.

From American Psychiatric Association. *Diagnostic and Statistical Manual of Mental Disorders*, 4th ed.
Text rev. Washington, DC: American Psychiatric Association, 2000, with permission.

   b. Can begin as early as 3 years of age and typically noted by 8 years of age and usually not later than adolescence.

   c. More common in males prior to puberty; sex ratio equal after puberty.

3. **Etiology**

   a. Possible result of unresolved conflicts.

   b. May be a reinforced, learned behavior.

4. **Differential diagnosis**

   a. Developmental-stage oppositional behavior. Duration is shorter and is not as frequent or intense.

   b. Adjustment disorder. Oppositional defiant behavior occurs temporarily in reaction to stress.

   c. Conduct disorder. The basic rights of others are violated.

5. **Course and prognosis.** Course depends on severity of symptoms in the child and the ability of the child to develop more adaptive responses to authority. The stability over time is variable. Persistence of symptoms poses an increased risk of additional disorders such as conduct disorder and substance use disorders. Prognosis depends on the degree of functioning in the family and the development of comorbid psychopathology.

6. **Treatment**

   a. Psychotherapy. Primary treatment is family intervention utilizing both direct training of parents in child management skills and careful assessment of family interactions. Behavior therapy focuses on selectively reinforcing and praising appropriate behavior and ignoring or not reinforcing undesired behavior. Individual psychotherapy is focused on adaptive responses.

   b. Pharmacotherapy. Comorbid disorders (i.e., anxiety or depression) treated with pharmacologic agents.

B. **Conduct disorder.** Characterized by aggression and violations of the rights of others. *DSM-IV-TR* requires three specific behaviors out of a list of 15, which include bullying and threatening or intimidating others, beginning before age 13 years.

1. **Diagnosis.** Patients show a repetitive pattern in which the basic rights of others or major societal norms or rules are violated. Antisocial behavior includes bullying, physical aggression, and cruel behavior toward peers. Children may be hostile, verbally abusive, and defiant. Persistent lying, truancy, and vandalism are also common. Severe cases demonstrate stealing and physical violence. Promiscuity and use of tobacco and illegal drugs begin unusually early. Suicidal thoughts, gestures, and acts are frequent (Table 26–22).

2. **Epidemiology**

   a. Prevalence ranges from 1% to 10% in studies.

   b. Male-to-female ratio ranges from 4:1 to 12:1.

3. **Etiology**

   a. Multifactorial.

Table 26–22
DSM-IV-TR Diagnostic Criteria for Conduct Disorder

A. A repetitive and persistent pattern of behavior in which the basic rights of others or major age-appropriate societal norms or rules are violated, as manifested by the presence of three (or more) of the following criteria in the past 12 months, with at least one criterion present in the past 6 months:

Aggression to people and animals
1. often bullies, threatens, or intimidates others
2. often initiates physical fights
3. has used a weapon that can cause serious physical harm to others (e.g., a bat, brick, broken bottle, knife, gun)
4. has been physically cruel to people
5. has been physically cruel to animals
6. has stolen while confronting a victim (e.g., mugging, purse snatching, extortion, armed robbery)
7. has forced someone into sexual activity

Destruction of property
8. has deliberately engaged in fire setting with the intention of causing serious damage
9. has deliberately destroyed others' property (other than by fire setting)

Deceitfulness or theft
10. has broken into someone else's house, building, or car
11. often lies to obtain goods or favors or to avoid obligations (i.e., "cons" others)
12. has stolen items of nontrivial value without confronting a victim (e.g., shoplifting, but without breaking and entering; forgery)

Serious violations of rules
13. often stays out at night despite parental prohibitions, beginning before age 13 years
14. has run away from home overnight at least twice while living in parental or parental surrogate home (or once without returning for a lengthy period)
15. is often truant from school, beginning before age 13 years

B. The disturbance in behavior causes clinically significant impairment in social, academic, or occupational functioning.

C. If the individual is age 18 years or older, criteria are not met for antisocial personality disorder.

Specify type based on age at onset:

Childhood-onset type: onset of at least one criterion characteristic of conduct disorder prior to age 10 years

Adolescent-onset type: absence of any criteria characteristic of conduct disorder prior to age 10 years

Unspecified type: age of onset is not known

Specify severity:

Mild: few if any conduct problems in excess of those required to make the diagnosis and conduct problems cause only minor harm to others

Moderate: number of conduct problems and effect on others are intermediate between "mild" and "severe"

Severe: many conduct problems in excess of those required to make the diagnosis or conduct problems cause considerable harm to others

From American Psychiatric Association. *Diagnostic and Statistical Manual of Mental Disorders*, 4th ed. Text rev. Washington, DC: American Psychiatric Association, 2000, with permission.

    b. Maladaptive aggressive behaviors are associated with family instability, physical and sexual victimization, socioeconomic factors, and negligent conditions.

    c. Often coexists with ADHD, learning disorders, or communication disorders.

    d. A subset may have low plasma levels of dopamine and B-hydroxylase. Abnormal serotonin levels have been implicated.

  4. Differential diagnosis

    a. Oppositional defiant disorder. Hostility and negativism fall short of seriously violating the rights of others.

Table 26–23
DSM-IV-TR Diagnostic Criteria for Disruptive Behavior Disorder
Not Otherwise Specified

This category is for disorders characterized by conduct or oppositional defiant behaviors that do not meet the criteria for conduct disorder or oppositional defiant disorder. For example, include clinical presentations that do not meet full criteria either for oppositional defiant disorder or conduct disorder, but in which there is clinically significant impairment.

From American Psychiatric Association. *Diagnostic and Statistical Manual of Mental Disorders*, 4th ed. Text rev. Washington, DC: American Psychiatric Association, 2000, with permission.

    b. Mood disorders. Often present in those children who exhibit irritability and aggressive behavior.

    c. Major depressive disorder and bipolar I disorder. Must be ruled out.

    d. ADHD. Impulsive and aggressive behavior is not as severe.

5. Course and prognosis. Prognosis is guarded in younger age groups, those who exhibit a greater number of symptoms, and those who express symptoms more frequently. Severe cases are most vulnerable to comorbid disorders later in life, such as substance use disorders and mood disorders. Good prognosis is predicted in mild cases in the absence of coexisting psychopathology and normal intellectual functioning.

6. Treatment

    a. Psychotherapy. Includes individual or family therapy, parenting classes, tutoring, and emphasis of special interests. Placement away from home may be necessary in some circumstances.

    b. Pharmacotherapy. Antipsychotics such as haloperidol (Haldol), risperidone, and olanzapine help control severe aggressive and assaultive behavior. Lithium (Eskalith) is helpful for some aggressive children with or without comorbid bipolar disorders. Stimulants may be used in comorbid ADHD.

C. Disruptive disorder not otherwise specified. Disorders of conduct or oppositional defiant behavior that does not meet the diagnostic criteria for conduct or oppositional defiant disorders but in which there is notable impairment (Table 26–23).

IX. Feeding and Eating Disorders of Infancy or Early Childhood

Persistent symptoms of inadequate food intake, recurrent regurgitating and rechewing of food, or repeated ingestion of nonnutritive substances. Includes pica, rumination disorder, and feeding disorder of infancy or early childhood.

A. Pica. Repeated ingestion of a nonnutritive substance for at least 1 month. The behavior must be developmentally inappropriate, not culturally sanctioned, and sufficiently severe to merit clinical attention.

    1. Diagnosis. Ingestion of nonedible substances after 18 months of age. Nonedible substances include paint, plaster, string, hair, cloth, dirt, feces, stones, and paper. Onset is usually between the ages of 12 and 24 months, and incidences decline with age. The clinical implication

Table 26–24
DSM-IV-TR Diagnostic Criteria for Pica

A. Persistent eating of nonnutritive substances for a period of at least 1 month.
B. The eating of nonnutritive substances is inappropriate to the developmental level.
C. The eating behavior is not part of a culturally sanctioned practice.
D. If the eating behavior occurs exclusively during the course of another mental disorder (e.g., mental retardation, pervasive developmental disorder, schizophrenia), it is sufficiently severe to warrant independent clinical attention.

From American Psychiatric Association. *Diagnostic and Statistical Manual of Mental Disorders,* 4th ed. Text rev. Washington, DC: American Psychiatric Association, 2000, with permission.

can be benign or life threatening depending on the objects ingested (Table 26–24).

2. **Epidemiology**
   a. More common in preadolescents.
   b. Occurs in up to 15% of those with severe mental retardation.
   c. Affects both sexes equally.
3. **Etiology**
   a. Associated with mental retardation, neglect, and nutritional deficiencies (e.g., iron or zinc).
   b. Onset usually between 1 and 2 years of age.
   c. Higher-than-expected incidences occur in relatives.
4. **Differential diagnosis**
   a. Iron and zinc deficiencies.
   b. Can occur in conjunction with schizophrenia, autistic disorder, Kleine–Levin syndrome, and anorexia nervosa.
5. **Course and prognosis.** Prognosis is variable. Children of normal intelligence remit spontaneously. In children, pica usually resolves with increasing age; in pregnant women, it is usually limited to the term of pregnancy. In some adults, especially those who are mentally retarded, pica may continue for years.
6. **Treatment.** In cases of neglect or maltreatment, such circumstances should be altered. Exposure to toxic substances (i.e., lead) should be eliminated. Treatments emphasize psychosocial, environmental, behavioral, and family guidance approaches. Mild aversion therapy or negative reinforcement (i.e., a mild electric shock, an unpleasant noise, or an emetic drug) has been successful. Positive reinforcement, modeling, behavioral shaping, and overcorrection treatment have also been used.

B. **Rumination disorder.** Repeated regurgitation and rechewing of food after a period of normal eating. Symptoms last at least 1 month, are not caused by a medical condition, and are severe enough for clinical attention.
   1. **Diagnosis.** Essential feature is the repeated regurgitation of food occurring at least 1 month following a period of normal eating. It is not due to a gastrointestinal condition or secondary to anorexia nervosa or

Table 26–25
DSM-IV-TR Diagnostic Criteria for Rumination Disorder

A. Repeated regurgitation and rechewing of food for a period of at least 1 month following a period of normal functioning.
B. The behavior is not due to an associated gastrointestinal or other general medical condition (e.g., esophageal reflux).
C. The behavior does not occur exclusively during the course of anorexia nervosa or bulimia nervosa. If the symptoms occur exclusively during the course of mental retardation or a pervasive developmental disorder, they are sufficiently severe to warrant independent clinical attention.

From American Psychiatric Association. *Diagnostic and Statistical Manual of Mental Disorders*, 4th ed. Text rev. Washington, DC: American Psychiatric Association, 2000, with permission.

bulimia nervosa. Swallowed food is forced back into the mouth without nausea, retching, or disgust. Subsequently it is ejected, or rechewed and swallowed (Table 26–25).

2. **Epidemiology**
   a. Rare. Occurs between 3 and 12 months.
   b. May be more common in males.
3. **Etiology**
   a. Associated with immature, emotionally neglectful mothers.
   b. Implication of a dysfunctional autonomic nervous system.
   c. Possible link to gastroesophageal reflux or hiatal hernia.
   d. Overstimulation and tension have been suggested.
4. **Differential diagnosis.** Pyloric stenosis is associated with projectile vomiting and typically manifests prior to 3 months.
5. **Course and prognosis.** There are high rates of spontaneous remission. Course may also include malnutrition, failure to thrive, and even death.
6. **Treatment.** Often involves parental guidance and behavioral techniques. Evaluation of the mother–child relationship may reveal deficits that can be influenced by offering guidance to the mother. Behavioral interventions, such as squirting lemon juice into the infant's mouth, can be effective in diminishing the behavior. Medications such as metoclopramide (Reglan), cimetidine (Tagamet), and antipsychotics (i.e., haloperidol) have seen success.

C. **Feeding disorder of infancy or early childhood.** Persistent failure to eat adequately for at least 1 month.
   1. **Diagnosis.** Failure to eat adequately for at least 1 month in the absence of a general medical or mental condition with a subsequent failure to gain weight or subsequent loss of weight (Table 26–26).
   2. **Epidemiology**
      a. Occurs in 1.5% of infants, 3% of infants with failure to thrive syndromes, and 50% of infants with feeding disorders.
      b. Onset is before 6 years of age.
   3. **Etiology.** Genetic studies indicate a high concordance among monozygotic twins.
   4. **Differential diagnosis.** Must be differentiated from gastrointestinal structural abnormalities contributing to discomfort during feeding.

Table 26–26
***DSM-IV-TR* Diagnostic Criteria for Feeding Disorder of Infancy or Early Childhood**

A. Feeding disturbance as manifested by persistent failure to eat adequately with significant failure to gain weight or significant loss of weight over at least 1 month.
B. The disturbance is not due to an associated gastrointestinal or other general medical condition (e.g., esophageal reflux).
C. The disturbance is not better accounted for by another mental disorder (e.g., rumination disorder) or by lack of available food.
D. The onset is before age 6 years.

From American Psychiatric Association. *Diagnostic and Statistical Manual of Mental Disorders*, 4th ed. Text rev. Washington, DC: American Psychiatric Association, 2000, with permission.

5. **Course and prognosis.** With intervention, failure to thrive may not develop. Children with later onset may develop deficits in growth and development when the disorder lasts for several months. Seventy percent persistent with the disorder in their first year will continue to have some feeding problems during childhood.
6. **Treatment.** Counseling of the caregiver is crucial if there are comorbid developmental delays or difficult temperament. Cognitive behavioral intervention can be useful.

X. Tic Disorders

A group of neuropsychiatric disorders that begin in childhood or adolescence and may be constant or wax and wane over time. *DSM-IV-TR* includes Tourette's disorder, chronic motor or vocal tic disorder, transient tic disorder, and tic disorder not otherwise specified under this category.

A. **Tourette's disorder.** Multiple motor tics and one or more vocal tics that occur several times a day for more than 1 year.
1. **Diagnosis.** Multiple motor tics and one or more vocal tics; these can be simple or complex. Simple motor tics appear first in the face and neck and include eye blinking, head jerking, and facial grimacing. These progress downwardly. Complex motor tics include hitting oneself and jumping. Simple vocal tics include coughing, grunting, or sniffing. Complex vocal tics include coprolalia (use of vulgar words), palilalia (repeating own words), and echolalia (repeating another's words). ADHD, learning problems, and obsessive–compulsive symptoms are associated with the disorder and are increased in first-degree relatives (Table 26–27).
2. **Epidemiology**
   a. Four to five cases per 10,000.
   b. Motor component generally occurs by 7 years; vocal tics emerge by 11 years, on average.
   c. Male-to-female ratio is 3:1.
3. **Etiology**
   a. Genetic contribution strongly supported by increased prevalence in first-degree relatives and higher concordance rates in monozygotic than dizygotic twins.

Table 26–27
DSM-IV-TR **Diagnostic Criteria for Tourette's Disorder**

A. Both multiple motor and one or more vocal tics have been present at some time during the illness, although not necessarily concurrently. (A tic is a sudden, rapid, recurrent, nonrhythmic, stereotyped motor movement or vocalization.)
B. The tics occur many times a day (usually in bouts) nearly every day or intermittently throughout a period of more than 1 year, and during this period there is never a tic-free period of more than 3 consecutive months.
C. The onset is before age 18 years.
D. The disturbance is not due to the direct physiologic effects of a substance (e.g., stimulants) or a general medical condition (e.g., Huntington's disease or postviral encephalitis).

From American Psychiatric Association, *Diagnostic and Statistical Manual of Mental Disorders*, 4th ed. Text rev. Washington, DC: American Psychiatric Association, 2000, with permission.

b. There is evidence of neurobiologic substrate–nonspecific electroencephalogram (EEG) abnormalities as well as abnormal computed tomography (CT) findings.
c. Abnormal dopamine levels may be implicated as dopamine antagonists generally diminish tics and stimulants worsen or precipitate tics. Additionally, abnormal levels of homovanillic acid in the CSF have been demonstrated.

4. **Differential diagnosis.** In stereotypic movement disorders, tics seem to be voluntary and often produce a sense of comfort.
5. **Course and prognosis.** Untreated, the disorder is usually chronic with waxing and waning symptoms. Severely affected persons may have serious emotional problems, including major depressive disorder.
6. **Treatment**
a. **Psychotherapy.** Includes family and patient education and learning behavioral techniques. Behavioral techniques and pharmacotherapy may have a synergistic effect.
b. **Pharmacotherapy.** High-potency antipsychotics, such as haloperidol (Haldol), lead to improvement in 85% of patients but are associated with acute dystonic reactions and parkinsonian symptoms. Pimozide is also effective, but it prolongs the QT interval and thus requires electrocardiographic (ECG) monitoring These drugs are being replaced with atypicals such as risperidone and olanzapine with similar success. Clonidine, a noradrenergic antagonist, has shown benefit in 40% to 70% of patients, although it is not presently approved for use in Tourette's disorder. Another α-adrenergic agonist, guanfacine (Tenex), is also used.

B. **Chronic motor or vocal tic disorder.** Rapid and repetitive involuntary muscle contractions resulting in movements or vocalizations. The disorder must have onset before the age of 18 years.
1. **Diagnosis.** Same as Tourette's disorder except that the patient has either single or multiple motor tics or vocal tics, but not both. Chronic vocal tics are less conspicuous than in Tourette's disorder and much rarer than chronic motor tics. Vocal tics are not loud or intense and

Table 26–28
DSM-IV-TR Diagnostic Criteria for Chronic Motor or Vocal Tic Disorder

A. Single or multiple motor or vocal tics (i.e., sudden, rapid, recurrent, nonrhythmic, stereotyped motor movements or vocalizations), but not both, have been present at some time during the illness.
B. The tics occur many times a day nearly every day or intermittently throughout a period of more than 1 year, and during this period there is never a tic-free period of more than 3 consecutive months.
C. The onset is before age 18 years.
D. The disturbance is not due to the direct physiologic effects of a substance (e.g., stimulants) or a general medical condition (e.g., Huntington's disease or postviral encephalitis).
E. Criteria have never been met for Tourette's disorder.

From American Psychiatric Association. *Diagnostic and Statistical Manual of Mental Disorders,* 4th ed. Text rev. Washington, DC: American Psychiatric Association, 2000, with permission.

are primarily produced by the vocal cords. Onset is usually in early childhood (Table 26–28).

2. Epidemiology

a. It is 100 to 1,000 times more frequent than Tourette's disorder; estimate is 1% to 2%.

b. School-aged males are at higher risk.

3. Etiology

a. Chronic motor or vocal tic disorder and Tourette's disorder aggregate in some families.

b. High concordance in monozygotic twins.

4. Differential diagnosis. Chronic motor tics must be differentiated from other motor movements such as choreiform movements, myoclonus, restless legs syndrome, akathisia, and dystonias. Involuntary vocal utterances can occur in neurologic disorders, such as Huntington's disease and Parkinson's disease.

5. Course and prognosis. Children whose tics begin between the ages of 6 and 8 years have the best outcomes. Symptoms usually last for 4 to 6 years and stop in early adolescence. Children whose tics involve the limbs or trunk tend to do less well than those with facial tics.

6. Treatment

a. Psychotherapy. Treatment depends on the severity and the frequency of the tics; the patient's subjective distress; the effects of the tics on school, work, or job performance and socialization; and the presence of any other concomitant mental disorder. Psychotherapy may be used to minimize the secondary emotional problems caused by the tics. Behavioral techniques, particularly habit reversal treatment, are effective.

b. Pharmacotherapy. Antipsychotic medication has been helpful in some cases, but the risk must be weighed against the possible clinical benefits because of adverse effects, including development of tardive dyskinesia.

Table 26-29
DSM-IV-TR Diagnostic Criteria for Transient Tic Disorder

A. Single or multiple motor and/or vocal tics (i.e., sudden, rapid, recurrent, nonrhythmic, stereotyped motor movements or vocalizations).
B. The tics occur many times a day, nearly every day for at least 4 weeks, but for no longer than 12 consecutive months.
C. The onset is before age 18 years.
D. The disturbance is not due to the direct physiologic effects of a substance (e.g., stimulants) or a general medical condition (e.g., Huntington's disease or postviral encephalitis).
E. Criteria have never been met for Tourette's disorder or chronic motor or vocal tic disorder.
Specify if:
Single episode or **recurrent**

From American Psychiatric Association. *Diagnostic and Statistical Manual of Mental Disorders*, 4th ed. Text rev. Washington, DC: American Psychiatric Association, 2000, with permission.

C. **Transient tic disorder.** Rapid and repetitive involuntary muscle contractions resulting in movements and/or vocalizations for a duration of less than 12 months.
   1. **Diagnosis.** Tics are single or multiple motor or vocal tics and occur many times a day nearly every day for at least 4 weeks, but for no longer than 12 consecutive months. The patient must have no history of Tourette's disorder or chronic motor or vocal tic disorder (Table 26–29).
   2. **Epidemiology**
      a. Transient ticlike movement and muscular twitches are common in children.
      b. Five percent to 24% of school-aged children have a history of tics.
      c. Onset is prior to age 18.
      d. Three times more common in males.
   3. **Etiology**
      a. Origins are psychogenic and/or organic. Most cases are psychogenic and increase during stress with spontaneous remission.
      b. Some tics progress to Tourette's disorder or chronic motor or vocal tic disorder; these are more likely to be associated with both psychogenic and organic causes.
   4. **Differential diagnosis.** Can be distinguished from Tourette's disorder and chronic motor or vocal tic disorder only by observing the symptoms' progression over time.
   5. **Course and prognosis.** Most do not progress to a more serious tic disorder. The tics either disappear permanently or recur during stressful periods.
   6. **Treatment.** Mild tics usually require no treatment. Severe tics require a complete psychiatric and pediatric neurologic examination. Behavioral techniques or psychotherapy are recommended for severe cases and depend on the results of the evaluations. Medication is reserved only for disabling cases.

Table 26–30
DSM-IV-TR Diagnostic Criteria for Tic Disorder Not Otherwise Specified

This category is for disorders characterized by tics that do not meet criteria for a specific tic disorder. Examples include tics lasting less than 4 weeks or tics with an onset after age 18 years.

From American Psychiatric Association. *Diagnostic and Statistical Manual of Mental Disorders*, 4th ed. Text rev. Washington, DC: American Psychiatric Association, 2000, with permission.

   D. Tic disorder not otherwise specified. Refers to disorders characterized by tics but not otherwise meeting the criteria for a specific tic disorder (Table 26–30).

XI. Elimination Disorders
   These disorders are considered when a child is chronologically and developmentally beyond the point at which it is expected that elimination functions can be mastered. These include encopresis and enuresis.
   A. Encopresis. An involuntary or intentional pattern of passing feces into inappropriate places.
      1. Diagnosis. Repeated passage of feces into inappropriate places whether involuntary or intentional, occurring at least 4 years of age on a regular basis (at least once a month) for 3 months. *DSM-IV-TR* includes two types: with constipation and overflow incontinence and without constipation and overflow incontinence (Table 26–31).
      2. Epidemiology
         a. Prevalence is about 1% of 5-year-old children.
         b. It is three to four times more common in males in all age groups.
      3. Etiology
         a. Constipation with overflow incontinence can be caused by faulty nutrition; structural disease of the anus, rectum, or colon; medical side effects; or endocrine disorders.
         b. Children without constipation and overflow incontinence (with control) often have oppositional defiant or conduct disorder.

Table 26–31
DSM-IV-TR Diagnostic Criteria for Encopresis

A. Repeated passage of feces into inappropriate places (e.g., clothing or floor) whether involuntary or intentional.
B. At least one such event a month for at least 3 months.
C. Chronologic age is at least 4 years (or equivalent developmental level).
D. The behavior is not due exclusively to the direct physiologic effects of a substance (e.g., laxatives) or a general medical condition except through a mechanism involving constipation.
Code as follows:
   With constipation and overflow incontinence
   Without constipation and overflow incontinence

From American Psychiatric Association. *Diagnostic and Statistical Manual of Mental Disorders*, 4th ed. Text rev. Washington, DC: American Psychiatric Association, 2000, with permission.

Table 26–32
***DSM-IV-TR* Diagnostic Criteria for Enuresis**

A. Repeated voiding of urine into bed or clothes (whether involuntary or intentional).
B. The behavior is clinically significant as manifested by either a frequency of twice a week for at least 3 consecutive months or the presence of clinically significant distress or impairment in social, academic (occupational), or other important areas of functioning.
C. Chronologic age is at least 5 years (or equivalent developmental level).
D. The behavior is not due exclusively to the direct physiologic effect of substance (e.g., diuretic) or a general medical condition (e.g., diabetes, spina bifida, or seizure disorder).
Specify type:
   Nocturnal only
   Diurnal only
   Nocturnal and diurnal

From American Psychiatric Association. *Diagnostic and Statistical Manual of Mental Disorders*, 4th ed. Text rev. Washington, DC: American Psychiatric Association, 2000, with permission.

    c. Inadequate training or emotional reasons may contribute to inefficient sphincter control. This can be precipitated by birth of a sibling or parental separation.
  4. Differential diagnosis
    a. Hirschsprung's disease. Patient may have an empty rectum and have no desire to defecate, but still have an overflow of feces; shows symptoms shortly after birth.
    b. Physiologic effects of a substance such as a laxative.
  5. Course and prognosis. Outcome depends on the cause, the chronicity of the symptoms, and coexisting behavioral problems. Many cases are self-limiting, rarely continuing beyond mid-adolescence.
  6. Treatment. Individual psychotherapy and relaxation techniques are used to address the cause and embarrassment. Behavioral techniques may be useful. Parental guidance and family therapy often are needed. Conditions such as impaction and anal fissures require a consultation with a pediatrician.
B. Enuresis. Repeated voiding of urine into bed or clothing.
  1. Diagnosis. Repeated voiding of urine into bed or clothes whether involuntary or intentional, occurring at at least 5 years of age. Behavior must occur twice weekly for a period of at least 3 months. Is broken down into three types: nocturnal only, diurnal only, and nocturnal and diurnal (Table 26–32).
  2. Epidemiology
    a. By age 5, 7%; age 10, 3%; age 18, 1%.
    b. Much more common in males.
    c. The diurnal subtype is least prevalent and more common in females.
    d. Mental disorders are present in 20% of patients.
  3. Etiology
    a. Strong genetic component; concordance is greater in monozygotic than dizygotic twins.
    b. Toilet training may be inadequate and some may have small bladders requiring frequent voiding.

   c. Psychosocial stressors such as birth of a sibling or parental separation may precipitate cases.

 4. Differential diagnosis

   a. Genitourinary pathology such as obstructive uropathy, spina bifida occulta, and cystitis.

   b. Diabetes insipidus and diabetes mellitus.

   c. Seizures, sleepwalking disorder, and side effects of medication, such as antipsychotics or diuretics.

 5. Course and prognosis. Usually self-limited; remissions are frequent between 6 and 8 years and puberty.

 6. Treatment

   a. **Behavioral therapy.** Classic conditioning with a bell or pad apparatus is the most effective treatment. Other approaches include rewards for delaying micturition and restricting fluids before bed.

   b. **Psychotherapy.** Not an effective treatment alone, but can be useful in dealing with coexisting psychiatric problems and emotional and family difficulties.

   c. **Pharmacotherapy.** Medications are not first line considering the high rate of spontaneous remissions and success of behavioral approaches. Imipramine (Tofranil) and desmopressin (DDAVP) have shown success in reducing or eliminating bed-wetting.

XII. Other Disorders of Infancy, Childhood, or Adolescence

 A. Separation anxiety disorder

  1. Diagnosis. Must be characterized by three of the following symptoms for at least 4 weeks: (1) persistent and excessive worry about losing or possible harm befalling major attachment figures, (2) persistent and excessive worry that an untoward event can lead to separation from a major attachment figure, (3) persistent reluctance to be without attachment figures (i.e., refusal to go to school), (4) persistent and excessive fear or reluctance to be alone or without major attachment figures, (5) repeated nightmares involving the theme of separation, (6) repeated complaints of physical symptoms (i.e., headaches, stomachaches) in anticipation of separation, and (7) recurrent excessive distress when separation is anticipated or involved. Anticipation of separation can manifest as nausea, vomiting, stomachaches, dizziness, faintness, or flulike symptoms (Table 26–33).

  2. Epidemiology

   a. Estimated prevalence is 4% of school-aged children.

   b. More common in 7- and 8-year-olds than adolescents or preschoolers.

   c. It found in equal rates among females and males.

  3. Etiology

   a. Clusters in families but genetic transmission is unclear.

   b. Biological offspring of adults with anxiety disorders and panic disorder with agoraphobia are prone to separation anxiety disorder.

Table 26–33
DSM-IV-TR **Diagnostic Criteria for Separation Anxiety Disorder**

A. Developmentally inappropriate and excessive anxiety concerning separation from home or from those to whom the individual is attached, as evidenced by three (or more) of the following:
   1. recurrent excessive distress when separation from home or major attachment figures occurs or is anticipated
   2. persistent and excessive worry about losing, or about possible harm befalling, major attachment figures
   3. persistent and excessive worry that an untoward event will lead to separation from a major attachment figure (e.g., getting lost or being kidnapped)
   4. persistent reluctance or refusal to go to school or elsewhere because of fear of separation
   5. persistent and excessive fear or reluctance to be alone or without major attachment figures at home or without significant adults in other settings
   6. persistent reluctance or refusal to go to sleep without being near a major attachment figure or to sleep away from home
   7. repeated nightmares involving the theme of separation
   8. repeated complaints of physical symptoms (such as headaches, stomachaches, nausea, or vomiting) when separation from major attachment figures occurs or is anticipated
B. The duration of the disturbance is at least 4 weeks.
C. The onset is before age 18 years.
D. The disturbance causes clinically significant distress or impairment in social, academic (occupational), or other important areas of functioning.
E. The disturbance does not occur exclusively during the course of a pervasive developmental disorder, schizophrenia, or other psychotic disorder, and in adolescents and adults, is not better accounted for by panic disorder with agoraphobia.
Specify if:
   Early onset: If onset occurs before age 6 years

From American Psychiatric Association. *Diagnostic and Statistical Manual of Mental Disorders*, text revision, 4th ed. Washington, DC: American Psychiatric Association, Copyright 2000, with permission.

  c. There is a neurophysiologic correlation of behavioral inhibition (extreme shyness).
  d. Increased autonomic nervous system activity has been demonstrated.
4. **Differential diagnosis**
  a. **Generalized anxiety disorder (GAD).** Anxiety is not focused on separation.
  b. **Panic disorder with agoraphobia.** Typically does not manifest until 18 years of age.
5. **Course and prognosis.** Course and prognosis are variable and are related to age of onset, the duration of the symptoms, and the development of comorbid anxiety and depressive disorders. Slower recovery found in those with earlier onset and later age at diagnosis. Prognosis is guarded when there is coexistent depression.
6. **Treatment**
  a. **Psychotherapy.** Cognitive–behavioral therapy is widely recommended as a first-line treatment. Attitudes and feelings about exaggerated environmental dangers are focused on. Family intervention is crucial, especially in children who refuse to attend school. Behavioral modification includes gradual adjustment strategies to achieve a return to school and separation from parents.

Table 26–34
DSM-IV-TR Diagnostic Criteria for Selective Mutism

A. Consistent failure to speak in specific social situations (in which there is an expectation for speaking, e.g., at school) despite speaking in other situations.
B. The disturbance interferes with educational or occupational achievement or with social communication.
C. The duration of the disturbance is at least 1 month (not limited to the first month of school).
D. The failure to speak is not due to a lack of knowledge of, or comfort with, the spoken language required in the social situation.
E. The disturbance is not better accounted for by a communication disorder (e.g., stuttering) and does not occur exclusively during the course of a pervasive developmental disorder, schizophrenia, or other psychotic disorder.

From American Psychiatric Association. *Diagnostic and Statistical Manual of Mental Disorders,* 4th ed. Text rev. Washington, DC: American Psychiatric Association, 2000, with permission.

  b. Pharmacotherapy. SSRIs are currently recommended as first-line medications in the treatment of childhood anxiety disorders. Diphenhydramine (Benadryl) may be used in the short-term to control sleep disturbances but with caution because some children show a paradoxical reaction of excitement. The benzodiazepine alprazolam (Xanax) may be helpful in controlling anxiety symptoms. Clonazepam (Klonopin) may be used in controlling symptoms of panic.

B. Selective mutism. A childhood condition in which a child who can speak and understand refuses to talk in social situations for at least 1 month.

  1. Diagnosis. Failure to speak in social situations for a duration of at least 1 month when it is clear that the child has adequate language skills in other environments. Mutism may develop gradually or suddenly after a disturbing experience. It is most commonly manifested in school and rarely at home. Child will commonly demonstrate social anxiety, separation anxiety disorder, and delayed language acquisition (Table 26–34).

  2. Epidemiology

    a. Prevalence estimated to range between three and eight per 10,000 children but may be as high as 0.5%.

    b. More common in females and young children.

    c. Begins between ages 4 and 8.

  3. Etiology

    a. Many children have histories of delayed onset of speech or speech abnormalities.

    b. Ninety percent met the criteria of social phobia, making it a possible subtype of social phobia.

  4. Differential diagnosis

    a. Shyness. Child exhibits a transient muteness in new, anxiety-provoking situations and has a history of not speaking in the presence of strangers and clinging to his or her mother.

    b. Mutism. Child improves spontaneously upon entering school.

c. **Mental retardation, pervasive developmental disorders, and expressive language disorder.** Symptoms are widespread and the child is unable to communicate normally.

d. **Mutism secondary to conversion disorder.** The mutism is pervasive.

5. **Course and prognosis.** The disorder usually remits with or without treatment. Most cases last for only a few weeks or months. Children who do not improve by age 10 have a long-term course and a worse prognosis. One third of children with the disorder, with or without treatment, may develop other psychiatric disorders, particularly other anxiety disorders and depression.

6. **Treatment**

a. **Psychotherapy.** A multimodal approach using individual, cognitive–behavioral, and family interventions is recommended. A therapeutic nursery is beneficial for preschool children. Individual cognitive–behavioral therapy is a first-line treatment for school-aged children. Family education and cooperation are beneficial.

b. **Pharmacotherapy.** SSRIs were an accepted component of treatment; however, their use in children is no longer warranted.

C. **Reactive attachment disorder of infancy or early childhood.** An inappropriate social relatedness that occurs in most contexts. Includes two subtypes: the inhibited type, in which the disturbance takes the form of constantly failing to initiate and respond to most social interactions, and the disinhibited type, in which the disturbance takes the form of undifferentiated, unselective social readiness.

1. **Diagnosis.** Markedly disturbed social relatedness in a child younger than 5 years old in the context of persistent disregard of physical or emotional needs or repeated change of caretaker. Expected social interaction and liveliness are not present. Infants demonstrate nonorganic failure to thrive. Physically, head circumference is normal, weight very low, and height somewhat short. Associated with low socioeconomic status and mothers who are depressed or isolated or have experienced abuse (Table 26–35).

2. **Epidemiology.** There is no specific data on prevalence, sex ratio, or familial pattern. Often diagnosed and treated by pediatricians.

3. **Etiology.** Linked to maltreatment, including neglect and physical abuse.

4. **Differential diagnosis**

a. **Autistic disorder.** The child is typically well nourished, of age-appropriate size and weight, alert and active, and does not improve rapidly if removed from home.

b. **Mental retardation.** Children show appropriate social readiness for their mental age and a sequence of development similar to that of normal children.

Table 26–35
DSM-IV-TR Diagnostic Criteria for Reactive Attachment Disorder of Infancy or Early Childhood

A. Markedly disturbed and developmentally inappropriate social relatedness in most contexts, beginning before age 5 years, as evidenced by either (1) or (2):
1. persistent failure to initiate or respond in a developmentally appropriate fashion to most social interactions, as manifest by excessively inhibited, hypervigilant, or highly ambivalent and contradictory responses (e.g., the child may respond to caregivers with a mixture of approach, avoidance, and resistance to comforting, or may exhibit frozen watchfulness)
2. diffuse attachments as manifest by indiscriminate sociability with marked inability to exhibit appropriate selective attachments (e.g., excessive familiarity with relative strangers or lack of selectivity in choice of attachment figures)
B. The disturbance in Criterion A is not accounted for solely by developmental delay (as in mental retardation) and does not meet criteria for a pervasive developmental disorder.
C. Pathogenic care as evidenced by at least one of the following:
1. persistent disregard of the child's basic emotional needs for comfort, stimulation, and affection
2. persistent disregard of the child's basic physical needs
3. repeated changes of primary caregiver that prevent formation of stable attachments (e.g., frequent changes in foster care)
D. There is a presumption that the care in Criterion C is responsible for the disturbed behavior in Criterion A (e.g., the disturbances in Criterion A began following the pathogenic care in Criterion C).
Specify type:
 Inhibited type: if Criterion A1 predominates in the clinical presentation
 Disinhibited type: if Criterion A2 predominates in the clinical presentation

From American Psychiatric Association. *Diagnostic and Statistical Manual of Mental Disorders*, 4th ed. Text rev. Washington, DC: American Psychiatric Association, 2000, with permission.

5. **Course and prognosis.** Course and prognosis depend on the duration and severity of the neglectful and pathogenic parenting and on associated complications such as failure to thrive. Outcomes range from the extremes of death to the developmentally healthy child. Generally, the earlier the intervention the more reversible is the disorder.
6. **Treatment.** Removal of the child is necessary in most cases. Malnourishment and other medical problems may require hospitalization. Parent education and provision of a homemaker or financial aid may improve conditions so child can return.

D. **Stereotypic movement disorder.** A repetitive, nonfunctional motor behavior that seems to be compulsive.
1. **Diagnosis.** Diagnostically, repetitive, seemingly nonfunctional behaviors that last for at least 4 weeks and interfere with normal activities or cause physical injury. Common behaviors include hand shaking, head banging, nail biting, nose picking, and hair pulling. In extreme cases, severe mutilation and life-threatening injuries may result, and secondary infection and septicemia may follow self-inflicted trauma (Table 26–36).
2. **Epidemiology**
   a. Ten percent to 20% of mentally retarded children are affected by symptoms.
   b. More prevalent in males than females.

Table 26–36
***DSM-IV-TR* Diagnostic Criteria for Stereotypic Movement Disorder**

A. Repetitive, seemingly driven, and nonfunctional motor behavior (e.g., hand shaking or waving, body rocking, head banging, mouthing of objects, self-biting, picking at skin or bodily orifices, hitting own body).

B. The behavior markedly interferes with normal activities or results in self-inflicted bodily injury that requires medical treatment (or would result in an injury if preventive measures were not used).

C. If mental retardation is present, the stereotypic or self-injurious behavior is of sufficient severity to become a focus of treatment.

D. The behavior is not better accounted for by a compulsion (as in obsessive-compulsive disorder), a tic (as in tic disorder), a stereotypy that is part of a pervasive developmental disorder, or hair pulling (as in trichotillomania).

E. The behavior is not due to the direct physiologic effects of a substance or a general medical condition.

F. The behavior persists for 4 weeks or longer.

Specify if:

With self-injurious behavior: if the behavior results in bodily damage that requires specific treatment (or that would result in bodily damage if protective measures were not used)

From American Psychiatric Association. *Diagnostic and Statistical Manual of Mental Disorders*, 4th ed. Text rev. Washington, DC: American Psychiatric Association, 2000, with permission.

3. **Etiology**
   a. Seems to be associated with an increase in dopamine activity.
   b. Common in mental retardation and blindness.

4. **Differential diagnosis**
   a. **Tic disorders.** Tics are often associated with distress.
   b. **Obsessive–compulsive disorder (OCD).** The compulsions must be ego-dystonic.

5. **Course and prognosis.** The duration and course are variable, as the symptoms may wax and wane. When present later in childhood or in a noncomforting manner, symptoms range from brief episodes occurring under stress to an ongoing pattern in the context of a chronic condition (i.e., mental retardation or pervasive development disorder).

6. **Treatment**
   a. **Behavioral.** Techniques including reinforcement and behavioral shaping are successful in some cases.
   b. **Pharmacotherapy.** Dopamine antagonists and opiate antagonists have reduced self-injurious behaviors. Fenfluramine (Pondimin) can diminish stereotypic behaviors in autistic children. Clomipramine (Anafranil) and fluoxetine can decrease self-injurious and other stereotypic movements.

E. **Disorders of infancy, childhood, or adolescence not otherwise specified.** Disorders with onset in infancy, childhood, or adolescence that do not meet the criteria for any specific disorder (Table 26–37).

XIII. Mood Disorders in Children and Adolescents

Core features are similar to those in adults with expression of features modified to match the age and maturity of the individual.

Table 26–37
DSM-IV-TR Diagnostic Criteria for Disorder of Infancy, Childhood, or Adolescence Not Otherwise Specified

This category is a residual category for disorders with onset in infancy, childhood, or adolescence that do not meet criteria for any specific disorder in the classification.

From American Psychiatric Association. *Diagnostic and Statistical Manual of Mental Disorders*, 4th ed. Text rev. Washington, DC: American Psychiatric Association, 2000, with permission.

A. Diagnosis

1. **Major depressive disorder.** It is most easily diagnosed in children when it is acute and occurs in a child without previous psychiatric symptoms. Onset is usually insidious, and the disorder occurs in a child who has had several years of difficulties with hyperactivity, separation anxiety disorder, or intermittent depressive symptoms. Symptoms include depressed or irritable mood, loss of interest or pleasure, failure to gain weight, daily insomnia or hypersomnia, psychomotor agitation or retardation, diminished ability to think or concentrate, and recurrent thoughts of death. Anhedonia, hopelessness, psychomotor retardation, and delusions are more common in adolescents and adults.

2. **Dysthymic disorder.** Onset in children and adolescents consists of a depressed or irritable mood for most of the day, for more days than not, over a period of at least 1 year. Patients may have a previous major depressive episode. The average age of onset is several years earlier than that of major depressive disorder.

3. **Bipolar I disorder.** Diagnostic criteria in children and adolescents are the same as for adults. Features include extreme mood variability, intermittent aggressive behavior, high levels of distractibility, and poor attention span. Patients may function poorly, require hospitalization, exhibit symptoms of depression, and often have a history of ADHD. When mania appears in adolescents, there is a higher incidence than in adults of psychotic features.

B. Epidemiology

1. Extremely rare in preschool children. Prevalence increases with increasing age.

2. Mania typically appears for the first time in adolescence.

C. Etiology

1. Increased incidence among children of parents with mood disorder and relatives of children with mood disorder.

2. Increased secretion of growth hormones during sleep in children with depressive disorder.

3. Possible link to a decrease in thyroid hormones and depression.

4. A dysfunction in the hypothalamic pituitary axis may contribute to depression in adolescents.

D. Differential diagnosis

1. Differentiate psychotic forms of mood disorders from schizophrenia.

2. Distinguish between agitated depressive or manic episodes and ADHD, which demonstrates persistent and excessive activity.

E. Course and prognosis. A young age of onset and multiple disorders predict a poorer prognosis. The mean length of an episode of major depression in children and adolescents is about 9 months. Recurrence of a major depressive episode is 40% by 2 years and 70% by 5 years. Dysthymic episodes last on average 4 years and are associated with major depression (70%), bipolar disorder (13%), substance abuse (15%), and suicide (12%).

F. Treatment

1. **Hospitalization.** Hospitalization is indicated when a patient is suicidal or has a coexisting substance abuse or dependence.

2. **Psychotherapy.** Cognitive–behavioral therapy for moderately severe depression aims to challenge maladaptive beliefs and enhance problem-solving abilities and social competence. "Active" treatments such as relaxation techniques are helpful for mild or moderate depression. Family education and participation are necessary for depression. Modeling and role-playing techniques can be useful in fostering good problem-solving skills.

3. **Pharmacotherapy.** The SSRIs currently are the drugs of choice in the pharmacological treatment of depressive disorders in children and adolescents. Given the FDA placement of the "black-box" warning in 2004 on all antidepressants used in children and adolescents because of the slightly increased risk of suicidal behaviors, it is imperative that close monitoring of suicidal ideation and behavior is achieved by all clinicians who prescribe these medications. Bupropion (Wellbutrin) is useful for depression as well as ADHD. Venlafaxine (Effexor) is used in treating adolescent depression. Lithium (Eskalith) has been used in the treatment of bipolar I and bipolar II disorder in childhood and adolescents. Divalproex (Depakote) is currently used frequently to treat bipolar disorder in children and adolescents. Few case reports and open label studies of atypical antipsychotics support the effectiveness of these medications in pediatric bipolar disorder. Many double and open label studies of olanzapine, risperidone, and quetiapine have demonstrated efficacy of these medications.

XIV. Early-Onset Schizophrenia

Onset is usually in late adolescence or early adulthood, but rarely presents in children 10 years of age or younger. Childhood onset is conceptually the same as that of adolescents and adults.

A. Diagnosis. Delusions, hallucinations, and thought disorders are difficult to diagnose in children. Onset is insidious, and all symptoms included in adult-onset schizophrenia may be found. The child may experience deterioration in function along with emergence of psychotic symptoms and might not reach developmental milestones. Auditory hallucinations, visual hallucinations, and delusions are frequent. The child may hear several voices making ongoing critical commentary, or command hallucinations may tell children to kill themselves. Visual hallucinations are often frightening.

B. Epidemiology
1. Less frequent than autistic disorder (0.05%).
2. More common in males.

C. Etiology
1. Prevalence is greater in first-degree relatives, and monozygotic twins demonstrate higher concordance rates than dizygotic twins.
2. Psychosocial stressors may also interact with mechanisms of biologic vulnerability to produce symptoms.

D. Differential diagnosis
1. **Schizotypal personality disorder.** Overt psychotic symptoms are not present.
2. **Major depressive disorder.** Delusions and hallucinations are not as bizarre.
3. **Pervasive developmental disorders.** Hallucinations, delusions, and formal thought disorder are not present.

E. Course and prognosis. Children with developmental delays, learning disorders, and premorbid behavioral disorders such as ADHD and conduct disorder are poor responders to medication treatment of schizophrenia and are more likely to have guarded prognoses. Some children given a diagnosis of schizophrenia will later be diagnosed with mood disorder when followed to adolescence.

F. Treatment
1. **Psychotherapy.** Family education and ongoing family interventions are critical. Proper educational setting is also important. Long-term intensive and supportive psychotherapy combined with pharmacotherapy is the most effective form of treatment. Psychotherapists must take into account a child's developmental level. They must continually support the child's good reality testing and have sensitivity to the child's sense of self.
2. **Pharmacotherapy.** Serotonin–dopamine agonists, including risperidone, olanzapine, and clozapine (Clozaril), have replaced dopamine receptor antagonists in the treatment of early-onset schizophrenia.

XV. Adolescent Substance Abuse
A. Diagnosis. Includes substance dependence, substance abuse, substance intoxication, and substance withdrawal diagnosed in adulthood. Diagnosis is made through careful interview, laboratory findings, and history provided by a reliable source.

B. Epidemiology
1. **Alcohol**
a. A significant problem in 10% to 20% of adolescents.
b. By 12th grade, 88% of high school students reported drinking, with the gap between male and female consumers decreasing.

2. **Marijuana**
   a. The strongest predictor of cocaine use.
   b. Ten percent, 23%, and 36% reported use in 8th, 10th, and 12th grade, respectively.
   c. Prevalence rates are highest among Native American and white males and females. The lowest rates are seen in Latin American females, African American females, and Asian American males and females.
3. **Cocaine**
   a. Annual cocaine use for high school seniors decreased more than 30% between 1990 and 2000.
   b. Daily use of 0.1% and 0.05% was reported for cocaine and crack, respectively.
4. **Lysergic acid diethylamide (LSD)**
   a. Current LSD rates are the lowest in 2 decades.
   b. Among 8th-, 10th-, and 12th-grade students, 2.7%, 5.6%, and 8.8%, respectively, reported use at some time.
5. **Inhalants**
   a. More common in younger than older adolescents.
   b. Among 8th-, 10th-, and 12th-grade students, 17.6%, 15.7% and 17.6%, respectively, reported use.

C. **Etiology**
1. Concordance for alcoholism is higher in monozygotic than dizygotic twins.
2. Low parental supervision has also been associated with earlier drug use.

D. **Treatment**
1. **Psychotherapy.** Treatment setting and strategy should be decided after a screening process determines type and severity of substance(s) abused. Treatment settings include inpatient units, residential treatment facilities, halfway houses, group homes, partial hospital programs, and outpatient settings. Basic components include individual psychotherapy, drug-specific counseling, self-help groups (e.g., Alcoholics Anonymous [AA], Narcotics Anonymous [NA]), substance abuse education and relapse prevention programs, and random urine drug testing. Cognitive–behavioral therapy generally requires that adolescents be motivated to participate in treatment and refrain from further substance use. Family therapy may be added.
2. **Pharmacotherapy.** When mood disorders are present, antidepressants can be used. In some cases, medication can be administered to block the reinforcing effect of the illicit drug (i.e., naltrexone [ReVia] for opioid abuse). Clonidine (Catapres) has been used in heroin withdrawal. Efficacious treatments for cigarette smoking cessation include nicotine-containing gum, patches, or nasal spray or inhaler. Bupropion (Zyban) is beneficial for smoking cessation.

XVI. Other Childhood Issues

A. **Child abuse and neglect.** An estimated 1 million children are abused or neglected annually in the United States, a problem that results in 2,000 to 4,000 deaths per year. The abused are apt to be of low birth weight or born prematurely (50% of all abused children), handicapped (e.g., mental retardation, cerebral palsy), or troubled (e.g., defiant, hyperactive). The abusing parent is usually the mother, who likely was abused herself. Abusing parents often are impulsive, substance abusers, depressed, antisocial, or narcissistic.

Each year, 150,000 to 200,000 new cases of sexual abuse are reported. Of these allegations, 2% to 8% appear to be false, and many other allegations cannot be substantiated. In 8 of 10 sexually abused children, the perpetrator, usually male, is known to the child. In 50%, the offender is a parent, parent surrogate, or relative.

B. **Borderline intellectual functioning.** A child has an IQ in the range of 71 to 84 and presents impaired adaptive functioning.

C. **Academic problem.** A child or adolescent has significant academic difficulties that are not deemed to be due to a specific learning or communication disorder or directly related to a mental or psychiatric disorder.

D. **Childhood or adolescent antisocial behavior.** A child or adolescent presents behavior that is not caused by a mental disorder and includes isolated antisocial acts, not a pattern of behavior. The acts violate the rights of others, such as overt acts of aggression and violence and covert acts of lying, stealing, truancy, and running away from home.

E. **Identity problem.** *DSM-IV-TR* does not recognize this as a mental disorder, but it can manifest in mental disorders such as mood disorders, psychotic disorders, and borderline personality disorders. It refers to uncerainty about issues relating to identity, such as goals, career choice, friendships, sexual behavior, moral values, and group loyalties.

F. **Obesity.** Present in 5% to 20% of children and adolescents. A small percentage present with an obesity–hypoventilation syndrome that is similar to adult Pickwickian syndrome. These children can have dyspnea, and their sleep is characterized by snoring, stridor, perhaps apnea, and hypoxia with oxygen desaturation. Death can result. Other conditions, such as hypothyroidism or Prader–Willi syndrome, should be ruled out.

G. **AIDS.** AIDS has presented child and adolescent psychiatrists with a multitude of difficult problems. For example, the care of young patients from lower socioeconomic groups, already grossly inadequate because of insufficient resources, is further burdened by HIV-related illness or the death of parents and relatives. Young psychiatric patients who have concomitant nonsymptomatic positive serology and require residential treatment are rejected for fear of transmission of the disease. In adolescence, AIDS has further complicated sexuality and the problem of substance abuse.

Table 26–38
***DSM-IV-TR* Diagnostic Criteria for Mental Retardation**

A. Significantly subaverage intellectual functioning: An IQ of aproximately 70 or below on an individually administered IQ test (for infants, a clinical judgment of significantly subaverage intellectual functioning).
B. Concurrent deficits or impairments in present adaptive functioning (i.e., the person's effectiveness in meeting the standards expected for his or her age by his or her cultural group) in at least two of the following areas: communication, self-care, home living, social/interpersonal skills, use of community resources, self-direction, functional academic skills, work, leisure, health, and safety.
C. The onset is before age 18 years.
Code based on degree of severity reflecting level of intellectual impairment:
Mild mental retardation: IQ level 50–55 to approximately 70
Moderate mental retardation: IQ level 35–40 to 50–55
Severe mental retardation: IQ level 20–25 to 35–40
Profound mental retardation: IQ level below 20 or 25
Mental retardation severity unspecified: When there is strong presumption of mental retardation but the person's intelligence is untestable by standard tests.

From American Psychiatric Association. *Diagnostic and Statistical Manual of Mental Disorders,* 4th ed. Text rev. Washington, DC: American Psychiatric Association, 2000, with permission.

XVII. Mental Retardation (MR)

A. Diagnosis. Diagnosis can be made after the history, a standardized intellectual assessment, and a measure of adaptive functioning indicate that a child's current behavior is significantly below the expected level (Table 26–38). In about 85% of persons with MR, the condition is mild, and they are considered educable, being able to attain about a sixth-grade education. About 10% have a moderate type and are considered trainable, being able to attain about a second-grade education. About 3% to 4% have a severe type, and about 1% to 2% have a profound type.

B. Epidemiology

1. Occurs in 1% of the population.
2. The male-to-female ratio is 1.5:1.

C. Etiology

1. **Genetic**

   a. Inborn errors of metabolism (e.g., phenylketonuria, Tay–Sachs disease).

   b. Presence of three of chromosome 21 (Down syndrome [trisomy 21]).

   c. A mutation on the X chromosome (Fragile X syndrome).

   d. A small deletion involving chromosome 15 (Prader–Willi syndrome).

   e. A simple recessive autosomal Mendelian trait (phenylketonuria [PKU]).

   f. Rett's disorder.

   g. A deficiency of an enzyme involved in purine metabolism (Lesch–Nyhan syndrome).

2. **Psychosocial.** Mild MR may be caused by chronic lack of intellectual stimulation.

Text continues on page 403.

Table 26-39
Common Psychoactive Drugs in Childhood and Adolescence

Drug	Indications	Dosage^a	Reactions and Monitoring
Antipsychotics-also known as *major tranquilizers, neuroleptics* 1. typical, conventional a. high potency, low dosage (e.g. haloperidol (Haldol), pimozide (Orap).) b. low potency, high dosage (more sedating) (e.g. chlorpromazine (Thorazine); thioridazine (Mellaril)) 2. atypicals (e.g., clozapine (Clozaril), risperidone (Risperdal), olanzapine (Zyprexa), quetiapine (Seroquel), ziprasidone (Geodon), and aripiprazole (Abilify))	Schizophrenia; bipolar disorder; agitated, aggressive, or self injurious behaviors in MR, PDD's, CD, and Tourette's disorder—haloperidol and pimozide Clozapine—refractory schizophrenia in adolescence.	All can be in divided doses or combined into one dose after gradual buildup. Haloperidol—child 0.5–6 mg/day, adolescent 0.5–16 mg/day Clozapine—dosage not determined in children; <600 mg/day in adolescents. Risperidone—0.5–3 mg/day Olanzapine—2.5–10 mg/day Quetiapine—25–500 mg/day Ziprasidone—up to 40 mg/day Aripiprazole—2.5–15 mg/day	In all: sedation; extrapyramidal symptoms, tardive dyskinesia (possibly less with atypicals), dysthymic reactions, hepatotoxicity, neuroleptic malignant syndrome. In some: weight gain, diabetes, metabolic syndrome, QT prolongation (above all in thioridazine and ziprasidone), agranulocytosis (clozapine), hyperprolectonemia (especially in risperidone), low seizure threshold (above all in clozapine). **Monitor** In all: CBC; liver enzymes, fasting glucose, lipids, and cholesterol. In some: ECG, EEG, retinal exam with high dosages of thioridazine for pigmentary retinopathy. With clozapine absolute neutrophil count and follow strict guidelines.
Stimulants Divided into amphetamines and methylphenidate and further divided into short acting (4 hours) and long acting (8 and 12 hours) Dextroamphetamine (Dexedrine), amphetamine salt combinations (Adderall, Adderall XR), lisdexamphetamine (Vyvanse) Methylphenidate (Ritalin, Ritalin SR, Ritalin LA, Metadate CD, Concerta), dextromethylphenidate (Focalin, Focalin XR), Skin Patch (Daytrana)	In ADHD for hyperactivity, impulsivity, and inattentiveness. Narcolepsy.	Short acting dextroamphetamine and methylphenidate are generally given at 8 AM and noon. Dextroamphetamine and Adderall— about half the dosage of methylphenidate is lisdexamphetamine 30 mg = 10 mg of Adderall XR. Methylphenidate—10 mg–60 mg/day or up to about 0.5 mg/kg per dose. Patch-follow guidelines in PDR for dosing.	Insomnia, anorexia, weight loss (possibly growth delay), rebound hyperactivity, headache, stomachache, tachycardia, precipitation, or exacerbation of tic disorders. Patch-skin irritation.
Atomoxitine (Strattera)—so called "non-stimulant", effects last all day		Start low, up to 1.2 mg/kg per day; not to exceed 100 mg/day.	Similar to tricyclic antidepressants.

Modafinal (Provigil)	ADHD, but studies are few; narcolepsy.	Insomnia, nausea, headache, tachycardia, Stevens-Johnson Syndrome (rare).
Mood stabilizers		
Lithium–also has anti-aggression properties	Bipolar disorder. MR and CD for explosive outburst; can be used for same in PDD.	Nausea, vomiting, polyuria, headache, tremor, weight gain, hypothyroid. Monitor thyroid. Experience with adults suggests renal function monitoring.
Divalproex (Depakote)—an anticonvulsant	Bipolar disorder, aggression.	Up to about 20 mg/kg per day; therapeutic blood level ranger appears to be 50–100 g/mL.	Monitor CBC and LFTs for possible blood dycrasias and hepatotoxicity in all anticonvulsants.
Carbamazepine (Tegretol)—an anticonvulsant	Aggression or dyscontrol in MR or CD. Bipolar disorder if other mood stabilizers fail.	Start with 10 mg/kg per day, can build to 20–30 mg/kg per day; therapeutic blood level range appears to be 4–12 mg per day.	Nausea, vomiting, sedation, hair loss, weight gain, possibly polycystic ovaries, pancreatitis. Drowsiness, nausea, rash, vertigo, irritability. Monitor CBC and LFTs, obtain blood levels.
Lamotrigine (Lamictal)—an anticonvulsant	Bipolar disorder, especially with recurrent depressions.	Follow closely PDR titration guidelines.	Stevens-Johnson Syndrome: Monitor CBC and LFTs.
Antidepressants		
SSRIs–fluoxetine (Prozac), sertraline (Zoloft), fluvoxamine (Luvox), paroxetine (Paxil), citalopram (Celexa), escitalopram (Lexapro)	Major depressive disorder, dysthymic disorder, OCD, anorexia nervosa, bulimia nervosa, repetitive behaviors in MR or PDD. Anxiety Disorders: GAD, SAD, SP, other phobias, OCD.	Less than adult dosages: Start low depending on age (e.g., fluoxetine 5 mg/day; sertraline 12.5 mg/day) and titrate up.	Nausea, headache, nervousness, insomnia, dry mouth, diarrhea, drowsiness, disinhibition (e.g., agitation, hostility), mania, suicide phenomena (rare), sexual dysfunction, nose bleed (rare), bruising (rare).
Buprorion (Wellbutrin)—short acting and sustained release	Depression, ADHD (second line).	Start low and titrate up to between 100 and 300 mg/day.	Disinhibition, insomnia, dry mouth, gastrointestinal problems, tremor, and lower seizure threshold (dose dependent).
Tricyclic antidepressants—imipramine (Tofranil), nortriptyline (Pamelor), clomipramine (Anafranil)	Major depressive disorder, separation anxiety disorder, bulimia nervosa, enuresis; sometimes used in ADHD, sleepwalking disorder, and sleep terror disorder. Clomipramine is effective in childhood OCD and sometimes in PDD.	Imipramine—start with divided doses totalling about 1.5 mg/kg per day; can build up to not more than 5 mg/kg per day and eventually combine in one dose, which is usually 50–100 mg before sleep. Clomipramine—start at 50 mg/day; can rise to not more than 3 mg/kg/day or 200 mg/day.	Dry mouth, constipation, tachycardia, arrhythmia, disinhibition. Clomipramine lowers seizure threshold. Monitor ECG.

(continued)

Table 26-39—continued

Common Psychoactive Drugs in Childhood and Adolescence

Drug	Indications	Dosage[a]	Reactions and Monitoring
Anxiolytics: (Divided into Benzodiazepines and SSRIs)			
Clonazepam (Klonopin)	GAD, panic disorder	Start low; titrate up to 0.5 mg–2.0 mg/day.	For all: Drowsiness, disinhibition. Potential for abuse or addiction.
lorazepam (Ativan)	GAD, SAD	Start low; titrate up to 1.5 mg/day.	
Diazepam (Valium)	Pavor nocturnus, somnambulism	Start low; titrate up to 0.5 mg–2.0 mg/day.	
SSRIs	GAD, SAD, SP. Other phobias, OCD	See under antidepressants	See under antidepressants
α₂-Adrenergic receptor agonists			
Clonidine (Catapres)	ADHD (second line), Tourette's disorder, severe disruptive behaviors.	0.5–0.4 mg/day	Sedation, bradycardia, arrhythmia, hypotension, withdrawal hypertension.
Guanfacine (Tenex) (Intuniv-extended release)	Same as clonidine	0.5–4.0 mg/day 1.0–4.0 mg/day	Same as with clonidine (but less sedative) plus headache, stomachache.
β-Adrenergic receptor antagonist (beta blocker)			
Propranolol (Inderal)	Impulsive aggression when other medications fail.	20–200 mg/day.	Contraindicated in asthma, hypoglycemia, and diabetes. Sedation, dizziness, bronchoconstriction. Bradycardia and hypotension require close monitoring. Reduce medication if pulse is <60 bpms, systematic blood pressure is <90 bpms or diabolic blood pressure is <60 bpms.
Other agents			
Naltrexone (ReVia)	Self-injurious behavior in autism or MR.	0.5–1.0 mg/kg per day.	Drowsiness, vomiting, anorexia, headache, nasal congestion, hyponatremic seizures.
Desmopressin (DDAVP)	Nocturnal enuresis.	20–40 μg in tablet or intranasal spray before bed.	Headache, nasal congestion, hyponatremic seizures (rare).
Sleep medications: No clear guidelines exist for children but clonidine, benzodiazepines, and melatonin can be tried.			

[a]The newer the drug, the less established the dosage range.

[b]Black-box warning on antidepressants in children and adolescents: Antidepressants increase the risk of suicidal thinking and behavior (suicidality) in children and adolescents with major depressive disorder (MDD) and other psychiatric disorders. Anyone considering the use of any antidepressant in a child or adolescent must balance this risk with the clinical need.

*MR, mental retardation; PDD, pervasive developmental disorder; CD, conduct disorder; CBC, complete blood count; LFT, liver function test; WBC, white blood cell; ECG, electrocardiogram; EEG, electroencephalogram; ADHD, attention-deficit/hyperactivity disorder; OCD, obsessive–compulsive disorder; ODD, oppositional defiant disorder; GAD, generalized anxiety disorder; SAD, separation anxiety disorder; SP, social phobia.

Table by Richard Perry, M.D.

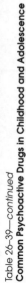

3. **Other.** Sequelae of infection, toxin, or brain trauma sustained prenatally, perinatally, or later (e.g., congenital rubella or fetal alcohol syndrome [microcephaly, midfacial hypoplasia, short palpebral fissure, pectus excavatum, possible cardiac defects, short stature]).

D. **Treatment**

1. **Educational.** Special schools or classes providing (as needed) remediation, tutoring, vocational training, and social skills training. Parents may benefit from continuous counseling and family therapy and should be allowed opportunities to express their feeling of guilt, despair, anguish, recurring denial, and anger about the disorder and their child's future.

2. **Psychotherapy.** Behavior therapy is used to shape and enhance social behaviors and to control and minimize aggressive and destructive behavior. Cognitive therapy, such as dispelling false beliefs and relaxation exercises with self-instruction, is recommended for those who are able to follow instructions. Psychodynamic therapy is used to decrease conflicts about expectations that result in persistent anxiety, rage, and depression.

   Mildly impaired persons with good verbal skills may profit from other psychotherapies for concomitant disorders.

3. **Pharmacotherapy.** A concomitant mental disorder, such as ADHD or depression, may require treatment with stimulants or antidepressants, respectively. Agitation, aggression, and tantrums often respond to antipsychotics. Atypical antipsychotics (e.g., risperidone [Risperdal], olanzapine [Zyprexa]) are preferred because they are less likely to cause extrapyramidal symptoms and dyskinesia. Many institutionalized MR patients are poorly monitored on medication. Lithium (Eskalith) is useful for aggressive or self-abusive behaviors. Carbamazepine (Tegretol), valproate (Depakene), and propranolol (Inderal) can be tried for aggressive behavior or tantrums. Their efficacy is less proven than that of antipsychotics and lithium (Table 26–39).

For a more detailed discussion of this topic, see Child Psychiatry, Ch 32, p. 3335; Psychiatric Examination of the Infant, Child, and Adolescent, Ch 33, p. 3366; Intellectual Disability, Ch 37, p. 3444; Learning Disorders, Ch 38, p. 3475; Motor Skills Disorder: Developmental Coordination Disorder, Ch 39, p. 3501; Communication Disorders, Ch 40, p. 3509; Pervasive Developmental Disorders, Ch 41, p. 3540; Attention-Deficit Disorders, Ch 42, p. 3560; Disruptive Behavior Disorders, Ch 43, p. 3580; Feeding and Eating Disorders of Infancy and Early Childhood, Ch 44, p. 3597; Tic Disorders, Ch 45, p. 3609; Elimination Disorders, Ch 46, p. 3624; Other Disorders of Infancy, Childhood, and Adolescence, Ch 47, p. 3636; Mood Disorders in Children and Adolescents, Ch 48, p. 3652; Anxiety Disorders in Children, Ch 49, p. 3671; Early-Onset Schizophrenia, Ch 50, p. 3699; Child Psychiatry: Psychiatric Treatment, Ch 51, p. 3707; and Child Psychiatry: Special Areas of Interest, Ch 52, p. 3784, in CTP/IX.

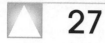

27
Geriatric Psychiatry

I. Introduction
Old age is not a disease. It is a phase of the life cycle characterized by its own developmental issues, many of which are concerned with loss of physical agility and mental acuity, friends and loved ones, and status and power. However, there are elderly persons with mental or physical disorders, or both, that impair their ability to function or even survive, known as the sick-old. Geriatric psychiatry is concerned with preventing, diagnosing, and treating psychological disorders in older adults and promoting longevity. Persons with a healthy mental adaptation to life have been found to live longer than those stressed with emotional problems.

II. Demographics
A. Late adulthood or old age is considered to begin at age 65. Divided into young-old, ages 65 to 74; old-old, ages 75 to 84; and oldest-old, age 85 and beyond. Also divided into well-old (those who are healthy) and sick-old (persons with an infirmity that interferes with daily functioning and that requires medical or psychiatric care).

B. The life expectancy in the United States is approaching 80 years, with an average of 74 for men and 81 for women. Women outlive men by about 7 years. People at least 85 years old now constitute 10% of those 65 and older and is the most rapidly growing segment of the older population.

III. Biology of Aging
A. The aging process (senescence) is characterized by a gradual decline in the functioning of all the body's systems—cardiovascular, respiratory, endocrine, and immune, among others. An overview of all the biological changes is given in Table 27–1.

B. **Cognition**
1. Mild memory loss common—called benign senescent forgetfulness. New material can be learned; however, it requires more repetition and practice than in younger persons. IQ does not decrease.
2. Persons of low socioeconomic status are at a higher risk for cognitive decline than persons in higher groups. Cognitive decline slowed in persons who are involved in continual learning and stimulation.

IV. Medical Illness
The leading five causes of death in the elderly are heart disease, cancer, stroke, Alzheimer's disease, and pneumonia. Central nervous system (CNS) changes and psychopathology are frequent causes of morbidity, as are arthritis and related symptoms. Benign prostatic hyperplasia affects three fourths of men over age 75. Urinary incontinence is believed to occur in as many as one fifth of

Table 27–1
Biological Changes Associated with Aging

Cellular level

Change in cellular DNA and RNA structures: intracellular organelle degeneration

Neuronal degeneration in central nervous system, primarily in superior temporal precentral and inferior temporal gyri; no loss in brainstem nuclei

Receptor sites and sensitivity altered

Decreased anabolism and catabolism of cellular transmitter substances

Intercellular collagen and elastin increase

Immune system

Impaired T-cell response to antigen

Increase in function of autoimmune bodies

Increased susceptibility to infection and neoplasia

Leukocytes unchanged, T lymphocytes reduced

Increased erythrocyte sedimentation (nonspecific)

Musculoskeletal

Decrease in height because of shortening of spinal column (2-inch loss in both men and women from the second to the seventh decade)

Reduction in lean muscle mass and muscle strength; deepening of thoracic cage

Increase in body fat

Elongation of nose and ears

Loss of bone matrix, leading to osteoporosis

Degeneration of joint surfaces may produce osteoarthritis

Risk of hip fracture is 10%–25% by age 90

Continual closing of cranial sutures (parietomastoid suture does not attain complete closure until age 80)

Men gain weight until about age 60, then lose; women gain weight until age 70, then lose

Integument

Graying of hair results from decreased melanin production in hair follicles (by age 50, 50% of all persons male and female are at least 50% gray; pubic hair is last to turn gray)

General wrinkling of skin

Less active sweat glands

Decrease in melanin

Loss of subcutaneous fat

Nail growth slowed

Genitourinary and reproductive

Decreased glomerular filtration rate and renal blood flow

Decreased hardness of erection, diminished ejaculatory spurt

Decreased vaginal lubrication

Enlargement of prostate

Incontinence

Special senses

Thickening of optic lens, reduced peripheral vision

Inability to accommodate (presbyopia)

High-frequency sound hearing loss (presbyacusis)—25% show loss by age 60, 65% by age 80

Yellowing of optic lens

Reduced acuity of taste, smell, and touch

Decreased light–dark adaption

Neuropsychiatric

Takes longer to learn new material, but complete learning still occurs

IQ remains stable until age 80

Verbal ability maintained with age

Psychomotor speed declines

Memory

Tasks requiring shifting attentions performed with difficulty

Encoding ability diminishes (transfer of short-term to long-term memory and vice versa)

Recognition of right answer on multiple-choice tests remains intact

Simple recall declines

Neurotransmitters

Norepinephrine decreases in central nervous system

Increased monoamine oxidase and serotonin in brain

(continued)

Table 27–1—*continued*
Biological Changes Associated with Aging

Brain
  Decrease in gross brain weight, about 17% by age 80 in both sexes
  Widened sulci, smaller convolutions, gyral atrophy
  Ventricles enlarge
  Increased transport across blood–brain barrier
  Decreased cerebral blood flow and oxygenation
Cardiovascular
  Increase in size and weight of heart (contains lipofuscin pigment derived from lipids)
  Decreased elasticity of heart valves
  Increased collagen in blood vessels
  Increased susceptibility to arrhythmias
  Altered homeostasis of blood pressure
  Cardiac output maintained in absence of coronary heart disease
Gastrointestinal (GI) system
  At risk for atrophic gastritis, hiatal hernia, diverticulosis
  Decreased blood flow to gut, liver
  Diminished saliva flow
  Altered absorption from GI tract (at risk for malabsorption syndrome and avitaminosis)
  Constipation
Endocrine
  Estrogen levels decrease in women
  Adrenal androgen decreases
  Testosterone production declines in men
  Increase in follicle-stimulating hormone (FSH) and luteinizing hormone (LH) in postmenopausal women
  Serum thyroxine (T_4) and thyroid-stimulating hormone (TSH) normal, triiodothyronine (T_3) reduced
  Glucose tolerance test result decreases
Respiratory
  Decreased vital capacity
  Diminished cough reflex
  Decreased bronchial epithelium ciliary action

the elderly, sometimes in association with dementia. These common disorders result in behavior modification. Arthritis, for example, may restrict activity and alter lifestyle. The elderly, like other adults, are profoundly embarrassed by urinary difficulties and will restrict activities and hide or deny their disability to maintain self-esteem. Cardiovascular disease is a prominent cause of morbidity and mortality in the elderly. Hypertension may be present in 40% of the elderly, many of whom are receiving diuretics or antihypertensive medications. Hypertension itself can result in CNS effects ranging from headaches to stroke, and pharmacotherapy for this condition can result in mood and cognitive disorders (e.g., electrolyte disturbances due to diuretic treatment). Atherosclerosis, associated with both cardiovascular disease and hypertension, has been related to the occurrence of the major forms of dementia—not only vascular dementia but also Alzheimer's disease. Sensory changes also accompany the aging process. One third of the aged have some degree of auditory disability. In one study, nearly one half of persons 75 to 85 years of age had lens cataracts, and more than 70% had glaucoma. Difficulties with convergence, accommodation, and macular degeneration also are sources of visual disability in the aged. These sensory changes frequently interact with psychopathological disabilities, serving to magnify psychopathological deficit and color symptoms.

V. Psychiatric Illness

Prevalence data for mental disorders in elderly persons vary widely, but a conservatively estimated 25% have significant psychiatric symptoms. The most common disorders of old age are depressive disorder, cognitive disorders (dementia), phobic disorders, and alcohol use disorders. Older adults (over age 75) also have one of the highest risks for suicide. Many mental disorders of old age can be prevented, ameliorated, or even reversed. Of special importance are the reversible causes of delirium and dementia; if not diagnosed accurately and treated in a timely fashion, these conditions can progress to an irreversible state requiring a patient's institutionalization.

A. **Dementing disorders.** About 5% of persons in the United States older than age 65 years have severe dementia, and 15% have mild dementia. Of persons older than age 80, about 20% have severe dementia. Known risk factors for dementia are age, family history, and female sex. Characteristic changes of dementia involve cognition, memory, language, and visuospatial functions, but behavioral disturbances are common as well and include agitation, restlessness, wandering, rage, violence, shouting, social and sexual disinhibition, impulsiveness, sleep disturbances, and delusions. Delusions and hallucinations occur during the course of the dementias in nearly 75% of patients. About 10% to 15% of all patients who exhibit symptoms of dementia have potentially treatable conditions. For a thorough discussion of dementia and delirium see Chapter 7.

1. **Dementia of the Alzheimer's type** (Also discussed in Chapter 7)

    a. **Diagnosis, signs, and symptoms.** Most common type of dementia. It is higher in women than in men. Characterized by the gradual onset and progressive decline of cognitive functions. Memory is impaired, and at least one of the following is seen: aphasia, apraxia, agnosia, and disturbances in executive functioning. Neurological defects (e.g., gait disturbances, aphasia, apraxia, and agnosia) eventually appear. About 50% of patients with Alzheimer's disease experience psychotic symptoms. See Table 27–2 to differentiate the two.

Table 27–2
Psychosis of AD Versus Schizophrenia in the Elderly: Clinical Characteristics

Characteristic	Schizophrenia	Psychosis of AD
Prevalence	1% of general population	50% of AD patients
Bizarre or complex delusions	Frequent	Rare
Common hallucinations	Auditory	Visual
First-rank symptoms	Frequent	Rare
Active suicidal ideation	Frequent	Rare
Past history of psychosis	Very common	Rare
Family history of psychosis	Sometimes	Uncommon
Eventual remission of psychosis	Uncommon	Frequent
Need for years of antipsychotic use	Very common	Uncommon
Optimal antipsychotic dose (% of dose for young adult with schizophrenia)	50%	20%

AD, Alzheimer's disease.
Forester BP, Dukoff R. Recognition and management of late-life psychosis. *Primary Psychiatry.* 2004;11:51–55, with permission.

    b. Etiology. Selective loss of cholinergic neurons. Reduced gyral volume in the frontal and temporal lobes. Microscopic alterations include senile plaques and neurofibrillary tangles.

    c. Treatment. There is no known prevention or cure. Treatment is palliative. Some patients with dementia of the Alzheimer's type show improvement in cognitive and functional measures when treated with donepezil (Aricept). Drugs such as memantine (Namenda) that project neurons from excessive glutamate stimulation are also of use.

  2. Vascular dementia. The second most common type of dementia is vascular dementia. It has focal neurological signs and symptoms as well as an abrupt onset and a stepwise, deteriorating course.

  3. Other dementias. Dementias due to Huntington's disease, dementia due to normal pressure hydrocephalus, Parkinson's disease, and other causes are covered in Chapter 7.

B. Depressive disorders. Present in about 15% of all older adult community residents and nursing home patients. Common signs and symptoms of depressive disorders include reduced energy and concentration, sleep problems (especially early morning awakening and multiple awakenings), decreased appetite, weight loss, and somatic complaints. Cognitive impairment in depressed geriatric patients is referred to as the *dementia syndrome of depression* (*pseudodementia*), which can be confused easily with true dementia. Pseudodementia occurs in about 15% of depressed older patients, and 25% to 50% of patients with dementia are depressed. See Chapter 14 for a thorough discussion of mood disorders.

C. Schizophrenia (late-onset). Psychopathology becomes less marked as the patient ages. Signs and symptoms include emotional blunting, social withdrawal, eccentric behavior, and illogical thinking. Delusions and hallucinations are uncommon.

    Women are more likely to have a late onset of schizophrenia than men. About 20% of persons with schizophrenia show no active symptoms by age 65, and 80% show varying degrees of impairments.

    Older persons with schizophrenic symptoms respond well to antipsychotic drugs. Medication must be administered judiciously, and lower-than-usual dosages are often effective for older adults. See Table 12–7 for commonly used antipsychotic medications.

D. Other disorders

  1. Delusional disorder

    a. Diagnosis, signs, and symptoms. Can occur under physical or psychological stress and may be precipitated by the death of a spouse, loss of a job, retirement, social isolation, adverse financial circumstances, debilitating medical illness or surgery, visual impairment, and deafness.

    b. Epidemiology. Usually occurs between ages 40 and 55. Delusions take many forms; the most common delusions are persecutory— patients believe that they are being spied on, followed, poisoned, or harassed in some way.

  c. **Etiology.** May result from prescribed medications or be early signs of a brain tumor.
2. **Anxiety disorder**
  a. **Diagnosis, signs, and symptoms.** Signs and symptoms of phobia in older adults are less severe than in those that occur in younger persons, but the effects are equally, if not more, debilitating for older patients. Obsessions and compulsions may appear for the first time in older adults, although older adults with obsessive–compulsive disorder usually had demonstrated evidence of the disorder (e.g., being orderly, perfectionistic, punctual, and parsimonious) when they were younger. When symptomatic, patients become excessive in their desire for orderliness, rituals, and sameness.
  b. **Epidemiology.** Anxiety disorders begin in early or middle adulthood, but some appear for the first time after age 60. The most common disorders are phobias (4% to 8%). The rate for panic disorder is 1%.
  c. **Treatment.** Treatment must be tailored to individual patients and must take into account the biopsychosocial interplay producing the disorder. Both pharmacotherapy and psychotherapy are required.
3. **Alcohol and other substance use disorders**
  a. **Diagnosis, signs, and symptoms.** Older adults with alcohol dependence usually give a history of excessive drinking that began in young or middle adulthood. They usually are medically ill, primarily with liver disease, and are either divorced, widowers, or men who never married. The clinical presentation of older patients with alcohol and other substance use disorders varies and includes confusion, poor personal hygiene, depression, malnutrition, and the effects of exposure and falls. Unexplained gastrointestinal, psychological, and metabolic problems should alert clinicians to over-the-counter substance abuse.
  b. **Epidemiology.** Twenty percent of nursing home patients have alcohol dependence. Alcohol and other substance use disorders account for 10% of all emotional problems in older persons, and dependence on such substances such as hypnotics, anxiolytics, and narcotics is more common in old age than is generally recognized. Thirty-five percent use over-the-counter analgesics, and 30% use laxatives.
4. **Sleep disorders**
  a. **Diagnosis, signs, and symptoms.** As a result of the decreased length of their daily sleep–wake cycle, older persons without daily routines, especially patients in nursing homes, may experience an advanced sleep phase, in which they go to sleep early and awaken during the night.
  b. **Epidemiology.** Reported more frequently by older rather than by younger adults are sleeping problems, daytime sleepiness, daytime napping, and the use of hypnotic drugs. Among the primary sleep disorders, dyssomnias are the most frequent, especially primary insomnia, nocturnal myoclonus, restless legs syndrome, and sleep apnea.

    c. Etiology. Deterioration in the quality of sleep in older persons is due to the altered timing and consolidation of sleep. Causes of sleep disturbances in older persons include primary sleep disorders, other mental disorders, general medical disorders, and social and environmental factors. Alcohol usage can also interfere with the quality of sleep and can cause sleep fragmentation and early morning awakening.

5. Suicide risk

    a. Diagnosis, signs, and symptoms. Older patients with major medical illnesses or a recent loss should be evaluated for depressive symptomatology and suicidal ideation or plans. There should be no reluctance to question patients about suicide because there is no evidence that such questions increase the likelihood of suicidal behavior.

    b. Epidemiology. Elderly persons have a higher risk for suicide than any other population. The suicide rate for white men over the age of 65 is five times higher than that of the general population. One third of elderly persons report loneliness as the principal reason for considering suicide. Approximately 10% of elderly individuals with suicide ideation report financial problems, poor medical health, or depression as reasons for suicidal thoughts. Seventy percent of suicide attempters take a drug overdose, and 20% cut or slash themselves. More elderly suicide victims are widowed and fewer are single, separated, or divorced than is true of younger adults.

6. Other conditions of old age

    a. Vertigo. Feelings of vertigo or dizziness, a common complaint of older adults, cause many older adults to become inactive because they fear falling. The causes of vertigo vary and include anemia, hypotension, cardiac arrhythmia, cerebrovascular disease, basilar artery insufficiency, middle ear disease, acoustic neuroma, and Ménière's disease. The overuse of anxiolytics can cause dizziness and daytime somnolence. Treatment with meclizine (Antivert), 25 to 100 mg daily, has been successful in many patients with vertigo.

    b. Syncope. The sudden loss of consciousness associated with syncope results from a reduction of cerebral blood flow and brain hypoxia. A thorough medical workup is required after an episode of syncope in the aged.

    c. Hearing loss. About 30% of persons over age 65 have significant hearing loss (presbycusis). After age 65, that figure rises to 50%. Causes vary. Clinicians should be sensitive to hearing loss in patients who complain they can hear but cannot understand what is being said or who ask that questions be repeated. Most elderly patients with hearing loss can be treated with hearing aids.

    d. Elder abuse. An estimated 10% of persons above 65 years of age are abused. *Elder abuse* is defined by the American Medical Association as "an act or omission which results in harm or threatened harm to the health or welfare of an elderly person." Mistreatment includes abuse and neglect—physically, psychologically, financially, and materially. Sexual abuse does occur.

e. **Spousal bereavement.** Demographic data suggest that 51% of women and 14% of men over the age of 65 will be widowed at least once. Spousal loss is among the most stressful of all life experiences. Elderly survivors of spouses who committed suicide are especially vulnerable, as are those with psychiatric illness.

VI. Psychotherapy in the Elderly

Common issues in therapy include evolving and changing relationships of the elderly with their adult children. For example, in the presence of disease, the elderly may have both a desire for independence and, in the present social context, unrealistic expectations with regard to their adult children. Adult children, in turn, may harbor resentments toward their parents continued from childhood, or, conversely, they may experience unrealistic feelings of guilt in regard to what they should be doing for their parents in the event of illness or other traumatic events.

Other goals of individual therapy particular to the elderly include the maintenance of self-esteem, despite physical, marital, and social change; the meaningful use of unaccustomed leisure time; and clarification of options in the context of more or less overwhelming physical and social change. In general, psychotherapy in the elderly is relatively situation and problem oriented and seeks solutions within the established personality framework rather than overwhelming personality change. Many elderly persons, however, respond remarkably well to seemingly overwhelming changes and personal tragedies (e.g., loss of health, loss of a spouse) and display hitherto unseen social strengths and adaptive capacities.

VII. Psychopharmacological Treatment in the Elderly

The major goals of the pharmacological treatment of older persons are to improve the quality of life, maintain persons in the community, and delay or avoid their placement in nursing homes. Individualization of dosing is the basic tenet of geriatric psychopharmacology. Alterations in drug doses are required because of the physiological changes that occur as a person ages. Renal disease is associated with decreased renal clearance of drugs, liver disease results in a decreased ability to metabolize drugs, cardiovascular disease and reduced cardiac output can affect both renal and hepatic drug clearance, and gastrointestinal disease and decreased gastric acid secretion influence drug absorption. As a general rule, the lowest possible dose should be used to achieve the desired therapeutic response. Clinicians must know the pharmacodynamics, pharmacokinetics, and biotransformation of each drug prescribed and the effects of the interaction of the drug with other drugs that a patient is taking.

See Chapter 30 for a complete discussion of pharmacological and other biological treatment.

For more detailed discussion of this topic, see Geriatric Psychiatry, Ch 54, p. 3932, in CTP/IX.

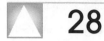

28

End-of-Life Care, Death, Dying, and Bereavement

I. End-of-Life Care

End-of-life refers to all those issues involved in caring for the terminally ill, and it begins when curative therapy ceases. Palliative care is the most important part of end-of-life care. Also included are other complex issues such as euthanasia, physician-assisted suicide, and ethical issues.

A. Palliative care. Palliative care (from Latin *palliere*, "to cloak") is concerned with treating the dying patient. It is geared to the relief of pain and suffering; it is not designed to cure. While this is most commonly associated with analgesic drug administration, many other medical interventions and surgical procedures fall under the umbrella of palliative care because they can make the patient more comfortable. Such care provides pain relief and emotional, social, and spiritual support, including psychiatric treatment if indicated. Psychiatric consultation is indicated for patients who become severely anxious, suicidal, depressed, or overtly psychotic. In each instance, appropriate psychiatric medication can be prescribed to provide relief. Palliative care physicians must also be skilled in pain management, especially in the use of powerful opioids—the gold standard of drugs used for pain relief. Pain management is discussed in further detail at the end of this chapter.

B. Euthanasia and physician-assisted suicide. Euthanasia is defined as a physician's deliberate act to cause a patient's death by directly administering a lethal dose of medication or other agent (sometimes called *mercy killing*). It is illegal and unethical. Physician-assisted suicide is defined as a physician's imparting information or providing means that enable a person to take his or her own life deliberately. Physician-assisted suicide and euthanasia should not be confused with palliative care designed to alleviate the suffering of dying patients.

C. Ethical issues. Euthanasia and physician-assisted suicide are opposed by the American Medical Association and the American Psychiatric Association. In Oregon, physicians are legally permitted to prescribe lethal medication for patients who are terminally ill (1994 Oregon Death with Dignity Law [Table 28–1]).

D. End-of-life decisions. The principle of patient autonomy requires that physicians respect the decision of a patient to forego life-sustaining treatment. Life-sustaining treatment is defined as any medical treatment that serves to prolong life without reversing the underlying medical condition. It includes, but is not limited to, mechanical ventilation, renal dialysis, blood transfusions, chemotherapy, antibiotics, and artificial nutrition and hydration.

Table 28–1
Oregon's Assisted Suicide Law

- Oregon residents whose physicians determine they have less than 6 months to live are eligible to ask for suicide medication.
- A second doctor must determine if the patient is mentally competent to make the decision and is not suffering from mental illness such as depression.
- The law does not compel doctors to comply with patients' requests for suicide medication.
- Doctors who agree to provide medication must receive a request in writing from the patient, signed by two witnesses. The written request must be made 48 hours before the doctor delivers the prescription. A second oral request is made just before the doctor writes the prescription.
- Pharmacists who are opposed to suicide may refuse to fill the prescriptions.
- The law does not specify which medication may be used. Supporters of the law say an overdose of barbiturates combined with antinausea medication would probably be used.

Patients *in extremis* should never be forced to endure intolerable, prolonged suffering in an effort to prolong life.

II. Grief, Mourning, and Bereavement

Grief, mourning, and bereavement are generally synonymous terms that describe a syndrome precipitated by the loss of a loved one. Attempts have been made to characterize the stages of grief, which are listed in Table 28–2.

Table 28–2
Grief and Bereavement

Stage	John Bowlby	Stage	CM Parkes
1	**Numbness or protest.** Characterized by distress, fear, and anger. Shock may last moments, days, or months.	1	**Alarm.** A stressful state characterized by physiological changes (e.g., rise in blood pressure and heart rate); similar to Bowlby's first stage.
2	**Yearning and searching for the lost figure.** World seems empty and meaningless, but self esteem remains intact. Characterized by preoccupation with lost person, physical restlessness, weeping, and anger. May last several months or even years.	2	**Numbness.** Person appears superficially affected by loss but is actually protecting himself or herself from acute distress.
3	**Disorganization and despair.** Restlessness and aimlessness. Increase in somatic preoccupation, withdrawal, introversion, and irritability. Repeated reliving of memories.	3	**Pining (searching).** Person looks for or is reminded of the lost person. Similar to Bowlby's second stage.
4	**Reorganization.** With establishment of new patterns, objects, and goods, grief recedes and is replaced by cherished memories. Healthy identification with deceased occurs.	4	**Depression.** Person feels hopeless about future, cannot go on living, and withdraws from family and friends.
		5	**Recovery and reorganization.** Person realizes that his or her life will continue with new adjustments and different goods.

Table 28–3
Grief Versus Depression

Grief	Depression
Normal identification with deceased. Little ambivalence toward deceased.	Abnormal overidentification with deceased. Increased ambivalence and unconscious anger toward deceased.
Crying, weight loss, decreased libido, withdrawal, insomnia, irritability, decreased concentration and attention.	Similar.
Suicidal ideas rare.	Suicidal ideas common.
Self-blame relates to how deceased was treated.	Self-blame is global. Person thinks he or she is generally bad or worthless.
No global feelings of worthlessness.	
Evokes empathy and sympathy.	Usually evokes interpersonal annoyance or irritation.
Symptoms abate with time. Self-limited. Usually clears within 6 months to 1 year.	Symptoms do not abate and may worsen. May still be present after years.
Vulnerable to physical illness.	Vulnerable to physical illness.
Responds to reassurance and social contacts.	Does not respond to reassurance and pushes away social contacts.
Not helped by antidepressant medication.	Helped by antidepressant medication.

Grief can occur for reasons other than the actual death of a loved one. These reasons include (1) loss of a loved one through separation, divorce, or incarceration; (2) loss of an emotionally charged object or circumstance (e.g., a prized possession or valued job or position); (3) loss of a fantasized love object (e.g., therapeutic abortion or death of an intrauterine fetus); and (4) loss resulting from narcissistic injury (e.g., amputation, mastectomy).

Grief is normal and differs from depression in a number of ways, described in Table 28–3. Risk factors for a major depressive episode after the death of a spouse are listed in Table 28–4. Complications of bereavement are listed in Table 28–5.

 CLINICAL HINTS: GRIEF MANAGEMENT AND THERAPY
- *Encourage the ventilation of feelings. Allow the patient to talk about loved ones. Reminiscing about positive experiences can be helpful.*
- *Do not tell a bereaved person not to cry or get angry.*
- *Try to have a small group of people who knew the deceased talk about him or her in the presence of the grieving person.*

Table 28–4
Risk Factors for Major Depressive Episode After Death of a Spouse

History of depression, major depressive disorder, dysthymic disorder, depressive personality disorder, bipolar disorder
Under 30 years of age
Poor general health
Limited social support system
Unemployment
Poor adaptation to the loss

Table 28–5
Complications of Bereavement

Disturbance in the process of grief
   Absent or delayed grief
   Exaggerated grief
   Prolonged grief
Increased vulnerability to adverse effects
   General medical morbidity
   Mortality
   Psychiatric disorders
      Anxiety disorders
      Substance use disorders
      Depressive disorders

Adapted from and courtesy of Sidney Zisook, M.D.

- *Do not prescribe antianxiety or antidepressant medication on a regular basis. If the person becomes acutely agitated, it is better to offer verbal comfort than a pill. However, small doses of medications (5 mg of diazepam [Valium]) may help in the short term.*
- *Frequent short visits are better than a few long visits.*
- *Be aware of delayed grief reaction, which occurs some time after a death and may be marked by behavioral changes, agitation, lability of mood, and substance abuse. Such reactions may occur close to the anniversary of a death (anniversary reaction).*
- *An anticipatory grief reaction occurs in advance of loss and can mitigate acute grief reaction at the actual time of loss. This can be a useful process if it is recognized when occurring.*
- *Be aware that the person grieving for a family member who died by suicide may not want to talk about his or her feelings of being stigmatized.*

III. Death and Dying

The reactions of patients to being told by a physician that they have a terminal illness vary. The reactions are described as a series of stages by thanatologist Elisabeth Kübler-Ross (Table 28–6).

Be aware that stages do not always occur in sequence. Shifts from one stage to another may occur. Moreover, children under 5 years of age do not appreciate death; they see it as a separation, similar to sleep. Between 5 and 10 years of age, they become increasingly aware of death as something that happens to others, particularly parents. After 10 years of age, children conceptualize death as something that can happen to them. Table 28–7 summarizes some essential features in the management of the dying patient.

CLINICAL HINTS: BREAKING BAD NEWS
- *Do not have a rigid attitude (e.g., "I always tell the patient"); let the patient be your guide. Many patients will want to know the diagnosis, whereas others will not. Determine what the patient already knows and understands about the prognosis.*

Table 28–6
Death and Dying (Reactions of Dying Patients): Elisabeth Kübler-Ross

Stage 1	**Shock and denial.** Patient's initial reaction is shock, followed by denial that anything is wrong. Some patients never pass beyond this state and may go doctor shopping until they find one who supports their position.
Stage 2	**Anger.** Patients become frustrated, irritable, and angry that they are ill; they ask "Why me?" Patients in this stage are difficult to manage because their anger is displaced onto doctors, hospital staff, and family. Sometimes anger is directed at themselves in the belief that illness has occurred as punishment for wrongdoing.
Stage 3	**Bargaining.** Patient may attempt to negotiate with physicians, friends, or even God, that in return for a cure, he or she will fulfill one or many promises (e.g., give to charity, attend church regularly).
Stage 4	**Depression.** Patient shows clinical signs of depression, withdrawal, psychomotor retardation, sleep disturbances, hopelessness, and possibly suicidal ideation. The depression may be a reaction to the effects of illness on his or her life (e.g., loss of job, economic hardship, isolation from friends and family), or it may be in anticipation of the actual loss of life that will occur shortly.
Stage 5	**Acceptance.** Person realizes that death is inevitable and accepts its universality.

- *Do not stifle hope or break through a patient's denial if that is the major defense. If the patient refuses to obtain help as a result of denial, gently and gradually help the patient to understand that help is necessary and available.*
- *Reassure the patient that he or she will be taken care of regardless of behavior.*
- *Stay with the patient for a period of time after informing him or her of the condition or diagnosis. Encourage the patient to ask questions and provide truthful answers. Indicate that you will return to answer any questions that the patient or family may have.*
- *Make a return visit after a few hours, if possible, to check on the patient's reaction. If the patient exhibits anxiety that cannot be coped with, 5 mg of diazepam can be prescribed as needed for 24 to 48 hours.*

Table 28–7
Essential Features in the Management of the Dying Patient

- **Concern:** Empathy, compassion, and involvement are essential; concern is ranked as the quality most appreciated by patients.
- **Competence:** Skills and knowledge can be as reassuring as warmth and concern. In particular, health care providers must adeptly manage the main medical and psychiatric complications of terminal illness: pain, nausea, shortness of breath, and hopelessness. Patients benefit immeasurably from the reassurance that their providers will not allow them to live or die in pain.
- **Communication:** Open lines of communication are essential in every stage of illness and dying, without exception.
- **Children:** Allowing children or family members who want to visit the dying patient to do so is generally advisable; family provides consolation to dying patients.
- **Cohesion:** Cohesion between the patient, family members, and caretakers maximizes patient support and helps the family through bereavement.
- **Cheerfulness:** A gentle, appropriate sense of humor can be palliative; a somber or anxious demeanor should be avoided.
- **Consistency:** Continuing, persistent attention is highly valued by patients, who often fear that they are a burden and will be abandoned; consistent physician involvement mitigates these fears.

- *Advise family members of the medical facts. Encourage them to visit and allow the patient to talk of his or her fears.*
- *Always check for the presence of living will or do not resuscitate (DNR) wishes of the patient or family. Try to anticipate their wishes regarding life-sustaining procedures.*
- *Alleviate pain and suffering. There is no reason for withholding narcotics for fear of dependence in a dying patient. Pain management should be vigorous.*

IV. Pain

Pain is a complex symptom consisting of a sensation underlying potential disease and an associated emotional state. Acute pain is a reflex biological response to injury. By definition, chronic pain is pain that lasts at least 6 months. A physiological classification of pain is listed in Table 28–8, and characteristics of pain are listed in Table 28–9.

V. Pain Management

Patients who fear death fear pain most of all. Those who fear death less also wish for a painless (i.e., peaceful) death. Thus, it cannot be overemphasized that pain management is essential. A good pain regimen may require several drugs or the same drug used in different ways and administered via different routes. For example, intravenous morphine may be supplemented by self-administered oral "rescue" doses, or a continuous epidural drip may be supplemented by bolus

Table 28–8
Physiological Classification of Pain

Type	Subtypes	Example	Comment
Nociceptive	Somatic Visceral	Bone metastasis Intestinal obstruction	Caused by activation of pain-sensitive fibers; usually aching or pressure.
Neuropathic	Peripheral Central Somatic Visceral Sympathetic-dependent Non–sympathetic- dependent	Causalgia Thalamic pain Causalgia Visceral pain in paraplegics Postherpetic pain Phantom pain	Caused by interruption of afferent pathways. Pathophysiology poorly understood, with most syndromes probably involving both peripheral and central nervous system changes. Usually dysesthetic, often burning and lancinating.
Psychogenic	Somatization disorder Psychogenic pain Hypochondriasis Specific pain diagnoses with organic contribution	Failed low back Atypical facial pain Chronic headache	Does not include factitious disorders (i.e., malingering, Munchausen's syndrome).

Adapted from Berkow R, ed. *Merck Manual*, 15th ed. Rahway, NJ: Merck, Sharp & Dohme Research Laboratories, 1987:1341, with permission.

Table 28–9
Characteristics of Somatic and Neuropathic Pain

Somatic Pain	Neuropathic Pain
Nociceptive stimulus usually evident	No obvious nociceptive stimulus
Usually well localized; visceral pain may be referred	Often poorly localized
Similar to other somatic pains in patient's experience	Unusual, dissimilar from somatic pain
Relieved by anti-inflammatory or narcotic analgesics	Only partially relieved by narcotic analgesics

Adapted from Braunwald E, Isselbacher K, Petersdorf RG, et al. *Harrison's Principles of Internal Medicine*, 11th ed., *Companion Handbook*. New York, McGraw-Hill, 1988:1.

intravenous doses. Transdermal patches may provide baseline concentrations in patients for whom intravenous or oral intake is difficult.

VI. Analgesia

Analgesia is the loss or absence of pain. The most effective analgesics are the narcotics (drugs derived from opium or an opiumlike substance), which relieve pain, alter mood and behavior, and have the potential to cause dependence and tolerance. *Opioids* is a generic term that includes drugs that bind to opioid receptors and produce a narcotic effect. They are most useful in the short-term management of severe, acute, serious pain. A goal should be to lower the pain level so that the patient can eat and sleep with minimal upset. A guideline should be to give the drug at the request of the patient. The self-administration by patients with pain of measured amounts of narcotics through an intravenous pump, when carried out in a hospital, is a new approach to pain control that is proving effective. The major opioid analgesics are listed in Table 28–10.

A. **Nonnarcotic analgesics.** Typical of this group is aspirin. Unlike narcotic analgesics, which act on the central nervous system (CNS), salicylates act at the peripheral or local level—the site of origin of the pain—and are usually taken every 3 hours.

With most analgesics, peak plasma concentrations occur in 45 minutes, and analgesic effects last 3 to 4 hours. Other nonsteroidal anti-inflammatory drugs (NSAIDs) can also be used for analgesia (200 to 400 mg of ibuprofen every 4 hours). Drug equivalents: 650 mg of aspirin = 32 mg of codeine = 65 mg of propoxyphene (Darvon) = 50 mg of oral pentazocine (Talwin).

B. **Placebos.** Placebos are substances with no known pharmacological activity that act through suggestion rather than biological action. It has recently been demonstrated, however, that naloxone (Narcan), an opioid antagonist, can block the analgesic effects of a placebo, which suggests that a release of endogenous opioids may explain some placebo effects.

Long-term treatment with placebos should never be undertaken when patients have clearly stated an objection to such treatment. Furthermore,

Table 28–10
Opioid Analgesics for Management of Cancer Pain

Drug and Equianalgesic Dose Relative Potency	Dose (mg IM or oral)	Plasma Half-Life (hr)	Starting Oral Dose[a] (mg)	Commercial Available Preparations
Opioid agonists				
Morphine	10 IM 60 oral	3–4	30–60	Oral: tablet, liquid, slow-release tablet Rectal: 5–30 mg Injectable: SC, IM, IV, epidural, intrathecal
Hydromorphone	1.5 IM 7.5 oral	2–3	2–48	Oral: tablets—1, 2, 4 mg Injectable: SC, IM, IV 2, 3, and 10 mg/mL
Methadone	10 IM 20 oral	12–24	5–10	Oral: tablets, liquid Injectable: SC, IM, IV
Levorphanol	2 IM 4 oral	12–16	2–4	Oral: tablets Injectable: SC, IM, IV
Oxymorphone	1 IM	2–3	NA	Rectal: 10 mg Injectable: SC, IM, IV
Heroin	5 IM 60 oral	3–4	NA	NA
Meperidine	75 IM 300 oral	3–4 (normeperidine 12–16)	75	Oral: tablets Injectable: SC, IM, IV
Codeine	30 IM 200 oral	3–4	60	Oral: tablets and combination with acetylsalicylic acid, acetaminophen, liquid
Oxycodone	15 oral 30 oral 80 oral	— Long-acting (12-hr OxyContin)	5	Oral: tablets, liquid, oral formulation in combination with acetaminophen (tablet and liquid) and aspirin (tablet)

The times of peak analgesia in nontolerant patients ranges from ½ to 1 hr, and the duration from 4 to 6 hr. The peak analgesic effect is delayed, and the duration is prolonged after oral administrations.
[a]Recommended starting IM doses; the optimal dose for each patient is determined by titration, and the maximal dose is limited by adverse effects.
Adapted from Foley K. Management of cancer pain. In: DeVita VT, Hellmon S, Rosenberg SA, eds. *Cancer: Principles and Practice of Oncology*, 4th ed. Philadelphia: Lippincott, 1993:22, with permission.

deceptive treatment with placebos seriously undermines patients' confidence in their physicians. Finally, placebos should not be used when an effective therapy is available.

For a more detailed discussion of this topic, see End-of-Life and Palliative Care, Sec 24.9, p. 2353; and Death, Dying, and Bereavement, Sec 24.10, p. 2378, in CTP/IX.

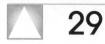

29
Psychotherapy

I. Definition

Psychotherapy is the treatment for mental illness and behavioral disturbances in which a trained person establishes a professional contract with the patient and through definite therapeutic communication, both verbal and nonverbal, attempts to alleviate the emotional disturbance, reverse or change maladaptive patterns of behavior, and encourage personality growth and development. It is distinguished from other forms of psychiatric treatment such as somatic therapies (e.g., psychopharmacology and convulsive therapies).

II. Psychoanalysis and Psychoanalytic Psychotherapy

These two forms of treatment are based on Sigmund Freud's theories of a dynamic unconscious and psychological conflict. The major goal of these forms of therapy is to help the patient develop insight into unconscious conflicts, based on unresolved childhood wishes and manifested as symptoms, and to develop more adult patterns of interacting and behaving.

A. Psychoanalysis. Psychoanalysis is a theory of human mental phenomena and behavior, a method of psychic investigation and research, and a form of psychotherapy originally formulated by Freud. As a method of treatment, it is the most intensive and rigorous of this type of psychotherapy. The patient is seen three to five times a week, generally for a minimum of several hundred hours over a number of years. The patient lies on a couch with the analyst seated behind, out of the patient's visual range. The patient attempts to say freely and without censure whatever comes to mind, to associate freely, so as to follow as deeply as possible the train of thoughts to their earliest roots. As a technique for exploring the mental processes, psychoanalysis includes the use of free association and the analysis and interpretation of dreams, resistances, and transferences. The analyst uses interpretation and clarification to help the patient work through and resolve conflicts that have been affecting the patient's life, often unconsciously. Psychoanalysis requires that the patient be stable, highly motivated, verbal, and psychologically minded. The patient also must be able to tolerate the stress generated by analysis without becoming overly regressed, distraught, or impulsive. As a form of psychotherapy, it uses the investigative technique, guided by Freud's libido and instinct theories and by ego psychology, to gain insight into a person's unconscious motivations, conflicts, and symbols and thus to effect a change in maladaptive behavior.

B. Psychoanalytically oriented psychotherapy. Based on the same principles and techniques as classic psychoanalysis, but less intense. There are two types: (1) insight-oriented or expressive psychotherapy and (2) supportive or relationship psychotherapy. Patients are seen one to two times a week and sit up facing the psychiatrist. The goal of resolution of unconscious psychological conflict is similar to that of psychoanalysis, but a greater emphasis is placed on day-to-day reality issues and a lesser emphasis on the development of transference issues. Patients suitable for psychoanalysis are suitable for this therapy, as are patients with a wider range of symptomatic and characterological problems. Patients with personality disorders are also suitable for this therapy. A comparison of psychoanalysis and psychoanalytically oriented psychotherapy is presented in Table 29–1.

In supportive psychotherapy, the essential element is support rather than the development of insight. This type of therapy often is the treatment of choice for patients with serious ego vulnerabilities, particularly psychotic patients. Patients in a crisis situation, such as

Table 29–1
Scope of Psychoanalytic Practice: A Clinical Continuum[a]

Feature	Psychoanalysis	Psychoanalytic Psychotherapy	
		Expressive Mode	Supportive Mode
Frequency	Regular, four to five times a week, 30–50 minute session.	Regular, one to three times a week, half to full hour.	Flexible, once a week or less or as needed, half to full hour.
Duration	Long-term, usually 3 to 5+ years.	Short term or long term, several sessions to months to years.	Short term or intermittent long term; single session to lifetime.
Setting	Patient primarily on couch with analyst out of view.	Patient and therapist face to face; occasional use of couch.	Patient and therapist face to face; couch contraindicated.
Modus operandi	Systematic analysis of all (positive and negative) transference and resistance; primary focus on analyst and intrasession events; transference neurosis facilitated; regression encouraged.	Partial analysis of dynamics and defenses; focus on current interpersonal events and transference to others outside sessions; analysis of negative transference; positive transference left unexplored unless it impedes progress; limited regression encouraged.	Formation of therapeutic alliance and real object relationship; analysis of transference contraindicated with rare exceptions; focus on conscious external events; regression discouraged.
Analyst–therapist role	Absolute neutrality; frustration of patient; reflector–minor role.	Modified neutrality; implicit gratification of patient and great activity.	Neutrality suspended; limited explicit gratification, direction, and disclosure.
Putative change agents	Insight predominates within relatively deprived environment.	Insight within empathic environment; identification with benevolent object.	Auxiliary or surrogate ego as temporary substitute; holding environment; insight to degree possible.
Patient population	Neuroses; mild character psychopathology.	Neuroses; mild to moderate character psychopathology, especially narcissistic and borderline personality disorders.	Severe character disorders; latent or manifest psychoses; acute crises; physical illness.

(continued)

Table 29–1—*continued*
Scope of Psychoanalytic Practice: A Clinical Continuum[a]

Feature	Psychoanalysis	Psychoanalytic Psychotherapy	
		Expressive Mode	Supportive Mode
Patient requisites	High motivation; psychological-mindedness; good previous object relationships; ability to maintain transference neurosis; good frustration tolerance.	High to moderate motivation and psychological-mindedness; ability to form therapeutic alliance; some frustration tolerance.	Some degree of motivation and ability to form therapeutic alliance.
Basic goals	Structural reorganization of personality; resolution of unconscious conflicts; insight into intrapsychic events; symptom relief an indirect result.	Partial reorganization of personality and defenses; resolution of preconscious and conscious derivatives of conflicts; insight into current interpersonal events; improved object relations; symptom relief a goal or prelude to further exploration.	Reintegration of self and ability to cope; stabilization or restoration of pre-existing equilibrium; strengthening of defenses; better adjustment or acceptance of pathology; symptom relief and environmental restructuring as primary goals.
Major techniques	Free association method predominates; fully dynamic interpretation (including confrontation, clarification, and working through), with emphasis on genetic reconstruction.	Limited free association; confrontation, clarification, and partial interpretation predominate, with emphasis on here-and-now interpretation and limited genetic interpretation.	Free association method contraindicated; suggestion (advice) predominates; abreaction useful; confrontation, clarification, and interpretation in the here-and-now secondary; genetic interpretation contraindicated.
Adjunct treatment	Primarily avoided; if applied, all negative and positive meanings and implications thoroughly analyzed.	May be necessary (e.g., psychotropic drugs as temporary adjunct); if applied, negative implications explored and diffused.	Often necessary (e.g., psychotropic drugs, family therapy, rehabilitative therapy, or hospitalization); if applied, positive implications are emphasized.

[a]This division is not categoric; all practice resides on a clinical continuum.
Table by Toksoz Byram Karasu, M.D.

acute grief, are also suitable. This therapy can be continued on a long-term basis and last many years, especially in the case of patients with chronic problems. Support can take the form of limit setting, increasing reality testing, reassurance, advice, and help with developing social skills.

C. **Brief dynamic psychotherapy.** A short-term treatment, generally consisting of 10 to 40 sessions during a period of less than 1 year. The goal, based on psychodynamic theory, is to develop insight into underlying conflicts; such insight leads to psychological and behavioral changes.

This therapy is more confrontational than the other insight-oriented therapies in that the therapist is very active in repeatedly directing the patient's associations and thoughts to conflictual areas. The number of hours is explicitly agreed on by the therapist and patient before the beginning of therapy, and a specific, circumscribed area of conflict is chosen to be the focus of treatment. More extensive change is not attempted. Patients suitable for this therapy must be able to define a specific central problem to be addressed and must be highly motivated, psychologically minded, and able to tolerate the temporary increase in anxiety or sadness that this type of therapy can evoke. Patients who are not suitable include those with fragile ego structures (e.g., suicidal or psychotic patients) and those with poor impulse control (e.g., borderline patients, substance abusers, and antisocial personalities).

III. Behavior Therapy

Behavior therapy focuses on overt and observable behavior and uses various conditioning techniques derived from learning theory to directly modify the patient's behavior. This therapy is directed exclusively toward symptomatic improvement, without addressing psychodynamic causation. Behavior therapy is based on the principles of learning theory, including operant and classical conditioning. Operant conditioning is based on the premise that behavior is shaped by its consequences; if behavior is positively reinforced, it will increase; if it is punished, it will decrease; and if it elicits no response, it will be extinguished. Classical conditioning is based on the premise that behavior is shaped by being coupled with or uncoupled from anxiety-provoking stimuli. Just as Ivan Pavlov's dogs were conditioned to salivate at the sound of a bell once the bell had become associated with meat, a person can be conditioned to feel fear in neutral situations that have come to be associated with anxiety. Uncouple the anxiety from the situation, and the avoidant and anxious behavior will decrease.

Behavior therapy is believed to be most effective for clearly delineated, circumscribed maladaptive behaviors (e.g., phobias, compulsions, overeating, cigarette smoking, stuttering, and sexual dysfunctions). In the treatment of conditions that can be strongly affected by psychological factors (e.g., hypertension, asthma, pain, and insomnia), behavioral techniques can be used to induce relaxation and decrease aggravating stresses (Table 29–2). There are several behavior therapy techniques.

A. **Token economy.** A form of *positive reinforcement* used with inpatients who are rewarded with various tokens for performing desired behaviors (e.g., dressing in street clothes, attending group therapy). Token economy has been used to treat schizophrenia, especially in hospital settings. The tokens can be exchanged for a variety of positive reinforcers such as food, television time, or a weekend pass.

B. **Aversion therapy.** A form of conditioning that involves the repeated coupling of an unpleasant or painful stimulus, such as an electric shock, with an undesirable behavior. In a less controversial form of aversion therapy, the patient couples imagining something unpleasant with the undesired behavior. Aversion therapy has been used to treat substance abuse.

Table 29–2
Some Common Clinical Applications of Behavior Therapy

Disorder	Comments
Agoraphobia	Graded exposure and flooding can reduce the fear of being in crowded places. About 60% of patients so treated are improved. In some cases, the spouse can serve as the model while accompanying the patient into the fear situation; however, the patient cannot get a secondary gain by keeping the spouse nearby and displaying symptoms.
Alcohol dependence	Aversion therapy, in which the alcohol-dependent patient is made to vomit (by adding an emetic to the alcohol) every time a drink is ingested, is effective in treating alcohol dependence. Disulfiram (Antabuse) can be given to alcohol-dependent patients when they are alcohol-free. Such patients are warned of the severe physiological consequences of drinking (e.g., nausea, vomiting, hypotension, collapse) with disulfiram in the system.
Anorexia nervosa	Observe eating behavior; contingency management; record weight.
Bulimia nervosa	Record bulimic episodes; log moods.
Hyperventilation	Hyperventilation test; controlled breathing; direct observation.
Other phobias	Systematic desensitization has been effective in treating phobias such as fears of heights, animals, and flying. Social skills training has also been used for shyness and fear of other people.
Paraphilias	Electric shocks or other noxious stimuli can be applied at the time of a paraphilic impulse, and eventually the impulse subsides. Shocks can be administered by either the therapist or the patient. The results are satisfactory but must be reinforced at regular intervals.
Schizophrenia	The token economy procedure, in which tokens are awarded for desirable behavior and can be used to buy ward privileges, has been useful in treating schizophrenic inpatients. Social skills training teaches schizophrenic patients how to interact with others in a socially acceptable way so that negative feedback is eliminated. In addition, the aggressive behavior of some schizophrenic patients can be diminished through those methods.
Sexual dysfunctions	Sex therapy, developed by William Masters and Virginia Johnson, is a behavior therapy technique used for various sexual dysfunctions, especially male erectile disorder, orgasm disorders, and premature ejaculation. It uses relaxation desensitization, and graded exposure as the primary techniques.
Shy bladder	Inability to void in a public bathroom; relaxation exercises.
Type A behavior	Physiological assessment, muscle relaxation, biofeedback (on electromyogram).

C. **Systematic desensitization.** This technique is based on the behavioral principle of countercon-ditioning, whereby a person overcomes maladaptive anxiety elicited by a situation or object by approaching the feared situation gradually and in a psychophysiological state that inhibits anx-iety. Rather than use actual situations or objects that elicit fear, patients and therapists prepare a graded list or hierarchy of anxiety-provoking scenes associated with a patient's fears. The learned relaxation state and the anxiety-provoking scenes are systematically paired in treatment. Thus, the three steps are relaxation training, hierarchy construction, and desensitization of the stimulus. When this procedure is performed in real life rather than in the imagination, it is called *graded exposure*.

D. **Flooding.** A technique in which the patient is exposed immediately to the most anxiety-provoking stimulus (e.g., the top of a tall building if he or she is afraid of heights) instead of being exposed gradually or systematically to a hierarchy of feared situations. If this technique is carried out in the imagination rather than in real life, it is called *implosion*. Flooding is thought to be an effective behavioral treatment of such disorders as phobias, provided the patient can tolerate the associated anxiety. A great deal of experimental work is being done with exposure to the feared situations using virtual reality. Beneficial effects have been reported with computer-generated virtual reality exposure of patients with height phobia, fear of flying, arachnophobia, and claustrophobia.

E. **Assertiveness training.** A variety of techniques, including role modeling, desensitization, and positive reinforcement, are used to increase assertiveness. To be assertive requires that people have confidence in their judgment and sufficient self-esteem to express their opinions. Social skills training deals with assertiveness but also attends to a variety of real-life tasks, such as food shopping, looking for work, interacting with other people, and overcoming shyness.

F. **Eye movement desensitization and reprocessing (EMDR).** Saccadic eye movements are rapid oscillations of the eyes that occur when a person tracks an object that is moved back and forth across a line of vision. If the saccades are induced while the person is imagining or thinking about an anxiety-producing event, a few studies have demonstrated that a positive thought or image can be induced that results in decreased anxiety.

IV. Cognitive–Behavioral Therapy

This therapy is based on the theory that behavior is determined by the way in which people think about themselves and their roles in the world. Maladaptive behavior is secondary to ingrained, stereotyped thoughts, which can lead to cognitive distortions or errors in thinking. The theory is aimed at correcting cognitive distortions and the self-defeating behaviors that result from them. Therapy is on a short-term basis, generally lasting for 15 to 20 sessions during a period of 12 weeks. Patients are made aware of their own distorted cognitions and the assumptions on which they are based. Homework is assigned; patients are asked to record what they are thinking in certain stressful situations (e.g., "I'm no good" or "No one cares about me") and to ascertain the underlying, often relatively unconscious, assumptions that fuel the negative cognitions. This process has been referred to as "recognizing and correcting automatic thoughts." The cognitive model of depression includes the cognitive triad, which is a description of the thought distortions that occur when a person is depressed. The triad includes (1) a negative view of the self, (2) a negative interpretation of present and past experience, and (3) a negative expectation of the future (Table 29–3).

Cognitive therapy has been most successfully applied to the treatment of mild to moderate nonpsychotic depressions. It also has been effective as an adjunctive treatment in substance abuse and in increasing compliance with medication. It has been used recently to treat schizophrenia.

Table 29–3
General Assumptions of Cognitive Therapy

Perception and experiencing in general are active processes that involve both inspective and introspective data.
The patient's cognitions represent a synthesis of internal and external stimuli.
How persons appraise a situation is generally evident in their cognitions (thoughts and visual images).
Those cognitions constitute their stream of consciousness or phenomenal field, which reflects their configuration of themselves, their world, their past, and their future.
Alterations in the content of their underlying cognitive structures affect their affective state and behavioral pattern.
Through psychological therapy, patients can become aware of their cognitive distortions.
Correction of those faulty dysfunctional constructs can lead to clinical improvement.

Adapted from Beck AT, Rush AJ, Shaw BF, et al. *Cognitive Therapy of Depression.* New York: Guilford, 1979:47, with permission.

V. Family Therapy

Family therapy is based on the theory that a family is a system that attempts to maintain homeostasis, regardless of how maladaptive the system may be. This theory has been referred to as a "family systems orientation," and the techniques include focusing on the family rather than on the identified patient. The family, therefore, becomes the patient, rather than the individual family member who has been identified as sick. One of the major goals of a family therapist is to determine what homeostatic role, however pathological, the identified patient is serving in the particular family system. A family therapist's goal is to help a family understand that the identified patient's symptoms in fact serve the crucial function of maintaining the family's homeostasis. One example is the triangulated child—the child who is identified by the family as the patient is actually serving to maintain the family system by becoming involved in a marital conflict as a scapegoat, referee, or even surrogate spouse. The therapist's job is to help the family understand the triangulation process and address the deeper conflict that underlies the child's apparent disruptive behavior. Techniques include reframing and positive connotation (a relabeling of all negatively expressed feelings or behaviors as positive); for example, "This child is impossible" becomes "This child is desperately trying to distract and protect you from what he or she perceives is an unhappy marriage."

Other goals of family therapy include changing maladaptive rules that govern a family, increasing awareness of cross-generational dynamics, balancing individuation and cohesiveness, increasing one-on-one direct communication, and decreasing blaming and scapegoating.

VI. Interpersonal Therapy

This is a short-term psychotherapy, lasting 12 to 16 weeks, developed specifically for the treatment of nonbipolar, nonpsychotic depression. Intrapsychic conflicts are not addressed. Emphasis is on current interpersonal relationships and on strategies to improve the patient's interpersonal life. Antidepressant medication is often used as an adjunct to interpersonal therapy. The therapist is very active in helping to formulate the patient's predominant interpersonal problem areas, which define the treatment focus (Table 29–4).

VII. Group therapy

Group therapies are based on as many theories as are individual therapies. Groups range from those that emphasize support and an increase in social skills, to those that emphasize specific symptomatic relief, to those that work through unresolved intrapsychic conflicts. Compared with individual therapies, two of the main strengths of group therapy are the opportunity for immediate feedback from a patient's peers and the chance for both patient and therapist to observe a patient's psychological, emotional, and behavioral responses to a variety of people who elicit a variety of transferences. Both individual and interpersonal issues can be resolved.

Groups tend to meet one to two times a week, usually for 1.5 hours. They may be homogeneous or heterogeneous, depending on the diagnosis. Examples

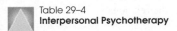

Table 29–4
Interpersonal Psychotherapy

Goal	Improvement in current interpersonal skills
Selection criteria	Outpatient, nonbipolar disorder, nonpsychotic depressive disorder
Duration	12–16 weeks, usually once-weekly meetings
Technique	Reassurance
	Clarification of feeling states
	Improvement of interpersonal communication
	Testing perceptions
	Development of interpersonal skills
	Medication

From Ursano RJ, Silberman EK. Individual psychotherapies. In: Talbott JA, Hales RE, Yudofsky SC, eds. *The American Psychiatric Press Textbook of Psychiatry.* Washington, DC: American Psychiatric Press, 1988:868, with permission.

of homogeneous groups include those for patients attempting to lose weight or stop smoking and groups whose members share the same medical or psychiatric problem (e.g., AIDS, posttraumatic stress disorder, substance use disorders). Certain types of patients do not do well in certain types of groups. Psychotic patients, who require structure and clear direction, do not do well in insight-oriented groups. Paranoid patients, antisocial personalities, and substance abusers can benefit from group therapy but do not do well in heterogeneous, insight-oriented groups. In general, acutely psychotic or suicidal patients do not do well in groups.

A. **Alcoholics Anonymous (AA).** An example of a large, highly structured, peer-run group that is organized around persons with a similar central problem. AA emphasizes sharing experiences, role models, ventilation of feelings, and a strong sense of community and mutual support. Similar groups include Narcotics Anonymous (NA) and Sex Addicts Anonymous (SAA).

B. **Milieu therapy.** The multidisciplinary therapeutic approach used on inpatient psychiatric wards. The term *milieu therapy* reflects the idea that all activities on a ward are oriented toward increasing a patient's ability to cope in the world and relate appropriately to others. The treatment emphasizes appropriate socioenvironmental manipulation for the benefit of the patient.

C. **Multiple family groups.** Composed of families of schizophrenic patients. The groups discuss issues and problems related to having a schizophrenic person in the family and share suggestions and means of coping. Multiple family groups are an important factor in decreasing relapse rates among the schizophrenic patients whose families participate in the groups.

VIII. **Couple and Marital Therapy**
As many as 50% of patients are estimated to enter psychotherapy primarily because of marital problems; another 25% experience marital problems along with their other presenting problems. Couple or marital therapy is designed to psychologically modify the interaction of two people who are in conflict with each other over one parameter or a variety of parameters—social, emotional,

sexual, or economic. As in family therapy, the relationship rather than either of the individuals is viewed as the patient.

IX. Dialectical Behavior Therapy

This form of therapy has been used successfully in patients with borderline personality disorder and parasuicidal behavior. It is eclectic, drawing on methods from supportive, cognitive, and behavioral therapies. Some elements are derived from Franz Alexander's view of therapy as a corrective emotional experience, and also from certain Eastern philosophical schools (e.g., Zen). Patients are seen weekly, with the goal of improving interpersonal skills and decreasing self-destructive behavior by means of techniques involving advice, use of metaphor, storytelling, and confrontation, among many others. Borderline patients especially are helped to deal with the ambivalent feelings that are characteristic of the disorder.

X. Hypnosis

Hypnosis is a complex mental state in which consciousness is altered in such a way that the subject is amenable to suggestion and receptive to direction by the therapist. When hypnotized, the patient is in a trance state, during which memories can be recalled and events experienced. The material can be used to gain insight into the makeup of a personality. Hypnosis is used to treat many disorders, including obesity, substance-related disorders (especially nicotine dependence), sexual disorders, and dissociative states.

XI. Guided Imagery

Used alone or with hypnosis. The patient is instructed to imagine scenes with associated colors, sounds, smells, and feelings. The scene may be pleasant (used to decrease anxiety) or unpleasant (used to master anxiety). Imagery has been used to treat patients with generalized anxiety disorders, posttraumatic stress disorder, and phobias, and as an adjunct therapy for medical or surgical disease.

XII. Biofeedback

Biofeedback provides information to a person about his or her physiological functions, usually related to the autonomic nervous system (e.g., blood pressure), with the goal of producing a relaxed, euthymic mental state. It is based on the idea that the autonomic nervous system can be brought under voluntary control through operant conditioning. It is used in the management of tension states associated with medical illness (e.g., to increase hand temperature in patients with Raynaud's syndrome and to treat headaches and hypertension) (Table 29–5).

XIII. Paradoxical Therapy

In this approach, the therapist suggests that the patient intentionally engages in an unwanted or undesirable behavior (called *paradoxical injunction*)—for example, avoiding a phobic object or performing a compulsive ritual. This approach can create new insights for some patients.

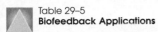

Table 29–5
Biofeedback Applications

Condition	Effects
Asthma	Both frontal EMG and airway resistance biofeedback have been reported as producing relaxation from the panic associated with asthma, as well as improving airflow rate.
Cardiac arrhythmias	Specific biofeedback of the ECG has permitted patients to lower the frequency of premature ventricular contractions.
Fecal incontinence and enuresis	The timing sequence of internal and external anal sphincters has been measured with triple–lumen rectal catheters providing feedback to incontinent patients for them to re-establish normal bowel habits in a relatively small number of biofeedback sessions. An actual precursor of biofeedback dating to 1938 was the sounding of a buzzer for sleeping enuretic children at the first sign of moisture (the pad and bell).
Grand mal epilepsy	A number of EEG biofeedback procedures have been used experimentally to suppress seizure activity prophylactically in patients not responsive to anticonvulsant medication. The procedures permit the patient to enhance the sensorimotor brain wave rhythm or to normalize brain activity, as computed in real-time power spectrum displays.
Hyperactivity	EEG biofeedback procedures have been used on children with attention-deficit/hyperactivity disorder to train them to reduce their motor restlessness.
Idiopathic hypertension and orthostatic hypotension	A variety of specific (direct) and nonspecific biofeedback procedures—including blood pressure feedback, galvanic skin response, and foot–hand thermal feedback combined with relaxation procedures—have been used to teach patients to increase or decrease their blood pressure. Some follow-up data indicate that the changes may persist for years and often permit the reduction or elimination of antihypertensive medications.
Migraine	The most common biofeedback strategy with classic or common vascular headaches has been thermal biofeedback from a digit accompanied by autogenic self-suggestive phrases encouraging hand warming and head cooling. The mechanism is thought to help prevent excessive cerebral artery vasoconstriction, often accompanied by an ischemic prodromal symptom, such as scintillating scotomata, followed by rebound engorgement of arteries and stretching of vessel wall pain receptors.
Myofascial and temporomandibular joint pain	High levels of EMG activity over the powerful muscles associated with bilateral temporomandibular joints have been decreased by means of biofeedback in patients who are jaw clenchers or have bruxism.
Neuromuscular rehabilitation	Mechanical devices or an EMG measurement of muscle activity displayed to a patient increases the effectiveness of traditional therapies, as documented by relatively long clinical histories in peripheral nerve–muscle damage, spasmodic torticollis, selected cases of tardive dyskinesia, cerebral palsy, and upper motor neuron hemiplegias.
Raynaud's syndrome	Cold hands and cold feet are frequent concomitants of anxiety and also occur in Raynaud's syndrome, caused by vasospasm of arterial smooth muscle. A number of studies report that thermal feedback from the hand, an inexpensive and benign procedure compared with surgical sympathectomy, is effective in about 70% of cases of Raynaud's syndrome.
Tension headaches	Muscle contraction headaches are most frequently treated with two large active electrodes spaced on the forehead to provide visual or auditory information about the levels of muscle tension. The frontal electrode placement is sensitive to EMG activity in the frontalis and occipital muscles, which the patient learns to relax.

ECG, electrocardiogram; EMG, electromyogram.

XIV. Sex Therapy

In sex therapy, the therapist discusses the psychological and physiological aspects of sexual functioning in great detail. Therapists adopt an educative attitude, and aids such as models of the genitalia and videotapes may be used. Treatment is on a short-term basis and behaviorally oriented. Specific exercises are prescribed, depending on the disorder being treated (e.g., graduated dilators for vaginismus). Usually, the couple is treated, but individual sex therapy is also effective.

XV. Social Skills Training

Most used in patients with schizophrenia or schizophreniclike disorders, this type of therapy improves social skills. Social dysfunction is normalized by teaching the patient how to accurately read or decode social inputs. Role-playing is used to decrease social anxiety and improve social and conversational skills. It is usually done in groups.

For a more detailed discussion of this topic, see Psychotherapies, Ch 30, p. 2746, in CTP/IX.

30
Psychopharmacology and Other Biological Therapies

I. Introduction

Since the last edition, many psychotropic medications have received approval by the U.S. Food and Drug Administration (FDA) to treat a range of psychiatric disorders. The use of terminology that classified these medicines belonging to a certain class of drugs like antipsychotic and mood stabilizers is becoming obsolete. All second-generation drugs have received approval to be used as monotherapy or adjunctive therapy in the treatment of bipolar disorder while some have also been approved for major depression, and their wider application in generalized anxiety disorder (GAD) is on the horizon. This is a fundamental shift in psychiatric thinking and conceptualization, and hence, it is preferable to think of drugs in terms of their pharmacological actions rather than their therapeutic indications, which often change and overlap. This wider application is, however, mostly restricted to serotonin–dopamine antagonists (SDAs), and hence in this chapter, the drugs are grouped in an outline format according to their primary therapeutic indications: anxiolytics and hypnotics, antipsychotics, antidepressants, antimanics and mood stabilizers, stimulants, cholinesterase inhibitors (cognitive enhancers), and other drugs.

II. Basic Principles of Psychopharmacology

A. **Pharmacological actions.** Pharmacological actions are divided into two categories: pharmacokinetic and pharmacodynamic. In simple terms, *pharmacokinetics* describes *what the body does to the drug* and *pharmacodynamics* describes *what the drug does to the body*. Pharmacokinetic data trace the absorption, distribution, metabolism, and excretion of a drug in the body. Pharmacodynamic data measure the effects of a drug on cells in the brain and other tissues of the body.

1. **Pharmacokinetics**

   a. **Absorption.** Orally administered drugs dissolve in the fluid of the gastrointestinal (GI) tract and then reach the brain through the blood-stream. Some drugs are available in *depot* preparations, which are injected intramuscularly (IM) once every 1 to 4 weeks. Intravenous (IV) administration is the quickest route for achieving therapeutic blood concentrations, but it also carries the highest risk for sudden and life-threatening adverse effects. Few drugs, however, are given in IV form.

   b. **Distribution and bioavailability.** Drugs that circulate bound to plasma proteins are *protein-bound,* and those that circulate unbound are said to be *free.* Only the free fraction can pass through the blood–brain barrier. The *distribution* of a drug to the brain is promoted

Table 30–1
Representative Psychotropic Drug Substrates of Human Cytochromes P450, Along with Representative Inhibitors

CYP 3A	CYP 2D6	CYP 2C19
Substrates	Substrates	Substrates
Triazolam (Halcion)	Desipramine (Norpramin)	Diazepam^a
Alprazolam (Xanax)	Nortriptyline (Aventyl)	Amitriptyline^a
Midazolam (Versed)	Paroxetine (Paxil)	Citalopram^a
Quetiapine (Seroquel)	Tramadol (Ultram)	Inhibitors
Nefazodone (Serzone)	Venlafaxine (Effexor)	Fluvoxamine
Buspirone (BuSpar)	Fluoxetine^a (Prozac)	Omeprazole (Prilosec)
Trazodone (Desyrel)	Citalopram^a	
Zolpidem^a (Ambien)	Inhibitors	
Amitriptyline^a (Endep)	Quinidine (Cardioquin)	
Imipramine^a (Tofranil)	Fluoxetine	
Haloperidol^a (Haldol)	Paroxetine	
Citalopram^a (Celexa)	Bupropion (Wellbutrin)	
Clozapine^a (Clozaril)	Terbinafine (Lamisil)	
Diazepam^a (Valium)	Diphenhydramine (Benadryl)	
Inhibitors		
Ritonavir (Norvir)		
Ketoconazole (Nizoral)		
Itraconazole (Sporanox)		
Nefazodone		
Fluvoxamine (Luvox)		
Erythromycin (E-Mycin)		
Clarithromycin (Biaxin)		

^{a}Indicates partial substrate.

by high rates of cerebral blood flow, lipid solubility, and receptor affinity.

Bioavailability refers to the fraction of administered drug that can eventually be recovered from the bloodstream.

  c. **Metabolism and excretion.** The four metabolic routes—*oxidation, reduction, hydrolysis,* and *conjugation*—usually produce metabolites that are readily excreted. Metabolism usually yields inactive metabolites that are more polar and, therefore, more readily excreted. However, metabolism also transforms many inactive prodrugs into therapeutically active metabolites. The liver is the principal site of *metabolism* (Table 30–1), and bile, feces, and urine are the major routes of *excretion*. Psychotherapeutic drugs are also excreted in body fluids, such as sweat and saliva.

 CLINICAL HINT:
Drugs are excreted in breast milk, an important fact to be considered for mothers who want to nurse their children.

The *half-life* of a drug is the amount of time it takes for its plasma concentration to be reduced by half during metabolism and excretion. A greater number of daily doses are required for drugs with shorter half-lives than for drugs with longer half-lives. Drug interactions or disease states that inhibit the metabolism of psychoactive drugs can produce toxicity.

d. **Cytochrome P450 enzymes.** Most psychotherapeutic drugs are oxidized by the hepatic cytochrome P450 (CYP) enzyme system, which is so named because it absorbs light strongly at a wavelength of 450 nm.

The CYP enzymes are responsible for the inactivation of most psychotherapeutic drugs (see Table 30–1). Expression of the CYP genes may be induced by alcohol, by certain drugs (barbiturates, anticonvulsants), or by smoking. For example, an inducer of CYP 3A4, such as cimetidine, may increase the metabolism and decrease the plasma concentrations of a substrate of 3A4, such as alprazolam (Xanax). Administration of a CYP 2D6 inhibitor, such as fluoxetine (Prozac), may inhibit the metabolism and thus raise the plasma concentrations of CYP 2D6 substrates, including amitriptyline (Elavil).

2. **Pharmacodynamics.** The major pharmacodynamic considerations include the molecular site of action, dose–response curve, therapeutic index, and development of tolerance, dependence, and withdrawal symptoms.

a. **Molecular site of action.** The *molecular site of action* is determined in laboratory assays and may or may not correctly identify the drug–receptor interactions responsible for a drug's clinical effects, which are identified empirically in clinical trials.

b. **Dose–response curve.** The *dose–response curve* plots the effects of a drug against its plasma concentration. *Potency* refers to the ratio of drug dosage to clinical effect. For example, risperidone (Risperdal) is more potent than olanzapine (Zyprexa) because about 4 mg of risperidone is required to achieve the comparable therapeutic effect of 20 mg of olanzapine. However, because both are capable of eliciting a similar beneficial response at their respective optimal dosages, the *clinical efficacies* of risperidone and olanzapine are equivalent.

c. **Therapeutic index.** The *therapeutic index* is the ratio of a drug's toxic dosage to its maximally effective dosage.

 CLINICAL HINT:
Lithium has a low therapeutic index, so close monitoring of plasma concentrations is required to avoid toxicity.

---

d. **Tolerance, dependence, and withdrawal symptoms.** When a person becomes less responsive to a particular drug with time, *tolerance* to the effects of the drug has developed. The development of tolerance can be associated with the appearance of physical *dependence,* which is the need to continue taking a drug to prevent the appearance of *withdrawal symptoms.*

III. Clinical Guidelines

Optimizing the results of psychotropic drug therapy involves consideration of the six *D*s: diagnosis, drug selection, dosage, duration, discontinuation, and dialogue.

A. The six *D*s

1. **Diagnosis.** A careful diagnostic investigation should identify specific target symptoms with which the drug response can be objectively assessed.

2. **Drug selection.** Factors that determine drug selection include diagnosis, past personal and family history of response to a particular agent, and the overall medical status of the patient. Certain drugs will be excluded because concurrent drug treatment of medical and other psychiatric disorders creates a risk for drug–drug interactions. Other drugs will be excluded because they have unfavorable adverse effect profiles. A choice of the ideal drug should emerge based on the clinician's experience and preferences.

    The Drug Enforcement Administration (DEA) has classified drugs according to their potential for abuse (Table 30–2), and clinicians are advised to use caution when prescribing controlled substances.

3. **Dosage.** The two most common causes of failure of psychotropic drug treatment are inadequate dosing and an incomplete therapeutic trial of a drug.

4. **Duration.** For antipsychotic, antidepressant, and mood-stabilizing drugs, a therapeutic trial should continue for 4 to 6 weeks. In the treatment of these conditions, drug efficacy tends to improve with time, whereas drug discontinuation is frequently associated with relapses. In contrast, for most anxiolytic and stimulant drugs, the maximum therapeutic benefit is usually evident within an hour of administration.

5. **Discontinuation.** Many psychotropic agents are associated with a discontinuation syndrome when they are stopped. Drugs with a short half-life are most prone to causing these withdrawal symptoms, especially if they are stopped abruptly after extended use. Thus, it is important to discontinue all drugs as slowly as possible, if clinical circumstances permit.

6. **Dialogue.** Informing patients about likely side effects at the outset of treatment, as well as the reasons they are taking a specific drug, serves to improve treatment compliance. Clinicians should distinguish between probable or expected adverse effects and rare or unexpected adverse effects.

B. Special considerations

1. **Children.** Begin with a small dosage and increase until clinical effects are observed. Do not hesitate to use adult dosages in children if the dosage is effective and no adverse effects develop. Some children need higher doses because their livers metabolize drugs more quickly than adults. Special caution should be used when prescribing selective

Table 30–2
Characteristics of Drugs at Each Drug Enforcement Agency Level

DEA Control Level (Schedule)	Characteristics of Drug at Each Control Level	Examples of Drugs at Each Control Level
I	High abuse potential No accepted use in medical treatment in the United States at the present time and, therefore, not for prescription use Can be used for research	Lysergic acid diethylamide (LSD), heroin, marijuana, peyote, 3, 4-methylenedioxymethamphetamine (MDMA), methcathinone, gamma hydroxybutyrate (GHB), phencyclidine (PCP), mescaline, psilocybin, nicocodeine, nicomorphine
II	High abuse potential Severe physical dependence liability Severe psychological dependence liability No refills; no telephone prescriptions	Amphetamine, opium, morphine, codeine, hydromorphone, phenmetrazine, amobarbital, secobarbital, pentobarbital, methylphenidate, ketamine
III	Abuse potential less than levels I and II Moderate or low physical dependence liability High psychological liability Prescriptions must be rewritten after 6 months or five refills	Glutethimide, methyprylon, nalorphine, sulfonmethane, benzphetamine, phendimetrazine, chlorphentermine; compounds containing codeine, morphine, opium, hydrocodone, dihydrocodeine, naltrexone, diethylpropion, dronabinol
IV	Low abuse potential Limited physical dependence liability Limited psychological dependence Prescriptions must be rewritten after 6 months or five refills	Phenobarbital, benzodiazepines,[a] chloral hydrate, ethchlorvynol, ethinamate, meprobamate, paraldehyde, phentermine
V	Lowest abuse potential of all controlled substances	Narcotic preparations containing limited amounts of nonnarcotic active medicinal ingredients

[a]In New York State, benzodiazepines are treated as schedule II substances, which require a triplicate prescription for a maximum of 1 month's supply.

serotonin reuptake inhibitors (SSRIs) in children because of the risk of suicidality, which is discussed in the following text.

2. **The elderly.** Begin treating elderly patients with a small dosage, usually approximately one-half the usual dosage. The dosage should be increased in small amounts, until either a clinical benefit is achieved or unacceptable adverse effects appear.

3. **Pregnant and nursing women.** Clinicians are best advised to avoid administering any drug to a woman who is pregnant (particularly during the first trimester) or nursing a child. This rule, however, occasionally needs to be broken when the mother's psychiatric disorder is severe. It has been suggested that withdrawing a drug during pregnancy could cause a discontinuation syndrome in both mother and fetus. Most psychotropic drugs have not been linked to an increased rate of specific birth defects.

4. **Medically ill persons.** Medically ill persons should be treated conservatively, which means beginning with a small dosage, increasing it slowly,

and watching for both clinical and adverse effects. If applicable, plasma drug concentrations are helpful during the treatment of these persons.

IV. Anxiolytics and Hypnotics
A. Treatment recommendations
1. **Treatment of acute anxiety.** Acute anxiety responds best to either oral or parenteral administration of benzodiazepines. In the presence of mania or psychosis, a benzodiazepine in combination with antipsychotics is appropriate.
2. **Treatment of chronic anxiety**
   a. **Antidepressants.** SSRIs and venlafaxine (Effexor) are antidepressants that are used for the control of chronic anxiety disorders, including obsessive–compulsive disorder (OCD). All antidepressants may increase anxiety when they are started.
   b. **Benzodiazepines.** Benzodiazepines may be used on a long-term basis for the treatment of generalized anxiety symptoms and panic disorder, but are generally used on a short-term basis.

 CLINICAL HINT:
Careful monitoring of benzodiazepine use should be done with long-term use. If the patient starts to increase the dose, tolerance and dependence should be considered.

   c. **Buspirone (BuSpar).** Buspirone is approved by the FDA for the treatment of anxiety disorders, specifically GAD.
   d. **Mirtazapine (Remeron).** Mirtazapine is effective for the treatment of anxiety symptoms, but its utility is limited by its marked sedative qualities and the tendency for increased appetite and weight gain.
   e. **Other treatments.** Monoamine oxidase inhibitors (MAOIs) and tricyclic and tetracyclic drugs are effective in treating anxiety, but are not used as first-line agents because of side effects and safety concerns.
3. **Treatment of insomnia**
   a. **Nonbenzodiazepines.** The nonbenzodiazepine agents zolpidem (Ambien), eszopiclone (Lunesta), and zaleplon (Sonata) have a rapid onset of action, specifically target insomnia, lack muscle relaxant and anticonvulsant properties, are completely metabolized within 4 or 5 hours, and rarely cause withdrawal symptoms or rebound insomnia. The usual bedtime dose of each is 10 mg. Zolpidem is said to be effective for 5 hours and zaleplon for 4 hours. The usual dose for eszopiclone is 2 mg, which can be increased to 3 mg. Adverse events may include dizziness, nausea, and somnolence.
   b. **Benzodiazepines.** Benzodiazepines shorten sleep latency and increase sleep continuity, so they are useful for the treatment of insomnia. The five benzodiazepines used primarily as hypnotics are

flurazepam (Dalmane), temazepam (Restoril), quazepam (Doral), estazolam (ProSom), and triazolam (Halcion).

Benzodiazepines also curtail sleep stages III and IV (deep or slow-wave sleep) and are useful for sleepwalking and night terrors, which occur in those stages of sleep. Benzodiazepines suppress disorders related to rapid eye movement (REM) sleep, most notably violent behavior during REM sleep (REM behavior disorder).

c. **Trazodone (Desyrel).** Low-dose trazodone, 25 to 100 mg at bedtime, is widely used to treat insomnia. It has a favorable effect on sleep architecture.

d. **Quetiapine (Seroquel).** This SDA is often used as an off-label medicine in a dosage of 25 to 100 mg for insomnia but may cause daytime somnolence and sedation.

e. **Ramelteon (Rozerem).** Ramelteon is an orally active hypnotic, and is indicated for the treatment of insomnia characterized by difficulty with sleep onset. It is a melatonin receptor agonist, with high binding affinity at the melatonin MT1 and MT2 receptors, and mimics and enhances the action of endogenous melatonin, which has been associated with maintenance of circadian sleep rhythm. The usual starting and maintenance dose is 8 mg, but some patients may need up to 16 mg.

It is available in an 8-mg strength tablet, and the usual dose is 8 mg taken within 30 minutes of going to bed.

B. **Benzodiazepine agonists and antagonists.** The benzodiazepines available for clinical use in the United States are listed in Table 30–3. They are widely prescribed, with at least 10% of the population using one of these drugs each year. They are safe, effective, and well tolerated in both short- and long-term use. The pharmacological effects of the benzodiazepines are listed in Table 30–4.

1. **Indications.** Benzodiazepines are often used to augment the effects of antidepressant drugs during the first month of use, before the antidepressant drug has begun to exert its anxiolytic effects; they are then tapered once the antidepressant becomes effective.

2. **Choice of drug.** The most important differences among the benzodiazepines relate to potency and elimination half-life.

a. **Potency.** High-potency benzodiazepines, such as alprazolam (Xanax), alprazolam XR, and clonazepam (Klonopin), are effective in suppressing panic attacks. In general, at doses needed to control panic attacks, low-potency benzodiazepines such as diazepam may produce unwanted sedation.

b. **Duration of action.** Diazepam (Valium) and triazolam (Halcion) are readily absorbed and have a rapid onset; chlordiazepoxide (Librium) and oxazepam (Serax) work more slowly.

Compounds with a long half-life tend to accumulate with repeated dosing so that the risk for excessive daytime sedation, difficulties with concentration and memory, and falls is increased. Rates

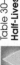

Table 30-3
Half-Lives, Doses, and Preparations of Benzodiazepine Receptor Agonists and Antagonists

Drug	Dose Equivalents	Half-Life (hr)	Rate of Absorption	Usual Adult Dosage	Dose Preparations
Agonists					
Clonazepam	0.5	Long (metabolite, >20)	Rapid	1–6 mg b.i.d.	0.5-, 1.0-, and 2.0-mg tablets
Diazepam	5	Long (>20) (nordiazepam—long, >20)	Rapid	4–40 mg b.i.d. to q.i.d.	2-, 5-, and 10-mg tablets (slow-release 15-mg capsules)
Alprazolam	0.25	Intermediate (6–20)	Medium	0.5–10 mg b.i.d. to q.i.d.	0.25-, 0.5-, 1.0-, and 2.0-mg tablets
Lorazepam	1	Intermediate (6–20)	Medium	1–6 mg t.i.d.	0.5-, 1.0-, and 2.0-mg tablets, 2 mg/mL, 4 mg/mL parenteral
Oxazepam	15	Intermediate (6–20)	Slow	30–120 mg t.i.d. or q.i.d.	10-, 15-, and 30-mg capsules (15-mg)
Temazepam	5	Intermediate (6–20)	Medium	7.5–30 mg hs	7.5-, 15-, and 30-mg capsules
Chlordiazepoxide	10	Intermediate (6–20) (desmethyl-chlordiazepoxide—intermediate, 6–20) (demoxapam—long, >20) (nordiazepam—long, >20)	Medium	10–150 mg t.i.d. or q.i.d.	5-, 10-, and 25-mg tablets and capsules
Flurazepam	5	Short (<6) (N-hydroxyethyl-flurazepam—short, <6) (N-desalkylflurazepam—long, >20)	Rapid	15–30 mg hs	15- and 30-mg capsules
Triazolam	0.1–0.03	Short (<6)	Rapid	0.125 mg or 0.250 mg hs	0.125- or 0.250-mg tablets
Clorazepate	7.5	Short (<6) (nordiazepam—long, >20)	Rapid	15–60 mg b.i.d. or q.i.d.	3.75-, 7.5-, and 15-mg tablets (slow-release 11.25- and 22.5-mg tablets)
Halazepam	20	Short (<6) (nordiazepam—long, >20)	Medium	60–160 mg t.i.d. or q.i.d.	20- and 40-mg tablets
Prazepam	10	Short (<6) (nordiazepam—long, >20)	Slow	30 mg (20–60 mg) q.i.d. or t.i.d.	5-, 10-, or 20-mg capsules
Estazolam	0.33	Intermediate (6–20) (4-hydroxy-estazolam—intermediate, 6–20)	Rapid	1.0 or 2.0 hs	1- and 2-mg tablets
Quazepam	5	Long (>20) (2-oxoquazepam-N-desalkylflurazepam—long, >20)	Rapid	7.5 or 15 mg hs	7.5- and 15-mg tablets
Midazolam	1.25–1.3	Short (<6)	Rapid	5–50 mg parenteral	5 mg/mL parenteral, 1-, 2-, 5-, and 10-mL vials
Zolpidem	2.5	Short (<6)	Rapid	5 mg or 10 mg hs	5- and 10-mg tablets
Zaleplon	2	Short (1)	Rapid	10 mg hs	5- and 10-mg capsules
Antagonist					
Flumazenil	0.06	Short (<6)	Rapid	0.2–0.5 mg/min injection over 3–10 min (total, 1–5 mg)	0.1 mg/mL (5 mL, and 10-mL vials)

Table 30–4
Pharmacological Effects of Benzodiazepines

Effects	Clinical Application/Consequences
Therapeutic effects	
Sedative	Insomnia, conscious sedation, alcohol withdrawal
Anxiolytic	Panic attacks, generalized anxiety
Anticonvulsant	Seizures
Muscle relaxant	Muscle tension, muscle spasm
Amnestic	Adjunct to chemotherapy or anesthesia
Antistress	Mild hypertension, irritable bowel syndrome, angina
Adverse effects	
Sedative	Daytime sleepiness, impaired concentration
Amnestic	Mild forgetfulness, anterograde memory impairment
Psychomotor	Accidents, falls
Behavioral	Depression, agitation
Decreased CO_2 response	Worsening of sleep apnea and other obstructive pulmonary disorders
Withdrawal syndrome	Dependence—anxiety, insomnia, excess sensitivity to light, excess sensitivity to sound, tachycardia, mild systolic hypertension, tremor, headache, sweating, abdominal distress, craving, seizures

of hip fractures resulting from falls are higher in elderly persons taking long-acting drugs than in those taking more rapidly eliminated compounds. Benzodiazepines with short half-lives also have the advantage of causing less impairment with regular use. However, they appear to produce a more severe withdrawal syndrome. Drugs affecting the rate of elimination of benzodiazepines are listed in Table 30–5.

c. **Dependence and withdrawal symptoms.** A major concern with long-term benzodiazepine use is the development of dependence, particularly with high-potency agents. Not only can discontinuation of benzodiazepines result in symptom recurrence and rebound, but it can also precipitate withdrawal symptoms. Several factors contribute to the development of benzodiazepine withdrawal symptoms (Table 30–6). Drug type and duration of use are the most significant

Table 30–5
Drugs Affecting the Rate of Elimination of Oxidized Benzodiazepines

Increase Elimination Half-Life	Decrease Elimination Half-Life
Cimetidine	Chronic ethyl alcohol use
Propranolol	Rifampin
Oral contraceptives (estrogens)	
Chloramphenicol	
Propoxyphene	
Isoniazid	
Disulfiram	
Allopurinol	
Tricyclic antidepressants	
Acute ethyl alcohol use	

Table 30–6
Key Factors in the Development of Benzodiazepine Withdrawal Symptoms

Factor	Explanation
Drug type	High-potency, short half-life compounds (e.g., alprazolam, triazolam, lorazepam)
Duration of use	Risk increases with time
Dose level	Higher doses increase risk
Rate of discontinuation	Abrupt withdrawal instead of taper increases risk for severe symptoms, including seizures
Diagnosis	Panic disorder patients more prone to withdrawal symptoms
Personality	Patients with passive-dependent, histrionic, somatizing, or asthenic traits more likely to experience withdrawal

factors, but other considerations such as personality makeup are also important.

 CLINICAL HINT:
Withdrawal symptoms can mimic signs and symptoms of the underlying disorder. Do not unnecessarily continue the drug when this occurs.

3. **Benzodiazepine antagonist.** Flumazenil (Romazicon) is a benzodiazepine antagonist used to reverse the effects of benzodiazepine receptor agonists in overdose and in clinical situations such as sedation or anesthesia. It has also been used to reverse benzodiazepine effects immediately before the administration of electroconvulsive therapy (ECT). Adverse effects include nausea, vomiting, and agitation. Flumazenil can precipitate seizures, particularly in persons who have seizure disorders, who are dependent on benzodiazepines, or who have taken large overdoses. The usual regimen is to give 0.2 mg intravenously over 30 seconds. If consciousness is not regained, an additional 0.3 mg can be given intravenously over 30 seconds. Most persons respond to a total of 1 to 3 mg. Doses larger than 3 mg are unlikely to add benefit.

V. **Antipsychotic Drugs**

These are classified into first-generation (conventional) antipsychotics or second-generation antipsychotics (SDAs, novel or atypical). Historically, conventional antipsychotics were efficacious for treating the positive symptoms of schizophrenia with worsening of negative, cognitive, and mood symptoms. Atypical antipsychotics have been suggested to show improvement in (1) positive symptoms such as hallucinations, delusions, disordered thoughts, and agitation, and (2) negative symptoms such as withdrawal, flat affect, anhedonia, poverty of speech, catatonia, and cognitive impairment. There has been controversy regarding the benefits of atypical antipsychotics compared to conventional antipsychotics. NIMH funded research studies like the CATIE Trial has brought attention to the long-term metabolic complications of atypical antipsychotics and showing no significant advantages over conventional antipsychotics. Overall, atypical antipsychotic agents represent a major advance in the pharmacological treatment for schizophrenia. The clinicians are advised to determine the best course of treatment based on each individual patient, taking into account risk benefit analysis in the long-term.

A. **Second-generation antipsychotic drugs (SDAs, atypical antipsychotic drugs).** The second-generation antipsychotic drugs include risperidone (Risperdal, Risperidal Consta [long acting]), olanzapine, quetiapine (Seroquel), quetiapine XR (Seroquel XR), ziprasidone (Geodon), aripiprazole (Abilify), paliperidone (Invega), asenapine (Saphris), iloperadone (Fanapt) and clozapine (Clozaril). These drugs improve three classes of disability typical of schizophrenia: (1) positive symptoms (hallucinations, delusions, disordered thoughts, agitation), (2) negative symptoms (withdrawal, flat affect, anhedonia, catatonia), and (3) cognitive impairment (perceptual distortions, memory deficits, inattentiveness). Second-generation drugs have largely replaced the typical antipsychotics (dopamine receptor antagonists) because they are associated with a lower risk of extrapyramidal symptoms and eliminate the need for anticholinergic drugs. Second-generation drugs are also effective for the treatment of bipolar disorder and mood disorders with psychotic or manic features. A few are also approved for the treatment of major depressive disorder (MDD) and will also have an indication in GAD. All of these drugs except clozapine are FDA approved for the treatment of bipolar I mania. Olanzapine is approved for bipolar I maintenance therapy. Elderly patients with dementia-related psychosis treated with atypical antipsychotic drugs are at an increased risk of death compared to placebo. Although the causes of death in clinical trials were varied, most of the deaths appeared to be either cardiovascular (e.g., heart failure, sudden death) or infectious (e.g., pneumonia) in nature. Observational studies are not clear as to what extent these mortality findings may be attributed to the antipsychotic drug as opposed to patient characteristics. Asenapine is not approved for the treatment of patients with dementia-related psychosis.

1. **Pharmacological actions**
    a. **Risperidone.** About 80% of risperidone is absorbed from the GI tract, and the combined half-life of risperidone averages 20 hours so that it is effective in once-daily dosing. Risperidal Consta is given once every two weeks because of its long half life.
    b. **Olanzapine.** Approximately 85% of olanzapine is absorbed from the GI tract, and its half-life averages 30 hours. Therefore, it is also effective in once-daily dosing.
    c. **Quetiapine.** Quetiapine is rapidly absorbed from the GI tract. Its half-life is about 6 hours, so dosing two or three times per day is necessary. Quetiapine XR has a comparable bioavailability to equivalent dose of quetiapine administered two to three times daily. Quetiapine XR is given once daily preferably in the evening.

    d. Ziprasidone. Ziprasidone is well absorbed. Its half-life is 5 to 10 hours, so twice-daily dosing is optimal.

    e. Clozapine. Clozapine is absorbed from the GI tract. Its half-life is 10 to 16 hours, and it is taken twice daily.

    f. Aripiprazole. Aripiprazole is well absorbed from the GI tract. It has a long half-life of about 75 hours and can be given as a single daily dose.

    g. Paliperidone. Paliperidone has a peak plasma concentration of approximately 24 hours after dosing. It is available only in extended release tablets, usually prescribed at 3 mg once daily.

    h. Asenapine. Asenapine is well absorbed sublingually with a half life of 24 hours. It is prescribed at a daily dose of 5 mg sublingually twice a day. Steady state is reached in three days.

    i. Iloperidone. Well absorbed. Ninety-six percent bioavailability. Peak plasma level in 2 to 4 hours. Starting dose 1 mg b.i.d. Target dose is 12 to 24 mg given as 6 to 12 mg b.i.d.

2. Therapeutic indications. Second-generation drugs are effective for initial and maintenance treatment of psychosis in schizophrenia and schizoaffective disorders in both adults and adolescents. They are also effective in the acute treatment of manic or mixed episodes in bipolar disorder and for psychoses of all types—secondary to head trauma, dementia, and drug-induced psychosis. Aripiprazole (Abilify) is the first medication approved by the FDA for add-on treatment to antidepressants for adults with MDD. Other SDAs are in the process of receiving this indication and extending it to GAD as well. Second-generation drugs are effective in acutely ill and treatment-refractory persons and prevent relapses. By comparison to persons treated with dopamine receptor antagonists, persons treated with second-generation drugs require less frequent hospitalization, fewer emergency room visits, less phone contact with mental health professionals, and less treatment in day programs.

    The parenteral form of olanzapine is indicated for the treatment of acute agitation associated with schizophrenia and bipolar disorder, while ziprasidone is indicated for the treatment of agitation related to schizophrenia. Aripiprazole (Abilify) injection is indicated for the acute treatment of agitation associated with schizophrenia or bipolar disorder, manic or mixed in adults. Quetiapine (Seroquel, Seroquel XR) is indicated in the treatment of bipolar depression.

 CLINICAL HINT:
Because clozapine can cause severe agranulocytosis, it should be used only in refractory cases of schizophrenia. Clozapine provides a therapeutic niche for patients with severe tardive dyskinesias, unmanageable extrapyramidal symptoms, refractory bipolar disorder, and psychosis secondary to antiparkinsonian drugs.

3. **Clinical guidelines.** Dosing for the second-generation drugs vary considerably. Table 30–7 summarizes the usual dosing recommendations for these agents.

   a. **Risperidone.** Risperidone is available in 0.25-, 0.5-, 1-, 2-, 3-, and 4-mg tablets, in M-tab form (rapidly dissolving), and as an oral solution with a concentration of 1 mg/mL. The initial dosage is usually 1 to 2 mg/day, taken at night. It can then be raised gradually (by 1 mg every 2 or 3 days) to 4 to 6 mg at night. Dosages higher than 6 mg/day are associated with increased adverse effects. Dosages below 6 mg/day have generally not been associated with extrapyramidal symptoms, but dystonic and dyskinetic reactions have been seen at dosages of 4 to 16 mg/day.

   Risperidal Consta is available in dosages of 25-, 37.5- or 50-mg risperidone provided as a dose-pack and a prefilled syringe. The recommended dosage is 25 mg IM every two weeks which can be titrated upward to 50 mg if needed. Fluoxetine and paroxetine double the plasma concentration of risperidone.

   b. **Olanzapine.** Olanzapine is available in 2.5-, 5-, 7.5-, 10-, 15- and 20-mg oral and Zydis form (orally disintegrating) tablets. The initial dosage is usually 10 to 15 mg once daily. A starting dosage of 5 mg/day is recommended for elderly and medically ill persons and for persons with hepatic impairment or hypotension. The dosage can be raised to 20 mg/day after 5 to 7 days. Dosages in clinical use range from 5 to 20 mg/day, but benefit in both schizophrenia and bipolar mania is noted in most people at dosages of 10 to 15 mg/day. The IM formulation for the treatment of agitation associated with schizophrenia and bipolar disorder is 10 mg. Coadministration with benzodiazepines is not approved. The higher dosages are occasionally associated with increased extrapyramidal and other adverse effects. Assessment of transaminases in patients with significant hepatic disease should be done periodically.

   c. **Quetiapine.** Quetiapine is available in 25-, 100-, 200-, and 300-mg tablets. The dosage should begin at 25 mg twice daily and can be raised by 25 to 50 mg per dose every 2 to 3 days up to a target dosage of 400 to 500 mg/day, divided into two daily doses. Studies have shown efficacy in the range of 300 to 800 mg/day, with most people receiving maximum benefit at 300 to 500 mg/day. Quetiapine XR is given once daily preferably in the evening without food or a light meal to prevent increase in Cmax. The usual starting dosage is 300 mg and may be increased to 400 to 800 mg.

   d. **Ziprasidone.** Ziprasidone is available in 20-, 40-, 60-, and 80-mg capsules. Dosing should be initiated at 40 mg/day, divided into two daily doses. Studies have shown efficacy in the range of 40 to 200 mg, divided into two daily doses; taken with meals, the absorption is increased up to twofold.

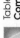

Table 30–7

Comparison of Usual Dosing^a for the Currently Available Second-Generation Antipsychotics in Schizophrenia

Antipsychotic	Typical Starting Dosage	Maintenance Therapy Dose Range	Titration	Maximum Recommended Dosage
Clozapine (tablets)	12.5 mg once or twice a day	150–300 mg/day in divided doses, or 200 mg as a single dose in the evening	The dosage should be increased to 25–50 mg on the second day. Further increases may be made in daily increments of 25–50 mg per day. Subsequent dosage increases should be made no more than once or twice weekly in increments of no more than 100 mg.	900 mg/day
Risperidone (tablets and oral solution)	1 mg once a day	2–6 mg once a day	Increase to 2 mg once a day on the second day and 4 mg once a day on the third day. In some patients, a slower titration may be appropriate. When dosage adjustments are necessary, further dosage increments of 1–2 mg/day at intervals of not less than 1 week are recommended.	16 mg/day
Risperidone IM long acting	25–50 mg every 2 weeks	Start with oral risperidone for 3 weeks	Starting dose: 25 mg every 2 weeks	50 mg for 2 weeks
Olanzapine (tablets and orally disintegrating tablets)	5–10 mg/day	10–20 mg/day	Dosage increments of 5 mg once a day are recommended when required, at intervals of not less than 1 week.	20 mg/day
Quetiapine (tablets)	25 mg twice a day	Lowest dose needed to maintain remission	Increase in increments of 25–50 mg two or three times a day on the second and third day, as tolerated, to a target dosage of 500 mg daily by the fourth day (given in two or three doses/day). Further dosage adjustments, if required, should be of 25–50 mg twice a day and occur at intervals of not fewer than 2 days.	800 mg/day
Ziprasidone (capsules)	20 mg twice a day with food	20–80 mg b.i.d.	Dosage adjustments based on individual clinical status may be made at intervals of not fewer than 2 days.	80 mg b.i.d.
Ziprasidone (intramuscular)	For acute agitation: 10–20 mg, as required, up to a maximum of 40 mg/day.	Not applicable	For acute agitation: Dosages of 10 mg may be administered every 2 hr, and dosages of 20 mg may be administered every 4 hr up to a maximum of 40 mg/day.	For acute agitation: 40 mg/day, for not more than 3 consecutive days
Aripiprazole (tablets)	10–15 mg once a day	10–30 mg/day	Dosage increases should not be made before 2 weeks.	30 mg/day
Paliperidone (extended-release tablets)	3–9 mg once a day	3–6 mg/day	Plasma concentration rises to a peak approximately 24 hr after dosing.	12 mg/day
Asenapine	5 mg sublingual twice a day	5–10 mg sublingual twice a day	For bipolar I manic patients: dosage is started at 10 mg and decreased eventually to 5 mg twice a day.	10 mg twice a day sublingual
Iloperidone	1 mg b.i.d.	12–24 mg in divided doses	Acute schizophrenia.	24 mg in divided doses

Note: Information taken from U.S. Prescribing Information for individual agents.
^aDosage adjustments may be required in special populations.

e. **Clozapine.** Clozapine is available in 25- and 100-mg tablets. The initial dosage is usually 25 mg one or two times daily, although a conservative initial dosage is 12.5 mg twice daily. The dosage can then be raised gradually (by 25 mg every 2 or 3 days) to 300 mg/day, usually divided into two daily doses, with the higher dose in the evening. Dosages of up to 900 mg/day can be used, although most patients respond in the 600 mg/day range.

f. **Aripiprazole.** Aripiprazole is available in 2-, 5-, 10-, 15-, 20-, and 30-mg tablets. The recommended starting and target dose is 10 to 15 mg/day given once a day. Dosages higher than 10 to 15 mg/day have not shown increased efficacy in clinical trials. The recommended starting dose for aripiprazole as adjunctive treatment for patients already taking an antidepressant is 2 to 5 mg/day. The efficacy of aripiprazole as an adjunctive therapy for MDD was established within a dose range of 2 to 15 mg/day. Dose adjustments of up to 5 mg/day should occur gradually, at intervals of no less than 1 week. The most commonly reported dose-related adverse effect is somnolence.

g. **Paliperidone.** Paliperidone is available in 3-, 6-, and 9-mg extended-release tablets. The usual dose is 3 to 6 mg/day. The maximum recommended dose is 12 mg/day.

h. **Asenapine.** Asenapine is available in 5- and 10-mg sublingual tablets. The recommended starting dose is 5 mg twice daily except for mania when 10 mg twice daily should be used and then reduced to 5 mg after the patient is stabilized. Do not use in demented patients because of increased mortality.

i. **Iloperidone.** Available in 1-, 2-, 4-, 6-, 8-, 10-, 12-, and 24-mg non-scored tablets. Usual dose is 12 to 24 mg per day.

4. **Pretreatment evaluation.** Before the initiation of treatment, an informed consent procedure should be documented. The patient's history should include information about blood disorders, epilepsy, cardiovascular disease, hepatic and renal diseases, and drug abuse. The presence of a hepatic or renal disease necessitates the use of low starting dosages. The physical examination should include supine and standing blood pressure measurements to screen for orthostatic hypotension. The laboratory examination should include an electrocardiogram (ECG); several complete blood cell counts including white blood cell counts, which can then be averaged; and tests of hepatic and renal function.

As second-generation drugs and SDAs have become the first-line treatment for various disorders, new controversies have arisen regarding their role in causing metabolic abnormalities (hyperglycemia, insulin resistance, and dyslipidemias). At this time, the American Psychiatric Association (APA) and American Diabetic Association (ADA) have developed a consensus guideline to help physicians monitor their patients. Olanzapine and clozapine have been the agents most often reported to be associated with treatment-emergent diabetes mellitus, a fact that may be linked to their propensity to cause marked weight gain.

The prevalence of diabetes in patients with schizophrenia and bipolar disorder is thought to be two to four times that of the general population. This is further complicated by the fact that obesity is on the rise and schizophrenics have an elevated risk of premature death from numerous medical problems. Obesity poses a serious health risk, contributing to such disorders as hypertension, dyslipidemia, cardiovascular disease, non–insulin-dependent diabetes, gallbladder disease, respiratory problems, gout, and osteoarthritis. Metabolic syndrome (disturbed glucose and insulin metabolism, obesity, dyslipidemia, and hypertension) is also more prevalent in patients with schizophrenia and numerous studies have suggested causal linkage to the use of antipsychotics, particularly the second generations. There are differences among the antipsychotics in regards to the risk for weight gain and diabetes, but the FDA has recommended the following guidelines for all second-generation antipsychotics.

a. **Baseline monitoring**
   (1) Personal and family history of obesity, diabetes, dyslipidemia, hypertension, and cardiovascular disease.
   (2) Weight and height (so that body mass index [BMI] can be calculated).
   (3) Waist circumference (at the level of the umbilicus).
   (4) Blood pressure.
   (5) Fasting plasma glucose.
   (6) Fasting lipid profile.

   Patients with pre-existing diabetes should have regular monitoring including HgA1C and, in some cases, insulin levels. The oral glucose tolerance test (OGTT) is not recommended for routine clinical use, but it may be required in the evaluation of patients with impaired fasting glucose or when diabetes is suspected despite normal fasting plasma glucose.

   It is recommended that clinicians screen, evaluate, and monitor patients for metabolic changes irrespective of the antipsychotic class, as these patients have an increased risk of metabolic syndrome and diabetes.

5. **Monitoring during treatment.** All patients on second-generation drugs should be routinely monitored for side effects. Although these drugs are presumed to have a lowered risk of tardive dyskinesia, some risk remains, so patients should be assessed for any movement abnormalities. According to FDA recommendations, all patients should have their blood glucose levels monitored, especially early in treatment or if weight gain occurs.

Clozapine requires special monitoring. During treatment with clozapine, weekly white blood cell counts are indicated for the first 6 months to monitor for the development of agranulocytosis; they should be obtained every 2 weeks thereafter. Although monitoring is expensive, early detection of agranulocytosis can prevent a fatal outcome. Probably more important than screening blood cell counts is educating persons to seek immediate medical evaluation if fever or any signs of infection develop. If the white cell count is less than $2,000/mm^3$ or the granulocyte count is less than $1,000/mm^3$, clozapine should be discontinued, a hematological consultation should be obtained, and a bone marrow biopsy should be considered. Persons with agranulocytosis should not be re-exposed to the drug. Clinicians can monitor the white blood cell count through any laboratory. Proof of monitoring must be presented to the pharmacist to obtain the medication. See Table 30–8 for guidelines of clinical management of clozapine-associated hematological abnormalities.

a. **Maintenance monitoring for SDAs.** Patients maintained on SDAs for prolonged periods should be monitored periodically as illustrated in Table 30–9.

6. **Switching from and to another antipsychotic drug.** The transition from a dopamine receptor antagonist to an SDA can be accomplished easily but should be done slowly. It is wise to overlap administration of the new drug with the old drug, lowering the dose of the former while raising the dose of the latter.

   Because the SDAs such as risperidone, quetiapine, asenapine, and ziprasidone lack anticholinergic effects, the abrupt transition from a dopamine receptor antagonist to one of these agents may cause cholinergic rebound, which consists of excessive salivation, nausea, vomiting, and diarrhea. The risk for cholinergic rebound can be mitigated by initially augmenting the SDA with an anticholinergic drug, which is then tapered slowly.

   With depot formulations of a dopamine receptor antagonist, the first dose of the SDA is given on the day the next injection is due. At present, the only SDA available in long-acting formulation is risperidone.

7. **Adverse effects**

   a. **All second-generation drugs**

      (1) **Neuroleptic malignant syndrome.** The development of neuroleptic malignant syndrome is considerably rarer with second-generation drugs than with dopamine receptor antagonists. This syndrome consists of muscular rigidity, fever, dystonia, akinesia, mutism, oscillation between obtundation and agitation, diaphoresis, dysphagia, tremor, incontinence, labile blood pressure, leukocytosis, and elevated creatine phosphokinase. Clozapine, especially if combined with lithium, and risperidone have been associated with neuroleptic malignant syndrome.

Table 30–8
Clinical Management of Reduced White Blood Cell (WBC) Count, Leukopenia, and Agranulocytosis

Problem Phase	WBC Findings	Clinical Findings	Treatment Plan
Reduced WBC	WBC count reveals a significant drop (even if WBC count is still in normal range). "Significant Drop" = 1) drop of over 3,000 cells from prior test, or 2) three or more consecutive drops in WBC counts	No symptoms of infection	1. Monitor patient closely 2. Institute twice-weekly complete blood cell (CBC) tests with differentials, if deemed appropriate by attending physician 3. Clozaril therapy may continue
Mild leukopenia	WBC = 3,000–3,500	Patient may or may not show clinical symptoms such as lethargy, fever, sore throat, weakness	1. Monitor patient closely 2. Institute a minimum of twice-weekly CBC tests with differentials 3. Clozaril therapy may continue
Leukopenia or granulocytopenia	WBC = 2,000–3,000 or granulocytes = 1,000–1,500	Patient may or may not show clinical symptoms such as fever, sore throat, lethargy, weakness	1. Interrupt Clozaril (clozapine) at once 2. Institute daily CBC tests with differentials 3. Increase surveillance, consider hospitalization 4. Clozaril therapy may be reinstituted after normalization of WBC count
Agranulocytosis (uncomplicated)	WBC count below 2,000 or granulocytes below 1,000	The patient may or may not show clinical symptoms such as fever, sore throat, lethargy, weakness	1. Discontinue Clozaril (clozapine) at once 2. Place patient in protective isolation in a medical unit with modern facilities 3. Consider a bone marrow specimen to determine if progenitor cells are being suppressed 4. Monitor patient every 2 days until WBC and differential counts return to normal (about 2 weeks) 5. Avoid use of concomitant medications with bone marrow-suppressing potential
Agranulocytosis (with complications)	WBC count below 2,000 or granulocytes below 1,000	Definite evidence of infection such as fever, sore throat, lethargy, weakness, malaise, skin ulcerations, etc.	6. Consult with hematologist or other specialist to determine appropriate antibiotic regimen 7. Start appropriate therapy; monitor closely
Recovery	WBC count over 4,000 and granulocytes over 2,000	No symptoms of infection	1. Once-weekly CBC with differential counts for four consecutive normal values 2. Clozaril (clozapine) must not be restarted

WBC, white blood cell.

Table 30–9
Maintenance Monitoring for SDAs

Parameters	Weeks
Weight	4, 8, 12, 16, 52
Waist circumference	52
Blood pressure	12, 52
Fasting glucose	12, 52
Fasting lipid	12; 5 years

    (2) **Tardive dyskinesias.** Second-generation drugs are significantly less likely than dopamine receptor antagonists to be associated with treatment-emergent tardive dyskinesias. Moreover, second-generation drugs, especially clozapine, relieve the symptoms of tardive dyskinesias and are especially indicated for psychotic persons with pre-existing tardive dyskinesias. For this reason, long-term maintenance treatment with dopamine receptor antagonists has become a questionable practice.

  b. Risperidone. Risperidone causes few adverse effects at the usual therapeutic dosages of 6 mg/day or less. The most common adverse effects include anxiety, insomnia, somnolence, dizziness, constipation, nausea, dyspepsia, rhinitis, rash, and tachycardia. At the rarely used higher dosages, it causes dosage-dependent extrapyramidal effects, hyperprolactinemia, sedation, orthostatic hypotension, palpitations, weight gain, decreased libido, and erectile dysfunction. Rare adverse effects associated with long-term use include neuroleptic malignant syndrome, priapism, thrombocytopenic purpura, and seizures in persons with hyponatremia.

  c. Olanzapine. Olanzapine is generally well tolerated except for moderate somnolence and weight gain of 10 to 25 pounds in up to 50% of persons on long-term therapy. Infrequent adverse effects include constipation, dizziness, hyperglycemia, orthostatic hypotension, transaminase elevations, and rarely extrapyramidal symptoms. More than other atypical antipsychotics, diabetes mellitus and acute-onset diabetic ketoacidosis have been reported in patients using olanzapine.

  d. Quetiapine. The most common adverse effects of quetiapine are somnolence, dry mouth, asthenia, postural hypotension, and dizziness, which are usually transient and are best managed with initial gradual upward titration of the dose. Quetiapine appears no more likely than placebo to cause extrapyramidal symptoms. Quetiapine is associated with modest transient weight gain, transient rises in liver transaminases, small increases in heart rate, and constipation.

  e. Ziprasidone. Adverse effects are unusual with ziprasidone. In particular, it is the only SDA not associated with weight gain. The most common adverse effects are somnolence, dizziness, nausea, and light-headedness. Ziprasidone causes almost no significant effects outside the central nervous system (CNS), but it does have the capacity to prolong the QT/QTc interval and the associated risk of developing torsades de pointes.

f. Clozapine. Significant potential for the development of serious adverse effects is the reason that clozapine is reserved for use in only the most treatment-refractory persons. The most common adverse effects are sedation, seizures, dizziness, syncope, tachycardia, hypotension, ECG changes, nausea, vomiting, leukopenia, granulocytopenia, agranulocytosis, and fever. Weight gain can be marked. Diabetes mellitus has been linked to clozapine, regardless of any weight gain. Patients exhibiting symptoms of chest pain, shortness of breath, fever, or tachypnea should be immediately evaluated for myocarditis or cardiomyopathy, an infrequent but serious adverse effect ending in death. Serial CPK with MB fractions, troponin levels, and EKG are recommended with immediate discontinuation of clozapine. Other common adverse effects include fatigue, sialorrhea, various GI symptoms (most commonly constipation), anticholinergic effects, and subjective muscle weakness. Clozapine is best used in a structured setting.

Because of additive risks of agranulocytosis, clozapine should not be combined with carbamazepine (Tegretol) or other drugs known to cause bone marrow suppression.

g. Aripiprazole. Aripiprazole is well tolerated, and the discontinuation rate is similar to placebo. The most common treatment-emergent events are headache, nausea, vomiting, insomnia, lightheadedness, and somnolence. In short-term clinical trials, the incidence of extra pyramidal symptoms was similar to placebo. In clinical practice, some patients experience marked agitation and akathisia with aripiprazole.

h. Paliperidone. Paliperidone is well tolerated. Common side effects include dizziness, constipation, and lethargy. Akathisia may occur. The drug should be avoided in persons with a history of chronic arrhythmias.

i. Asenapine. Asenapine can cause movement disorders similar to other second-generation drugs and is associated with weight gain. About 10% of patients discontinued the drug because of anxiety and oral hypoesthesia (1%). Otherwise the drug is well tolerated.

j. Iloperidone. Iloperidone is well tolerated with the most common side effect being weight gain and orthostasis.

8. Drug interactions. CNS depressants, alcohol, or tricyclic drugs coadministered with second-generation drugs may increase the risk for seizures, sedation, and cardiac effects. Antihypertensive medications may exacerbate the orthostatic hypotension caused by second-generation drugs. The coadministration of benzodiazepines and second-generation drugs may be associated with an increased incidence of orthostasis, syncope, and respiratory depression. Risperidone, olanzapine, quetiapine, and ziprasidone can antagonize the effects of levodopa and dopamine agonists. Long-term use of second-generation drugs together with drugs that induce CYP metabolic enzymes (e.g., carbamazepine, barbiturates, omeprazole [Prilosec], rifampin [Rifadin, Rifamate], glucocorticoids) may increase the clearance of second-generation drugs by 50% or more. Some significant drug–drug interactions are described below.

a. **Risperidone.** The concurrent use of risperidone and phenytoin or SSRIs may produce extrapyramidal symptoms. The use of risperidone by persons with opioid dependence may precipitate opioid withdrawal symptoms. The addition of risperidone to the regimen of a person taking clozapine can raise clozapine plasma concentrations by 75%.

b. **Olanzapine.** Fluvoxamine (Luvox) increases the serum concentrations of olanzapine.

c. **Quetiapine.** Phenytoin increases quetiapine clearance fivefold, and thioridazine (Mellaril) increases quetiapine clearance by 65%. Cimetidine reduces quetiapine clearance by 20%. Quetiapine reduces lorazepam (Ativan) clearance by 20%. A high-fat meal (800 to 1,000 calories) causes a significant increase in C_{max} of quetiapine XR. It is suggested that quetiapine be taken without food or a light meal (300 calories).

d. **Ziprasidone.** Ziprasidone has a low potential for causing clinically significant drug interactions.

e. **Clozapine.** Clozapine should not be used with any other drug that can cause bone marrow suppression. Such drugs include carbamazepine, phenytoin, propylthiouracil, sulfonamides, and captopril (Capoten). The addition of paroxetine (Paxil) may precipitate clozapine-associated neutropenia. Lithium combined with clozapine may increase the risk for seizures, confusion, and movement disorders. Lithium should not be used in combination with clozapine by persons who have experienced an episode of neuroleptic malignant syndrome. Risperidone, fluoxetine, paroxetine, and fluvoxamine increase serum concentrations of clozapine.

f. **Aripiprazole.** Carbamazepine may lower the blood levels of aripiprazole. Fluoxetine and paroxetine can inhibit the metabolism and hence elimination of aripiprazole.

g. **Paliperidone.** Drugs such as paroxetine, fluoxetine, and other SSRIs can block the action of paliperidone. Combined use of SSRIs and paliperidone can result in significant elevation of prolactin in men and women.

h. **Asenapine.** Asenapine can double the level of paroxetine and fluoxetine in the blood. It is excreted in milk and nursing mothers should not take the drug.

i. **Iloperidone.** Some SSRIs, such as fluoxetine and paroxetine, can elevate levels of iloperidone.

B. Dopamine receptor antagonists. The dopamine receptor antagonists are presently second-line agents for the treatment of schizophrenia and other psychotic disorders. Because of their immediate calming effects, however, dopamine receptor antagonists are often used for the management of acute psychotic episodes.

1. **Choice of drug.** Although dopamine receptor antagonist potency varies widely (Table 30–10), all available typical dopamine receptor antagonists are equally efficacious in the treatment of schizophrenia. The dopamine receptor antagonists are available in a wide range of formulations and doses (Table 30–11).

   a. **Short-term treatment.** The equivalent of 5 to 10 mg of haloperidol is a reasonable dose for an adult person in an acute psychotic state. An elderly person may benefit from as little as 1 mg of haloperidol.

   IM administration of the dopamine receptor antagonists results in peak plasma concentrations in about 30 minutes, versus 90 minutes with the oral route. Doses of dopamine receptor antagonists for IM administration are about half the doses given by the oral route. The patient should be observed for 1 hour after the first dose. After that time, most clinicians administer a second dose or a sedative agent (e.g., a benzodiazepine) to achieve effective behavioral control. Possible sedatives include 2 mg of lorazepam IM and 50 to 250 mg of amobarbital (Amytal) IM. There have been reports of sudden death, QT-prolongation, and torsades de pointes in patients receiving Haldol. Higher and IV dosages appear to be associated with increased risk of QT-prolongation and torsades de pointes.

 CLINICAL HINT:
The administration of more than 50 mg of chlorpromazine in one injection may result in serious hypotension. It is safer to start with a dose of 25 mg.

There are two short-acting IM formulations of atypical antipsychotics available that can be used in the treatment of acute agitation associated with schizophrenia or bipolar disorder (manic or mixed episode).

(1) **Olanzapine.** Available in 10-mg injection form and can be administered in a single dose to be repeated in 2 hours. A third dose can be given 4 hours after the second injection. It has a rapid onset of action occurring within 15 minutes in agitated schizophrenic patients and within 30 minutes in agitated bipolar patients. The most common observed side effect is somnolence.

 CLINICAL HINT:
The coadministration of lorazepam and olanzapine should be avoided because fatalities have occurred.

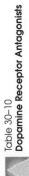

Table 30-10
Dopamine Receptor Antagonists

Drug Name	Chemical Classification	Therapeutic Dose Equivalent Oral Dosage (mg)	Relative Potency	Therapeutically (mg/day)[a]	Side Effects Sedation	Side Effects Autonomic[b]	Side Effects Extrapyramidal Reactions[c]
Acetophenazine (Tindal)	Phenothiazine: piperazine compound	20	Med	20–100	++	+	++/+++
Chlorpromazine (Thorazine)	Phenothiazine: aliphatic compound	100	Low	150–2,000	+++	+++	++
Chlorprothixene (Taractan)	Thioxanthene	100	Low	100–600	+++	+++	+/++
Fluphenazine (Permitil) (Prolixin)	Phenothiazine: piperazine compound	2	High	5–60	+	+	+++
Haloperidol (Haldol)	Butyrophenone	2	High	2–100	+	+	+++
Loxapine (Loxitane)	Dibenzoxazepine	10	Med	30–250	++	+/++	++/+++
Mesoridazine (Serentil)	Phenothiazine: piperidine compound	50	—	—	+++	++	+
Molindone (Moban)	Dihydroindolone	10	—	—	+++	+	+
Perphenazine (Trilafon)	Phenothiazine: piperazine compound	8	Med	8–64	++	+	++/+++
Pimozide (Orap)[d]	Diphenylbutylpiperidine	1.5	High	2–20	+	+	+++
Prochlorperazine (Compazine)	Phenothiazine: piperazine compound	15	—	—	++	+	+++
Thioridazine (Mellaril)	Phenothiazine: piperidine compound	100	Low	100–800	+++	+++	+
Thiothixene (Navane)	Thioxanthene	4	High	5–60	+	+	+++
Trifluoperazine (Stelazine)	Phenothiazine: piperazine compound	5	Med	5–60	++	+	++
Triflupromazine (Vesprin)	Phenothiazine: aliphatic compound	25	High	20–150	+++	++/+++	++

[a]Extreme range.
[b]Anti-α-adrenergic and anticholinergic effects.
[c]Excluding tardive dyskinesia, which appears to be produced to the same degree and frequency by all agents with equieffective antipsychotic dosages.
[d]Pimozide is used principally in the treatment of Tourette's syndrome; prochlorperazine is used rarely, if ever, as an antipsychotic agent.
Adapted from American Medical Association. AMA Drug Evaluations: Annual 1992. Chicago: Author; 1992.

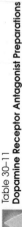

Table 30-1
Dopamine Receptor Antagonist Preparations

Drug Name	Tablets (mg)	Capsules (mg)	Solution	Parenteral	Rectal Suppositories (mg)
Chlorpromazine	10, 25, 50, 100, 200	30, 75, 150, 200, 300	10 mg/5 mL, 30 mg/mL, 100 mg/mL	25 mg/L	25, 100
Chlorprothixene	10, 25, 50, 100	—	100 mg/5 mL (suspension)	12.5 mg/mL	—
Droperidol	—	—	—	2.5 mg/mL	—
Fluphenazine	1, 2.5, 5, 10	—	2.5 mg/5 mL, 5 mg/mL	2.5 mg/mL (IM only)	—
Fluphenazine decanoate	—	—	—	25 mg/mL	—
Fluphenazine enanthate	—	—	—	25 mg/mL	—
Haloperidol	0.5, 1, 2, 5, 10, 20	—	2 mg/mL	5 mg/mL (IM only)	—
Haloperidol decanoate	—	—	—	50 mg/mL, 100 mg/mL (IM only)	—
Loxapine	—	5, 10, 25, 50	25 mg/5 mL	50 mg/mL	—
Molindone	5, 10, 25, 50, 100	—	20 mg/mL	—	—
Perphenazine	2, 4, 8, 16	—	16 mg/5 mL	5 mg/mL	—
Pimozide	2	—	—	—	—
Prochlorperazine	5, 10, 25	10, 15, 30	5 mg/5 mL	5 mg/mL	2.5, 5, 25
Thioridazine	10, 15, 25, 50, 100, 150, 200	—	25 mg/5 mL, 100 mg/5 mL, 30 mg/mL, 100 mg/mL	—	—
Thiothixene	—	1, 2, 5, 10, 20	5 mg/mL	5 mg/mL (IM only), 2 mg/mL (IM only)	—
Trifluoperazine	1, 2, 5, 10	—	10 mg/mL	2 mg/mL	—

IM, intramuscular.

(2) **Ziprasidone.** Indicated for the treatment of acute agitation associated with psychoses. It is available in 20-mg injection form and is administered in 10 to 20 mg as required to a maximum dose of 40 mg/day. Doses of 10 mg may be administered every 2 hours; doses of 20 mg may be given every 4 hours up to a maximum of 40 mg/day. The peak serum concentration typically occurs at approximately 60 minutes postdose, and the mean half-life ranges from 2 to 5 hours. The most common adverse effects are somnolence, nausea, and headache.

(3) **Aripiprazole.** The recommended dose in agitation associated with schizophrenia or bipolar mania (IM injection) is 9.75 mg. The effectiveness of aripiprazole injection in controlling agitation in schizophrenia and bipolar mania was demonstrated over a dose range of 5.25 mg to 15 mg.

b. **Long-acting depot medications.** Because some persons with schizophrenia do not comply with oral dopamine receptor antagonist regimens, long-acting depot preparations may be needed. A clinician usually administers the IM preparations once every 1 to 4 weeks. Depot dopamine receptor antagonists may be associated with an increase in adverse effects, including tardive dyskinesia.

(1) **Risperidone Consta.** Risperidone Consta is the only SDA available in a long-acting formulation. It is administered every 2 weeks, and the recommended starting dose is 25 mg. To start the patient on Consta, the patient needs to receive 3 weeks of oral antipsychotic supplementation. It is also available in doses of 37.5 and 50 mg. Dosing adjustment should not be made more frequently than once a month, and the maximum dose should not exceed 50 mg over 2 weeks. The FDA recently approved deltoid administration of Risperdal Consta for the treatment of schizophrenia. This mode of administration is supposedly less painful than the gluteal administration, as the needle is only 1 inch long as compared to the 2-inch needle. The most common adverse events reported are somnolence, akathisia, parkinsonism, dyspepsia, constipation, dry mouth, fatigue, and weight gain.

(2) **Precautions and adverse reactions.** Low-potency dopamine receptor antagonists are most likely to cause nonneurological adverse effects, and high-potency dopamine receptor antagonists are most likely to cause neurological (i.e., extrapyramidal) adverse effects. Second-generation drugs are more likely to cause metabolic disturbances. Recent studies have suggested that atypical antipsychotic drugs had a similar, dose-related increased risk of sudden cardiac death as conventional antipsychotics. Clinicians should appropriately screen and monitor patients maintained on atypical antipsychotics for long periods of time.

Table 30–12
Antipsychotic Drug Interaction

Drug	Consequences
Tricyclic antidepressants	Increased concentration of both
Anticholinergics	Anticholinergic toxicity, decreased absorption of antipsychotics
Antacids	Decreased absorption of antipsychotics
Cimetidine	Decreased absorption of antipsychotics
Food	Decreased absorption of antipsychotics
Buspirone	Elevation of haloperidol levels
Barbiturates	Increased metabolism of antipsychotics, excessive sedation
Phenytoin	Decreased phenytoin metabolism
Guanethidine	Reduced hypotensive effect
Clonidine	Reduced hypotensive effect
α-Methyldopa	Reduced hypotensive effect
Levodopa	Decreased effects of both
Succinylcholine	Prolonged muscle paralysis
Monoamine oxidase inhibitors	Hypotension
Halothane	Hypotension
Alcohol	Potentiation of central nervous system depression
Cigarettes	Decreased plasma levels of antipsychotics
Epinephrine	Hypotension
Propranolol	Increased plasma concentration of both
Warfarin	Decreased plasma concentration of warfarin

2. **Drug interactions.** Because they produce numerous receptor effects and are for the most part metabolized in the liver, the dopamine receptor antagonists are associated with many pharmacokinetic and pharmacodynamic drug interactions (Table 30–12).

VI. **Antidepressants**

This section describes various antidepressants along with their indications, dosing guidelines, and adverse reactions.

A. **SSRIs.** Six SSRIs are now first-line agents for the treatment of depression. Fluoxetine (Prozac) was introduced in 1988, and it has since become the single most widely prescribed antidepressant in the world. During the subsequent decade, sertraline (Zoloft) and paroxetine (Paxil) became nearly as widely prescribed as fluoxetine. Citalopram (Celexa), paroxetine CR (Paxil CR), and escitalopram (Lexapro) are the other SSRIs approved for depression. A seventh SSRI, fluvoxamine (Luvox), while also effective as an antidepressant, is FDA approved only as a treatment for obsessive–compulsive disorder. The SSRIs also are effective for a broad range of anxiety disorders.

1. **Pharmacological actions**

a. **Pharmacokinetics.** All SSRIs are well absorbed after oral administration and reach their peak concentrations in 4 to 8 hours. Fluoxetine has the longest half-life, 2 to 3 days; its active metabolite norfluoxetine has a half-life of 7 to 9 days. The half-life of sertraline is 26 hours, and its significantly less active metabolite has a half-life of 3 to 5 days. The half-lives of the other three SSRIs, which do not have metabolites with significant pharmacological activity, are

Table 30–13
Pharmacokinetic Profiles of the Selective Serotonin Reuptake Inhibitors

Drug	Time to Peak Plasma Concentration	Half-Life	Half-Life Metabolite	Time to Steady State (days)	Plasma Protein Binding (percentage)
Citalopram (Celexa)	4 hr	35 hr	3 hr	7	80
Escitalopram (Lexapro)	5 hr	27–32 hr	—	7	56
Fluoxetine (Prozac)	6–8 hr	4–6 days	4–16 days	28–35	95
Fluvoxamine (Luvox)	3–8 hr	15 hr	—	5–7	80
Paroxetine (Paxil)	5–6 hr	21 hr	—	5–10	95
Paroxetine CR (Paxil CR)	6–10 hr	15–20 hr	—	<14	95
Sertraline (Zoloft)	4.5–8.5 hr	26 hr	62–104 hr	7	95

35 hours for citalopram and escitalopram, 21 hours for paroxetine and paroxetine CR, and 15 hours for fluvoxamine. (See Table 30–13).

The administration of SSRIs with food has little effect on absorption and may reduce the incidence of nausea and diarrhea.

b. **Pharmacodynamics.** The clinical benefits of SSRIs are attributed to the relatively selective inhibition of serotonin reuptake, with little effect on the reuptake of norepinephrine and dopamine. The same degree of clinical benefit can usually be achieved through either steady use of a low dosage or more rapid escalation of the dosage. However, the clinical response varies considerably from person to person.

2. **Therapeutic indications**

a. **Depression.** Fluoxetine, sertraline, paroxetine, citalopram, paroxetine CR, and escitalopram are indicated for the treatment of depression in the general population, the elderly, the medically ill, and pregnant women. For severe depression and melancholia, several studies have found that the maximum efficacy of serotonin–norepinephrine reuptake inhibitors, such as venlafaxine, duloxetine (Cymbalta), or tricyclic drugs, may exceed that of SSRIs.

(1) **Choice of drug.** Direct comparisons of the benefits of specific SSRIs have not shown any one to be generally superior to the others. However, responses to the various SSRIs can vary considerably within a given patient. A number of reports indicate that more than 50% of people who respond poorly to one SSRI will respond favorably to another. Thus, it is most reasonable to try other agents in the SSRI class for patients who do not respond to their first SSRI before shifting to non-SSRI antidepressants.

(2) **Comparison with tricyclic antidepressants.** The efficacy of the SSRIs is similar to that of the tricyclic antidepressants, but their adverse effect profile is markedly better. Some degree of nervousness or agitation, sleep disturbances, GI symptoms, and

perhaps sexual adverse effects are more common in persons treated with SSRIs than in those treated with tricyclic drugs.

b. Suicide. In the overwhelming majority of people at risk for suicide, SSRIs reduce the risk. Some persons become especially anxious and agitated when given fluoxetine. The appearance of these symptoms in a suicidal person could conceivably aggravate the seriousness of their suicidal ideation.

 CLINICAL HINT:

Suicidal persons often act out their suicidal thoughts more effectively as they recover from their depression. Thus, potentially suicidal persons should be closely monitored during the first few weeks of SSRI therapy.

---

c. Depression during and after pregnancy. The use of fluoxetine during pregnancy is not associated with increases in perinatal complications, congenital fetal anomalies, learning disabilities, language delays, or specific behavioral problems. Emerging data for sertraline, paroxetine, and fluvoxamine indicate that these agents are probably similarly safe when taken during pregnancy.

d. Depression in the elderly and medically ill. All SSRIs are useful for elderly, medically frail persons.

e. Chronic depression. Because discontinuation of SSRIs within 6 months after a depressive episode is associated with a high rate of relapse, a person with chronic depression should remain on SSRI therapy for several years. SSRIs are well tolerated in long-term use.

f. Depression in children. SSRIs are increasingly prescribed to treat childhood depression and to forestall efforts by children and adolescents to self-medicate their depressed feelings with alcohol or illicit drugs. The adverse effect profile of SSRIs in children includes GI symptoms, insomnia, motor restlessness, social disinhibition, mania, hypomania, and psychosis. An FDA warning was issued to physicians regarding the potential risks of suicide in adolescents who are prescribed these antidepressants. Close monitoring of these medications by the physician is recommended.

g. Premenstrual dysphoric disorder. SSRIs reduce the debilitating mood and behavioral changes that occur in the week preceding menstruation in women with premenstrual dysphoric disorder. Scheduled administration of SSRIs either throughout the cycle or only during the luteal phase (the 2-week period between ovulation and menstruation) is equally effective for this purpose.

3. Clinical guidelines

a. Dosage and administration. See Table 30–14.

(1) Fluoxetine. Fluoxetine is available in 10- and 20-mg capsules, in a scored 10-mg tablet, and as a liquid (20 mg/5 mL). For

Table 30–14
SSRI Dosage

	Starting (mg)	Maintenance (mg)	High Dosage (mg)
Paroxetine	5–10	20–60	>60
Paroxetine CR	25	25–62.5	>62.5
Fluoxetine	2–5	20–60	>80
Sertraline	12.5–25	50–200	>300
Citalopram	10	20–40	>60
Escitalopram	5	10–30	>30
Fluvoxamine	25	50–100	>300

the treatment of depression, the initial dosage is usually 10 or 20 mg/day orally. The drug is generally taken in the morning because insomnia is a potential adverse effect. Fluoxetine may be taken with food to minimize possible nausea. Because of the long half-lives of the drug and its metabolite, a 4-week period is required to reach steady-state concentrations. As with all available antidepressants, the antidepressant effects of fluoxetine may be seen in the first 1 to 3 weeks, but the clinician should wait until the patient has been taking the drug for 4 to 6 weeks before definitively evaluating its antidepressant activity.

Several studies indicate that 20 mg may be as effective as higher doses for the treatment of depression. The maximum daily dosage recommended by the manufacturer is 80 mg/day, and higher dosages may cause seizures. A reasonable strategy is to maintain a patient on 20 mg/day for 3 weeks. If the patient shows no signs of clinical improvement at that time, an increase to 40 mg/day may be warranted.

 CLINICAL HINT:
To minimize the early adverse effects of anxiety and restlessness, initiate fluoxetine at 5 to 10 mg/day, with use of the scored 10-mg tablets. Alternatively, because of the long half-life of fluoxetine, the drug can be initiated with an every-other-day administration schedule.

At least 2 weeks should elapse between the discontinuation of MAOIs and the initiation of fluoxetine. Fluoxetine must be discontinued for at least 5 weeks before the initiation of MAOI treatment.

(2) **Sertraline.** Sertraline is available in scored 25-, 50-, and 100-mg tablets. For the initial treatment of depression, sertraline should be initiated at a dosage of 50 mg taken once daily. To limit the GI effects, some clinicians begin at 25 mg/day and increase the dosage to 50 mg/day after 3 weeks. Persons who do not respond after 1 to 3 weeks may benefit from increases of

50 mg every week up to a maximum dosage of 200 mg taken once daily. Sertraline is generally given in the evening because it is somewhat more likely to cause sedation than insomnia. Persons who experience GI symptoms may benefit by taking the drug with food.

(3) Paroxetine. Paroxetine is available in scored 20-mg tablets, unscored 10-, 30-, and 40-mg tablets, and an orange-flavored oral suspension with a concentration of 10 mg/5 mL. Paroxetine is usually initiated for the treatment of depression at a dosage of 10 or 20 mg/day. An increase should be considered when an adequate response is not seen in 1 to 3 weeks. At that point, the clinician can initiate upward titration in 10-mg increments at weekly intervals to a maximum dosage of 50 mg/day. Dosages of up to 80 mg/day may be tolerated. Persons who experience GI symptoms may benefit by taking the drug with food.

Paroxetine should be taken initially as a single daily dose in the evening. Higher dosages may be divided into two doses per day. Persons with melancholic features may require dosages greater than 20 mg/day. The suggested therapeutic dosage range for elderly persons is 10 to 20 mg/day.

 CLINICAL HINT:
Paroxetine is the SSRI most likely to produce a discontinuation syndrome. To limit the development of symptoms of abrupt discontinuation, the dosage of paroxetine should be reduced by 10 mg each week until it is 10 mg/day, at which point it may be decreased to 5 mg/day and stopped after one more week.

(4) Citalopram. Citalopram is available in scored 20- and 40-mg tablets. The usual starting dosage is 20 mg/day for the first week, after which it is generally increased to 40 mg/day. Some persons may require 60 mg/day. For elderly persons or persons with hepatic impairment, a dosage of 20 mg/day is recommended, with an increase to 40 mg/day only if no response is noted at 20 mg/day. Tablets should be taken once daily, either in the morning or evening, with or without food.

(5) Paroxetine CR. Paroxetine CR (Paxil CR) is available as an enteric-coated tablet in 12.5-, 25-, and 37.5-mg doses. Paroxetine CR should be administered as a single daily dose, usually in the morning, with or without food. The recommended initial dose is 25 mg/day. Some patients not responding to a 25-mg dose may benefit from dose increases, in 12.5-mg/day increments, up to a maximum of 62.5 mg/day. Dose changes should occur at intervals of at least 1 week. Patients should be cautioned that paroxetine CR should not be chewed or crushed and should be swallowed whole.

(6) **Escitalopram.** Escitalopram (Lexapro) is available in 10- and 20-mg scored tablets. The medication should be initiated at 10 mg/day, taken in a single daily dose, with or without food. Patients not responding to this dosage may be increased to 20 mg/day after a minimum of 1 week.

b. **Strategies for limiting adverse effects.** Most adverse effects of SSRIs appear within the first 1 to 2 weeks and generally subside or resolve spontaneously if the drugs are continued at the same dosage. However, up to 15% of patients are not able to tolerate the lowest dosage. One approach for such persons is to fractionate the dose over a week, with one dose taken every 2, 3, or 4 days. Some people may tolerate a different SSRI or, if not, may have to take another class of antidepressant, such as a tricyclic drug.

c. **Augmentation strategies.** In depressed people with a partial response to SSRIs, augmentation strategies may be used. One such drug combination, SSRIs plus bupropion, has demonstrated marked added benefits. Some patients have also responded favorably to the addition of lithium, levothyroxine (Levoxine, Levothroid, Synthroid), or amphetamine (5 to 15 mg/day).

d. **Loss of efficacy.** Potential methods to manage attenuation of the response to an SSRI include increasing or decreasing the dosage; tapering the drug, then rechallenging with the same medication; switching to another SSRI or non-SSRI antidepressant; and augmenting with bupropion, thyroid hormone, lithium, sympathomimetics, buspirone, anticonvulsants, naltrexone (ReVia), or another non-SSRI antidepressant. A change in response to an SSRI should be explored in psychotherapy, which may reveal the underlying conflicts causing an increase in depressive symptoms.

4. **Precautions and adverse reactions**

a. **Sexual dysfunction.** Sexual inhibition is the most common adverse effect of SSRIs and may occur in up to 80% of patients. The most common complaints are inhibited orgasm and decreased libido, which are dosage dependent. Unlike most of the other adverse effects of SSRIs, sexual inhibition does not resolve within the first few weeks of use but usually continues as long as the drug is taken.

Treatment for SSRI-induced sexual dysfunction includes decreasing the dosage or switching to bupropion, which does not cause sexual dysfunction. Other options include adding bupropion once or twice per day or adding sildenafil (Viagra). Small doses of amphetamines (2.5 mg) may also be of use.

b. **GI adverse effects.** The most common GI complaints are nausea, diarrhea, anorexia, vomiting, and dyspepsia. The nausea and loose stools are dosage related and transient, usually resolving within a few weeks. Paroxetine CR is better tolerated due to its enteric coating, which delays dissolution until passing into the small intestine and hence potentially minimizes nausea. Anorexia is most common with fluoxetine, but some people gain weight while taking fluoxetine. Fluoxetine-induced loss of appetite and loss of weight begin as soon as the drug is taken and peak at 20 weeks, after which weight often returns to baseline.

c. **Weight gain.** Up to one third of people taking SSRIs gain weight, sometimes more than 20 pounds. Paroxetine is the SSRI most often associated with weight gain, but it can occur with any agent.

d. **Headaches.** The incidence of headache with SSRIs is about 18% to 20%. Fluoxetine is the most likely to cause headache. On the other hand, all SSRIs are effective prophylaxis against both migraine and tension-type headaches in many people.

 CLINICAL HINT:
Headaches usually occur in the morning and can be treated with aspirin or acetaminophen. They usually subside spontaneously after a few weeks.

e. **CNS adverse effects**

(1) **Anxiety.** Fluoxetine is the most likely to cause anxiety, agitation, and restlessness, particularly in the first few weeks. These initial effects usually give way to an overall reduction in anxiety after the first month of use. Five percent of people discontinue taking fluoxetine because of increased nervousness. An increase in anxiety is caused considerably less frequently by the other SSRIs.

 CLINICAL HINT:
It may be useful to provide patients with a few 5-mg diazepam tablets that they can take if anxiety occurs when they first start the SSRI.

(2) **Insomnia and sedation.** The major effect in this area attributable to SSRIs is improved sleep resulting from the treatment of depression and anxiety. However, as many as one fourth of people taking SSRIs note either trouble sleeping or excessive somnolence. Fluoxetine is the most likely to cause insomnia, for which reason it is often taken in the morning. Sertraline is about equally likely to cause insomnia or somnolence; citalopram and especially paroxetine are more likely to cause somnolence than insomnia. With the latter agents, people usually report that taking the dose before retiring helps them sleep better and does not cause residual daytime somnolence.

SSRI-induced insomnia can be treated with benzodiazepines, trazodone (clinicians must explain the risk for priapism), or other sedating medicines. The presence of significant SSRI-induced somnolence often requires switching to another SSRI or to bupropion.

(3) **Vivid dreams and nightmares.** A minority of people taking SSRIs report recalling extremely vivid dreams or nightmares. A patient experiencing such dreams with one SSRI may derive the same therapeutic benefit without disturbing dream images by switching to another SSRI. This adverse effect often resolves spontaneously during several weeks.

(4) **Seizures.** Seizures have been reported in 0.1% to 0.2% of all persons treated with SSRIs. This incidence is comparable with the incidence reported with other antidepressants and is not significantly different from that noted with placebo. Seizures are more frequent at the highest dosages of SSRIs (100 mg or more of fluoxetine per day).

(5) **Extrapyramidal symptoms.** Tremor is seen in 5% to 10% of people taking SSRIs. SSRIs may rarely cause akathisia, dystonia, tremor, cogwheel rigidity, torticollis, opisthotonos, gait disorders, and bradykinesia. People with well-controlled Parkinson's disease may experience acute worsening of their motor symptoms when they take SSRIs. Extrapyramidal adverse effects are most closely associated with the use of fluoxetine; they are particularly noted at dosages in excess of 40 mg/day but may occur at any time during the course of therapy.

f. **Anticholinergic effects.** Paroxetine has mild anticholinergic activity that causes dry mouth, constipation, and sedation in a dosage-dependent fashion. However, the anticholinergic activity of paroxetine is perhaps only one-fifth that of nortriptyline, and most persons taking paroxetine do not experience cholinergic adverse effects. Although not considered to have anticholinergic activity, the other SSRIs are associated with dry mouth in about 20% of patients. This complaint may disappear with time.

g. **Hematological adverse effects.** SSRIs affect platelet function but are rarely associated with increased bruisability. Paroxetine and fluoxetine are rarely associated with the development of reversible neutropenia, particularly if administered concurrently with clozapine.

h. **Electrolyte and glucose disturbances.** SSRIs are rarely associated with a decrease in glucose concentrations; therefore, persons with diabetes should be carefully monitored and the dosage of their hypoglycemic drug decreased as necessary. Rare cases of SSRI-associated hyponatremia and the secretion of inappropriate antidiuretic hormone (SIADH) have been seen in persons treated with diuretics who are also water deprived.

i. **Rash and allergic reactions.** Various types of rashes may appear in about 4% of all persons; in a small subset, generalization of the allergic reaction and involvement of the pulmonary system result rarely in fibrotic damage and dyspnea. SSRI treatment may have to be discontinued in persons with drug-related rashes.

j. Galactorrhea. SSRIs may cause reversible galactorrhea, presumably a consequence of interference with dopaminergic regulation of prolactin secretion.

k. Serotonin syndrome. Serotonin syndrome is rare. Concurrent administration of an SSRI with an MAOI can raise plasma serotonin concentrations to toxic levels and produce a constellation of symptoms called *serotonin syndrome*. This serious and possibly fatal syndrome of serotonin overstimulation comprises, in order of appearance as the condition worsens, (1) diarrhea; (2) restlessness; (3) extreme agitation, hyperreflexia, and autonomic instability with possible rapid fluctuations of vital signs; (4) myoclonus, seizures, hyperthermia, uncontrollable shivering, and rigidity; and (5) delirium, coma, status epilepticus, cardiovascular collapse, and death.

Treatment of serotonin syndrome consists of removing the offending agents and promptly instituting comprehensive supportive care with nitroglycerine, cyproheptadine, methysergide (Sansert), cooling blankets, chlorpromazine (Thorazine), dantrolene (Dantrium), benzodiazepines, anticonvulsants, mechanical ventilation, and paralyzing agents.

l. SSRI discontinuation syndrome. The abrupt discontinuance of an SSRI, especially one with a relatively short half-life, such as paroxetine, has been associated with a syndrome that may include dizziness, weakness, nausea, headache, rebound depression, anxiety, insomnia, poor concentration, upper respiratory symptoms, paresthesias, and migrainelike symptoms. It usually does not appear until after at least 6 weeks of treatment and generally resolves spontaneously in 3 weeks. Persons who experience transient adverse effects in the first weeks of SSRI therapy are more likely to experience discontinuation symptoms. Fluoxetine is the least likely to be associated with this syndrome because the half-life of its metabolite is more than 1 week and it effectively tapers itself. Fluoxetine, therefore, has been used in some cases to treat the discontinuation syndrome associated with the termination of therapy with other SSRIs, although the syndrome itself is self-limited.

5. **Drug interactions.** See Table 30–15. SSRIs do not interfere with most other drugs. Serotonin syndrome can develop with concurrent administration of MAOIs, L-tryptophan, lithium, or other antidepressants that inhibit the reuptake of serotonin. Fluoxetine, sertraline, and paroxetine can raise the plasma concentrations of tricyclic antidepressants to levels that can cause clinical toxicity.

The combination of lithium and all serotonergic drugs should be used with caution because of the possibility of precipitating seizures.

Table 30–15
Interactions of Drugs with the SSRIs

SSRI	Other Drugs	Effect	Clinical Importance
Fluoxetine	Desipramine	Inhibits metabolism	Possible
	Carbamazepine	Inhibits metabolism	Possible
	Diazepam	Inhibits metabolism	Not important
	Haloperidol	Inhibits metabolism	Possible
	Warfarin	No interaction	
	Tolbutamide	No interaction	
Fluvoxamine	Antipyrine	Inhibits metabolism	Not important
	Propranolol	Inhibits metabolism	Unlikely
	Tricyclics	Inhibits metabolism	Unlikely
	Warfarin	Inhibits metabolism	Possible
	Atenolol	No interaction	
	Digoxin	No interaction	
Paroxetine	Phenytoin	AUC increases by 12%	Possible
	Procyclidine	AUC increases by 39%	Possible
	Cimetidine	Paroxetine AUC increases by 50%	Possible
	Antipyrine	No interaction	
	Digoxin	No interaction	
	Propranolol	No interaction	
	Tranylcypromine	No interaction	Caution with combined treatment
Sertraline	Warfarin	No interaction	Not important
	Antipyrine	Increased clearance	
	Diazepam	Clearance decreased by 13%	Not important
	Tolbutamide	Clearance decreased by 16%	Not important
	Digoxin	No interaction	
	Lithium	No pharmacokinetic interaction	Caution with combined treatment
	Desipramine	No interaction	
	Atenolol	No pharmacokinetic interaction	
Citalopram	Cimetidine	Citalopram AUC increases	
	Metoprolol	May double blood concentration	

Adapted from Warrington SJ. Clinical implications of the pharmacology of serotonin reuptake inhibitors. *Int Clin Psychopharmacol* 1987;7(Suppl 2):13, with permission.
AUC, area under curve.

SSRIs may increase the duration and severity of zolpidem-induced hallucinations. Some significant interactions are discussed below.

a. **Fluoxetine.** Fluoxetine may slow the metabolism of carbamazepine, antineoplastic agents, diazepam, and phenytoin.

b. **Sertraline.** Sertraline may displace warfarin from plasma proteins and may increase the prothrombin time.

c. **Paroxetine.** Because of the potential for interference with the CYP 2D6 enzyme, the coadministration of paroxetine with other antidepressants, phenothiazine, and antiarrhythmic drugs should be undertaken with caution. Paroxetine may increase the anticoagulant effect of warfarin. Coadministration of paroxetine and tramadol (Ultram) may precipitate a serotonin syndrome in elderly persons.

d. **Citalopram.** Concurrent administration of cimetidine increases concentrations of citalopram by about 40%.

B. **Venlafaxine (Effexor) and Desvenlafaxine (Pristiq).** Venlafaxine and desvenlafaxine are effective antidepressant drugs with a rapid onset of action. Venlafaxine is among the most efficacious drugs for the treatment of severe depression with melancholic features.

1. **Pharmacological actions.** Venlafaxine is well absorbed from the GI tract and reaches peak plasma concentrations within 2.5 hours. It has a half-life of about 3.5 hours, and its one active metabolite, O-desmethylvenlafaxine, has a half-life of 11 hours. Therefore, venlafaxine must be taken two to three times daily. Desvenlafaxine is an extended release tablet and an active metabolite of venlafaxine. The peak plasma concentration is reached within 7.5 hours and has a half-life of 11 hours. It is formulated for once-a-day administration, and the usual dose is 50 mg with no further benefit seen at higher doses.

   Venlafaxine and desvenlafaxine are nonselective inhibitors of the reuptake of three biogenic amines—serotonin, norepinephrine, and, to a lesser extent, dopamine. They have no activity at muscarinic, nicotinic, histaminergic, opioid, or adrenergic receptors, and are not active as an MAOI.

2. **Therapeutic efficacy.** Venlafaxine is approved for the treatment of MDD and GAD, while desvenlafaxine is indicated for the treatment of MDD. Many severely depressed persons respond to venlafaxine at a dosage of 200 mg/day and desvenlafaxine at a dosage of 50 mg/day within 2 weeks, a period of time somewhat shorter than the 2 to 4 weeks usually required for SSRIs to take effect. Therefore, venlafaxine at high dosages may become a preferred drug for seriously ill persons in whom a rapid response is desired. However, sympathomimetics (e.g., amphetamines) and ECT appear to have the most rapid onset of antidepressant action, usually taking effect within 1 week. In direct comparison with fluoxetine for the treatment of seriously depressed persons with melancholic features, venlafaxine is considered superior.

3. **Clinical guidelines.** Venlafaxine is available in 25-, 37.5-, 50-, 75-, and 100-mg immediate-release tablets and in 37.5-, 75-, and 150-mg extended-release capsules (Effexor XR). The immediate-release tablets should be given in two or three daily doses, and the extended-release capsules are taken in a single dose before sleep up to a maximum dosage of 225 mg/day. The tablets and the extended-release capsules are equally potent, and persons stabilized with one can switch to an equivalent dosage of the other. Desvenlafaxine is available in 50- and 100-mg tablets. They are taken in a single dose of 50 mg with no further benefit observed at higher doses.

   The usual starting dosage for venlafaxine in depressed persons is 75 mg/day, given as tablets in two to three divided doses or as extended-release capsules in a single dose before sleep. Some persons require a starting dosage of 37.5 mg/day for 4 to 7 days to minimize adverse effects, particularly nausea, before titration up to 75 mg/day. In persons with depression, the dosage can be raised to 150 mg/day, given as tablets in two or three divided doses or as extended-release capsules once at night, after an appropriate period of clinical assessment at the lower dosage (usually 2 to 3 weeks). The dosage can be raised in increments of 75 mg/day every 4 days or more. Moderately depressed persons probably do not require dosages in excess of 225 mg/day, whereas severely depressed persons may require dosages of 300 to 375 mg/day for a satisfactory response.

A rapid antidepressant response—within 1 to 2 weeks—may result from the administration of a dosage of 200 mg/day from the beginning. The maximum dosage of venlafaxine is 375 mg/day. The dosage of venlafaxine should be halved in persons with significant diminished hepatic or renal function. If discontinued, venlafaxine should be gradually tapered during 2 to 4 weeks.

4. **Precautions and adverse reactions.** Venlafaxine and desvenlafaxine are generally well tolerated. The most common adverse reactions are nausea, somnolence, dry mouth, dizziness, and nervousness. The incidence of nausea is reduced somewhat with use of the extended-release capsules. The sexual adverse effects of these medicines can be treated like those of the SSRIs. Abrupt discontinuation may produce a discontinuation syndrome consisting of nausea, somnolence, and insomnia. Therefore, they should be tapered gradually during 2 to 4 weeks. The most potentially worrisome adverse effect associated with venlafaxine is an increase in blood pressure in some persons, particularly those treated with more than 300 mg/day. Thus, the drug should be used cautiously by persons with pre-existing hypertension, and then only at lower dosages.

   Information about the use of venlafaxine by pregnant and nursing women is not available at this time. However, clinicians should avoid prescribing all newly introduced drugs to pregnant and nursing women until more clinical experience has been acquired.

5. **Drug interactions.** Venlafaxine may raise plasma concentrations of concurrently administered haloperidol. Like all antidepressant medications, venlafaxine and desvenlafaxine should not be used within 14 days of the use of MAOIs, and they may potentiate the sedative effects of other drugs that act on the CNS.

C. **Bupropion.** Bupropion is used for the treatment of depression and for smoking cessation. It generally is more effective against symptoms of depression than of anxiety, and it is quite effective in combination with SSRIs. Despite early warnings that it could cause seizures, clinical experience now shows that when used at recommended dosages, bupropion is no more likely to cause seizures than any other antidepressant drug. Smoking cessation is most successful when bupropion (called Zyban for this indication) is used in combination with behavioral modification techniques.

   Bupropion is unique among antidepressants because of a highly favorable profile of adverse effects. Of particular note among antidepressants, the rates of sedation, sexual dysfunction, and weight gain are minor with this drug. Some patients, however, experience severe anxiety or agitation when starting bupropion.

1. **Pharmacological actions.** Bupropion is well absorbed from the GI tract. Peak plasma concentrations of the immediate-release formulation of bupropion are usually reached within 2 hours of oral administration, and peak concentrations of the sustained-release formulation are seen after 3 hours. The half-life of the compound ranges from 8 to 40 hours (mean, 12 hours). The extended-release form reaches peak plasma concentration in about 5 hours and has a half-life of about 35 hours.

2. **Therapeutic efficacy.** The therapeutic efficacy of bupropion in depression is well established in both outpatient and inpatient settings.

3. **Dosage and administration.** There are three preparations of bupropion: (1) immediate-release bupropion is available in 75- and 100-mg tablets; (2) sustained-release bupropion (Wellbutrin SR) is available in 100-, 150-, and 200-mg tablets; and (3) extended-release bupropion is available in 150- and 300-mg tablets. Treatment in the average adult person should be initiated at 100 mg of the immediate-release version orally twice a day, or 150 mg of the sustained-release and extended-release version once a day. On the fourth day of treatment, the dosage can be raised to 100 mg of the immediate-release preparation orally three times a day, or 150 mg of the sustained-release preparation orally twice a day. The extended-release version can be raised to 300 mg once a day. Alternatively, 300 mg of the sustained-release version can be taken once each morning. The dosage of 300 mg/day should be maintained for several weeks before it is increased further. Because of the risk for seizures, increases in dosage should never exceed 100 mg in a 3-day period; a single dose of immediate-release bupropion should never exceed 150 mg, and a single dose of sustained-release bupropion should never exceed 300 mg; the total daily dose should not exceed 450 mg (immediate release or extended release) or 400 mg (sustained release).

4. **Precautions and adverse reactions.** The most common adverse effects associated with the use of bupropion are headache, insomnia, upper respiratory complaints, and nausea. Restlessness, agitation, and irritability may also occur. Most likely because of its potentiating effects on dopaminergic neurotransmission, bupropion has rarely been associated with psychotic symptoms (e.g., hallucinations, delusions, and catatonia) and delirium. Most notable about bupropion is the absence of significant drug-induced orthostatic hypotension, weight gain, daytime drowsiness, and anticholinergic effects. Some persons, however, may experience dry mouth or constipation, and weight loss may occur in about 25% of persons. Bupropion causes no significant cardiovascular or clinical laboratory changes.

A major advantage of bupropion over SSRIs is that bupropion is virtually devoid of any adverse effects on sexual functioning, whereas SSRIs are associated with such effects in up to 80% of all persons. Some people taking bupropion experience an increase in sexual responsiveness and even spontaneous orgasm.

At dosages of 300 mg/day or less, the incidence of seizures is about 0.1%, which is no worse, and in some cases superior, to the incidence of seizures with other antidepressants. The risk for seizures increases to about 5% in dosages between 450 and 600 mg/day. Risk factors for seizures, such as a past history of seizures, abuse of alcohol, recent benzodiazepine withdrawal, organic brain disease, head trauma, or epileptiform discharges on electroencephalogram (EEG), warrant critical examination of the decision to use bupropion.

Because high dosages (>450 mg/day) of bupropion may be associated with a euphoric feeling, bupropion may be relatively contraindicated in persons with a history of substance abuse. The use of bupropion by pregnant women has not been studied and is not recommended. Because bupropion is secreted in breast milk, its use in nursing women is not recommended.

Overdoses of bupropion are associated with a generally favorable outcome, except in cases of huge doses and overdoses of mixed drugs. Seizures occur in about one third of all cases of overdose, and fatalities may result from uncontrollable seizures, bradycardia, and cardiac arrest. In general, however, overdoses of bupropion are less harmful than overdoses of other antidepressants, except perhaps SSRIs.

5. **Drug interactions.** Bupropion should not be used concurrently with MAOIs because of the possibility of inducing a hypertensive crisis, and at least 14 days should pass after an MAOI is discontinued before treatment with bupropion is initiated. Delirium, psychotic symptoms, and dyskinetic movements may be associated with the coadministration of bupropion and dopaminergic agents (e.g., levodopa [Larodopa], pergolide [Permax], ropinirole [Requip], pramipexole [Mirapex], amantadine [Symmetrel], and bromocriptine [Parlodel]).

D. **Duloxetine.** Duloxetine is a selective serotonin and norepinephrine reuptake inhibitor (SSNRI) effective in the treatment of MDD.

1. **Pharmacological actions.** Duloxetine is well absorbed from the GI tract and reaches peak plasma concentration within 6 hours. Food delays the time to peak concentration from 6 to 10 hours and marginally decreases the extent of absorption by about 10%. It has a half-life of about 12 hours and steady-state plasma concentrations are achieved after 3 days. It is mainly metabolized through P450 isoenzymes, CYP 2D6, and CYP 1A2, and is highly protein bound (>90%).

It is a potent inhibitor of neuronal serotonin and norepinephrine reuptake and a less potent inhibitor of dopamine reuptake.

2. **Therapeutic efficacy.** Duloxetine is approved for the treatment of MDD and diabetic peripheral neuropathic pain.

3. **Clinical guidelines.** Duloxetine is available in 20-, 30-, and 60-mg delayed-release capsules. The capsule should be administered preferably once a day without regard to meals, starting at a total dose of

40 mg/day (given as 20 mg b.i.d.) to 60 mg/day (given either once a day or as 30 mg b.i.d.). If starting at 30 to 40 mg/day, the dose should be titrated quickly to 60 mg/day. There is no evidence that doses greater than 60 mg/day are more beneficial. There is no need for dosage adjustment based on age or gender.

4. **Precautions and adverse reactions.** Duloxetine is usually well tolerated. The most common adverse events reported were nausea, dry mouth, and insomnia. Of those reporting nausea, 60% had mild symptoms that lasted about 1 week.

Sexual dysfunction may occur, more frequently in males who have difficulty in attaining orgasm. Duloxetine can also affect urethral resistance, and this should be considered if symptoms develop. Discontinuation symptoms can develop, and gradual dose reduction is recommended.

There is a mean increase in blood pressure, averaging 2 mm Hg systolic and 0.5 mm Hg diastolic. Periodic measurements are recommended. It can cause mydriasis and should be used cautiously in patients with narrow-angle glaucoma.

There are no adequate studies in pregnant women, and duloxetine should only be used if the benefit justifies the risk.

5. **Drug interactions.** Duloxetine is metabolized through both CYP 1A2 and CYP 2D6. When used concomitantly with fluvoxamine, a potent CYP 1A2 inhibitor, the dose of duloxetine should be decreased. Similarly, CYP 2D6 inhibitors can cause elevated duloxetine levels.

E. **Mirtazapine.** Mirtazapine is effective in lifting mood, yet it lacks the anticholinergic effects of tricyclic antidepressants and the GI and anxiogenic effects of SSRIs. However, it is rarely used because it is no more efficacious than other antidepressants and causes somnolence.

F. **Reboxetine (Vestra).** Reboxetine is not yet approved for sale in the United States. It selectively inhibits norepinephrine reuptake and has little effect on serotonin reuptake. It is thus a mirror image of SSRIs, which inhibit the reuptake of serotonin but not of norepinephrine. In direct clinical comparison with fluoxetine, reboxetine was a more effective treatment for persons with severe depression, poor self-image, and little motivation.

1. **Therapeutic efficacy.** Reboxetine is effective for the treatment of acute and chronic depressive disorders, such as MDD and dysthymia. Reboxetine can also produce a relatively rapid decrease in the symptoms of social phobia. Reboxetine increases sleep efficiency, unlike fluoxetine, yet is not associated with daytime somnolence.

2. **Clinical guidelines.** Most persons respond at 4 mg twice a day; the maximum dosage is 10 mg/day. The dosage of reboxetine should be lowered for elderly persons and those with severe renal impairment.

3. **Precautions and adverse reactions.** The most common adverse effects are urinary hesitancy, headache, constipation, nasal congestion, diaphoresis, dizziness, dry mouth, and decreased libido. In long-term

use, persons taking reboxetine experience no more adverse effects than those taking a placebo.

G. **Nefazodone.** Nefazodone has antidepressant effects comparable with those of SSRIs, yet unlike SSRIs, nefazodone improves sleep continuity and has little effect on sexual functioning. It is chemically related to trazodone but causes less sedation. Among the more serious side effects is liver toxicity; because of this, it is not commonly used.

1. **Clinical guidelines.** Nefazodone is available in 50-, 200-, and 250-mg unscored and 100- and 150-mg scored tablets. The recommended starting dosage of nefazodone is 100 mg twice daily, but 50 mg twice daily may be better tolerated, especially in elderly persons. To limit the development of adverse effects, the daily dose should be slowly increased in increments of 100 to 200 mg, with intervals of no less than 1 week between each increase. Elderly patients should receive about two-thirds the usual nongeriatric dosages, with a maximum of 400 mg/day. The clinical benefits of nefazodone, like those of other antidepressants, usually become apparent after 2 to 4 weeks of treatment.

2. **Precautions and adverse reactions.** In preclinical trials, 16% of persons discontinued nefazodone because of an adverse event. Liver impairment precludes its use.

   A summary of dosages and pharmacokinetics of the non-SSRI antidepressants discussed above is presented in Table 30–16.

H. **Tricyclic and tetracyclic drugs.** Tricyclic and tetracyclic antidepressants (Table 30–17) are rarely used because of their adverse effects.

I. **MAOIs.** MAOIs (Table 30–18) are highly effective antidepressants, but they are rarely used because of the dietary precautions that must be followed to avoid tyramine-induced hypertensive crises and because of harmful drug interactions.

J. **Selegiline transdermal patch (EMSAM).** EMSAM is a transdermally administered antidepressant. When applied to intact skin, EMSAM is designed to continuously deliver selegiline over a 24-hour period. EMSAM systems are transdermal patches that contain 1 mg of selegiline per cm^2 and

Table 30–16
Non-SSRI Antidepressants

Drugs	Time to Peak Plasma Concentration (hr)	Half-Life (hr)	Starting Dose (mg)	Maintenance Dose (mg)	High Dose (mg)
Venlafaxine	2.5	9	75	225	300–375
Venlafaxine XR	5	11	37.5–75	150	225
Bupropion	2	8	100	300	450
Bupropion SR	3	12	150	300	400
Bupropion XL	5	35	150	300	>300
Mirtazapine	2	20–40	15	45	60
Duloxetine	6	12	30–40	60	>60
Nefazodone	1	4–8	100–200	300–600	>600

Table 30–17
Clinical Information for the Tricyclic and Tetracyclic Drugs

Generic Name	Trade Name	Usual Adult Dosage Range (mg/day)[a]
Imipramine	Tofranil	150–300[b]
Desipramine	Norpramin	150–300[b]
Trimipramine	Surmontil	150–200
Amitriptyline	Elavil	150–300[b]
Nortriptyline	Pamelor, Aventyl	50–150
Protriptyline	Vivactil	15–60
Amoxapine	Asendin	150–400
Doxepin	Adapin, Sinequan	150–300[b]
Maprotiline	Ludiomil	150–225
Clomipramine	Anafranil	150–250

[a]Exact range may vary among laboratories.
[b]Includes parent compound and desmethyl metabolite.

deliver approximately 0.3 mg of selegiline per cm^2 over 24 hours. Selegiline (the drug substance of EMSAM) is an irreversible MAOI, and steady-state selegiline plasma concentrations are achieved within 5 days of daily dosing. In humans, selegiline is approximately 90% bound to plasma proteins. Transdermally absorbed selegiline (via EMSAM) is not metabolized in human skin and is extensively metabolized by several CYP450-dependent enzyme systems including CYP2B6, CYP2C9, and CYP3A4/5.

EMSAM is contraindicated with SSRIs, dual serotonin and norepinephrine reuptake inhibitors (SNRIs), TCAs, bupropion hydrochloride; meperidine and analgesic agents such as tramadol, methadone, and propoxyphene; the antitussive agent dextromethorphan; St. John's wort; mirtazapine; and cyclobenzaprine. EMSAM should not be used with oral selegiline or other MAOIs.

Even though EMSAM is an irreversible MAOI, the data for EMSAM 6 mg/24 hours support the recommendation that a modified (tyramine rich) diet is not required at this dose. If a hypertensive crisis occurs, EMSAM

Table 30–18
Available Preparations and Typical Dosages of MAOIs

Generic Name	Trade Name	Preparations	Usual Daily Dosage (mg)	Usual Maximum Daily Dosage (mg)
Isocarboxazid[a]	Marplan	10-mg tablets	20–40	60
Moclobemide[b]	Manerix	100- and150-mg tablets	300–600	600
Phenelzine	Nardil	15-mg tablets	30–60	90
Selegiline	Eldepryl, Altaryl	5-mg capsules, 5-mg tablets	10	30
Tranylcypromine	Parnate	10-mg tablets	20–60	60

[a]Available directly from the manufacturer.
[b]Not available in the United States.

should be discontinued immediately and therapy to lower blood pressure should be instituted immediately.

EMSAM should be applied to dry, intact skin on the upper torso (below the neck and above the waist), upper thigh, or the outer surface of the upper arm. A new application site should be selected with each new patch to avoid reapplication to the same site on consecutive days. Patches should be applied at approximately the same time each day.

EMSAM is supplied as 6 mg/24 hours (20 mg/20 cm^2), 9 mg/24 hours (30 mg/30 cm^2), and 12 mg/24 hours (40 mg/40 cm^2) transdermal systems.

VII. Antimanic Drugs

A. Lithium. Lithium is used for the short-term and prophylactic treatment of bipolar I disorder.

1. **Pharmacological actions.** After ingestion, lithium is completely absorbed by the GI tract. Serum concentrations peak in 1 to 1.5 hours for standard preparations and in 4 to 4.5 hours for controlled-release preparations. Lithium does not bind to plasma proteins, is not metabolized, and is excreted through the kidneys. The blood–brain barrier permits only slow passage of lithium, which is why a single overdose does not necessarily cause toxicity and why long-term lithium intoxication is slow to resolve. The half-life of lithium is about 20 hours, and equilibrium is reached after 5 to 7 days of regular intake. The renal clearance of lithium is decreased in persons with renal insufficiency (common in the elderly). The excretion of lithium is increased during pregnancy but decreased after delivery. Lithium is excreted in breast milk and in insignificant amounts in feces and sweat.

2. **Therapeutic efficacy**

   a. **Manic episodes.** Lithium controls acute mania. It prevents relapse in about 80% of persons with bipolar I disorder and in a somewhat smaller percentage of persons with mixed or dysphoric mania, rapid cycling bipolar disorder, comorbid substance abuse, or encephalopathy. Lithium alone at therapeutic concentrations exerts its antimanic effects in 1 to 3 weeks. To control mania acutely, therefore, a benzodiazepine (e.g., clonazepam or lorazepam) or a dopamine receptor agonist (e.g., haloperidol or chlorpromazine) should also be administered for the first few weeks.

   Lithium is effective as long-term prophylaxis for both manic and depressive episodes in about 70% to 80% of persons with bipolar I disorder.

   b. **Depressive episodes.** Lithium is effective in the treatment of MDD and depression associated with bipolar I disorder. Lithium exerts a partial or complete antidepressant effect in about 80% of persons with bipolar I disorder. Many persons take lithium and an antidepressant together as long-term maintenance for their bipolar disease. Augmentation of lithium therapy with valproate or carbamazepine is usually well tolerated, with little risk for the precipitation of mania.

When a depressive episode occurs in a person taking maintenance lithium, the differential diagnosis should include lithium-induced hypothyroidism, substance abuse, and lack of compliance with the lithium therapy. Treatment approaches include increasing the lithium concentration (up to 1 to 1.2 mEq/L); adding supplemental thyroid hormone (e.g., 25 mg of liothyronine [Cytomel] per day), even in the presence of normal findings on thyroid function tests; augmenting lithium with valproate or carbamazepine; and judiciously using antidepressants or ECT. Some experts report that administering ECT to a person taking lithium increases the risk for cognitive dysfunction, but this point is controversial. Once the acute depressive episode resolves, other therapies should be tapered in favor of lithium monotherapy, if clinically effective.

c. **Maintenance.** Maintenance treatment with lithium markedly decreases the frequency, severity, and duration of manic and depressive episodes in persons with bipolar I disorder. Lithium provides relatively more effective prophylaxis for mania than for depression, and supplemental antidepressant strategies may be necessary either intermittently or continuously.

Lithium maintenance is almost always indicated after a second episode of bipolar I disorder depression or mania. Lithium maintenance should be seriously considered after a first episode for adolescents or for persons who have a family history of bipolar I disorder, have poor support systems, had no precipitating factors for the first episode, had a serious first episode, are at high risk for suicide, are 30 years old or older, had a sudden onset of their first episode, had a first episode of mania, or are male. Lithium is also effective treatment for persons with severe cyclothymic disorder.

The wisdom of initiating maintenance therapy after a first manic episode is illustrated by several observations. First, each episode of mania increases the risk for subsequent episodes. Second, among people responsive to lithium, relapses are 28 times more likely to occur after lithium is discontinued. Third, case reports describe persons who were initially responsive to lithium, then stopped taking it and had a relapse, and were no longer responsive to lithium during subsequent episodes.

The response to lithium treatment is such that continued maintenance treatment is often associated with increasing efficacy and reduced mortality. It does not necessarily represent treatment failure, therefore, if an episode of depression or mania occurs after a relatively short period of lithium maintenance. However, lithium treatment alone may begin to lose its effectiveness after several years of successful use. If this occurs, then supplemental treatment with carbamazepine or valproate may be useful.

Maintenance lithium dosages often can be adjusted to achieve a serum or plasma concentration somewhat lower than that needed for

Table 30–19
Lithium

Initial Medical Workup
Physical examination
Laboratory workup
  Serum creatinine (or a 24-hr urine creatinine)
  Electrolytes
  Thyroid function (thyroid-stimulating hormone, T_3, and T_4)
  Complete blood count
  Electrocardiogram
  Pregnancy test (women of childbearing age)

---

the treatment of acute mania. If lithium use is to be discontinued, then the dosage should be slowly tapered. Abrupt discontinuation of lithium therapy is associated with an increased risk for rapid recurrence of manic or depressive episodes.

3. **Dosage and clinical guidelines**

   a. **Initial medical workup.** Before the clinician administers lithium, a physician should conduct a routine laboratory and physical examination (Table 30–19). The laboratory examination should include measurement of the serum creatinine concentration (or the 24-hour urine creatinine concentration if the clinician has any reason to be concerned about renal function), an electrolyte screen, thyroid function tests (thyroid-stimulating hormone, triiodothyronine, and thyroxine), a complete blood cell count, an ECG, and a pregnancy test in women of childbearing age.

   b. **Dosage recommendations.** In the United States, lithium formulations include 150-, 300-, and 600-mg regular-release lithium carbonate capsules (Eskalith, Lithonate); 300-mg regular-release lithium carbonate tablets (Lithotabs); 450-mg controlled-release lithium carbonate capsules (Eskalith CR); and lithium citrate syrup in a concentration of 8 mEq/5 mL.

   The starting dosage for most adult persons is 300 mg of the regular-release formulation three times daily. The starting dosage in elderly persons or persons with renal impairment should be 300 mg once or twice daily. An eventual dosage of between 900 and 1,200 mg/day usually produces a therapeutic concentration of 0.6 to 1 mEq/L, and a dosage of 1,200 to 1,800 mg/day usually produces a therapeutic concentration of 0.8 to 1.2 mEq/L. Maintenance dosing can be given either in two or three divided doses of the regular-release formulation or in a single dose of the sustained-release formulation that is equivalent to the combined daily doses of the regular-release formulation. The use of divided doses reduces gastric upset and avoids single high-peak lithium concentrations.

   c. **Serum and plasma concentrations.** The measurement of serum and plasma concentrations of lithium is a standard method of assessment, and these values serve as a basis for titration. Lithium concentrations

Table 30–20
Common Lithium Side Effects and Their Management

Side Effect	Possible Approaches (Most Not Based on Strong Evidence)
Tremor (C); usually worse under social scrutiny	Lower dose ++; use β-blocker, such as propranolol (Inderal) 10 mg four times daily ++
	Consider primidone (Mysoline) as alternative +
	Replace some of lithium (Eskalith) dose with dihydropyridine calcium channel blocker +
Gastrointestinal distress (O)	Lower dose +
	Switch lithium preparations ±
	Replace some of lithium dose with a calcium channel blocker ±
Weight gain (O)	Warn and treat in advance ±
	Avoid nondiet sodas +
	Consider weight loss adjuncts ++
Cognitive impairment (UC)	Treat residual depression +
	Check thyroid
	Even if euthyroid, consider treating with T_3 +++
Increased urination (C) (diabetes insipidus, i.e., blockage of vasopressin receptor response at level of decreased production of cyclic adenosine monophosphate)	If extreme or functionally impairing, treat with thiazide diuretics or amiloride (Midamor)
	Switch to other mood stabilizing agents
	Carbamazepine (Tegretol) does not cause diabetes insipidus but does not correct lithium-related diabetes insipidus
Kidney function impairment (UC)	Reduce dose ±
	Monitor closely
	Discontinue drug if rise in creatine is consistent ±
	Replace with other mood stabilizers +
Psoriasis (O, I)	Omega-3 fatty acid supplementation may help suppress lithium effect +
Acne (O)	Retinoic acid only for women not of childbearing age or men ++
	Tetracycline (Achromycin V), clindamycin (Cleocin) +
Hypothyroidism (O)	Replace with T_4 ++
	Use T_4 and T_3 combination if mood remains low +

+, likely works; ++, many case reports; +++, well supported, controlled data; ±, questionable or hypothetical; C, common; D, dose related; I, idiosyncratic; O, occasional; T_3, triiodothyronine; T_4, thyroxine; UC, uncommon; VC, very common; VR, very rare.

should be determined routinely every 2 to 6 months and promptly in persons who are suspected to be noncompliant with the prescribed dosage, who exhibit signs of toxicity, or who are undergoing a dosage adjustment.

The most common guidelines are 1.0 to 1.5 mEq/L for the treatment of acute mania and 0.4 to 0.8 mEq/L for maintenance treatment.

4. **Precautions and adverse reactions.** Significant adverse effects are experienced by at least 30% of those taking lithium. The most common adverse effects of lithium treatment are gastric distress, weight gain, tremor, fatigue, and mild cognitive impairment. Table 30–20 lists common lithium side effects and their management.

5. **Drug interactions.** Lithium drug interactions are summarized in Table 30–21.

Table 30–21
Drug Interactions with Lithium

Drug Class	Reaction
Antipsychotics	Case reports of encephalopathy, worsening of extrapyramidal adverse effects, and neuroleptic malignant syndrome. Inconsistent reports of altered red blood cell and plasma concentrations of lithium, antipsychotic drug, or both
Antidepressants	Occasional reports of a serotoninlike syndrome with potent serotonin reuptake inhibitors
Anticonvulsants	No significant pharmacokinetic interactions with carbamazepine or valproate; reports of neurotoxicity with carbamazepine; combinations helpful for treatment resistance
Nonsteroidal anti-inflammatory drugs	May reduce renal lithium clearance and increase serum concentration; toxicity reported (exception is aspirin)
Diuretics	
Thiazides	Well-documented reduced renal lithium clearance and increased serum concentration; toxicity reported
Potassium sparing	Limited data, may increase lithium concentration
Loop	Lithium clearance unchanged (some case reports of increased lithium concentration)
Osmotic (mannitol, urea)	Increase renal lithium clearance and decrease lithium concentration
Xanthine (aminophylline, caffeine, theophylline)	Increase renal lithium clearance and decrease lithium concentration
Carbonic anhydrase inhibitors (acetazolamide)	Increase renal lithium clearance
Angiotensin-converting enzyme (ACE) inhibitors	Reports of reduced lithium clearance, increased concentrations, and toxicity
Calcium channel inhibitors	Case reports of neurotoxicity; no consistent pharmacokinetic interactions
Miscellaneous	
Succinylcholine, pancuronium	Reports of prolonged neuromuscular blockade
Metronidazole	Increased lithium concentration
Methyldopa	Few reports of neurotoxicity
Sodium bicarbonate	Increased renal lithium clearance
Iodides	Additive antithyroid effects
Propranolol	Used for lithium tremor. Possible slight increase in lithium concentration.

B. Valproate. Valproate is a first-line drug in the treatment of acute manic episodes in bipolar I disorder, at least equal in efficacy and safety to lithium. Available formulations include valproic acid (Depakene), a 1:1 mixture of valproic acid and sodium valproate (Depakote), and injectable sodium valproate (Depacon). Each of these is therapeutically equivalent because at physiological pH valproic acid dissociates into valproate ion.

    1. Pharmacological actions. All valproate formulations are rapidly and completely absorbed after oral administration. The steady-state half-life of valproate is about 8 to 17 hours, and clinically effective plasma concentrations can usually be maintained with dosing once, twice, or three or four times per day. Protein binding becomes saturated and concentrations of therapeutically effective free valproate increase at serum concentrations above 50 to 100 μg/mL.

2. **Therapeutic efficacy**
    a. **Manic episodes.** Valproate effectively controls manic symptoms in about two thirds of persons with acute mania. Valproate also reduces overall psychiatric symptoms and the need for supplemental doses of benzodiazepines or dopamine receptor agonists. Persons with mania usually respond 1 to 4 days after valproate serum concentrations rise above 50 μg/mL. With the use of gradual dosing strategies, this serum concentration can be achieved within 1 week of initiation of dosing, but newer, rapid oral loading strategies achieve therapeutic serum concentrations in 1 day and can control manic symptoms within 5 days. The short-term antimanic effects of valproate can be augmented with the addition of lithium, carbamazepine, or dopamine receptor agonists. SDAs and gabapentin (Neurontin) may also potentiate the effects of valproate, albeit less rapidly. Because of its more favorable profile of cognitive, dermatologic, thyroid, and renal adverse effects, valproate is preferred to lithium for the treatment of acute mania in children and elderly persons.
    b. **Depressive episodes.** Valproate alone is less effective for the short-term treatment of depressive episodes in bipolar I disorder than for the treatment of manic episodes. In patients with depressive symptoms, valproate is a more effective treatment for agitation than for dysphoria.
    c. **Maintenance.** Valproate is not FDA approved for maintenance treatment of bipolar I disorder, but studies have found that long-term use of valproate is associated with fewer, less severe, and shorter manic episodes. In direct comparisons, valproate is at least as effective as lithium and is better tolerated than lithium. In comparison with lithium, valproate may be particularly effective in persons with rapid-cycling and ultrarapid-cycling bipolar I disorder, dysphoric or mixed mania, mania secondary to a general medical condition, and in persons who have comorbid substance abuse or panic attacks or who have not shown a completely favorable response to lithium treatment. The combination of valproate and lithium may be more effective than lithium alone.

    In persons with bipolar I disorder, maintenance valproate treatment markedly reduces the frequency and severity of manic episodes, but it is only mildly to moderately effective in the prevention of depressive episodes.

    The prophylactic effectiveness of valproate can be augmented by the addition of lithium, carbamazepine, dopamine receptor antagonists, second-generation drugs, antidepressant drugs, gabapentin, or lamotrigine (Lamictal).

3. **Clinical guidelines**
    a. **Pretreatment evaluation.** Pretreatment evaluation should routinely include white blood cell and platelet counts, measurement of hepatic transaminase concentrations, and pregnancy testing, if applicable.

Amylase and coagulation studies should be performed if baseline pancreatic disease or coagulopathy is suspected.

b. **Dosage and administration.** Valproate is available in a number of formulations and dosages. For treatment of acute mania, an oral loading strategy of 20 to 30 mg/kg/day can be used to accelerate control of symptoms. This regimen is usually well tolerated but can cause excessive sedation and tremor in elderly persons. Rapid stabilization of agitated behavior can be achieved with an IV infusion of valproate. If acute mania is absent, it is best to initiate the drug treatment gradually so as to minimize the common adverse effects of nausea, vomiting, and sedation. The dosage on the first day should be 250 mg administered with a meal. The dosage can be increased to 250 mg orally three times daily during the course of 3 to 6 days.

Plasma concentrations can be assessed in the morning before the first daily dose of the drug is administered. Therapeutic plasma concentrations for the control of seizures range between 50 to 150 mg/mL, but concentrations up to 200 mg/mL are usually well tolerated. It is reasonable to use the same range for the treatment of mental disorders; most of the controlled studies have used 50 to 100 mg/mL.

Most persons attain therapeutic plasma concentrations on a dosage of between 1,200 and 1,500 mg/day administered in divided doses. Once symptoms are well controlled, the full daily dose can be taken once before sleep.

c. **Laboratory monitoring.** White blood cell and platelet counts and hepatic transaminase concentrations should be determined 1 month after the initiation of therapy and every 6 to 24 months thereafter. However, because even frequent monitoring may not predict serious organ toxicity, it is prudent to emphasize the need for prompt evaluation of any illnesses when giving instructions to patients. Asymptomatic elevations of transaminase concentrations to up to three times the upper limit of normal are common and do not require any change in dosage.

4. **Precautions and adverse reactions.** Valproate treatment is generally well tolerated and safe. The most common adverse effects are nausea, vomiting, dyspepsia, and diarrhea (Table 30 22). The GI effects are generally most common during the first month of treatment, particularly if the dosage is increased rapidly. Unbuffered valproic acid is more likely than the enteric-coated "sprinkle" or the delayed-release divalproex formulations to cause GI symptoms. GI symptoms may respond to histamine H_2 receptor antagonists. Other common adverse effects involve the nervous system (e.g., sedation, ataxia, dysarthria, and tremor). Valproate-induced tremor may respond well to treatment with β-adrenergic receptor antagonists or gabapentin. To treat the other neurological adverse effects, the valproate dosage must be lowered.

Table 30–22
Valproate Side Effects

Side Effect	Treatment	Comment
GI distress (O)	Switch to enteric coated preparation ++	—
	Add histamine 2 blocker +	—
	Give with meals or all at night +	—
Tremor (O)	↓ Dose +	—
	Propranolol (Inderal) +	—
	Prophylactic diet and exercise instructions +	—
Weight gain (O)	Augment with topiramate (Topamax), sibutramine (Meridia) ++	—
Alopecia (UC)	Prophylaxis with zinc and selenium supplements ±	Straight hair may grow back curly
Polycystic ovary syndrome (UC)	Preventive treatment with oral contraceptives +	(May precede use of VPA)
	Switch to lamotrigine (Lamictal) ++	May be associated with ↑ testosterone
Hepatitic enzyme (O) Elevation >3× normal	Monitor direction of change D/C VPA	Patient should advise physician if right upper quadrant pain occurs or if fever, malaise, fatigue, colored urine, or jaundice occurs
Hepatitis	D/C VPA	—
Pancreatitis (VR)	D/C VPA, monitor amylase	Patient should advise physician if severe GI pain, nausea, or vomiting occurs
Asymptomatic ↑ ammonia	↓ Dose, add l-carnitine ±	
Coarse, flapping tremor	↓ Dose, add l-carnitine ±	—
Encephalopathy	D/C VPA	—
Spina bifida 1%–4% in in utero exposed fetus	Avoid pregnancy +	Avoid VPA and other anticonvulsants in combination (such as carbamazepine (Tegretol))
	Use birth control pill, other methods +	
	Use folate prophylactically in women of childbearing age +	

+, likely works; ++, many case reports; +++, well-supported, controlled data; ± , questionable or hypothetical; C, common; D, dose related; D/C, discontinue; GI, gastrointestinal; I, idiosyncratic; O, occasional; PCO, polycystic ovary; S, sensitivity may cross to other anticonvulsant; UC, uncommon; VC, very common; VPA, valproate; VR, very rare.

Weight gain is a common adverse effect, especially in long-term treatment, and can best be treated by recommending a combination of a reasonable diet and moderate exercise.

The two most serious adverse effects of valproate treatment involve the pancreas and liver. Table 30–23 lists black box warnings and other warnings involving valproate. If symptoms of lethargy, malaise, anorexia, nausea and vomiting, edema, and abdominal pain occur in a person treated with valproate, the clinician must consider the possibility of severe hepatotoxicity. Rare cases of pancreatitis have been reported; they occur most often in the first 6 months of treatment, and the condition occasionally results in death.

C. Lamotrigine

1. **Pharmacological actions.** Lamotrigine is completely absorbed, has bioavailability of 98%, and has a steady-state plasma half-life of

Table 30–23
Black Box Warnings and Other Warnings for Valproate

More Serious Side Effect	Management Considerations
Hepatotoxicity	Rare, idiosyncratic event Estimated risk 1:118,000 (adults) Greatest risk profile (polypharmacy, younger than 2 yr of age, mental retardation) → 1:800
Pancreatitis	Rare, similar pattern to hepatotoxicity Incidence in clinical trials data is 2 of 2,416 (0.0008%) Postmarketing surveillance shows no increased incidence Relapse with rechallenge Asymptomatic amylase not predictive
Hyperammonemia	Rare—more common in combination with carbamazepine (Tegretol) Associated with coarse tremor and may respond to l-carnitine administration
Associated with urea cycle disorders	Discontinue valproate and protein intake Assess underlying urea cycle disorder Divalproex is contraindicated in patients with urea cycle disorders
Teratogenicity	Neural tube defect: 1%–4% with valproate Preconceptual education and folate–vitamin B complex supplementation for all young women of childbearing potential
Somnolence in the elderly	Slower titration than conventional doses Regular monitoring of fluid and nutritional intake
Thrombocytopenia	Decrease dose if clinically symptomatic (i.e., bruising, bleeding gums) Thrombocytopenia more likely with valproate levels ≥ 110 μg/mL (women) and ≥ 135 μg/mL (men)

Adapted from *Physician's Desk Reference*. Oradell, NJ: Medical Economics Company: 2002.

25 hours. However, the rate of lamotrigine's metabolism varies over a sixfold range, depending on which other drugs are administered concomitantly. Dosing is escalated slowly to twice-a-day maintenance dosing. Food does not affect its absorption, and it is 55% protein-bound in the plasma; 94% of lamotrigine and its inactive metabolites are excreted in the urine. Among the better-delineated biochemical actions of lamotrigine are blockade of voltage-sensitive sodium channels, which in turn modulate release of glutamate and aspartate, and a slight effect on calcium channels. Lamotrigine modestly increases plasma serotonin concentrations, possibly through inhibition of serotonin reuptake, and is a weak inhibitor of serotonin 5-HT$_3$ receptors.

2. **Therapeutic efficacy**

a. **Bipolar disorder.** In currently or recently depressed, manic, or hypomanic bipolar I patients, lamotrigine prolongs the time between depressive and manic episodes. These findings were more robust for depression. While lamotrigine can be initiated while patients are in any mood state, effectiveness in the acute treatment of mood episodes has not been established.

b. **Depression.** Lamotrigine may possess acute antidepressant effects. Studies involving acute lamotrigine treatment of bipolar depression and rapid-cycling bipolar disorder have demonstrated therapeutic benefit from lamotrigine. Conversely, it does not appear to act as an acute antimanic agent.

Table 30–24
Gradual Introduction of Lamotrigine in Adults with Bipolar Disorder

	Lamotrigine with Valproate (mg/day)	Lamotrigine with Carbamazepine (mg/day)	Lamotrigine with Neither (mg/day)
Weeks 1 and 2 dose	12.5	50	25
Weeks 3 and 4 dose	25	100	50
Week 5 dose	50	200	100
Subsequent weekly dose increments	25–50	100	50–100
FDA target dose	100	400	200
Typical final dose range	100–200	400–800	200–400

FDA, U.S. Food and Drug Administration.

    c. Other indications. There is no well-established role for lamotrigine in treating other psychiatric disorders, although there have been reports of therapeutic benefit in the treatment of borderline personality disorder, and as a treatment for various pain syndromes.

3. Dosage and clinical guidelines. In the clinical trials leading to the approval of lamotrigine as a treatment for bipolar disorder, no consistent increase in efficacy was associated with doses above 200 mg/day. Most patients should take between 100 and 200 mg/day. In epilepsy, the drug is administered twice daily, but in bipolar disorder, the total dose can be taken once a day, either in the morning or night, depending on whether the patient finds the drug activating or sedating.

    Lamotrigine is available as unscored 25-, 100-, 150-, and 200-mg tablets. The major determinant of lamotrigine dosing is minimization of the risk of rash. Lamotrigine should not be taken by anyone under the age of 16 years. Because valproic acid markedly slows the elimination of lamotrigine, concomitant administration of these two drugs necessitates a much slower titration (Table 30–24). The schedule differs based on whether the patient is taking valproic acid, carbamazepine, or neither of these drugs.

    People with renal insufficiency should aim for a lower maintenance dosage. Appearance of any type of rash necessitates immediate discontinuation of lamotrigine administration. Lamotrigine should usually be discontinued gradually, over 2 weeks, unless a rash emerges, in which case it should be discontinued over 1 to 2 days.

    Chewable dispersible tablets of 2-, 5-, and 25-mg are also available.

4. Precautions and adverse events. Lamotrigine is remarkably well tolerated. The absence of sedation, weight gain, or other metabolic effects is noteworthy. The most common adverse effects reported in clinical trials were dizziness, ataxia, somnolence, headache, diplopia, blurred vision, and nausea and were typically mild. In actual practice, cognitive impairment and joint or back pain appear to be more common than found in studies. Only rash, which is common and occasionally very severe, is a source of concern.

About 8% of patients started on lamotrigine develop a benign maculopapular rash during the first 4 months of treatment. It is advised that the drug be discontinued if a rash develops and it is felt to be associated with the use of lamotrigine. Even though these rashes are benign, there is concern that in some cases, they may represent early manifestations of Stevens–Johnson syndrome or toxic epidermal necrolysis. Nevertheless, even if lamotrigine is discontinued immediately upon development of rash or other sign of hypersensitivity reaction, such as fever and lymphadenopathy, this may not prevent subsequent development of life-threatening rash or permanent disfiguration.

Lamotrigine has a large pregnancy registry that supports research data that lamotrigine is not associated with congenital malformations in humans.

5. **Drug interactions.** The most potentially serious lamotrigine drug interaction involves concurrent use of the anticonvulsant valproic acid, which doubles serum lamotrigine concentrations. Sertraline (Zoloft) also increases plasma lamotrigine concentrations, but to a lesser extent than does valproic acid. Combinations of lamotrigine and other anticonvulsants have complex effects on the time of peak plasma concentration and the plasma half-life of lamotrigine.

D. **Carbamazepine.** Carbamazepine is effective for the treatment of acute mania and for the prophylactic treatment of bipolar I disorder. It is a first-line agent, along with lithium and valproic acid.

1. **Therapeutic efficacy**

   a. **Manic episodes.** The efficacy of carbamazepine in the treatment of acute mania is comparable with that of lithium and antipsychotics. Carbamazepine is also effective as a second-line agent to prevent both manic and depressive episodes in bipolar I disorder, after lithium and valproic acid.

   b. **Depressive episodes.** Carbamazepine is an alternative drug for patients whose depressive episodes show a marked or rapid periodicity.

2. **Clinical guidelines**

   a. **Dosage and administration.** Carbamazepine is available in 100- and 200-mg tablets and as a suspension containing 100 mg/5 mL. The usual starting dosage is 200 mg orally two times a day; however, with titration, three-times-a-day dosing is optimal. An extended-release version suitable for twice-a-day dosing is available in 100-, 200-, and 400-mg tablets. The dosage should be increased by no more than 200 mg/day every 2 to 4 days to minimize the occurrence of adverse effects.

   b. **Blood concentrations.** The anticonvulsant blood concentration range of 4 to 12 mg/mL should be reached before it is determined that carbamazepine is not effective in the treatment of a mood disorder. The dosage necessary to achieve plasma concentrations in the usual therapeutic range varies from 400 to 1,600 mg/day, with a mean of about 1,000 mg/day.

3. **Precautions and adverse reactions.** The rarest but most serious adverse effects of carbamazepine are blood dyscrasias, hepatitis, and exfoliative dermatitis. Otherwise, carbamazepine is relatively well tolerated by persons except for mild GI and CNS effects that can be significantly reduced if the dosage is increased slowly and minimal effective plasma concentrations are maintained.

4. **Drug interactions.** Principally, because it induces several hepatic enzymes, carbamazepine may interact with many drugs, particularly other anticonvulsants whose plasma levels are lowered. There is an increased risk of neurotoxic effects with lithium.

E. **Atypical antipsychotics.** The atypical antipsychotics also act as mood stabilizers. They include the following drugs, which have been discussed in detail above.

1. **Aripiprazole.** Aripiprazole is the latest of the atypical antipsychotics approved for the treatment of acute manic and mixed episodes associated with bipolar disorder. The effectiveness of aripiprazole in maintenance treatment has not been established.

2. **Olanzapine.** Indicated for the acute treatment of manic and mixed episodes associated with bipolar disorder, as well as in the maintenance treatment of bipolar disorder. It can be used as monotherapy or in combination with lithium or divalproex. Olanzapine is the only atypical antipsychotic that also has an indication in the maintenance treatment of bipolar disorder along with lithium and lamotrigine.

3. **Risperidone.** Risperidone is approved for the short-term treatment of acute manic episodes, associated with bipolar I disorder as monotherapy, or in combination with lithium or divalproex.

4. **Quetiapine and Quetiapine XR.** Quetiapine is indicated for the short-term treatment of acute manic episodes associated with bipolar I disorder as either monotherapy or adjunct therapy to lithium or divalproex. It is also approved for bipolar depression.

5. **Ziprasidone.** Ziprasidone is approved for the short-term treatment of acute manic or mixed episodes associated with bipolar I disorder.

6. **Paliperidone.** Paliperidone is used for the treatment of bipolar disorder.

7. **Asenapine.** Indicated for bipolar I disorder.

F. **Other mood-stabilizing drugs**

1. **Symbyax.** Symbyax (olanzapine and fluoxetine) is indicated for the treatment of depressive episodes associated with bipolar disorder. Improvement occurs as early as week 1 in symptoms of sadness, sleep, lassitude, and suicidal thoughts.

   Symbyax exerts its antidepressant effects through multiple neurotransmitter systems. The activation of three monoaminergic neural systems (serotonin, norepinephrine, and dopamine) is responsible for its enhanced antidepressant effect. There is a synergistic increase in norepinephrine and dopamine release in the prefrontal cortex, as well as an increase in serotonin. It is available in 6 mg/25 mg, 12 mg/25 mg,

6 mg/50 mg, and 12 mg/50 mg, where 6 mg and 12 mg represent olanzapine, and 25 mg and 50 mg represent fluoxetine.

The half-life of olanzapine and fluoxetine is 30 hours and 9 days, respectively, requiring only once-daily dosing, usually in the evening. The starting dose is generally 6 mg/25 mg given in a single daily dose. Dosing should be adjusted in the elderly, smokers, and those with hepatic impairment. As with other atypical antipsychotics, the possibility of metabolic abnormalities should be entertained, and baseline and maintenance monitoring be done.

The most common adverse events are weight gain, sleepiness, diarrhea, dizziness, hyponatremia, dry mouth, and increased appetite. It should not be used with an MAOI or within at least 14 days of discontinuing an MAOI. If used concomitantly with fluvoxamine, dosage adjustment is needed secondary to CYP 1A2 inhibition.

2. **Levetiracetam (Keppra).** FDA-approved for multiple seizure disorders. Due to its molecular characteristics, there has been interest in its use in nonepileptic neurologic disorders and psychiatric disorders (e.g., anxiety, panic, stress, mood and bipolar, autism, and Tourette's syndrome). Oral absorption is rapid and peaks at 1 hour. Intravenous and oral are bioequivalent. Steady-state is achieved within 2 days. Its half-life is 6 to 8 hours. Mostly renal excretion (half-life increased in patients with renal impairment). It affects areas of the brain involved in mood disorders, including hippocampus and amygdala.

3. **Oxcarbazepine (Trileptal).** This is indicated for use as monotherapy or adjunctive therapy in the treatment of partial seizures in adults and as monotherapy in the treatment of children aged 4 years and above with epilepsy. The drug available is as 150-, 300- and 600 mg film-coated tablets for oral administration. It should not be used with oral contraceptive because it decreases the plasma level of hormones dramatically. It causes hyponatremia and should be used cautiously in patient with renal impairment. Sodium levels should be monitored during use. Common side effects are cognitive symptoms and somnolescence. Stevens-Johnson syndrome has been reported in children and adults in rare cases.

VIII. Stimulants

A. **Sympathomimetics** (also called *analeptics* and *psychostimulants*). The sympathomimetics are effective in the treatment of attention-deficit/hyperactivity disorder (ADHD). The first-line sympathomimetics are methylphenidate (Ritalin, Concerta), dextroamphetamine (Dexedrine), Lisdexamfetamine Dimesylate (Vyvanse), and a reformulation of existing dextroamphetamine and amphetamine (Adderall). Pemoline (Cylert) is now considered a second-line agent because of rare but potentially fatal hepatic toxicity.

1. **Pharmacological actions.** All the drugs are well absorbed from the GI tract. Dextroamphetamine and the reformulation reach peak plasma concentrations in 2 to 3 hours and have a half-life of about 6 hours, so

that once- or twice-daily dosing is necessary. Methylphenidate reaches peak plasma levels in 1 to 2 hours and has a short half-life of 2 to 3 hours, so that multiple daily dosing is necessary. A sustained-release formulation doubles the effective half-life of methylphenidate. A novel osmotic pump capsule (Concerta) may sustain the effects of methylphenidate for 12 hours. Lisdexamfetamine dimesylate is rapidly absorbed from the GI tract and converted to dextroamphetamine and L-lysine.

2. **Therapeutic efficacy.** Sympathomimetics are effective about 75% of the time. Methylphenidate and dextroamphetamine are generally equally effective and work within 15 to 30 minutes. The drugs decrease hyperactivity, increase attentiveness, and reduce impulsivity. They may also reduce comorbid oppositional behaviors associated with ADHD. Many persons take these drugs throughout their schooling and beyond. In responsive persons, the use of a sympathomimetic may be a critical determinant of scholastic success. Sympathomimetics improve the core ADHD symptoms—hyperactivity, impulsivity, and inattentiveness—and permit improved social interactions with teachers, family, other adults, and peers.

The success of long-term treatment of ADHD with sympathomimetics supports a model in which ADHD results from a genetically determined neurochemical imbalance that requires lifelong pharmacological management. A recent comparison between medication and psychosocial approaches for the treatment of ADHD found clear benefit with medication but little improvement with nonpharmacological treatments.

3. **Clinical guidelines**

   a. **Pretreatment evaluation.** The pretreatment evaluation should include an assessment of the patient's cardiac function, with particular attention to the presence of hypertension or tachyarrhythmias. The clinician should also examine the patient for the presence of movement disorders (e.g., tics and dyskinesia), because these conditions can be exacerbated by the administration of sympathomimetics. If tics are present, many experts do not use sympathomimetics but instead choose clonidine (Catapres) or antidepressants. However, recent data indicate that sympathomimetics may cause only a mild increase in motor tics and may actually suppress vocal tics.

   Hepatic and renal function should be assessed, and dosages of sympathomimetics should be reduced if the patient's metabolism is impaired. In the case of pemoline, any elevation of liver enzymes is a compelling reason to discontinue the medication.

   b. **Dosage and administration.** The dosage ranges and the available preparations for sympathomimetics are presented in Table 30–25.

      (1) **Methylphenidate.** Methylphenidate is the agent most commonly used initially, at a dosage of 5 to 10 mg every 3 to 4 hours. The dosage may be increased to a maximum of 20 mg four times daily. Use of the 20-mg sustained-release formulation, to provide 6 hours of benefit and eliminate the need

Table 30–25
Sympathomimetics Commonly Used in Psychiatry

Generic Name	Trade Name	Preparations	Initial Daily Dose	Usual Daily Dose for ADHD[a]	Usual Daily Dose for Narcolepsy	Maximal Daily Dose
Atomoxetine	Strattera	10-, 18-, 25-, 40-, 60-mg tablets	20 mg	40–80 mg	Not used	Children 80 mg, adults 100 mg
Amphetamine-dextroamphetamine	Adderall	5-, 10-, 20-, 30-mg tablets	5 to 10 mg	20–30 mg	5–60 mg	Children 40 mg, adults 60 mg
Armodafinil[b]	Nuvigil	150-, 250-mg tablets	150–250 mg	—	150–250 mg	250 mg
Dexmethylphenidate	Focalin	2.5-, 5-, 10-mg capsules	5 mg	5–20 mg	Not used	20 mg
Dextroamphetamine	Dexedrine, Dextrostat	5-, 10-, 15-mg ER capsules; 5-, 10-mg tablets	5 to 10 mg	20–30 mg	5–60 mg	Children 40 mg, adults 60 mg
Lisdexamfetamine	Vyvanse	30-, 50-, 70-mg, ER tablets	30 mg	30–70 mg	Not used	70 mg
Modafinil	Provigil	100-, 200-mg tablets	100 mg	Not used	400 mg	400 mg
Methamphetamine	Desoxyn	5-mg tablets; 5-, 10-, 15-mg ER tablets	5–10 mg	20–25 mg	Not generally used	45 mg
Methylphenidate	Ritalin, Methidate, Methylin, Attenade Concerta	5-, 10-, 20-mg tablets; 10-, 20-mg SR tablets; 18-, 36-mg ER tablets	5–10 mg	5–60 mg	20–30 mg	Children 80 mg, adults 90 mg
Pemoline	Cylert	13.75-, 37.5-, 75-mg tablets; 37.5-mg chewable tablets	18 mg	18–54 mg	Not yet established	54 mg
			37.5 mg	56.25–75 mg	Not used	112.5 mg

ADHD, attention-deficit/hyperactivity disorder; ER, extended release; SR, sustained released.
[a]For children 6 years of age or older.
[b]Not studied in children and not approved for ADHD.

for dosing at school, is sometimes recommended, but it may be less effective than the immediate-release formulation.

Children with ADHD can take immediate-release methylphenidate at 8 a.m. and 12 noon. The sustained-release preparation of methylphenidate may be taken once at 8 a.m. The starting dose of methylphenidate ranges from 2.5 mg (regular preparation) to 20 mg (sustained-release). If this is inadequate, the dosage may be increased to a maximum of 20 mg four times daily.

(2) **Dextroamphetamine.** The dosage of dextroamphetamine is 2.5 to 40 mg/day (up to 0.5 mg/kg/day). Dextroamphetamine is about twice as potent as methylphenidate on a per-milligram basis and provides 6 to 8 hours of benefit.

(3) **Lisdexamfetamine dimesylate.** Adults and children 6 to 12 years of age. Start with 30 mg once daily in the morning. Dosage may be adjusted in 10 or 20 mg/day increments at approximately weekly intervals (max, 70 mg/day).

(4) **Treatment failures.** Seventy percent of nonresponders to one sympathomimetic may benefit from another. All the sympathomimetic drugs should be tried before the patient is switched to a drug of a different class.

4. **Precautions and adverse reactions.** The most common adverse effects associated with amphetaminelike drugs are stomach pain, anxiety, irritability, insomnia, tachycardia, cardiac arrhythmias, and dysphoria. The treatment of common adverse effects in children with ADHD is usually straightforward (Table 30–26).

Less common adverse effects include the induction of movement disorders (e.g., tics, Tourette's disorder–like symptoms, and dyskinesias), which are often self-limited over 7 to 10 days. Small to moderate dosages of sympathomimetics may be well tolerated without causing an increase in the frequency and severity of tics. In severe cases, augmentation with risperidone is necessary.

Methylphenidate may worsen tics in one third of patients, who fall into two groups: those whose methylphenidate-induced tics resolve immediately after the dose has been metabolized, and a smaller group in whom methylphenidate appears to trigger tics that persist for several months but eventually resolve spontaneously.

The most limiting adverse effect of sympathomimetics is their association with psychological and physical dependence. Sympathomimetics may exacerbate glaucoma, hypertension, cardiovascular disorders, hyperthyroidism, anxiety disorders, psychotic disorders, and seizure disorders.

High doses of sympathomimetics can cause dry mouth, pupillary dilation, bruxism, formication, excessive ebullience, restlessness, and emotional lability. The long-term use of a high dosage can cause a delusional disorder that is indistinguishable from paranoid schizophrenia.

Table 30–26
Management of Common Stimulant-Induced Adverse Effects in Attention-Deficit/Hyperactivity Disorder

Adverse Effect	Management
Anorexia, nausea, weight loss	• Administer stimulant with meals. • Use calorie-enhanced supplements. Discourage forcing meals. • If using pemoline, check liver function tests.
Insomnia, nightmares	• Administer stimulants earlier in day. • Change to short-acting preparations. • Discontinue afternoon or evening dosing. • Consider adjunctive treatment (e.g., antihistamines, clonidine, antidepressants).
Dizziness	• Monitor blood pressure. • Encourage fluid intake. • Change to long-acting form.
Rebound phenomena	• Overlap stimulant dosing. • Change to long-acting preparation or combine long- and short-acting preparations. • Consider adjunctive or alternative treatment (e.g., clonidine, antidepressants).
Irritability	• Assess timing of phenomena (during peak or withdrawal phase). • Evaluate comorbid symptoms. • Reduce dose. • Consider adjunctive or alternative treatment (e.g., lithium, antidepressants, anticonvulsants).
Dysphoria, moodiness, agitation	• Consider comorbid diagnosis (e.g., mood disorder). • Reduce dose or change to long-acting preparation. • Consider adjunctive or alternative treatment (e.g., lithium, anticonvulsants, antidepressants).

Adapted from Wilens TE, Biederman J. The stimulants. In: Shaffer D, ed. *The Psychiatric Clinics of North America: Pediatric Psychopharmacology.* Philadelphia: Saunders, 1992, with permission.

Patients who have taken overdoses of sympathomimetics present with hypertension, tachycardia, hyperthermia, toxic psychosis, delirium, and occasionally seizures. Overdoses of sympathomimetics can also result in death, often caused by cardiac arrhythmias. Seizures can be treated with benzodiazepines, cardiac effects with β-adrenergic receptor antagonists, fever with cooling blankets, and delirium with dopamine receptor agonists.

5. **Atomoxetine.** Atomoxetine (Strattera) is indicated for the treatment of ADHD in children 6 years of age and older, adolescents, and adults. The precise mechanism of its therapeutic effects is unknown but is thought to be related to selective inhibition of the presynaptic norepinephrine transporter. Atomoxetine improves symptoms in both inattentive and hyperactive/impulsive domains in children, adolescents, and adults.

It has a half-life of about 5 hours and requires twice-daily dosing. It is available in 10-, 18-, 25-, 40-, and 60-mg capsules. For children and adolescents over 70 kg of body weight, it should be initiated at a dose of 40 mg/day and increased after a minimum of 3 days to a target dose of approximately 80 mg/day.

For adults, atomoxetine should be initiated at a total daily dose of 40 mg and increased after a minimum of 3 days to a target dose of 80 mg/day. Because of liver toxicity, atomoxetine is no longer a drug of first choice, and its use is diminishing.

6. **Modafinil (Provigil).** Modafinil is a unique drug with psychostimulant effects. Its specific mechanism of action is unknown but it may have some effect on blocking norepinephrine reuptake. Modafinil is used to improve wakefulness in patients with excessive daytime sleepiness associated with narcolepsy, obstructive sleep apnea, or shift work sleep disorder. It is supplied in 100 and 200 mg tablets and taken once daily. Maximum daily dose is 200 mg. Drug interactions are related to modafinil-inducing CYP 2C19 enzymes; thus, it may increase levels of diazepam, propranolol, or phenytoin. Adverse reactions include headache, nausea, anxiety, and insomnia.

IX. Cholinesterase Inhibitors

A. **Therapeutic efficacy.** Donepezil (Aricept), rivastigmine, (Exelon) and Memantine ([Namenda] discussed separately below) are among the few proven treatments for mild to moderate dementia of the Alzheimer's type. They reduce the intrasynaptic cleavage and inactivation of acetylcholine and thus potentiate cholinergic neurotransmission, which in turn tends to produce a modest improvement in memory and goal-directed thought. These drugs are considered most useful for persons with mild to moderate memory loss, who nevertheless still have enough preserved basal forebrain cholinergic neurons to benefit from an augmentation of cholinergic neurotransmission.

Donepezil is well tolerated and widely used. Rivastigmine appears more likely than donepezil to cause GI and neuropsychiatric adverse effects. An older cholinesterase inhibitor, tacrine (Cognex), is currently very rarely used because of its potential for hepatotoxicity. Cholinesterase inhibitors have been coadministered with vitamin E and gingko biloba extract.

The cholinesterase inhibitors slow the progression of memory loss and diminish apathy, depression, hallucinations, anxiety, euphoria, and purposeless motor behaviors. Some persons note immediate improvement in memory, mood, psychotic symptoms, and interpersonal skills. Others note little initial benefit but are able to retain their cognitive and adaptive faculties at a relatively stable level for many months. The use of cholinesterase inhibitors may delay or reduce the need for nursing home placement.

B. **Clinical guidelines**

1. **Pretreatment evaluation.** Before the initiation of treatment with cholinesterase inhibitors, potentially treatable causes of dementia should be ruled out with a thorough neurological evaluation. The psychiatric evaluation should focus on depression, anxiety, and psychosis.

2. **Dosage and administration**

   a. **Donepezil.** Donepezil is available in 5- and 10-mg tablets. Treatment should be initiated with a dosage of 5 mg/day, taken at night. If well tolerated and of some discernible benefit after 4 weeks, the dosage should be increased to a maintenance level of 10 mg/day. Donepezil absorption is unaffected by meals.

   b. Rivastigmine. Rivastigmine is available in 1.5-, 3-, 4.5-, and 6-mg capsules. The recommended initial dosage is 1.5 mg twice daily for a minimum of 2 weeks, after which increases of 1.5 mg/day can be made at intervals of at least 2 weeks to a target dosage of 6 mg/day, taken in two equal doses. If tolerated, the dosage may be further titrated upward to a maximum of 6 mg twice daily. The risk for adverse GI events can be reduced by taking rivastigmine with food.

C. Precautions and adverse reactions

   1. Donepezil. Donepezil is generally well tolerated at recommended dosages. Fewer than 3% of persons taking donepezil experience nausea, diarrhea, and vomiting. These mild symptoms are more common at the 10-mg than the 5-mg dose, and when present, they tend to resolve after 3 weeks of continued use. Donepezil may cause weight loss. Donepezil treatment has been infrequently associated with bradyarrhythmias, especially in persons with underlying cardiac disease. A small number of persons experience syncope.

   2. Rivastigmine. Rivastigmine is generally well tolerated, but recommended dosages may need to be scaled back in the initial period of treatment to limit GI and CNS adverse effects. These mild symptoms are more common at dosages above 6 mg/day, and when present, they tend to resolve once the dosage is lowered.

   The most common adverse effects associated with rivastigmine are nausea, vomiting, dizziness, and headache. Rivastigmine may cause weight loss.

X. Other Drugs

A. α_2-Adrenergic agonists (clonidine and guanfacine). Clonidine and guanfacine are used in psychiatry to control symptoms caused by withdrawal from opiates and opioids, treat Tourette's disorder, suppress agitation in posttraumatic stress disorder, and control aggressive or hyperactive behavior in children, especially those with autistic features.

   The most common adverse effects associated with clonidine are dry mouth and eyes, fatigue, sedation, dizziness, nausea, hypotension, and constipation. A similar but milder adverse effect profile is seen with guanfacine, especially at dosages of 3 mg/day or more. Adults with blood pressure below 90/60 mm Hg or with cardiac arrhythmias, especially bradycardia, should not take clonidine and guanfacine. Clonidine, in particular, is associated with sedation, and tolerance does not usually develop to this adverse effect. Uncommon CNS adverse effects of clonidine include insomnia, anxiety, and depression; rare CNS adverse effects include vivid dreams, nightmares, and hallucinations. Fluid retention associated with clonidine treatment can be treated with diuretics.

B. β-Adrenergic receptor antagonists. β-Adrenergic receptor antagonists (e.g., propranolol [Inderal], pindolol [Visken]) are effective peripherally and are centrally acting agents for the treatment of social phobia (e.g., performance anxiety), lithium-induced postural tremor, and neuroleptic-induced acute akathisia, and for the control of aggressive behavior.

The β-adrenergic receptor antagonists are contraindicated for use in people with asthma, insulin-dependent diabetes, congestive heart failure, significant vascular disease, persistent angina, and hyperthyroidism. The most common adverse effects of β-adrenergic receptor antagonists are hypotension and bradycardia.

 CLINICAL HINT:
Patients who must give a speech or perform publically can be given propanol (10 to 20 mg) 30 minutes beforehand and their signs of anxiety will diminish in many cases.

C. Anticholinergics and amantadine (Symmetrel). In the clinical practice of psychiatry, the anticholinergic drugs are primarily used to treat medication-induced movement disorders, particularly neuroleptic-induced parkinsonism, neuroleptic-induced acute dystonia, and medication-induced postural tremor.

D. N-methyl-D-aspartate (NMDA)-receptor antagonist. Memantine hydrochloride (Namenda) is approved for the treatment of moderate to severe Alzheimer's disease.

   1. Therapeutic efficacy. The NMDA-receptor antagonist memantine binds to NMDA-receptor–operated cation channels, which activate glutamate. Glutamate is a neurotransmitter essential for learning and memory; hence, increasing its activity may improve learning and memory.

   2. Dosage and administration. Memantine is rapidly and completely absorbed after oral administration. Peak plasma levels are attained in 3 to 7 hours, and the half-life is approximately 60 to 80 hours. Memantine is primarily excreted by the kidneys, so patients with renal impairment need dose reduction.

   It has minimal inhibition of CYP 450 enzyme system and low serum protein binding. As a result, the drug–drug interactions are low.

   Memantine is available in 5- and 10-mg tablets. The dosing schedule is illustrated in Table 30–27.

 Table 30–27
Memantine Dosing Schedule

Titration Schedule	Maintenance Dose
Week 1	5 mg once daily
Week 2	10 mg/day (5 mg b.i.d.)
Week 3	15 mg/day (10 mg in the morning and 5 mg in the evening)
Week 4	20 mg/day (10 mg b.i.d.)

3. **Adverse reactions.** Memantine is safe and well tolerated. The most commonly observed adverse events are dizziness, confusion, headache, and constipation. There are no clinically important changes in vital signs, and only minimal hemodynamic effects are observed.

E. **Pregabalin (Lyrica).** Pregabalin is the only drug approved for the management of fibromyalgia. It decreases excitatory neurotransmitter release (glutamate, substance P, and norepinephrine). It provides rapid relief as early as week 1 with reduction in pain and has shown sustained relief in a 6-month study. Common adverse effects include dizziness, somnolence, dry mouth, edema, weight gain, and constipation. It may cause life-threatening angioedema and should be immediately discontinued. It is available as 25-, 50-, 75-, 100-, 150-, 200-, 250-, and 300-mg tablets. The usual recommended dose is 300 mg/day in divided doses and may be increased to 450 mg/day. Some studies have suggested its efficacy in GAD, but it has not been approved by the FDA and is used mostly off label.

F. **Ropinirole (Requip).** Ropinirole is the first and only FDA-approved medicine indicated for the treatment of moderate-to-severe primary restless leg syndrome. The usual starting dose is 0.25 mg taken 1 to 3 hours before bedtime. The dose may be increased to 4 mg/day based on clinical response. The most common adverse effects include somnolence, vomiting, dizziness, and fatigue. More serious side effects include syncope or symptomatic hypotension, especially during initial treatment or dose titration.

XI. Electroconvulsive Therapy (ECT)
A. Indications
1. MDD (any type).
2. Bipolar disorder—depression.
3. Bipolar disorder—mania.
4. Schizophrenia.
5. Pregnancy with any of the above disorders.

B. Therapeutic efficacy
1. Does not cure any illness but can induce remissions in an acute episode.
2. Should be followed by other treatments.
3. Also may be used prophylactically to prevent recurrence.

C. Clinical guidelines
1. **Pretreatment evaluation**
   a. Pertinent history.
      (1) Hypertension.
      (2) Musculoskeletal injuries or osteoporosis.
      (3) Reserpine or anticholinesterases.
      (4) Lithium.
      (5) Tricyclic antidepressants.
      (6) Antipsychotics.
   b. Drugs that raise the seizure threshold should be discontinued.
   c. Preparing the patient.

        (1) Informed consent.

        (2) Alternative treatments.

        (3) Adverse effects.

        (4) Convalescent period.

  2. Procedure

    a. Medications.

      (1) Anticholinergics.

      (2) Anesthesia.

        (a) Methohexital (Brevital).

        (b) Ketamine (Ketalar) or etomidate (Amidate).

        (c) Propofol (Diprivan).

      (3) Muscle relaxants.

        (a) Succinylcholine (Anectine).

        (b) Curare.

    b. Types of electrical stimuli.

      (1) Sine wave.

      (2) Brief pulse.

    c. Electrode placement.

      (1) Bilateral.

      (2) Nondominant unilateral.

      (3) Other.

    d. Administering the stimulus.

      (1) Check vital signs (temperature, cardiac rhythm, blood pressure, pulse).

      (2) Apply electrodes and make sure treatment bed is not grounded.

      (3) Clear patient's mouth, remove any hearing aids.

      (4) Begin anesthesia (before muscle relaxants).

      (5) Administer muscle relaxants.

      (6) Ventilation.

      (7) Apply bite block.

      (8) Apply electrical stimulus.

      (9) Induce a seizure that is therapeutic.

    e. Monitoring.

      (1) ECG.

      (2) EEG.

D. Precautions and adverse effects

  1. Relative contraindications. There are no absolute contraindications, but consider the following:

    a. Fever.

    b. Significant arrhythmias.

    c. Extreme hypertension.

    d. Coronary ischemia.

  2. Adverse effects

    a. Cardiac.

    b. CNS.

    c. General.

XII. Transcranial Magnetic Stimulation (TMS)

In October 2008, the FDA approved the TMS therapy system for the treatment of depression. It involves the use of very short pulses of magnetic energy to stimulate nerve cells in the brain. It is specifically indicated for the treatment of MDD in adult patients who have failed to achieve satisfactory improvement from one prior antidepressant medication at or above the minimal effective dose and duration in the current episode.

Repetitive transcranial magnetic stimulation (rTMS) produces focal secondary electrical stimulation of targeted cortical regions. It is nonconvulsive, requires no anesthesia, has a safe side effect profile, and is not associated with cognitive side effects.

The patients do not require anesthesia or sedation and remain awake and alert. It is a 40-minute outpatient procedure that is prescribed by a psychiatrist and performed in a psychiatrist's office. The treatment is typically administered daily for 4 to 6 weeks. The most common adverse event related to treatment was scalp pain or discomfort.

TMS therapy is contraindicated in patients with implanted metallic devices or nonremovable metallic objects in or around the head.

XIII. Vagal Nerve Stimulation (VNS)

VNS therapy is a new modality indicated for use as an adjunctive long-term treatment of chronic or recurrent depression for patients 18 years of age or older who are experiencing a major depressive episode and have not had an adequate response to four or more adequate antidepressant treatments. VNS affects serotonin and norepinephrine neurotransmitters and brain structures thought to be involved in mood regulation.

Activation of the left vagus nerve has been shown to induce widespread bilateral effects in the areas of the brain implicated in depression, including in the inferior temporal structures (amygdala) and the prefrontal cortex.

There are no undesired drug interactions with VNS therapy and concurrent antidepressant medication. There are no systemic neurotoxic effects, and unlike ECT, there is no deterioration in any neurocognitive measures. The most common side effects with VNS therapy include temporary hoarseness or a slight change in voice tone, increased coughing, shortness of breath upon physical exertion, and a tickling in the throat.

The typical stimulation cycle is 30 seconds on, followed by 5 minutes off. Psychiatrists may adjust stimulation with handheld computer and telemetric wand during in-office visits. Frequent office visits (every 2 to 4 weeks) are suggested for the first several months to monitor patient tolerability and adjust device parameters.

For a more detailed discussion of this topic, see Biological Therapies, Ch 31, p. 2965, in CTP/IX.

31
Medication-Induced Movement Disorders

I. General Introduction
The typical antipsychotic drugs are associated with a number of uncomfortable and potentially serious neurological adverse effects. The drugs act by blocking the binding of dopamine to the dopamine receptors involved in the control of both voluntary and involuntary movements. The newer antipsychotics, the serotonin-dopamine antagonists, block binding to dopamine receptors to a much lesser degree and thereby, are less likely to produce such movement disorders. See Table 31–1 for selected medications associated with movement disorders and their impact on relevant neuroreceptors.

II. Neuroleptic-Induced Parkinsonism
A. Diagnosis, signs, and symptoms. Symptoms include muscle stiffness (lead pipe rigidity), cogwheel rigidity, shuffling gait, stooped posture, and drooling. The pill-rolling tremor of idiopathic parkinsonism is rare, but a regular, coarse tremor similar to essential tremor may be present. The so-called *rabbit syndrome* is a tremor affecting the lips and perioral muscles and is another parkinsonian effect seen with antipsychotics, although perioral tremor is more likely than other tremors to occur late in the course of treatment.
B. Epidemiology. Parkinsonian adverse effects occur in about 15% of patients who are treated with antipsychotics, usually within 5 to 90 days of the initiation of treatment. Patients who are elderly and female are at the highest risk for neuroleptic-induced parkinsonism, although the disorder can occur at all ages.
C. Etiology. Caused by the blockade of dopamine type 2 (D$_2$) receptors in the caudate at the termination of the nigrostriatal dopamine neurons. All antipsychotics can cause the symptoms, especially high-potency drugs with low levels of anticholinergic activity (e.g., trifluoperazine [Stelazine]). Chlorpromazine (Thorazine) and thioridazine (Mellaril) are not likely to be involved. The newer, atypical antipsychotics (e.g., aripiprazole [Abilify], olanzapine [Zyprexa], and quetiapine [Seroquel]) are less likely to cause parkinsonism.
D. Differential diagnosis. Includes idiopathic parkinsonism, other organic causes of parkinsonism, and depression, which can also be associated with parkinsonian symptoms.
E. Treatment. Can be treated with anticholinergic agents, benztropine (Cogentin), amantadine (Symmetrel), or diphenhydramine (Benadryl) (Table 31–2). Anticholinergics should be withdrawn after 4 to 6 weeks to assess whether tolerance to the parkinsonian effects has developed;

Table 31–1
Selected Medications Associated with Movement Disorders: Impact on Relevant Neuroreceptors

Type (Subtype)	Name (Brand)	D$_2$ Blockade	5-HT$_2$ Blockade	mACh Blockade
Antipsychotics				
Phenothiazine (Aliphatic)	Chlorpromazine (Thorazine)	Low	High	High
Phenothiazine (Piperidines)	Thioridazine (Mellaril)	Low	Med	High
	Mesoridazine (Serentil)	Low	Med	High
Phenothiazine (Piperazines)	Trifluoperazine (Stelazine)	Med	Med	Med
	Fluphenazine (Prolixin)	High	Low	Low
	Perphenazine (Trilafon)	High	Med	Low
Thioxanthenes	Thiothixene (Navane)	High	Med	Low
	Chlorprothixene (Taractan)	Med	High	Med
Dibenzoxazepines	Loxapine (Loxitane)	Med	High	Low
Butyrophenones	Haloperidol (Haldol)	High	Low	Low
	Droperidol (Inapsine)	High	Med	—
Diphenylbutylpiperidines	Pimozide (Orap)	High	Med	Low
Dihydroindolones	Molindone (Moban)	Med	Low	Low
Dibenzodiazepines	Clozapine (Clozaril)	Low	High	High
Benzisoxazole	Risperidone (Risperdal)	High	High	Low
Thienobenzodiazepines	Olanzapine (Zyprexa)	Low	High	High
Dibenzothiazepines	Quetiapine (Seroquel)	Low/med	Low/med	Low
Benzisothiazolyls	Ziprasidone (Geodon)	Med	High	Low
Quinolones	Aripiprazole (Abilify)	High (as partial agonist)	High	Low
Nonantipsychotic psychotropics				
Anticonvulsants	Lithium (Eskalith)	Low	Low	Low
Antidepressants	All	Low (except amoxapine)	(Varies)	(Varies)

D$_2$, dopamine type 2; 5-HT$_2$, 5-hydroxytryptamine type 2; mACh, muscarinic acetylcholine.
Adapted from Janicak PG, Davis JM, Preskorn SH, et al. *Principles and Practice of Psychopharmacotherapy*, 3rd ed. Philadelphia: Lippincott Williams & Wilkins; 2001.

about half of patients with neuroleptic-induced parkinsonism require continued treatment. Even after the antipsychotics are withdrawn, parkinsonian symptoms may last for up to 2 weeks and even up to 3 months in elderly patients. With such patients, the clinician may continue the anticholinergic drug after the antipsychotic has been stopped until the parkinsonian symptoms resolve completely.

III. Neuroleptic-Induced Acute Dystonia

    A. Diagnosis, signs, and symptoms. Dystonias are brief or prolonged contractions of muscles that result in obviously abnormal movements or postures, including oculogyric crises, tongue protrusion, trismus, torticollis, laryngeal–pharyngeal dystonias, and dystonic postures of the limbs and trunk. Other dystonias include blepharospasm and glossopharyngeal dystonia; the latter results in dysarthria, dysphagia, and even difficulty in breathing, which can cause cyanosis. Children are particularly likely to evidence opisthotonos, scoliosis, lordosis, and writhing movements. Dystonia can be painful and frightening and often results in noncompliance with future drug treatment regimens.

B. Epidemiology. The development of dystonic symptoms is characterized by their early onset during the course of treatment with neuroleptics and their high incidence in men, in patients younger than age 30, and in patients given high dosages of high-potency medications.

C. Etiology. Although it is most common with intramuscular doses of high-potency antipsychotics, dystonia can occur with any antipsychotic. It is least common with thioridazine and is uncommon with atypical antipsychotics. The mechanism of action is thought to be dopaminergic hyperactivity in the basal ganglia that occurs when central nervous system (CNS) levels of the antipsychotic drug begin to fall between doses.

D. Differential diagnosis. Includes seizures and tardive dyskinesia.

E. Course and prognosis. Dystonia can fluctuate spontaneously and respond to reassurance so that the clinician acquires the false impression that the movement is hysterical or completely under conscious control.

F. Treatment. Prophylaxis with anticholinergics or related drugs (Table 31–2) usually prevents dystonia, although the risks of prophylactic treatment weigh against that benefit. Treatment with intramuscular anticholinergics or intravenous or intramuscular diphenhydramine (50 mg) almost

Table 31–2
Drug Treatment of Extrapyramidal Disorders

Generic Name	Trade Name	Usual Daily Dosage	Indications
Anticholinergics			
Benztropine	Cogentin	PO 0.5–2 mg t.i.d.; IM or IV 1–2 mg	Acute dystonia, parkinsonism, akinesia, akathisia
Biperiden	Akineton	PO 2–6 mg t.i.d.; IM or IV 2 mg	
Procyclidine	Kemadrin	PO 2.5–5 mg b.i.d.–q.i.d.	
Trihexyphenidyl	Artane, Tremin	PO 2–5 mg t.i.d.	
Orphenadrine	Norflex, Disipal	PO 50–100 mg b.i.d.–q.i.d.; IV 60 mg	Rabbit syndrome
Antihistamine			
Diphenhydramine	Benadryl	PO 25 mg q.i.d.; IM or IV 25 mg	Acute dystonia, parkinsonism, akinesia, rabbit syndrome
Amantadine	Symmetrel	PO 100–200 mg b.i.d.	Parkinsonism, akinesia, rabbit syndrome
β-Adrenergic antagonist			
Propranolol	Inderal	PO 20–40 mg t.i.d.	Akathisia, tremor
α-Adrenergic antagonist			
Clonidine	Catapres	PO 0.1 mg t.i.d.	Akathisia
Benzodiazepines			
Clonazepam	Klonopin	PO 1 mg b.i.d.	Akathisia, acute dystonia
Lorazepam	Ativan	PO 1 mg t.i.d.	
Buspirone	BuSpar	PO 20–40 mg q.i.d.	Tardive dyskinesia
Vitamin E	—	PO 1,200–1,600 IU/day	Tardive dyskinesia

PO, oral; IM, intramuscular; IV, intravenous; b.i.d., twice a day; t.i.d., three times a day; q.i.d.; four times a day.

always relieves the symptoms. Diazepam (Valium) (10 mg intravenously), amobarbital (Amytal), caffeine sodium benzoate, and hypnosis have also been reported to be effective. Although tolerance for the adverse effect usually develops, it is sometimes prudent to change the antipsychotic if the patient is particularly concerned that the reaction may recur.

IV. Neuroleptic-Induced Acute Akathisia

A. **Diagnosis, signs, and symptoms.** Akathisia is subjective feelings of restlessness, objective signs of restlessness, or both. Examples include a sense of anxiety, inability to relax, jitteriness, pacing, rocking motions while sitting, and rapid alternation of sitting and standing. Akathisia has been associated with the use of a wide range of psychiatric drugs, including antipsychotics, antidepressants, and sympathomimetics. Once akathisia is recognized and diagnosed, the antipsychotic dose should be reduced to the minimal effective level. Akathisia may be associated with a poor treatment outcome.

B. **Epidemiology.** Middle-aged women are at increased risk of akathisia, and the time course is similar to that for neuroleptic-induced parkinsonism.

C. **Treatment.** Three basic steps in the treatment of akathisia are (1) reducing medication dosage, (2) attempting treatment with appropriate drugs, and (3) considering changing the neuroleptic. The most efficacious drugs are β-adrenergic receptor antagonists, although anticholinergic drugs, benzodiazepines, and cyproheptadine (Periactin) may benefit some patients. In some cases of akathisia, no treatment seems to be effective.

V. Neuroleptic-Induced Tardive Dyskinesia

A. **Diagnosis, signs, and symptoms.** Tardive dyskinesia is a delayed effect of antipsychotics; it rarely occurs until after 6 months of treatment. The disorder consists of abnormal, involuntary, irregular choreoathetoid movements of the muscles of the head, limbs, and trunk. The severity of the movements ranges from minimal—often missed by patients and their families—to grossly incapacitating. Perioral movements are the most common and include darting, twisting, and protruding movements of the tongue, chewing and lateral jaw movements, lip puckering, and facial grimacing. Finger movements and hand clenching are also common. Torticollis, retrocollis, trunk twisting, and pelvic thrusting occur in severe cases. In the most serious cases, patients may have breathing and swallowing irregularities that result in aerophagia, belching, and grunting. Respiratory dyskinesia has also been reported. Dyskinesia is exacerbated by stress and disappears during sleep. Twitching of the nose has been called *rabbit syndrome*.

B. **Epidemiology.** Tardive dyskinesia develops in about 10% to 20% of patients who are treated for more than a year. About 20% to 40% of patients undergoing long-term hospitalization have tardive dyskinesia. Women are more likely to be affected than men. Children, patients who are more than 50 years of age, and patients with brain damage or mood disorders are also at high risk.

C. **Course and prognosis.** Between 5% and 40% of all cases of tardive dyskinesia eventually remit, and between 50% and 90% of all mild cases remit. However, tardive dyskinesia is less likely to remit in elderly patients than in young patients.

D. **Treatment.** The three basic approaches to tardive dyskinesia are prevention, diagnosis, and management. Prevention is best achieved by using antipsychotic medications only when clearly indicated and in the lowest effective doses. The atypical antipsychotics are associated with less tardive dyskinesia than the typical antipsychotics. Clozapine is the only antipsychotic to have minimal risk of tardive dyskinesia, and can even help improve pre-existing symptoms of tardive dyskinesia. This has been attributed to its low affinity for D_2 receptors and high affinity for 5HT receptor antagonism. Patients who are receiving antipsychotics should be examined regularly for the appearance of abnormal movements, preferably with the use of a standardized rating scale (Table 31–3). Patients frequently experience an exacerbation of their symptoms when the dopamine receptor antagonist is withheld, whereas substitution of a serotonin–dopamine antagonist (SDA) may limit the abnormal movements without worsening the progression of the dyskinesia.

Table 31–3
Abnormal Involuntary Movement Scale (AIMS) Examination Procedure

Patient Identification	Date
Rated by	

Either before or after completing the examination procedure, observe the patient unobtrusively at rest (e.g., in waiting room).

The chair to be used in this examination should be a hard, firm one without arms.

After observing the patient, rate him or her on a scale of 0 (none), 1 (minimal), 2 (mild), 3 (moderate), and 4 (severe) according to the severity of the symptoms.

Ask the patient whether there is anything in his or her mouth (i.e., gum, candy, etc.) and, if so, to remove it.

Ask the patient about the current condition of his or her teeth. Ask patient if he or she wears dentures. Do teeth or dentures bother patient now?

Ask patient whether he or she notices any movement in mouth, face, hands, or feet. If yes, ask patient to describe and indicate to what extent they currently bother patient or interfere with his or her activities.

0 1 2 3 4 Have patient sit in chair with hands on knees, legs slightly apart, and feet flat on floor. (Look at entire body for movement while in this position.)

0 1 2 3 4 Ask patient to sit with hands hanging unsupported. If male, between legs; if female and wearing a dress, hanging over knees. (Observe hands and other body areas.)

0 1 2 3 4 Ask patient to open mouth. (Observe tongue at rest within mouth.) Do this twice.

0 1 2 3 4 Ask patient to protrude tongue. (Observe abnormalities of tongue movement.) Do this twice.

0 1 2 3 4 Ask the patient to tap thumb, with each finger, as rapidly as possible for 10 to 15 seconds: separately with right hand, then with left hand. (Observe facial and leg movements.)

0 1 2 3 4 Flex and extend patient's left and right arms. (One at a time.)

0 1 2 3 4 Ask patient to stand up. (Observe in profile. Observe all body areas again, hips included.)

0 1 2 3 4[a] Ask patient to extend both arms outstretched in front with palms down. (Observe trunk, legs, and mouth.)

0 1 2 3 4[a] Have patient walk a few paces, turn, and walk back to chair. (Observe hands and gait.) Do this twice.

[a]Activated movements.

Once tardive dyskinesia is recognized, the clinician should consider reducing the dose of the antipsychotic or even stopping the medication altogether. Alternatively, the clinician may switch the patient to clozapine or to one of the new dopamine receptor antagonists. In patients who cannot continue taking any antipsychotic medication, lithium, carbamazepine (Tegretol), or benzodiazepines may effectively reduce the symptoms of both the movement disorder and the psychosis.

VI. Neuroleptic Malignant Syndrome

A. **Diagnosis, signs, and symptoms.** Neuroleptic malignant syndrome is a life-threatening complication that can occur anytime during the course of antipsychotic treatment. The motor and behavioral symptoms include muscular rigidity and dystonia, akinesia, mutism, obtundation, and agitation. The autonomic symptoms include high fever, sweating, and increased pulse and blood pressure. Laboratory findings include an increased white blood cell count and increased levels of creatinine phosphokinase, liver enzymes, plasma myoglobin, and myoglobinuria, occasionally associated with renal failure.

B. **Epidemiology.** Men are affected more frequently than women, and young patients are affected more commonly than elderly patients. The mortality rate can reach 10% to 20% or even higher when depot antipsychotic medications are involved. The prevalence of the syndrome is estimated to range up to 2% to 2.4% of patients exposed to dopamine receptor antagonists.

C. **Pathophysiology.** Unknown.

D. **Course and prognosis.** The symptoms usually evolve over 24 to 72 hours, and the untreated syndrome lasts 10 to 14 days. The diagnosis is often missed in the early stages, and the withdrawal or agitation may mistakenly be considered to reflect an exacerbation of the psychosis.

E. **Treatment.** (See Table 31–4). In addition to supportive medical treatment, the most commonly used medications for the condition are dantrolene (Dantrium) and bromocriptine (Parlodel), although amantadine (Symmetrel) is sometimes used. Bromocriptine and amantadine possess direct dopamine receptor agonist effects and may serve to overcome the antipsychotic-induced dopamine receptor blockade. The lowest effective dosage of antipsychotic drug should be used to reduce the chance of neuroleptic malignant syndrome. Antipsychotic drugs with anticholinergic effects seem less likely to cause neuroleptic malignant syndrome.

VII. Medication-Induced Postural Tremor

A. **Diagnosis, signs, and symptoms.** Tremor is a rhythmic alteration in movement that is usually faster than one beat per second.

B. **Epidemiology.** Typically, tremors decrease during periods of relaxation and sleep and increase with stress or anxiety.

C. **Etiology.** Whereas all of the above diagnoses specifically include an association with a neuroleptic, a range of psychiatric medications can produce tremor—most notably lithium, antidepressants, and valproate (Depakene).

Table 31–4
Treatment of Neuroleptic Malignant Syndrome

Intervention	Dosing	Effectiveness
Amantadine	200–400 mg/day PO in divided doses	Beneficial as monotherapy or in combination; decreases death rate
Bromocriptine	2.5 mg PO b.i.d. or t.i.d. may increase to a total of 45 mg/day	Mortality reduced as a single or combined agent
Levodopa/carbidopa	Levodopa 50–100 mg/day IV as continuous infusion	Case reports of dramatic improvement
Electroconvulsive therapy	Reports of good outcome with both unilateral and bilateral treatments response may occur in as few as 3 treatments	Effective when medications have failed; also may treat underlying psychiatric disorder
Dantrolene	1 mg/kg/day for 8 days then continue as PO for 7 additional days	Benefits may occur in minutes or hours as a single agent or in combination
Benzodiazepines	1–2 mg IM as test dose; if effective, switch to PO; consider use if underlying disorder has catatonic symptoms	Has been reported effective when other agents have failed
Supportive measures	IV hydration Cooling blankets Ice packs Ice water enema Oxygenation Antipyretics	Often effective as initial approach early in the episode

Adapted from Davis IM, Caroff SN, Mann SC. Treatment of neuroleptic malignant syndrome. *Psychiatr Ann* 2000;30:325–331.
PO, oral; IM, intramuscular; IV, intravenous; b.i.d., twice a day; t.i.d., three times a day.

D. Treatment. The treatment involves four principles.
1. The lowest possible dose of the psychiatric drug should be taken.
2. Patients should minimize caffeine consumption.
3. The psychiatric drug should be taken at bedtime to minimize the amount of daytime tremor.
4. β-adrenergic receptor antagonists (e.g., propranolol [Inderal]) can be given to treat drug-induced tremors.

VIII. Other Disorders
A. Nocturnal myoclonus. Nocturnal myoclonus consists of highly stereotyped abrupt contractions of certain leg muscles during sleep. Patients lack any subjective awareness of the leg jerks. The condition may be present in about 40% of persons over age 65. It may accompany the use of selective serotonin reuptake inhibitors (SSRIs).

The repetitive leg movements occur every 20 to 60 seconds, with extension of the large toe and flexion of the ankle, the knee, and the hips. Frequent awakenings, unrefreshing sleep, and daytime sleepiness are major symptoms. No treatment for nocturnal myoclonus is universally effective. Treatments that may be useful include benzodiazepines, levodopa (Larodopa), quinine, and, in rare cases, opioids.

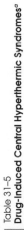

Table 31–5
Drug-Induced Central Hyperthermic Syndromes[a]

Condition (and Mechanism)	Common Drug Causes	Frequent Symptoms	Possible Treatment[b]	Clinical Course
Hyperthermia (↓ heat dissipation) (↑ heat production)	Atropine, lidocaine, meperidine NSAID toxicity, pheochromocytoma, thyrotoxicosis	Hyperthermia, diaphoresis, malaise	Acetaminophen per rectum (325 mg q4h), diazepam oral or per rectum (5 mg q8h) for febrile seizures	Benign, febrile seizures in children
Malignant hyperthermia (↑ heat production)	NMJ blockers (succinylcholine[c], halothane	Hyperthermia, **muscle rigidity, arrhythmias,** ischemia,[c] hypotension, **rhabdomyolysis;** disseminated intravascular coagulation	Dantrolene sodium (1–2 mg/kg/min IV infusion)[d]	Familial, 10% mortality if untreated
Tricyclic overdose (↑ heat production)	Tricyclic antidepressants, cocaine	Hyperthermia, confusion, visual hallucinations, agitation, **hyperreflexia, muscle relaxation, anticholinergic effects** (dry skin, pupil dilation), arrhythmias	Sodium bicarbonate (1 mEq/kg IV bolus) if arrhythmias are present, physostigmine (1–3 mg IV) with cardiac monitoring	Fatalities have occurred if untreated
Autonomic hyperreflexia (↑ heat production)	CNS stimulants (amphetamines)	Hyperthermia excitement, **hyperreflexia**	Trimethaphan (0.3–7 mg/min IV infusion)	Reversible
Lethal catatonia (↓ heat dissipation)	Lead poisoning	Hyperthermia, intense anxiety, **destructive behavior, psychosis**	Lorazepam (1–2 mg IV q4h), antipsychotics may be contraindicated	High mortality if untreated
Neuroleptic malignant syndrome (mixed: hypothalamic, ↓ heat dissipation, ↑ heat production)	Antipsychotics (neuroleptics), methyldopa, reserpine	Hyperthermia, **muscle rigidity, diaphoresis (60%),** leukocytosis, delirium, **rhabdomyolysis, elevated CPK,** autonomic deregulation, **extrapyramidal symptoms**	**Bromocriptine (2–10 mg q8h PO or nasogastric tube),** lisuride (0.02–0.1 mg/hr IV infusion), carbidopa-levodopa (Sinemet) (25/100 PO q8h), dantrolene sodium (0.3–1 mg/kg IV q6h)	Rapid onset, 20% mortality if untreated

[a]Boldface indicates features that may be used to distinguish one syndrome from another. NSAID, nonsteroidal anti-inflammatory drugs; PO, orally; MAOI, monoamine oxidase inhibitors; NMJ, neuromuscular junction; CNS, central nervous system; CPK, creatine phosphokinase; IV, intravenously.
[b]Gastric lavage and supportive measures, including cooling, are required in most cases.
[c]Oxygen consumption increases by 7% for every 1°F up in body temperature.
[d]Has been associated with idiosyncratic hepatocellular injury, as well as severe hypotension in one case.
From Theoharides TC, Harris RS, Weckstein D. Neuroleptic malignant-like syndrome due to cyclobenzaprine? (letter). *J Clin Psychopharmacol* 1995;15:80, with permission.

B. Restless legs syndrome. In restless legs syndrome, persons feel deep sensations of creeping inside the calves whenever sitting or lying down. The dysesthesias are rarely painful but are agonizingly relentless and cause an almost irresistible urge to move the legs; thus, this syndrome interferes with sleep and with falling asleep. It peaks in middle age and occurs in 5% of the population. It may occur with the use of selective serotonin reuptake inhibitors.

The syndrome has no established treatment. Symptoms of restless legs syndrome are relieved by movement and by leg massage. When pharmacotherapy is required, the benzodiazepines, levodopa, quinine, opioids, propranolol (Inderal), valproate (Depakene), and carbamazepine (Tegretol) are of some benefit.

IX. Hyperthermic Syndromes

All the medication-induced movement disorders may be associated with hyperthermia. Table 31–5 lists the various conditions associated with hyperthermia. Electroconvulsive therapy has been reported to be of use when other agents have failed.

For a more detailed discussion of this topic, see Neuropsychiatric Aspects of Movement Disorders, Sec 2.6, p. 481, Medication-Induced Movement Disorders, Sec 31.3, p. 2996; and First-Generation Antipsychotics, Sec 31.17, p. 3105, in CTP/IX.

Legal and Ethical Issues in Psychiatry

I. Introduction

There are four major factors that fall within the realm for forensic psychiatry: (1) the psychiatrist's professional, ethical, and legal duties are to provide competent care to patients; (2) the patient's rights of self-determination to receive or refuse treatment; (3) court decisions, legislative directives, governmental regulatory agencies, and licensure boards; and (4) the ethical codes and practice guidelines of professional organizations.

II. Medical Malpractice

To prove malpractice, the plaintiff (e.g., patient, family, or estate) must establish, by a preponderance of evidence that: **(1)** a doctor–patient relationship existed and created a duty of care; **(2)** a deviation from the standard of care occurred; **(3)** the patient was damaged; and **(4)** the deviation caused the damage.

These elements are often referred to as the *4 Ds* of malpractice (duty, deviation, damage, direct-causation). Each of the four elements of a malpractice claim must be present or there can be no liability. For example, a psychiatrist whose actions cause direct harm is not liable if no doctor–patient relationship has been established. In addition to negligence, psychiatrists may be sued for intentional torts such as assault, battery, false imprisonment, defamation, fraud, or misrepresentation in a case; invasion of privacy; and intentional infliction of emotional distress.

III. Split Treatment

A. In split treatment, the psychiatrist provides medication, and a nonmedical therapist conducts psychotherapy.

B. The psychiatrist retains full responsibility for the patient's care in a split treatment situation.

C. It is important that the psychiatrist does a thorough evaluation, including obtaining prior medical records.

D. Prescribing medication, outside of a working doctor–patient relationship, does not meet generally accepted standards of good clinical care and may lead to malpractice action.

E. It is important that the psychiatrist remain thoroughly informed of the patient's status and efficacy of any prescribed drug treatments. It is also imperative that the psychiatrist maintain a direct involvement in the patient's care.

IV. Privilege and Confidentiality

A. **Privilege.** The right to maintain secrecy and confidentiality in the face of a subpoena.

1. Privileged communications within a relationship, such as husband–wife, priest–penitent, doctor–patient, are protected from forced disclosure on the witness stand.
2. The right to privilege belongs to the patient, not the physician, and the patient can waive the right if they choose.
3. Privilege does not exist at all in military courts, regardless to whether or not the physician is military or civilian.

B. **Confidentiality.** The long held promise of medical ethics, which binds the physician to hold secret all information given by the patient.
   1. Confidentiality applies to a population sharing information without specific permission of the patient. The circle of confidentiality does not only include the physician, but also encompasses all staff members, clinical supervisors, and consultants involved in the patient's care.
   2. A subpoena can force a psychiatrist to breach confidentiality.
   3. Physicians are usually served with a *subpoena duces tecum*, which requires that they also produce their relevant records and documents.
   4. In bona fide emergencies, information may be released in as limited a way as possible in order to carry out the necessary interventions. Clinical practices dictate that, if at all possible, the psychiatrist should make an effort to obtain the patient's permission and should debrief the patient after the emergency situation has been resolved.
   5. Though oral permission is sufficient, it is always best to obtain written permission from the patient. It should be noted that each release is only good for one piece of information and permission should be obtained for each subsequent release, even to the same party.
   6. Finally, release constitutes permission and not obligation. If the psychiatrist feels that releasing said information would be destructive, the matter may be discussed, and the release may be refused, with some expectations.

C. **Child abuse.** Many states require that all physicians take a course on child abuse for medical licensure. All states legally require that psychiatrists, among others, who have reason to believe that a child has been abused, sexually or otherwise, immediately report their suspicions to the appropriate agency. In this situation, the potential harm to a child greatly outweighs the value of confidentiality in a psychiatric setting.

V. High-Risk Clinical Situations

A. **Suicidal Patients.** Psychiatrists can be sued if their patient commits suicide, particularly in the case of inpatient suicide, where psychiatrists are expected to have greater control of the patient's behavior. Suicide is a rare event, and the evaluation of a suicide risk is one of the most complex, dauntingly difficult clinical tasks, and as of now, there is no way to accurately predict whether or not a patient will commit suicide.

B. **Violent patients.** Psychiatrists treating violent or potentially violent patients can be sued for failure to control aggressive outpatients, for the discharge of violent inpatients, and for the failure to protect society from a patient's violent actions. In most states, if a patient threatens to harm another person, it is required that the physician intervene to prevent harm from occurring. The options to warn and protect include voluntary hospitalization, involuntary hospitalization, warning the victim of the threat, notifying the police, adjusting medication, and seeing the patient more frequently.

VI. Hospitalization: Procedures of Admission

The American Bar Association has specifically endorsed four procedures of admission to psychiatric facilities: informal admission, voluntary admission, temporary admission, and involuntary admission. These procedures are intended to safeguard civil liberties and to ensure that no person is railroaded into a mental hospital. Though each of the 50 states has the power to enact its own laws in regards to psychiatric hospitalization, the above-mentioned procedures are gaining much acceptance.

A. **Informal Admission.** Informal admission operates under the general hospital model, in which a psychiatric patient is admitted to the psychiatric unit in the same way that a medical or surgical patient is admitted to a medical ward.

B. **Voluntary Admission.** Patients who are voluntarily admitted to the psychiatric unit either do so under the advice of a physician or they seek treatment on their own. Such patients apply in writing for admission to the psychiatric unit and maintain an ordinary doctor–patient relationship, and are free to leave, even against medical advice.

C. **Temporary Admission.** A temporary form of involuntary commitment for patients who are senile, confused, or unable to make their own decisions. In an emergency admission, the patient cannot be hospitalized against his or her will for more than 15 days.

D. **Involuntary Admission.** If patients are a danger to themselves (suicidal) or others (homicidal), they may be admitted to a hospital after a friend or relative applies for admission and two physicians confirm the need for hospitalization. It allows the patient to be hospitalized for 60 days, after which a board consisting of psychiatrists, nonpsychiatric physicians, lawyers, and other impartial parties must review the case.

VII. Right to Treatment

The right of an involuntarily committed patient to active treatment has been enunciated by lower federal courts and enacted in some state statutes.

A. *Wyatt v. Stickney* (1971) set the pattern of reform by requiring treatment in addition to hospitalization. It also required specific changes in the operations of institutions and their programs, including changes in physical conditions, staffing, and quality of treatment provided.

B. *Donaldson v. O'Connor* (1976). The U.S. Supreme Court held that an involuntarily committed person who is not dangerous and who can survive by himself or herself with help must be released from the hospital.

VIII. Right to Refuse Treatment

The right to refuse treatment is a legal doctrine that holds that, except in emergencies, persons cannot be forced to accept treatment against their will. An emergency is defined as a condition in clinical practice that requires immediate intervention to prevent death or serious harm to the patient or another person or to prevent deterioration of the patient's clinical state.

A. *O'Connor v. Donaldson* (1976). The U.S. Supreme Court ruled that harmless mentally ill patients cannot be confined against their will without treatment if they can survive outside. According to the court, a finding of mental illness alone cannot justify a state's confining persons in a hospital against their will. Instead, involuntarily confined patients must be considered dangerous to themselves or others or possibly so unable to care for themselves that they cannot survive outside.

B. As a result of the 1979 case of *Rennie v. Klein*, patients have the right to refuse treatment and to use an appeal process.

C. As a result of the 1981 case of *Roger v. Oken*, patients have an absolute right to refuse treatment, but a guardian may authorize treatment.

IX. Seclusion and Restraint
Seclusion refers to placing and keeping an inpatient in a special room for the purpose of containing a clinical situation that may result in a state of emergency. *Restraint* involves measures designed to confine a patient's bodily movements, such as the use of leather cuffs and anklets or straitjackets. The doctrine of the least restrictive alternative is used (i.e., seclusion should be used only when no less-restrictive alternative is available). Additional restrictions include the following: (1) restraint and seclusion can only be implemented by a written order from an appropriate medical official; (2) orders are to be confined to specific, time-limited periods; (3) a patient's condition must be regularly reviewed and documented; and (4) any extension of an original order must be reviewed and reauthorized.

X. Informed Consent
A. **Informed consent form.** A written document outlining a patient's consent to a proposed procedure or treatment plan. It should include a fair explanation of procedures and their purposes, including the following: (1) identification of procedures that are experimental, (2) discomfort and risks to be expected, (3) disclosure of alternative procedures that may be advantageous, (4) an offer to answer any inquiries concerning the procedures, and (5) instructions that the patient is free to withdraw consent and discontinue participation at any time without prejudice.
B. **Exceptions to the rules of informed consent.**
   1. **Emergencies.** Usually defined in terms of imminent physical danger to the patient or others.
   2. **Therapeutic privilege.** Information that in the opinion of the psychiatrist would harm the patient or be antitherapeutic and that may be withheld on those grounds.

XI. Child Custody
In cases of disputed custody, the almost universally accepted criterion is "the best interest of the child." In that context, the task of the psychiatrist is to provide an expert opinion and supporting data regarding which party should be granted custody to best serve the interests of the child.

The mental disability of a parent can lead to the transfer of custody to the other parent or to a public agency. When the mental disability is chronic and the parent is incapacitated, a procedure for the termination of parental rights may result. That also is the case when evidence of child abuse is pervasive. In the Gault decision (1967), the U.S. Supreme Court held that a juvenile also has constitutional rights to due process and procedural safeguards (e.g., counsel, jury, trials).

XII. Testamentary and Contractual Capacity and Competence
A. **Mental competence.** Psychiatrists often are called on to give an opinion about a person's psychological capacity or competence to perform certain civil and legal functions (e.g., make a will, manage his or her financial affairs). Competence is context related (i.e., the ability to perform a certain function for a particular legal purpose). It is especially important to

emphasize that incompetence in one area does not imply incompetence in any or all areas. A person may have a mental disorder and still be competent.

B. Contracts. When a party to an otherwise legal contract is mentally ill and the illness directly and adversely affects the person's ability to understand what he or she is doing (called **contractual capacity**), the law may void the contract. The psychiatrist must evaluate the condition of the party seeking to void the contract at the time that the contract was supposedly entered into. The psychiatrist must then render an opinion as to whether the psychological condition of the party caused an incapacity to understand the important aspects or ramifications of the contract.

C. Wills. The criteria concerning wills (called *testamentary capacity*) are whether, when the will was made, the testator was capable of knowing without prompting (1) the nature of the act, (2) the nature and extent of his or her property, and (3) the natural objects of his or her bounty and their claims on him or her (e.g., heirs, relatives, family members). The mental health of the testator also will indicate whether he or she was in such a condition as to be subject to undue influence.

D. Marriage. A marriage may be void or voidable if one of the parties was incapacitated because of mental illness such that he or she could not reasonably understand the nature and consequences of the transaction (i.e., consent).

E. Guardianship. Guardianship involves a court proceeding for the appointment of a guardian in case of a formal adjudication of incompetence. The criterion is whether, by reason of mental illness, a person can manage his or her own affairs.

F. Durable power of attorney. Permits people to make provisions for their own anticipated loss of decision-making capacity. It permits the advance selection of a substitute decision maker.

G. Competence to inform. Involves a patient's interaction with a clinician. A clinician explains to the patient the value of being honest with the clinician and then determines whether the patient is competent to weigh the risks and benefits of withholding information about suicidal or homicidal intent.

XIII. Criminal Law

A. Competence to stand trial. At any point in the criminal justice process, the psychiatrist may be called on to assess a defendant's present competence to be arraigned, be tried, enter a plea, be sentenced, or be executed. The criteria for competence to be tried are whether, in the presence of a mental disorder, the defendant (1) understands the charges against him or her and (2) can assist in his or her defense.

B. Competence to be executed. Requirement for competence rests on three general principles: (1) a person's awareness of what is happening is supposed to heighten the retributive element of the punishment; (2) a competent person who is about to be executed is believed to be in the best position to make whatever peace is appropriate for his or her religious beliefs, including confession and absolution; and (3) a competent person who is about to be executed preserves, until the end, the possibility of recalling a forgotten detail of the events or the crime that may prove exonerating. It is unethical for any clinician to participate in state-mandated executions; a physician's duty to preserve life transcends all other competing requirements.

C. Criminal responsibility (the insanity defense). The criteria for criminal responsibility involve two separate aspects—whether, at the time of the act, as a consequence of mental disorder, the defendant (1) did not know what he or she was doing or that it was wrong (a cognitive test) or (2) could not conform his or her conduct to the requirements of the law (a volitional test).

1. **M'Naghten rule.** The most famous set of criteria for the insanity defense was developed by the House of Lords after the defendant was exculpated in the M'Naghten case (England, 1843). The M'Naghten rule states that the defendant is not guilty by means of insanity if he or she was unaware of the nature, the quality, and consequences of his or her actions due to a mental disease. The M'Naghten rule, therefore, is a cognitive test.

2. **Irresistible impulse.** In 1922, a committee of jurists suggested broadening the concept of insanity in criminal cases to include the irresistible impulse test, which rules that a person charged with a criminal offense is not responsible for an act that was committed under an impulse that the person was unable to resist because of mental illness. The court grants an impulse to be irresistible only when it can be determined that the accused would have committed the act even if a policeman had been at the elbow of the accused.

3. **Model Penal Code.** The American Law Institute incorporates both a cognitive and a volitional test in its Model Penal Code. The criterion for legal insanity set forth in the rule is that "a person is not responsible for criminal conduct if at the time of such conduct he lacks substantial capacity either to appreciate the criminality (wrongfulness) of his conduct (the cognitive prong) or to conform his conduct to the requirements of the law (the volitional prong)." To prevent the inclusion of antisocial behavior, the Model Penal Code adds, "As used in this article, the terms 'mental disease or defect' do not include an abnormality manifested only by repeated criminal or otherwise antisocial conduct."

4. **Durham rule.** The accused is not criminally responsible if his or her unlawful act was the product of mental disease or mental defect.

   a. This rule is derived from the case of *Durham v. United States,* where Judge Bazelon expressly stated that the purpose of the rule was to get good and complete psychiatric testimony. However, in cases using the Durham rule, there was confusion over the terms "product," "disease," and "defect."

   b. In 1972, the Court of Appeals for the District of Columbia, in the *United States v. Brawner* case, discarded the rule and adopted the American Law Institute's Model Penal Code, which is used in federal courts today.

5. **Other tests.** The American Medical Association has proposed limiting insanity exculpation to cases in which the person is so ill that he or she lacks the necessary criminal intent (*mens rea*), thereby all but eliminating the insanity defense and placing a burden on the prisons to accept a large number of persons who are mentally ill. The American Bar Association and the American Psychiatric Association proposed a defense of nonresponsibility, which focuses solely on whether the defendants, as a result of a mental disease or defect, are unable to appreciate the wrongfulness of their conduct. The American Psychiatric Association also urged that "mental illness" be limited to severely abnormal mental conditions.

XIV. Ethical Issues in Psychiatry

Ethics in psychiatry refers to the principles of conduct that govern the behavior of psychiatrists as well as other mental health professionals. As a discipline, ethics deals with what is good and what is bad, what is right and what is wrong, and moral duties, obligations, and responsibilities. See Table 32–1.

For a more detailed discussion of this topic, see Ethics and Forensic Psychiatry, Ch 57, p. 4427, in CTP/IX.

Table 32–1
Ethical Questions and Answers

Topic	Question	Answer
Abandonment	How can psychiatrists avoid being charged with patient abandonment upon retirement?	Retiring psychiatrists are not abandoning patients if they provide their patients with sufficient notice and make every reasonable effort to find follow-up care for the patients.
	Is it ethical to provide only outpatient care to a seriously ill patient who may require hospitalization?	This could constitute abandonment unless the outpatient practitioner or agency arranges for their patients to receive inpatient care from another provider.
Bequests	A dying patient bequeaths his or her estate to his or her treating psychiatrist. Is this ethical?	No. Accepting the bequest seems improper and exploitational of the therapeutic relationship. However, it may be ethical to accept a token bequest from a deceased patient who named his or her psychiatrist in the will without that psychiatrist's knowledge.
Competency	Is it ethical for psychiatrists to perform vaginal exams? Hospital physicals?	Psychiatrists may provide nonpsychiatric medical procedures if they are competent to do so and if the procedures do not preclude effective psychiatric treatment by distorting the transference. Pelvic exams carry a high risk of distorting the transference and would be better performed by another clinician.
	Can ethics committees review issues of physician competency?	Yes. Incompetency is an ethical issue.
Confidentiality	Must confidentiality be maintained after the death of a patient?	Yes. Ethically, confidences survive a patient's death. Exceptions include protecting others from imminent harm or proper legal compulsions.
	Is it ethical to release information about a patient to an insurance company?	Yes, if the information provided is limited to that which is needed to process the insurance claim.
	Can a videotaped segment of a therapy session be used at a workshop for professionals?	Yes, if informed, uncoerced consent has been obtained, anonymity maintained, the audience is advised that editing makes this an incomplete session, and the patient knows the purpose of the videotape.
	Should a physician report mere suspicion of child abuse in a state requiring reporting of child abuse?	No. A physician must make several assessments before deciding whether to report suspected abuse. One must consider whether abuse is ongoing, whether abuse is responsive to treatment, and whether reporting will cause potential harm. Check specific statutes. Make safety for potential victims the top priority.
Conflict of interest	Is there a potential ethical conflict if a psychiatrist has both psychotherapeutic and administrative duties in dealing with students or trainees?	Yes. You must define your role in advance to the trainees or students. Administrative opinions should be obtained from a psychiatrist who is not involved in a treatment relationship with the trainee or student.
Diagnosis without examination	Is it ethical to offer a diagnosis based only on review of records to determine, for insurance purposes, if suicide was the result of the illness?	Yes.

(continued)

Table 32–1—*continued*
Ethical Questions and Answers

Topic	Question	Answer
	Is it ethical for a supervising psychiatrist to sign a diagnosis on an insurance form for services when the psychiatrist has not examined the patient?	Yes, if the psychiatrist ensures that proper care is given and the insurance form clearly indicates the role of supervisor and supervisee.
Exploitation (also see Bequests)	What constitutes exploitation of the therapeutic relationship?	Exploitation occurs when the psychiatrist uses the therapeutic relationship for personal gain. This includes adopting or hiring a patient as well as sexual or financial relationships.
Fee splitting	What is fee splitting?	Fee splitting occurs when one physician pays another for a patient referral. This would also apply to lawyers giving a forensic psychiatrist referrals in exchange for a percentage of the fee. Fee splitting may occur in an office setting if the psychiatrist takes a percentage of his or her office mates' fees for supervision or expenses. Costs for such items or services must be arranged separately. Otherwise, it would appear that the office owner could benefit from referring patients to a colleague in the office. Fee splitting is illegal.
Informed consent	Is it ethical to refuse to divulge information about a patient who has agreed to give this information to those requesting it?	No. It is the patient's decision, not the therapist's.
	Is informed consent needed when presenting or writing about case material?	Not if the patient is aware of the supervisor/teaching process and confidentiality is preserved.
Moonlighting	Can psychiatric residents ethically "moonlight?"	They can if their duties are not beyond their ability, if they are properly supervised, and if the moonlighting does not interfere with their residency training.
Reporting	Should psychiatrists expose or report unethical behavior of a colleague or colleagues? Can a spouse bring an ethical complaint?	Psychiatrists are obligated to report colleagues' unethical behaviors. A spouse with knowledge of unethical behavior can bring an ethical complaint as well.
Research	How can ethical research be performed with subjects who cannot give informed consent?	Consent can be given by a legal guardian or via a living will. Incompetent persons have the right to withdraw from the research project at any time.
Retirement	See Abandonment.	
Supervision	What are the ethical requirements when a psychiatrist supervises other mental health professionals?	The psychiatrist must spend sufficient time to ensure that proper care is given and that the supervisees are not providing services that are outside the scope of their training. It is ethical to charge a fee for supervision.
Taping and recording	Can videotapes of patient interviews be used for training purposes on a national level (e.g., workshops, board exam preparation)?	Appropriate and explicit informed consent must be obtained. The purpose and scope of exposure of the tape must be emphasized in addition to the resulting loss of confidentiality.

Table by Eugene Rubin, M.D. Adapted from American Psychiatric Association: *Opinions of the Ethics Committee on the Principles of Medical Ethics with Annotation Especially Applicable to Psychiatry.* Washington, DC: 1995.

Glossary of Signs and Symptoms

Signs are objective. Symptoms are subjective. Signs are the clinician's observations, such as noting a agitation; symptoms are the patient's experiences, such as a complaint of feeling depressed. In psychiatry, signs and symptoms are not as clearly demarcated as in other fields of medicine; they often overlap. Because of this, disorders in psychiatry are often described as syndromes—a constellation of signs and symptoms that together make up a recognizable condition.

abreaction A process by which repressed material, particularly a painful experience or a conflict, is brought back to consciousness; in this process, the person not only recalls, but also relives the repressed material, which is accompanied by the appropriate affective response.

abstract thinking Thinking characterized by the ability to grasp the essentials of a whole, to break a whole into its parts, and to discern common properties. To think symbolically.

abulia Reduced impulse to act and to think, associated with indifference about consequences of action. Occurs as a result of neurological deficit, depression, and schizophrenia.

acalculia Loss of ability to do calculations; not caused by anxiety or impairment in concentration. Occurs with neurological deficit and learning disorder.

acataphasia Disordered speech in which statements are incorrectly formulated. Patients may express themselves with words that sound like the ones intended but are not appropriate to the thoughts, or they may use totally inappropriate expressions.

acathexis Lack of feeling associated with an ordinarily emotionally charged subject; in psychoanalysis, it denotes the patient's detaching or transferring of emotion from thoughts and ideas. Also called *decathexis*. Occurs in anxiety, dissociative, schizophrenic, and bipolar disorders.

acenesthesia Loss of sensation of physical existence.

acrophobia Dread of high places.

acting out Behavioral response to an unconscious drive or impulse that brings about temporary partial relief of inner tension; relief is attained by reacting to a present situation as if it were the situation that originally gave rise to the drive or impulse. Common in borderline states.

aculalia Nonsense speech associated with marked impairment of comprehension. Occurs in mania, schizophrenia, and neurological deficit.

adiadochokinesia Inability to perform rapid alternating movements. Occurs with neurological deficit and cerebellar lesions.

adynamia Weakness and fatigability, characteristic of neurasthenia and depression.

aerophagia Excessive swallowing of air. Seen in anxiety disorder.

affect The subjective and immediate experience of emotion attached to ideas or mental representations of objects. Affect has outward manifestations that may be classified as restricted, blunted, flattened, broad, labile, appropriate, or inappropriate. *See also* **mood.**

ageusia Lack or impairment of the sense of taste. Seen in depression and neurological deficit.

aggression Forceful, goal-directed action that may be verbal or physical; the motor counterpart of the affect of rage, anger, or hostility. Seen in neurological deficit, temporal lobe disorder, impulse-control disorders, mania, and schizophrenia.

agitation Severe anxiety associated with motor restlessness.

agnosia Inability to understand the import or significance of sensory stimuli; cannot be explained by a defect in sensory pathways or cerebral lesion; the term has also been used to refer to the selective loss or disuse of knowledge of specific objects because of emotional circumstances, as seen in certain schizophrenic, anxious, and depressed patients. Occurs with neurological deficit. For types of agnosia, see the specific term.

agoraphobia Morbid fear of open places or leaving the familiar setting of the home. May be present with or without panic attacks.

agraphia Loss or impairment of a previously possessed ability to write.

ailurophobia Dread of cats.

akathisia Subjective feeling of motor restlessness manifested by a compelling need to be in constant movement; may be seen as an extrapyramidal adverse effect of antipsychotic medication. May be mistaken for psychotic agitation.

akinesia Lack of physical movement, as in the extreme immobility of catatonic schizophrenia; may also occur as an extrapyramidal effect of antipsychotic medication.

akinetic mutism Absence of voluntary motor movement or speech in a patient who is apparently alert (as evidenced by eye movements). Seen in psychotic depression and catatonic states.

alexia Loss of the ability to understand written language; not explained by defective visual acuity. *Compare with* **dyslexia.**

alexithymia Inability or difficulty in describing or being aware of one's emotions or moods; elaboration of fantasies associated with depression, substance abuse, and posttraumatic stress disorder (PTSD).

algophobia Dread of pain.

alogia Inability to speak because of a mental deficiency or an episode of dementia.

ambivalence Coexistence of two opposing impulses toward the same thing in the same person at the same time. Seen in schizophrenia, borderline states, and obsessive–compulsive disorders (OCDs).

amimia Lack of the ability to make gestures or to comprehend those made by others.

amnesia Partial or total inability to recall past experiences; may be organic (*amnestic disorder*) or emotional (*dissociative amnesia*) in origin.

amnestic aphasia Disturbed capacity to name objects, even though they are known to the patient. Also called *anomic aphasia.*

anaclitic Depending on others, especially as the infant depends on the mother; anaclitic depression in children results from an absence of mothering.

analgesia State in which one feels little or no pain. Can occur under hypnosis and in dissociative disorder.

anancasm Repetitious or stereotyped behavior or thought usually used as a tension-relieving device; used as a synonym for obsession and seen in obsessive–compulsive (anankastic) personality.

androgyny Combination of culturally determined female and male characteristics in one person.

anergia Lack of energy.

anhedonia Loss of interest in, and withdrawal from, all regular and pleasurable activities. Often associated with depression.

anomia Inability to recall the names of objects.

anorexia Loss of or decrease in appetite. In *anorexia nervosa*, appetite may be preserved, but the patient refuses to eat.

anosognosia Inability to recognize a physical deficit in oneself (e.g., patient denies paralyzed limb).

anterograde amnesia Loss of memory for events subsequent to the onset of the amnesia; common after trauma. *Compare with* **retrograde amnesia.**

anxiety Feeling of apprehension caused by anticipation of danger, which may be internal or external.

apathy Dulled emotional tone associated with detachment or indifference; observed in certain types of schizophrenia and depression.

aphasia Any disturbance in the comprehension or expression of language caused by a brain lesion. For types of aphasia, see the specific term.

aphonia Loss of voice. Seen in conversion disorder.

apperception Awareness of the meaning and significance of a particular sensory stimulus as modified by one's own experiences, knowledge, thoughts, and emotions. *See also* **perception.**

appropriate affect Emotional tone in harmony with the accompanying idea, thought, or speech.

apraxia Inability to perform a voluntary purposeful motor activity; cannot be explained by paralysis or other motor or sensory impairment. In *constructional apraxia*, a patient cannot draw two- or three-dimensional forms.

astasia abasia Inability to stand or to walk in a normal manner, even though normal leg movements can be performed in a sitting or lying down position. Seen in conversion disorder.

astereognosis Inability to identify familiar objects by touch. Seen with neurological deficit. *See also* **neurological amnesia.**

asyndesis Disorder of language in which the patient combines unconnected ideas and images. Commonly seen in schizophrenia.

ataxia Lack of coordination, physical or mental. (1) In neurology, refers to loss of muscular coordination. (2) In psychiatry, the term *intrapsychic ataxia* refers to lack of coordination between feelings and thoughts; seen in schizophrenia and in severe OCD.

atonia Lack of muscle tone. *See* **waxy flexibility.**

attention Concentration; the aspect of consciousness that relates to the amount of effort exerted in focusing on certain aspects of an experience, activity, or task. Usually impaired in anxiety and depressive disorders.

auditory hallucination False perception of sound, usually voices, but also other noises, such as music. Most common hallucination in psychiatric disorders.

aura (1) Warning sensations, such as automatisms, fullness in the stomach, blushing, and changes in respiration, cognitive sensations, and mood states usually experienced before a seizure. (2) A sensory prodrome that precedes a classic migraine headache.

autistic thinking Thinking in which the thoughts are largely narcissistic and egocentric, with emphasis on subjectivity rather than objectivity, and without regard for reality; used interchangeably with autism and dereism. Seen in schizophrenia and autistic disorder.

behavior Sum total of the psyche that includes impulses, motivations, wishes, drives, instincts, and cravings, as expressed by a person's behavior or motor activity. Also called *conation.*

bereavement Feeling of grief or desolation, especially at the death or loss of a loved one.

bizarre delusion False belief that is patently absurd or fantastic (e.g., invaders from space have implanted electrodes in a person's brain). Common in schizophrenia. In nonbizarre delusion, content is usually within the range of possibility.

blackout Amnesia experienced by alcoholics about behavior during drinking bouts; usually indicates reversible brain damage.

blocking Abrupt interruption in train of thinking before a thought or idea is finished; after a brief pause, the person indicates no recall of what was being said or was going to be said (also known as *thought deprivation* or *increased thought latency*). Common in schizophrenia and severe anxiety.

blunted affect Disturbance of affect manifested by a severe reduction in the intensity of externalized feeling tone; one of the fundamental symptoms of schizophrenia, as outlined by Eugen Bleuler.

bradykinesia Slowness of motor activity, with a decrease in normal spontaneous movement.

bradylalia Abnormally slow speech. Common in depression.

bradylexia Inability to read at normal speed.

bruxism Grinding or gnashing of the teeth, typically occurring during sleep. Seen in anxiety disorder.

carebaria Sensation of discomfort or pressure in the head.

catalepsy Condition in which persons maintain the body position into which they are placed; observed in severe cases of catatonic schizophrenia. Also called *waxy flexibility* and *cerea flexibilitas. See also* **command automatism.**

cataplexy Temporary sudden loss of muscle tone, causing weakness and immobilization; can be precipitated by a variety of emotional states and is often followed by sleep. Commonly seen in narcolepsy.

catatonic excitement Excited, uncontrolled motor activity seen in catatonic schizophrenia. Patients in catatonic state may suddenly erupt into an excited state and may be violent.

catatonic posturing Voluntary assumption of an inappropriate or bizarre posture, generally maintained for long periods of time. May switch unexpectedly with catatonic excitement.

catatonic rigidity Fixed and sustained motoric position that is resistant to change.

catatonic stupor Stupor in which patients ordinarily are well aware of their surroundings.

cathexis In psychoanalysis, a conscious or unconscious investment of psychic energy in an idea, concept, object, or person. *Compare with* **acathexis.**

causalgia Burning pain that may be organic or psychic in origin.

cenesthesia Change in the normal quality of feeling tone in a part of the body.

cephalgia Headache.

cerea flexibilitas Condition of a person who can be molded into a position that is then maintained; when an examiner moves the person's limb, the limb feels as if it were made of wax. Also called *catalepsy* or *waxy flexibility.* Seen in schizophrenia.

chorea Movement disorder characterized by random and involuntary quick, jerky, purposeless movements. Seen in Huntington's disease.

circumstantiality Disturbance in the associative thought and speech processes in which a patient digresses into unnecessary details and inappropriate thoughts before communicating the central idea. Observed in schizophrenia, obsessional disturbances, and certain cases of dementia. *See also* **tangentiality.**

clang association Association or speech directed by the sound of a word rather than by its meaning; words have no logical connection; punning and rhyming may dominate the verbal behavior. Seen most frequently in schizophrenia or mania.

claustrophobia Abnormal fear of closed or confining spaces.

clonic convulsion An involuntary, violent muscular contraction or spasm in which the muscles alternately contract and relax. Characteristic phase in grand mal epileptic seizure.

clouding of consciousness Any disturbance of consciousness in which the person is not fully awake, alert, and oriented. Occurs in delirium, dementia, and cognitive disorder.

cluttering Disturbance of fluency involving an abnormally rapid rate and erratic rhythm of speech that impedes intelligibility; the affected individual is usually unaware of communicative impairment.

cognition Mental process of knowing and becoming aware; function is closely associated with judgment.

coma State of profound unconsciousness from which a person cannot be roused, with minimal or no detectable responsiveness to stimuli; seen in injury or disease of the brain, in systemic conditions such as diabetic ketoacidosis and uremia, and in intoxications with alcohol and other drugs. Coma may also occur in severe catatonic states and in conversion disorder.

coma vigil Coma in which a patient appears to be asleep but can be aroused (also known as *akinetic mutism*).

command automatism Condition associated with catalepsy in which suggestions are followed automatically.

command hallucination False perception of orders that a person may feel obliged to obey or unable to resist.

complex A feeling-toned idea.

complex partial seizure A seizure characterized by alterations in consciousness that may be accompanied by complex hallucinations (sometimes olfactory) or illusions. During the seizure, a state of impaired consciousness resembling a dreamlike state may occur, and the patient may exhibit repetitive, automatic, or semipurposeful behavior.

compulsion Pathological need to act on an impulse that, if resisted, produces anxiety; repetitive behavior in response to an obsession or performed according to certain rules, with no true end in itself other than to prevent something from occurring in the future.

conation That part of a person's mental life concerned with cravings, strivings, motivations, drives, and wishes, as expressed through behavior or motor activity.

concrete thinking Thinking characterized by actual things, events, and immediate experience, rather than by abstractions; seen in young children, in those who have lost or never developed the ability to generalize (as in certain cognitive mental disorders), and in schizophrenic persons. *Compare with* **abstract thinking.**

condensation Mental process in which one symbol stands for a number of components.

confabulation Unconscious filling of gaps in memory by imagining experiences or events that have no basis in fact, commonly seen in amnestic syndromes; should be differentiated from lying. *See also* **paramnesia.**

confusion Disturbances of consciousness manifested by a disordered orientation in relation to time, place, or person.

consciousness State of awareness, with response to external stimuli.

constipation Inability to defecate or difficulty in defecating.

constricted affect Reduction in intensity of feeling tone that is less severe than that of blunted affect.

constructional apraxia Inability to copy a drawing, such as a cube, clock, or pentagon, as a result of a brain lesion.

conversion phenomena The development of symbolic physical symptoms and distortions involving the voluntary muscles or special sense organs; not under voluntary control and not explained by any physical disorder. Most common in conversion disorder, but also seen in a variety of mental disorders.

convulsion An involuntary, violent muscular contraction or spasm. *See also* **clonic convulsion** *and* **tonic convulsion.**

coprolalia Involuntary use of vulgar or obscene language. Observed in some cases of schizophrenia and in Tourette's syndrome.

coprophagia Eating of filth or feces.

cryptographia A private written language.

cryptolalia A private spoken language.

cycloplegia Paralysis of the muscles of accommodation in the eye; observed, at times, as an autonomic adverse effect (anticholinergic effect) of antipsychotic or antidepressant medication.

decompensation Deterioration of psychic functioning caused by a breakdown of defense mechanisms. Seen in psychotic states.

déjà entendu Illusion that what one is hearing one has heard previously. *See also* **paramnesia.**

déjà pensé Condition in which a thought never entertained before is incorrectly regarded as a repetition of a previous thought. *See also* **paramnesia.**

déjà vu Illusion of visual recognition in which a new situation is incorrectly regarded as a repetition of a previous experience. *See also* **paramnesia.**

delirium Acute reversible mental disorder characterized by confusion and some impairment of consciousness; generally associated with emotional lability, hallucinations or illusions, and inappropriate, impulsive, irrational, or violent behavior.

delirium tremens Acute and sometimes fatal reaction to withdrawal from alcohol, usually occurring 72 to 96 hours after the cessation of heavy drinking; distinctive characteristics are marked autonomic hyperactivity (tachycardia, fever, hyperhidrosis, and dilated pupils), usually accompanied by tremulousness, hallucinations, illusions, and delusions. Called *alcohol withdrawal delirium* in *DSM-IV-TR. See also* **formication.**

delusion False belief, based on incorrect inference about external reality, that is firmly held despite objective and obvious contradictory proof or evidence and despite the fact that other members of the culture do not share the belief.

delusion of control False belief that a person's will, thoughts, or feelings are being controlled by external forces.

delusion of grandeur Exaggerated conception of one's importance, power, or identity.

delusion of infidelity False belief that one's lover is unfaithful. Sometimes called *pathological jealousy.*

delusion of persecution False belief of being harassed or persecuted; often found in litigious patients who have a pathological tendency to take legal action because of imagined mistreatment. Most common delusion.

delusion of poverty False belief that one is bereft or will be deprived of all material possessions.

delusion of reference False belief that the behavior of others refers to oneself or that events, objects, or other people have a particular and unusual significance, usually of a negative nature; derived from idea of reference, in which persons falsely feel that others are talking about them (e.g., belief that people on television or radio are talking to or about the person). *See also* **thought broadcasting.**

delusion of self-accusation False feeling of remorse and guilt. Seen in depression with psychotic features.

dementia Mental disorder characterized by general impairment in intellectual functioning without clouding of consciousness; characterized by failing memory, difficulty with calculations, distractibility, alterations in mood and affect, impaired judgment and abstraction, reduced facility with language, and disturbance of orientation. Although irreversible because of underlying progressive degenerative brain disease, dementia may be reversible if the cause can be treated.

denial Defense mechanism in which the existence of unpleasant realities is disavowed; refers to keeping out of conscious awareness of any aspects of external reality that, if acknowledged, would produce anxiety.

depersonalization Sensation of unreality concerning oneself, parts of oneself, or one's environment that occurs under extreme stress or fatigue. Seen in schizophrenia, depersonalization disorder, and schizotypal personality disorder.

depression Mental state characterized by feelings of sadness, loneliness, despair, low self-esteem, and self-reproach; accompanying signs include psychomotor retardation or, at times, agitation, withdrawal from interpersonal contact, and vegetative symptoms, such as insomnia and anorexia. The term refers to a mood that is so characterized or a mood disorder.

derailment Gradual or sudden deviation in train of thought without blocking; sometimes used synonymously with *loosening of association.*

derealization Sensation of changed reality or that one's surroundings have altered. Usually seen in schizophrenia, panic attacks, and dissociative disorders.

dereism Mental activity that follows a totally subjective and idiosyncratic system of logic and fails to take the facts of reality or experience into consideration. Characteristic of schizophrenia. *See also* **autistic thinking.**

detachment Characterized by distant interpersonal relationships and lack of emotional involvement.

devaluation Defense mechanism in which a person attributes excessively negative qualities to self or others. Seen in depression and paranoid personality disorder.

diminished libido Decreased sexual interest and drive.

dipsomania Compulsion to drink alcoholic beverages.

disinhibition (1) Removal of an inhibitory effect, as in the reduction of the inhibitory function of the cerebral cortex by alcohol. (2) In psychiatry, a greater freedom to act in accordance with inner drives or feelings and with less regard for restraints dictated by cultural norms or one's superego.

disorientation Confusion; impairment of awareness of time, place, and person (the position of the self in relation to other persons). Characteristic of cognitive disorders.

displacement Unconscious defense mechanism by which the emotional component of an unacceptable idea or object is transferred to a more acceptable one. Seen in phobias.

dissociation Unconscious defense mechanism involving the segregation of any group of mental or behavioral processes from the rest of the person's psychic activity; may entail the separation of an idea from its accompanying emotional tone, as seen in dissociative and conversion disorders. Seen in dissociative disorders.

distractibility Inability to focus one's attention; the patient does not respond to the task at hand but attends to irrelevant phenomena in the environment.

dread Massive or pervasive anxiety, usually related to a specific danger.

dreamy state Altered state of consciousness, likened to a dream situation, that develops suddenly and usually lasts a few minutes; accompanied by visual, auditory, and olfactory hallucinations. Commonly associated with temporal lobe lesions.

drowsiness State of impaired awareness associated with a desire or inclination to sleep.

dysarthria Difficulty in articulation, the motor activity of shaping phonated sounds into speech, not in word finding or in grammar.

dyscalculia Difficulty in performing calculations.

dysgeusia Impaired sense of taste.

dysgraphia Difficulty in writing.

dyskinesia Difficulty in performing movements. Seen in extrapyramidal disorders.

dyslalia Faulty articulation caused by structural abnormalities of the articulatory organs or impaired hearing.

dyslexia Specific learning disability syndrome involving an impairment of the previously acquired ability to read; unrelated to the person's intelligence. *Compare with* **alexia.**

dysmetria Impaired ability to gauge distance relative to movements. Seen in neurological deficit.

dysmnesia Impaired memory.

dyspareunia Physical pain in sexual intercourse, usually emotionally caused and more commonly experienced by women; may also result from cystitis, urethritis, or other medical conditions.

dysphagia Difficulty in swallowing.

dysphasia Difficulty in comprehending oral language (*reception dysphasia*) or in trying to express verbal language (*expressive dysphasia*).

dysphonia Difficulty or pain in speaking.

dysphoria Feeling of unpleasantness or discomfort; a mood of general dissatisfaction and restlessness. Occurs in depression and anxiety.

dysprosody Loss of normal speech melody (*prosody*). Common in depression.

dystonia Extrapyramidal motor disturbance consisting of slow, sustained contractions of the axial or appendicular musculature; one movement often predominates, leading to relatively sustained postural deviations; acute dystonic reactions (facial grimacing and torticollis) are occasionally seen with the initiation of antipsychotic drug therapy.

echolalia Psychopathological repeating of words or phrases of one person by another; tends to be repetitive and persistent. Seen in certain kinds of schizophrenia, particularly the catatonic types.

ego-alien Denoting aspects of a person's personality that are viewed as repugnant, unacceptable, or inconsistent with the rest of the personality. Also called *ego-dystonia. Compare with* **ego-syntonic.**

egocentric Self-centered; selfishly preoccupied with one's own needs; lacking interest in others.

ego-dystonic *See* **ego-alien.**

egomania Morbid self-preoccupation or self-centeredness. *See also* **narcissism.**

ego-syntonic Denoting aspects of a personality that are viewed as acceptable and consistent with that person's total personality. Personality traits are usually ego-syntonic. *Compare with* **ego-alien.**

eidetic image Unusually vivid or exact mental image of objects previously seen or imagined.

elation Mood consisting of feelings of joy, euphoria, triumph, and intense self-satisfaction or optimism. Occurs in mania when not grounded in reality.

elevated mood Air of confidence and enjoyment; a mood more cheerful than normal, but not necessarily pathological.

emotion Complex feeling state with psychic, somatic, and behavioral components; external manifestation of emotion is *affect.*

emotional insight A level of understanding or awareness that one has emotional problems. It facilitates positive changes in personality and behavior when present.

emotional lability Excessive emotional responsiveness characterized by unstable and rapidly changing emotions.

encopresis Involuntary passage of feces, usually occurring at night or during sleep.

enuresis Incontinence of urine during sleep.

erotomania Delusional belief, more common in women than in men, that someone is deeply in love with them (also known as *de Clérambault syndrome*).

erythrophobia Abnormal fear of blushing.

euphoria Exaggerated feeling of well-being that is inappropriate to real events. Can occur with drugs such as opiates, amphetamines, and alcohol.

euthymia Normal range of mood, implying absence of depressed or elevated mood.

evasion Act of not facing up to, or strategically eluding, something; consists of suppressing an idea that is next in a thought series and replacing it with another idea closely related to it. Also called *paralogia* and *perverted logic.*

exaltation Feeling of intense elation and grandeur.

excited Agitated, purposeless motor activity uninfluenced by external stimuli.

expansive mood Expression of feelings without restraint, frequently with an overestimation of their significance or importance. Seen in mania and grandiose delusional disorder.

expressive aphasia Disturbance of speech in which understanding remains, but ability to speak is grossly impaired; halting, laborious, and inaccurate speech (also known as *Broca's*, *nonfluent*, and *motor aphasias*).

expressive dysphasia Difficulty in expressing verbal language; the ability to understand language is intact.

externalization More general term than *projection* that refers to the tendency to perceive in the external world and in external objects elements of one's own personality, including instinctual impulses, conflicts, moods, attitudes, and styles of thinking.

extroversion State of one's energies being directed outside oneself. *Compare with* **introversion.**

false memory A person's recollection and belief of an event that did not actually occur. In *false memory syndrome*, persons erroneously believe that they sustained an emotional or physical (e.g., sexual) trauma in early life.

fantasy Daydream; fabricated mental picture of a situation or chain of events. A normal form of thinking dominated by unconscious material that seeks wish fulfillment and solutions to conflicts; may serve as the matrix for creativity. The content of the fantasy may indicate mental illness.

fatigue A feeling of weariness, sleepiness, or irritability after a period of mental or bodily activity. Seen in depression, anxiety, neurasthenia, and somatoform disorders.

fausse reconnaissance False recognition, a feature of paramnesia. Can occur in delusional disorders.

fear Unpleasurable emotional state consisting of psychophysiological changes in response to a realistic threat or danger. *Compare with* **anxiety.**

flat affect Absence or near absence of any signs of affective expression.

flight of ideas Rapid succession of fragmentary thoughts or speech in which content changes abruptly and speech may be incoherent. Seen in mania.

floccillation Aimless plucking or picking, usually at bedclothes or clothing, commonly seen in dementia and delirium.

fluent aphasia Aphasia characterized by inability to understand the spoken word; fluent but incoherent speech is present. Also called *Wernicke's*, *sensory*, and *receptive aphasias.*

folie à deux Mental illness shared by two persons, usually involving a common delusional system; if it involves three persons, it is referred to as *folie à trois*, and so on. Also called *shared psychotic disorder.*

formal thought disorder Disturbance in the form of thought rather than the content of thought; thinking characterized by loosened associations, neologisms, and illogical constructs; thought process is disordered, and the person is defined as psychotic. Characteristic of schizophrenia.

formication Tactile hallucination involving the sensation that tiny insects are crawling over the skin. Seen in cocaine addiction and delirium tremens.

free-floating anxiety Severe, pervasive, generalized anxiety that is not attached to any particular idea, object, or event. Observed particularly in anxiety disorders, although it may be seen in some cases of schizophrenia.

fugue Dissociative disorder characterized by a period of almost complete amnesia, during which a person actually flees from an immediate life situation and begins a different life pattern; apart from the amnesia, mental faculties and skills are usually unimpaired.

galactorrhea Abnormal discharge of milk from the breast; may result from the endocrine influence (e.g., prolactin) of dopamine receptor antagonists, such as phenothiazines.

generalized tonic–clonic seizure Generalized onset of tonic–clonic movements of the limbs, tongue biting, and incontinence followed by slow, gradual recovery of consciousness and cognition; also called *grand mal seizure.*

global aphasia Combination of grossly nonfluent aphasia and severe fluent aphasia.

glossolalia Unintelligible jargon that has meaning to the speaker but not to the listener. Occurs in schizophrenia.

grandiosity Exaggerated feelings of one's importance, power, knowledge, or identity. Occurs in delusional disorder and manic states.

grief Alteration in mood and affect consisting of sadness appropriate to a real loss; normally, it is self-limited. *See also* **depression** *and* **mourning.**

guilt Emotional state associated with self-reproach and the need for punishment. In psychoanalysis, refers to a feeling of culpability that stems from a conflict between the ego and the superego (conscience). Guilt has normal psychological and social functions, but special intensity or absence of guilt characterizes many mental disorders, such as depression and antisocial personality disorder, respectively. Psychiatrists distinguish shame as a less internalized form of guilt that relates more to others than to the self. *See also* **shame.**

gustatory hallucination Hallucination primarily involving taste.

gynecomastia Femalelike development of the male breasts; may occur as an adverse effect of antipsychotic and antidepressant drugs because of increased prolactin levels or anabolic–androgenic steroid abuse.

hallucination False sensory perception occurring in the absence of any relevant external stimulation of the sensory modality involved. For types of hallucinations, see the specific term.

hallucinosis State in which a person experiences hallucinations without any impairment of consciousness.

haptic hallucination Hallucination of touch.

hebephrenia Complex of symptoms, considered a form of schizophrenia, characterized by wild or silly behavior or mannerisms, inappropriate affect, and delusions and hallucinations that are transient and unsystematized. Hebephrenic schizophrenia is now called *disorganized schizophrenia.*

holophrastic Using a single word to express a combination of ideas. Seen in schizophrenia.

hyperactivity Increased muscular activity. The term is commonly used to describe a disturbance found in children that is manifested by constant restlessness, overactivity, distractibility, and difficulties in learning. Seen in *attention-deficit/hyperactivity disorder* (ADHD).

hyperalgesia Excessive sensitivity to pain. Seen in somatoform disorder.

hyperesthesia Increased sensitivity to tactile stimulation.

hypermnesia Exaggerated degree of retention and recall. It can be elicited by hypnosis and may be seen in certain prodigies; also may be a feature of OCD, some cases of schizophrenia, and manic episodes of bipolar I disorder.

hyperphagia Increase in appetite and intake of food.

hyperpragia Excessive thinking and mental activity. Generally associated with manic episodes of bipolar I disorder.

hypersomnia Excessive time spent asleep. May be associated with underlying medical or psychiatric disorder or narcolepsy, may be part of the Kleine–Levin syndrome, or may be primary.

hyperventilation Excessive breathing, generally associated with anxiety, which can reduce blood carbon dioxide concentration and can produce lightheadedness, palpitations, numbness, tingling periorally and in the extremities, and, occasionally, syncope.

hypervigilance Excessive attention to and focus on all internal and external stimuli; usually seen in delusional or paranoid states.

hypesthesia Diminished sensitivity to tactile stimulation.

hypnagogic hallucination Hallucination occurring while falling asleep, not ordinarily considered pathological.

hypnopompic hallucination Hallucination occurring while awakening from sleep, not ordinarily considered pathological.

hypnosis Artificially induced alteration of consciousness characterized by increased suggestibility and receptivity to direction.

hypoactivity Decreased motor and cognitive activity, as in psychomotor retardation; visible slowing of thought, speech, and movements. Also called *hypokinesis.*

hypochondria Exaggerated concern about health that is based not on real medical pathology, but on unrealistic interpretations of physical signs or sensations as abnormal.

hypomania Mood abnormality with the qualitative characteristics of mania but somewhat less intense. Seen in cyclothymic disorder.

idea of reference Misinterpretation of incidents and events in the outside world as having direct personal reference to oneself; occasionally observed in normal persons, but frequently seen in paranoid patients. If present with sufficient frequency or intensity or if organized and systematized, they constitute delusions of reference.

illogical thinking Thinking containing erroneous conclusions or internal contradictions; psychopathological only when it is marked and not caused by cultural values or intellectual deficit.

illusion Perceptual misinterpretation of a real external stimulus. *Compare with* **hallucination.**

immediate memory Reproduction, recognition, or recall of perceived material within seconds after presentation. *Compare with* **long-term memory** *and* **short-term memory.**

impaired insight Diminished ability to understand the objective reality of a situation.

impaired judgment Diminished ability to understand a situation correctly and to act appropriately.

impulse control Ability to resist an impulse, drive, or temptation to perform some action.

inappropriate affect Emotional tone out of harmony with the idea, thought, or speech accompanying it. Seen in schizophrenia.

incoherence Communication that is disconnected, disorganized, or incomprehensible. *See also* **word salad**.

incorporation Primitive unconscious defense mechanism in which the psychic representation of another person or aspects of another person are assimilated into oneself through a figurative process of symbolic oral ingestion; represents a special form of introjection and is the earliest mechanism of identification.

increased libido Increase in sexual interest and drive. Often associated with mania.

ineffability Ecstatic state in which persons insist that their experience is inexpressible and indescribable and that it is impossible to convey what it is like to one who never experienced it.

initial insomnia Falling asleep with difficulty; usually seen in anxiety disorder. *Compare with* **middle insomnia** *and* **terminal insomnia.**

insight Conscious recognition of one's own condition. In psychiatry, it refers to the conscious awareness and understanding of one's own psychodynamics and symptoms of maladaptive behavior; highly important in effecting changes in the personality and behavior of a person.

insomnia Difficulty in falling asleep or difficulty in staying asleep. It can be related to a mental disorder, can be related to a physical disorder or an adverse effect of medication, or can be primary (not related to a known medical factor or another mental disorder). *See also* **initial insomnia, middle insomnia,** *and* **terminal insomnia.**

intellectual insight Knowledge of the reality of a situation without the ability to use that knowledge successfully to effect an adaptive change in behavior or to master the situation. *Compare with* **true insight.**

intelligence Capacity for learning and ability to recall, to integrate constructively, and to apply what one has learned; the capacity to understand and to think rationally.

intoxication Mental disorder caused by recent ingestion or presence in the body of an exogenous substance producing maladaptive behavior by virtue of its effects on the central nervous system (CNS). The most common psychiatric changes involve disturbances of perception, wakefulness, attention, thinking, judgment, emotional control, and psychomotor behavior; the specific clinical picture depends on the substance ingested.

intropunitive Turning anger inward toward oneself. Commonly observed in depressed patients.

introspection Contemplating one's own mental processes to achieve insight.

introversion State in which a person's energies are directed inward toward the self, with little or no interest in the external world.

irrelevant answer Answer that is not responsive to the question.

irritability Abnormal or excessive excitability, with easily triggered anger, annoyance, or impatience.

irritable mood State in which one is easily annoyed and provoked to anger. *See also* **irritability.**

jamais vu Paramnestic phenomenon characterized by a false feeling of unfamiliarity with a real situation that one has previously experienced.

jargon aphasia Aphasia in which the words produced are neologistic, that is, nonsense words created by the patient.

judgment Mental act of comparing or evaluating choices within the framework of a given set of values for the purpose of electing a course of action. If the course of action chosen is consonant with reality or with mature adult standards of behavior, judgment is said to be *intact* or *normal*; judgment is said to be *impaired* if the chosen course of action is frankly maladaptive, results from impulsive decisions based on the need for immediate gratification, or is otherwise not consistent with reality as measured by mature adult standards.

kleptomania Pathological compulsion to steal.

la belle indifférence Inappropriate attitude of calm or lack of concern about one's disability. May be seen in patients with conversion disorder.

labile affect Affective expression characterized by rapid and abrupt changes, unrelated to external stimuli.

labile mood Oscillations in mood between euphoria and depression or anxiety.

laconic speech Condition characterized by a reduction in the quantity of spontaneous speech; replies to questions are brief and unelaborated, and little or no unprompted additional information is provided. Occurs in major depression, schizophrenia, and organic mental disorders. Also called *poverty of speech.*

lethologica Momentary forgetting of a name or proper noun. *See* **blocking.**

lilliputian hallucination Visual sensation that persons or objects are reduced in size; more properly regarded as an illusion. *See also* **micropsia.**

localized amnesia Partial loss of memory; amnesia restricted to specific or isolated experiences. Also called *lacunar amnesia* and *patch amnesia.*

logorrhea Copious, pressured, coherent speech; uncontrollable, excessive talking; observed in manic episodes of bipolar disorder. Also called *tachylogia, verbomania,* and *volubility.*

long-term memory Reproduction, recognition, or recall of experiences or information that was experienced in the distant past. Also called *remote memory. Compare with* **immediate memory** *and* **short-term memory.**

loosening of associations Characteristic schizophrenic thinking or speech disturbance involving a disorder in the logical progression of thoughts, manifested as a failure to communicate verbally adequately; unrelated and unconnected ideas shift from one subject to another. *See also* **tangentiality.**

macropsia False perception that objects are larger than they really are. *Compare with* **micropsia.**

magical thinking A form of dereistic thought; thinking similar to that of the preoperational phase in children (Jean Piaget), in which thoughts, words, or actions assume power (e.g., to cause or to prevent events).

malingering Feigning disease to achieve a specific goal, for example, to avoid an unpleasant responsibility.

mania Mood state characterized by elation, agitation, hyperactivity, hypersexuality, and accelerated thinking and speaking (flight of ideas). Seen in bipolar I disorder. *See also* **hypomania.**

manipulation Maneuvering by patients to get their own way, characteristic of antisocial personalities.

mannerism Ingrained, habitual involuntary movement.

melancholia Severe depressive state. Used in the term *involutional melancholia* as a descriptive term and also in reference to a distinct diagnostic entity.

memory Process whereby what is experienced or learned is established as a record in the CNS (registration), where it persists with a variable degree of permanence (retention) and can be recollected or retrieved from storage at will (recall). For types of memory, see **immediate memory, long-term memory,** and **short-term memory.**

mental disorder Psychiatric illness or disease whose manifestations are primarily characterized by behavioral or psychological impairment of function, measured in terms of deviation from some normative concept; associated with distress or disease, not just an expected response to a particular event or limited to relations between a person and society.

mental retardation Subaverage general intellectual functioning that originates in the developmental period and is associated with impaired maturation and learning, and social maladjustment. Retardation is commonly defined in terms of IQ: mild (between 50 and 55 to 70), moderate (between 35 and 40 to between 50 and 55), severe (between 20 and 25 to between 35 and 40), and profound (below 20 to 25).

metonymy Speech disturbance common in schizophrenia in which the affected person uses a word or phrase that is related to the proper one but is not the one ordinarily used; for example, the patient speaks of consuming a *menu* rather than a *meal*, or refers to losing the *piece of string* of the conversation, rather than the *thread* of the conversation. *See also* **paraphasia** *and* **word approximation.**

microcephaly Condition in which the head is unusually small as a result of defective brain development and premature ossification of the skull.

micropsia False perception that objects are smaller than they really are. Sometimes called *lilliputian hallucination. Compare with* **macropsia.**

middle insomnia Waking up after falling asleep without difficulty and then having difficulty in falling asleep again. *Compare with* **initial insomnia** *and* **terminal insomnia.**

mimicry Simple, imitative motion activity of childhood.

monomania Mental state characterized by preoccupation with one subject.

mood Pervasive and sustained feeling tone that is experienced internally and that, in the extreme, can markedly influence virtually all aspects of a person's behavior and perception of the world. Distinguished from affect, the external expression of the internal feeling tone. For types of mood, see the specific term.

mood-congruent delusion Delusion with content that is mood appropriate (e.g., depressed patients who believe that they are responsible for the destruction of the world).

mood-congruent hallucination Hallucination with content that is consistent with a depressed or manic mood (e.g., depressed patients hearing voices telling them that they are bad persons and manic patients hearing voices telling them that they have inflated worth, power, or knowledge).

mood-incongruent delusion Delusion based on incorrect reference about external reality, with content that has no association to mood or is mood inappropriate (e.g., depressed patients who believe that they are the new Messiah).

mood-incongruent hallucination Hallucination not associated with real external stimuli, with content that is not consistent with depressed or manic mood (e.g., in depression, hallucinations not involving such themes as guilt, deserved punishment, or inadequacy; in mania, not involving such themes as inflated worth or power).

mood swings Oscillation of a person's emotional feeling tone between periods of elation and periods of depression.

motor aphasia Aphasia in which understanding is intact, but the ability to speak is lost. Also called *Broca's, expressive,* or *nonfluent aphasias.*

mourning Syndrome following loss of a loved one, consisting of preoccupation with the lost individual, weeping, sadness, and repeated reliving of memories. *See also* **bereavement** *and* **grief.**

muscle rigidity State in which the muscles remain immovable; seen in schizophrenia.

mutism Organic or functional absence of the faculty of speech. *See also* **stupor.**

mydriasis Dilation of the pupil; sometimes occurs as an autonomic (anticholinergic) or atropinelike adverse effect of some antipsychotic and antidepressant drugs.

narcissism In psychoanalytic theory, divided into primary and secondary types: primary narcissism, the early infantile phase of object relationship development, when the child has not differentiated the self from the outside world, and all sources of pleasure are unrealistically recognized as coming from within the self, giving the child a false sense of omnipotence; secondary narcissism, when the libido, once attached to external love objects, is redirected back to the self. *See also* **autistic thinking.**

needle phobia The persistent, intense, pathological fear of receiving an injection.

negative signs In schizophrenia: flat affect, alogia, abulia, and apathy.

negativism Verbal or nonverbal opposition or resistance to outside suggestions and advice; commonly seen in catatonic schizophrenia in which the patient resists any effort to be moved or does the opposite of what is asked.

neologism New word or phrase whose derivation cannot be understood; often seen in schizophrenia. It has also been used to mean a word that has been incorrectly constructed but whose origins are nonetheless understandable (e.g., *headshoe* to mean *hat*), but such constructions are more properly referred to as *word approximations.*

neurological amnesia (1) Auditory amnesia: loss of ability to comprehend sounds or speech. (2) Tactile amnesia: loss of ability to judge the shape of objects by touch. *See also* **astereognosis.** (3) Verbal amnesia: loss of ability to remember words. (4) Visual amnesia: loss of ability to recall or to recognize familiar objects or printed words.

nihilism Delusion of the nonexistence of the self or part of the self; also refers to an attitude of total rejection of established values or extreme skepticism regarding moral and value judgments.

nihilistic delusion Depressive delusion that the world and everything related to it have ceased to exist.

noesis Revelation in which immense illumination occurs in association with a sense that one has been chosen to lead and command. Can occur in manic or dissociative states.

nominal aphasia Aphasia characterized by difficulty in giving the correct name of an object. *See also* **anomia** *and* **amnestic aphasia.**

nymphomania Abnormal, excessive, insatiable desire in a woman for sexual intercourse. *Compare with* **satyriasis.**

obsession Persistent and recurrent idea, thought, or impulse that cannot be eliminated from consciousness by logic or reasoning; obsessions are involuntary and ego-dystonic. *See also* **compulsion.**

olfactory hallucination Hallucination primarily involving smell or odors; most common in medical disorders, especially in the temporal lobe.

orientation State of awareness of oneself and one's surroundings in terms of time, place, and person.

overactivity Abnormality in motor behavior that can manifest itself as psychomotor agitation, hyperactivity (hyperkinesis), tics, sleepwalking, or compulsions.

overvalued idea False or unreasonable belief or idea that is sustained beyond the bounds of reason. It is held with less intensity or duration than a delusion but is usually associated with mental illness.

panic Acute, intense attack of anxiety associated with personality disorganization; the anxiety is overwhelming and accompanied by feelings of impending doom.

panphobia Overwhelming fear of everything.

pantomime Gesticulation; psychodrama without the use of words.

paramnesia Disturbance of memory in which reality and fantasy are confused. It is observed in dreams and in certain types of schizophrenia and organic mental disorders; it includes phenomena such as *déjà vu* and *déjà entendu*, which may occur occasionally in normal persons.

paranoia Rare psychiatric syndrome marked by the gradual development of a highly elaborate and complex delusional system, generally involving persecutory or grandiose delusions, with few other signs of personality disorganization or thought disorder.

paranoid delusions Includes persecutory delusions and delusions of reference, control, and grandeur.

paranoid ideation Thinking dominated by suspicious, persecutory, or grandiose content of less than delusional proportions.

paraphasia Abnormal speech in which one word is substituted for another, the irrelevant word generally resembling the required one in morphology, meaning, or phonetic composition; the inappropriate word may be a legitimate one used incorrectly, such as *clover* instead of *hand*, or a bizarre nonsense expression, such as *treen* instead of *train*. Paraphasic speech may be seen in organic aphasias and in mental disorders such as schizophrenia. *See also* **metonymy** *and* **word approximation.**

parapraxis Faulty act, such as a slip of the tongue or the misplacement of an article. Freud ascribed parapraxes to unconscious motives.

paresis Weakness or partial paralysis of organic origin.

paresthesia Abnormal spontaneous tactile sensation, such as a burning, tingling, or pins-and-needles sensation.

perception Conscious awareness of elements in the environment by the mental processing of sensory stimuli; sometimes used in a broader sense to refer to the mental process by which all kinds of data, intellectual, emotional, and sensory, are meaningfully organized. *See also* **apperception.**

perseveration (1) Pathological repetition of the same response to different stimuli, as in a repetition of the same verbal response to different questions. (2) Persistent repetition of specific words or concepts in the process of speaking. Seen in cognitive disorders, schizophrenia, and other mental illness. *See also* **verbigeration.**

phantom limb False sensation that an extremity that has been lost is, in fact, present.

phobia Persistent, pathological, unrealistic, intense fear of an object or situation; the phobic person may realize that the fear is irrational but, nonetheless, cannot dispel it. For types of phobias, see the specific term.

pica Craving and eating of nonfood substances, such as paint and clay.

polyphagia Pathological overeating.

positive signs In schizophrenia: hallucinations, delusions, and thought disorder.

posturing Strange, fixed, and bizarre bodily positions held by a patient for an extended time. *See also* **catatonia.**

poverty of content of speech Speech that is adequate in amount but conveys little information because of vagueness, emptiness, or stereotyped phrases.

poverty of speech Restriction in the amount of speech used; replies may be monosyllabic. *See also* **laconic speech.**

preoccupation of thought Centering of thought content on a particular idea, associated with a strong affective tone, such as a paranoid trend or a suicidal or homicidal preoccupation.

pressured speech Increase in the amount of spontaneous speech; rapid, loud, accelerated speech, as occurs in mania, schizophrenia, and cognitive disorders.

primary process thinking In psychoanalysis, the mental activity directly related to the functions of the id and characteristic of unconscious mental processes; marked by primitive, prelogical thinking and by the tendency to seek immediate discharge and gratification of instinctual demands. Includes thinking that is dereistic, illogical, and magical; normally found in dreams, abnormally in psychosis. *Compare with* **secondary process thinking.**

projection Unconscious defense mechanism in which persons attribute to another those generally unconscious ideas, thoughts, feelings, and impulses that are in themselves undesirable or unacceptable as a form of protection from anxiety arising from an inner conflict; by externalizing whatever is unacceptable, they deal with it as a situation apart from themselves.

prosopagnosia Inability to recognize familiar faces that is not due to impaired visual acuity or level of consciousness.

pseudocyesis Rare condition in which a nonpregnant patient has the signs and symptoms of pregnancy, such as abdominal distention, breast enlargement, pigmentation, cessation of menses, and morning sickness.

pseudodementia (1) Dementialike disorder that can be reversed by appropriate treatment and is not caused by organic brain disease. (2) Condition in which patients show exaggerated indifference to their surroundings in the absence of a mental disorder, also occurs in depression and factitious disorders.

pseudologia phantastica Disorder characterized by uncontrollable lying, in which patients elaborate extensive fantasies that they freely communicate and act on.

psychomotor agitation Physical and mental overactivity that is usually nonproductive and is associated with a feeling of inner turmoil, as seen in agitated depression.

psychosis Mental disorder in which the thoughts, affective response, ability to recognize reality, and ability to communicate and relate to others are sufficiently impaired to interfere grossly with the capacity to deal with reality; the classical characteristics of psychosis are impaired reality testing, hallucinations, delusions, and illusions.

psychotic (1) Person experiencing psychosis. (2) Denoting or characteristic of psychosis.

rationalization An unconscious defense mechanism in which irrational or unacceptable behavior, motives, or feelings are logically justified or made consciously tolerable by plausible means.

reaction formation Unconscious defense mechanism in which a person develops a socialized attitude or interest that is the direct antithesis of some infantile wish or impulse that is harbored consciously or unconsciously. One of the earliest and most unstable defense mechanisms, closely related to repression; both are defenses against impulses or urges that are unacceptable to the ego.

reality testing Fundamental ego function that consists of tentative actions that test and objectively evaluate the nature and limits of the environment; includes the ability to differentiate between the external world and the internal world and to accurately judge the relation between the self and the environment.

recall Process of bringing stored memories into consciousness. *See also* **memory.**

recent memory Recall of events over the past few days.

recent past memory Recall of events over the past few months.

receptive aphasia Organic loss of ability to comprehend the meaning of words; fluid and spontaneous, but incoherent and nonsensical, speech. *See also* **fluent aphasia** *and* **sensory aphasia.**

receptive dysphasia Difficulty in comprehending oral language; the impairment involves comprehension and production of language.

regression Unconscious defense mechanism in which a person undergoes a partial or total return to earlier patterns of adaptation; observed in many psychiatric conditions, particularly schizophrenia.

remote memory Recall of events in the distant past.

repression Freud's term for an unconscious defense mechanism in which unacceptable mental contents are banished or kept out of consciousness; important in normal psychological development and in neurotic and psychotic symptom formation. Freud recognized two kinds of repression: (1) repression proper, in which the repressed material was once in the conscious domain, and (2) primal repression, in which the repressed material was never in the conscious realm. *Compare with* **suppression.**

restricted affect Reduction in intensity of feeling tone that is less severe than in blunted affect but clearly reduced. *See also* **constricted affect.**

retrograde amnesia Loss of memory for events preceding the onset of the amnesia. *Compare with* **antero-grade amnesia.**

retrospective falsification Memory becomes unintentionally (unconsciously) distorted by being filtered through a person's present emotional, cognitive, and experiential state.

rigidity In psychiatry, a person's resistance to change, a personality trait.

ritual (1) Formalized activity practiced by a person to reduce anxiety, as in OCD. (2) Ceremonial activity of cultural origin.

rumination Constant preoccupation with thinking about a single idea or theme, as in OCD.

satyriasis Morbid, insatiable sexual need or desire in a man. *Compare with* **nymphomania.**

scotoma (1) In psychiatry, a figurative blind spot in a person's psychological awareness. (2) In neurology, a localized visual field defect.

secondary process thinking In psychoanalysis, the form of thinking that is logical, organized, reality oriented, and influenced by the demands of the environment; characterizes the mental activity of the ego. *Compare with* **primary process thinking.**

seizure An attack or sudden onset of certain symptoms, such as convulsions, loss of consciousness, and psychic or sensory disturbances; seen in epilepsy and can be substance induced. For types of seizures, see the specific term.

sensorium Hypothetical sensory center in the brain that is involved with clarity of awareness about oneself and one's surroundings, including the ability to perceive and to process ongoing events in light of past experiences, future options, and current circumstances; sometimes used interchangeably with *consciousness.*

sensory aphasia Organic loss of ability to comprehend the meaning of words; fluid and spontaneous, but incoherent and nonsensical, speech. *See also* **fluent aphasia** *and* **receptive aphasia.**

sensory extinction Neurological sign operationally defined as failure to report one of two simultaneously presented sensory stimuli, despite the fact that either stimulus alone is correctly reported. Also called *sensory inattention.*

shame Failure to live up to self-expectations; often associated with fantasy of how person will be seen by others. *See also* **guilt.**

short-term memory Reproduction, recognition, or recall of perceived material within minutes after the initial presentation. *Compare with* **immediate memory** *and* **long-term memory.**

simultanagnosia Impairment in the perception or integration of visual stimuli appearing simultaneously.

somatic delusion Delusion pertaining to the functioning of one's body.

somatic hallucination Hallucination involving the perception of a physical experience localized within the body.

somatopagnosia Inability to recognize a part of one's body as one's own (also called *ignorance of the body* and *autotopagnosia*).

somnolence Pathological sleepiness or drowsiness from which one can be aroused to a normal state of consciousness.

spatial agnosia Inability to recognize spatial relations.

speaking in tongues Expression of a revelatory message through unintelligible words; not considered a disorder of thought if associated with practices of specific Pentecostal religions. *See also* **glossolalia.**

stereotypy Continuous mechanical repetition of speech or physical activities; observed in catatonic schizophrenia.

stupor (1) State of decreased reactivity to stimuli and less than full awareness of one's surroundings; as a disturbance of consciousness, it indicates a condition of partial coma or semicoma. (2) In psychiatry, used synonymously with *mutism* and does not necessarily imply a disturbance of consciousness; in *catatonic stupor,* patients are ordinarily aware of their surroundings.

stuttering Frequent repetition or prolongation of a sound or syllable, leading to markedly impaired speech fluency.

sublimation Unconscious defense mechanism in which the energy associated with unacceptable impulses or drives is diverted into personally and socially acceptable channels; unlike other defense mechanisms, it offers some minimal gratification of the instinctual drive or impulse.

substitution Unconscious defense mechanism in which a person replaces an unacceptable wish, drive, emotion, or goal with one that is more acceptable.

suggestibility State of uncritical compliance with influence or of uncritical acceptance of an idea, belief, or attitude; commonly observed among persons with hysterical traits.

suicidal ideation Thoughts or act of taking one's own life.

suppression Conscious act of controlling and inhibiting an unacceptable impulse, emotion, or idea; differentiated from repression in that repression is an unconscious process.

symbolization Unconscious defense mechanism in which one idea or object comes to stand for another because of some common aspect or quality in both; based on similarity and association; the symbols formed protect the person from the anxiety that may be attached to the original idea or object.

synesthesia Condition in which the stimulation of one sensory modality is perceived as sensation in a different modality, as when a sound produces a sensation of color.

syntactical aphasia Aphasia characterized by difficulty in understanding spoken speech, associated with gross disorder of thought and expression.

systematized delusion Group of elaborate delusions related to a single event or theme.

tactile hallucination Hallucination primarily involving the sense of touch. Also called *haptic hallucination.*

tangentiality Oblique, digressive, or even irrelevant manner of speech in which the central idea is not communicated.

tension Physiological or psychic arousal, uneasiness, or pressure toward action; an unpleasurable alteration in mental or physical state that seeks relief through action.

terminal insomnia Early morning awakening or waking up at least 2 hours before planning to wake up. *Compare with* **initial insomnia** *and* **middle insomnia.**

thought broadcasting Feeling that one's thoughts are being broadcast or projected into the environment. *See also* **thought withdrawal.**

thought disorder Any disturbance of thinking that affects language, communication, or thought content; the hallmark feature of schizophrenia. Manifestations range from simple blocking and mild circumstantiality to profound loosening of associations, incoherence, and delusions; characterized by a failure to follow semantic and syntactic rules that is inconsistent with the person's education, intelligence, or cultural background.

thought insertion Delusion that thoughts are being implanted in one's mind by other people or forces.

thought latency The period of time between a thought and its verbal expression. Increased in schizophrenia (*see* **blocking**) and decreased in mania (*see* **pressured speech**).

thought withdrawal Delusion that one's thoughts are being removed from one's mind by other people or forces. *See also* **thought broadcasting.**

tic disorders Predominantly psychogenic disorders characterized by involuntary, spasmodic, stereotyped movement of small groups of muscles; seen most predominantly in moments of stress or anxiety, rarely as a result of organic disease.

tinnitus Noises in one or both ears, such as ringing, buzzing, or clicking; an adverse effect of some psychotropic drugs.

tonic convulsion Convulsion in which the muscle contraction is sustained.

trailing phenomenon Perceptual abnormality associated with hallucinogenic drugs in which moving objects are seen as a series of discrete and discontinuous images.

trance Sleeplike state of reduced consciousness and activity.

tremor Rhythmical alteration in movement, which is usually faster than one beat a second; typically, tremors decrease during periods of relaxation and sleep and increase during periods of anger and increased tension.

true insight Understanding of the objective reality of a situation coupled with the motivational and emotional impetus to master the situation or change behavior.

twilight state Disturbed consciousness with hallucinations.

twirling Sign present in autistic children who continually rotate in the direction in which their head is turned.

unconscious (1) One of three divisions of Freud's topographic theory of the mind (the others being the conscious and the preconscious) in which the psychic material is not readily accessible to conscious awareness by ordinary means; its existence may be manifest in symptom formation, in dreams, or under the influence of drugs. (2) In popular (but more ambiguous) usage, any mental material not in the immediate field of awareness. (3) Denoting a state of unawareness, with lack of response to external stimuli, as in a coma.

undoing Unconscious primitive defense mechanism, repetitive in nature, by which a person symbolically acts out in reverse something unacceptable that has already been done or against which the ego must defend itself; a form of magical expiatory action, commonly observed in OCD.

unio mystica Feeling of mystic unity with an infinite power.

vegetative signs In depression, denoting characteristic symptoms such as sleep disturbance (especially early morning awakening), decreased appetite, constipation, weight loss, and loss of sexual response.

verbigeration Meaningless and stereotyped repetition of words or phrases, as seen in schizophrenia. Also called *cataphasia. See also* **perseveration.**

vertigo Sensation that one or the world around one is spinning or revolving; a hallmark of vestibular dysfunction, not to be confused with dizziness.

visual agnosia Inability to recognize objects or persons.

visual amnesia *See* **neurological amnesia.**

visual hallucination Hallucination primarily involving the sense of sight.

waxy flexibility Condition in which a person maintains the body position into which they are placed. Also called *catalepsy.*

word approximation Use of conventional words in an unconventional or inappropriate way (metonymy or of new words that are developed by conventional rules of word formation) (e.g., *hand shoes* for *gloves* and *time measure* for *clock*); distinguished from a *neologism,* which is a new word whose derivation cannot be understood. *See also* **paraphasia.**

word salad Incoherent, essentially incomprehensible, mixture of words and phrases commonly seen in far-advanced cases of schizophrenia. *See also* **incoherence.**

xenophobia Abnormal fear of strangers.

zoophobia Abnormal fear of animals.

For further information please refer to Comprehensive Glossary of Psychiatry and Psychology by H.I. Kaplan. M.D. and B. J. Sadock, M.D. Williams & Wilkins, Baltimore, 1991.

Index

Page numbers followed by *t* indicate tables.

DSM-IV-TR Classification

NOS, not otherwise specified.

An *x* appearing in a diagnostic code indicates that a specific code number is required.

An ellipsis (. . .) is used in the names of certain disorders to indicate that the name of a specific mental disorder or general medical condition should be inserted when recording the name (e.g., 293.0 Delirium due to hypothyroidism).

If criteria are currently met, one of the following severity specifiers may be noted after the diagnosis:
> Mild
> Moderate
> Severe

If criteria are no longer met, one of the following specifiers may be noted:
> In partial remission
> In full remission
> Prior history

Disorders Usually First Diagnosed in Infancy, Childhood, or Adolescence

---

MENTAL RETARDATION
Note: *These are coded on Axis II.*
317   Mild mental retardation
318.0   Moderate mental retardation
318.1   Severe mental retardation
318.2   Profound mental retardation
319   Mental retardation, severity unspecified

LEARNING DISORDERS
315.00   Reading disorder
315.1   Mathematics disorder
315.2   Disorder of written expression
315.9   Learning disorder NOS

MOTOR SKILLS DISORDER
315.4   Developmental coordination disorder

COMMUNICATION DISORDERS
315.31   Expressive language disorder
315.32   Mixed receptive-expressive language disorder
315.39   Phonological disorder
307.0   Stuttering
307.9   Communication disorder NOS

PERVASIVE DEVELOPMENTAL DISORDERS
299.00   Autistic disorder
299.80   Rett's disorder
299.10   Childhood disintegrative disorder
299.80   Asperger's disorder
299.80   Pervasive developmental disorder NOS

ATTENTION-DEFICIT AND DISRUPTIVE BEHAVIOR DISORDERS
314.xx   Attention-deficit/hyperactivity disorder
     .01   Combined type
     .00   Predominantly inattentive type
     .01   Predominantly hyperactive-impulsive type
314.9   Attention-deficit/hyperactivity disorder NOS
312.xx   Conduct disorder
     .81   Childhood-onset type
     .82   Adolescent-onset type
     .89   Unspecified onset
313.81   Oppositional defiant disorder
312.9   Disruptive behavior disorder NOS

FEEDING AND EATING DISORDERS OF INFANCY OR EARLY CHILDHOOD
307.52   Pica
307.53   Rumination disorder
307.59   Feeding disorder of infancy or early childhood

TIC DISORDERS
307.23   Tourette's disorder
307.22   Chronic motor or vocal tic disorder
307.21   Transient tic disorder (115)
     Specify if: single episode/recurrent
307.20   Tic disorder NOS

ELIMINATION DISORDERS
——.—   Encopresis
787.6   With constipation and overflow incontinence
307.7   Without constipation and overflow incontinence
307.6   Enuresis (not due to a general medical condition)
     Specify type: nocturnal only/diurnal only/nocturnal and diurnal

OTHER DISORDERS OF INFANCY, CHILDHOOD, OR ADOLESCENCE
309.21   Separation anxiety disorder
     Specify if: early onset
313.23   Selective mutism

313.89 Reactive attachment disorder of infancy or early childhood *Specify type:* inhibited type/ disinhibited type

307.3 Stereotypic movement disorder *Specify if:* with self-injurious behavior

313.9 Disorder of infancy, childhood, or adolescence NOS

Delirium, Dementia, and Amnestic and Other Cognitive Disorders

---

DELIRIUM

293.0 Delirium due to . . . *[indicate the general medical condition]*

——.— Substance intoxication delirium *(refer to Substance-Related Disorders for substance-specific codes)*

——.— Substance withdrawal delirium *(refer to Substance-Related Disorders for substance-specific codes)*

——.— Delirium due to multiple etiologies *(code each of the specific etiologies)*

780.09 Delirium NOS

DEMENTIA

294.xx Dementia of the Alzheimer's type, with early onset *(also code 331.0 Alzheimer's disease on Axis III)*
.10 Without behavioral disturbance
.11 With behavioral disturbance

294.xx Dementia of the Alzheimer's type, with late onset *(also code 331.0 Alzheimer's disease on Axis III)*
.10 Without behavioral disturbance
.11 With behavioral disturbance

290.xx Vascular dementia
.40 Uncomplicated
.41 With delirium
.42 With delusions
.43 With depressed mood
Specify if: with behavioral disturbance

Code presence or absence of a behavioral disturbance in the fifth digit for dementia due to a general medical condition:

0 = Without behavioral disturbance
1 = With behavioral disturbance

294.1x Dementia due to HIV disease *(also code 042 HIV on Axis III)*

294.1x Dementia due to head trauma *(also code 854.00 head injury on Axis III)*

294.1x Dementia due to Parkinson's disease *(also code 332.0 Parkinson's disease on Axis III)*

294.1x Dementia due to Huntington's disease *(also code 333.4 Huntington's disease on Axis III)*

294.1x Dementia due to Pick's disease *(also code 331.1 Pick's disease on Axis III)*

294.1x Dementia due to Creutzfeldt-Jakob disease *(also code 046.1 Creutzfeldt-Jakob disease on Axis III)*

294.1x Dementia due to . . . *[indicate the general medical condition not listed above] (also code the general medical condition on Axis III)*

——.— Substance-induced persisting dementia *(refer to Substance-Related Disorders for substance-specific codes)*

——.— Dementia due to multiple etiologies *(code each of the specific etiologies)*

294.8 Dementia NOS

AMNESTIC DISORDERS

294.0 Amnestic disorder due to . . . *[indicate the general medical condition]*
Specify if: transient/chronic

——.— Substance-induced persisting amnestic disorder *(refer to Substance-Related Disorders for substance-specific codes)*

294.8 Amnestic disorder NOS

OTHER COGNITIVE DISORDERS

294.9 Cognitive disorder NOS

Mental Disorders Due to a General Medical Condition Not Elsewhere Classified

---

293.89 Catatonic disorder due to . . . *[indicate the general medical condition]*

310.1 Personality change due to . . . *[indicate the general medical condition]*
Specify type: labile type/ disinhibited type/aggressive type/apathetic type/paranoid type/other type/combined type/unspecified type

293.9 Mental disorder NOS due to . . . *[indicate the general medical condition]*

Substance-Related Disorders

The following specifiers apply to substance dependence as noted:
  [a] With physiological dependence/without physiological dependence
  [b] Early full remission/early partial remission/substained full remission/sustained partial remission
  [c] In a controlled environment
  [d] On agonist therapy

The following specifiers apply to substance-induced disorders as noted:

  [I] With onset during intoxication/[W] With onset during withdrawal

ALCOHOL-RELATED DISORDERS

Alcohol Use Disorders
303.90   Alcohol dependence[a,b,c]
305.00   Alcohol abuse

Alcohol-Induced Disorders
303.00   Alcohol intoxication
291.81   Alcohol withdrawal
         Specify if: with perceptual disturbances
291.0   Alcohol intoxication delirium
291.0   Alcohol withdrawal delirium
291.2   Alcohol-induced persisting dementia
291.1   Alcohol-induced persisting amnestic disorder
291.x   Alcohol-induced psychotic disorder
   .5   With delusions[I,W]
   .3   With hallucinations[I,W]
291.89   Alcohol-induced mood disorder[I,W]
291.89   Alcohol-induced anxiety disorder[I,W]
291.89   Alcohol-induced sexual dysfunction[I]
291.89   Alcohol-induced sleep disorder[I,W]
291.9   Alcohol-related disorder NOS

AMPHETAMINE-(OR AMPHETAMINE-LIKE)-RELATED DISORDERS

Amphetamine Use Disorders
304.40   Amphetamine dependence[a,b,c]
305.70   Amphetamine abuse

Amphetamine-Induced Disorders
292.89   Amphetamine intoxication
         Specify if: with perceptual disturbances
292.0   Amphetamine withdrawal
292.81   Amphetamine intoxication delirium

292.xx   Amphetamine-induced psychotic disorder
   .11   With delusions[I]
   .12   With hallucinations[I]
292.84   Amphetamine-induced mood disorder[I,W]
292.89   Amphetamine-induced anxiety disorder[I]
292.89   Amphetamine-induced sexual dysfunction[I]
292.89   Amphetamine-induced sleep disorder[I,W]
292.9   Amphetamine-related disorder NOS

CAFFEINE-RELATED DISORDER

Caffeine-Induced Disorders
305.90   Caffeine intoxication
292.89   Caffeine-induced anxiety disorder[I]
292.89   Caffeine-induced sleep disorder[I]
292.9   Caffeine-related disorder NOS

CANNABIS-RELATED DISORDERS

Cannabis Use Disorders
304.30   Cannabis dependence[a,b,c]
305.20   Cannabis abuse

Cannabis-Induced Disorders
292.89   Cannabis intoxication
         Specify if: with perceptual disturbances
292.81   Cannabis intoxication delirium
292.xx   Cannabis-induced psychotic disorder
   .11   With delusions[I]
   .12   With hallucinations[I]
292.89   Cannabis-induced anxiety disorder
292.9   Cannabis-related disorder NOS

COCAINE-RELATED DISORDERS

Cocaine Use Disorders
304.20   Cocaine dependence[a,b,c]
305.60   Cocaine abuse

Cocaine-Induced Disorders
292.89   Cocaine intoxication
         Specify if: with perceptual disturbances
292.0   Cocaine withdrawal
292.81   Cocaine intoxication delirium
292.xx   Cocaine-induced psychotic disorder
   .11   With delusions[I]
   .12   With hallucinations[I]
292.84   Cocaine-induced mood disorder[I,W]

292.89   Cocaine-induced anxiety
         disorder[l,w]
292.89   Cocaine-induced sexual
         dysfunction[l]
292.89   Cocaine-induced sleep disorder[l,w]
292.9   Cocaine-related disorder NOS

HALLUCINOGEN-RELATED DISORDERS

Hallucinogen Use Disorders
304.50   Hallucinogen dependence[b,c]
305.30   Hallucinogen abuse

Hallucinogen-Induced Disorders
292.89   Hallucinogen intoxication
292.89   Hallucinogen persisting perception
         disorder (flashbacks)
292.81   Hallucinogen intoxication delirium
292.xx   Hallucinogen-induced psychotic
         disorder
   .11   With delusions[l]
   .12   With hallucinations[l]
292.84   Hallucinogen-induced mood
         disorder[l]
292.89   Hallucinogen-induced anxiety
         disorder[l]
292.9   Hallucinogen-related disorder
         NOS

INHALANT-RELATED DISORDERS

Inhalant Use Disorders
304.60   Inhalant dependence[b,c]
305.90   Inhalant abuse

Inhalant-Induced Disorders
292.89   Inhalant intoxication
292.81   Inhalant intoxication delirium
292.82   Inhalant-induced persisting
         dementia
292.xx   Inhalant-induced psychotic
         disorder
   .11   With delusions[l]
   .12   With hallucinations[l]
292.84   Inhalant-induced mood disorder[l]
292.89   Inhalant-induced anxiety disorder[l]
292.9   Inhalant-related disorder NOS

NICOTINE-RELATED DISORDERS

Nicotine Use Disorder
305.1   Nicotine dependence[a,b]

Nicotine-Induced Disorder
292.0   Nicotine withdrawal
292.9   Nicotine-related disorder NOS

OPIOID-RELATED DISORDERS

Opioid Use Disorders
304.00   Opioid dependence[a,b,c,d]
305.50   Opioid abuse

Opioid-Induced Disorders
292.89   Opioid intoxication
         Specify if: with perceptual
         disturbances
292.0   Opioid withdrawal
292.81   Opioid intoxication delirium
292.xx   Opioid-induced psychotic disorder
   .11   With delusions[l]
   .12   With hallucinations[l]
292.84   Opioid-induced mood disorder[l]
292.89   Opioid-induced sexual dysfunction[l]
292.89   Opioid-induced sleep disorder[l,w]
292.9   Opioid-related disorder NOS

PHENCYCLIDINE- (OR PHENCYCLIDINE-LIKE)–RELATED DISORDERS

Phencyclidine Use Disorders
304.60   Phencyclidine dependence[b,c]
305.90   Phencyclidine abuse

Phencyclidine-Induced Disorders
292.89   Phencyclidine intoxication
         Specify if: with perceptual
         disturbances
292.81   Phencyclidine intoxication delirium
292.xx   Phencyclidine-induced psychotic
         disorder
   .11   With delusions[l]
   .12   With hallucinations[l]
292.84   Phencyclidine-induced mood
         disorder[l]
292.89   Phencyclidine-induced anxiety
         disorder[l]
292.9   Phencyclidine-related disorder
         NOS

SEDATIVE-, HYPNOTIC-, OR ANXIOLYTIC-RELATED DISORDERS

Sedative, Hypnotic, or Anxiolytic Use Disorders
304.10   Sedative, hypnotic, or anxiolytic
         dependence[a,b,c]
305.40   Sedative, hypnotic, or anxiolytic
         abuse

Sedative-, Hypnotic-, or Anxiolytic-Induced Disorders
292.89   Sedative, hypnotic, or anxiolytic
         intoxication
292.0   Sedative, hypnotic, or anxiolytic
         withdrawal

Specify if: with perceptual disturbances

292.81	Sedative, hypnotic, or anxiolytic intoxication delirium
292.81	Sedative, hypnotic, or anxiolytic withdrawal delirium
292.82	Sedative-, hypnotic-, or anxiolytic-induced persisting dementia
292.83	Sedative-, hypnotic-, or anxiolytic-induced persisting amnestic disorder
292.xx	Sedative-, hypnotic-, or anxiolytic-induced psychotic disorder
.11	With delusions[I,W]
.12	With hallucinations[I,W]
292.84	Sedative-, hypnotic-, or anxiolytic-induced mood disorder[I,W]
292.89	Sedative-, hypnotic-, or anxiolytic-induced anxiety disorder[W]
292.89	Sedative-, hypnotic-, or anxiolytic-induced sexual dysfunction[I]
292.89	Sedative-, hypnotic-, or anxiolytic-induced sleep disorder[I,W]
292.9	Sedative-, hypnotic-, or anxiolytic-related disorder NOS

POLYSUBSTANCE-RELATED DISORDER

304.80	Polysubstance dependence[a,b,c,d]

OTHER (OR UNKNOWN) SUBSTANCE-RELATED DISORDERS

Other (or Unknown) Substance Use Disorders

304.90	Other (or unknown) substance dependence[a,b,c,d]
305.90	Other (or unknown) substance abuse

Other (or Unknown) Substance-Induced Disorders

292.89	Other (or unknown) substance intoxication
	Specify if: with perceptual disturbances
292.0	Other (or unknown) substance withdrawal
	Specify if: with perceptual disturbances
292.81	Other (or unknown) substance-induced delirium
292.82	Other (or unknown) substance-induced persisting dementia
292.83	Other (or unknown) substance-induced persisting amnestic disorder
292.xx	Other (or unknown) substance-induced psychotic disorder
.11	With delusions[I,W]
.12	With hallucinations[I,W]
292.84	Other (or unknown) substance-induced mood disorder[I,W]
292.89	Other (or unknown) substance-induced anxiety disorder[I,W]
292.89	Other (or unknown) substance-induced sexual dysfunction[I]
292.89	Other (or unknown) substance-induced sleep disorder[I,W]
292.9	Other (or unknown) substance-related disorder NOS

Schizophrenia and Other Psychotic Disorders

295.xx Schizophrenia

The following classification of longitudinal course applies to all subtypes of schizophrenia:

Episodic with interepisode residual symptoms (*specify if:* with prominent negative symptoms)/episodic with no interepisode residual symptoms

Continuous (*specify if:* with prominent negative symptoms)

Single episode in partial remission (*specify if:* with prominent negative symptoms)/single episode in full remission

Other or unspecified pattern	
.30	Paranoid type
.10	Disorganized type
.20	Catatonic type
.90	Undifferentiated type
.60	Residual type
295.40	Schizophreniform disorder
	Specify if: without good prognostic features/with good prognostic features
295.70	Schizoaffective disorder
	Specify if: bipolar type/depressive type
297.1	Delusional disorder
	Specify if: erotomanic type/grandiose type/jealous type/persecutory type/somatic type/mixed type/unspecified type

298.8	Brief psychotic disorder	

298.8 Brief psychotic disorder
Specify if: with marked stressor(s)/without marked stressor(s)/with postpartum onset

297.3 Shared psychotic disorder

293.xx Psychotic disorder due to . . . *[indicate the general medical condition]*

   .81   With delusions

   .82   With hallucinations

——.— Substance-induced psychotic disorder (*refer to Substance-Related Disorders for substance-specific codes*)
Specify if: with onset during intoxication/with onset during withdrawal

298.9 Psychotic Disorder NOS

Mood Disorders
Code current state of major depressive disorder or bipolar I disorder in fifth digit:

1 = Mild

2 = Moderate

3 = Severe without psychotic features

4 = Severe with psychotic features
Specify: mood-congruent psychotic features/mood-incongruent psychotic features

5 = In partial remission

6 = In full remission

0 = Unspecified

The following specifiers apply (for current or most recent episode) to mood disorders as noted:

  [a]Severity/psychotic/remission specifiers/ [b]Chronic/[c]With catatonic features/[d]With melancholic features/[e]With atypical features/[f]With postpartum onset

The following specifiers apply to mood disorders as noted:

  [g]With or without full interepisode recovery/ [h]With seasonal pattern/[i]With rapid cycling

DEPRESSIVE DISORDERS
296.xx Major depressive disorder

   .2x   Single episode[a,b,c,d,e,f]

   .3x   Recurrent[a,b,c,d,e,f,g,h]

300.4 Dysthymic disorder
Specify if: early onset/late onset
Specify if: with atypical features

311 Depressive disorder NOS

BIPOLAR DISORDERS
296.xx Bipolar I disorder

   .0x   Single manic episode[a,c,f]
Specify if: mixed

   .40   Most recent episode hypomanic[g,h,i]

   .4x   Most recent episode manic[a,c,f,g,h,i]

   .6x   Most recent episode mixed[a,c,f,g,h,i]

   .5x   Most recent episode depressed[a,b,c,d,e,f,g,h,i]

   .7   Most recent episode unspecified[g,h,i]

296.89 Bipolar II disorder[a,b,c,d,e,f,g,h,i]
Specify (current or most recent episode): hypomanic/depressed

301.13 Cyclothymic disorder

296.80 Bipolar disorder NOS

293.83 Mood disorder due to . . . *[indicate the general/medical condition]*
Specify type: with depressive features/with major depressive-like episode/with manic features/with mixed features

——.— Substance-induced mood disorder (*refer to Substance-Related Disorders for substance-specific codes*)
Specify type: with depressive features/with manic features/with mixed features
Specify if: with onset during intoxication/with onset during withdrawal

296.90 Mood disorder NOS

Anxiety Disorders

300.01 Panic disorder without agoraphobia

300.21 Panic disorder with agoraphobia

300.22 Agoraphobia without history of panic disorder

300.29 Specific phobia
Specify type: animal type/natural environment type/blood-injection-injury type/situational type/other type

300.23 Social phobia
Specify if: generalized

300.3 Obsessive-compulsive disorder
Specify if: with poor insight

309.81 Posttraumatic stress disorder
Specify if: acute/chronic
Specify if: with delayed onset

308.3 Acute stress disorder

300.02 Generalized anxiety disorder

293.84 Anxiety disorder due to . . . *[Indicate the general medical condition]*
Specify if: with generalized anxiety/with panic attacks/with obsessive-compulsive symptoms

——.— Substance-induced anxiety disorder (refer to Substance-Related Disorders for substance-specific codes)

Specify if: with generalized anxiety/with panic attacks/with obsessive-compulsive symptoms/with phobic symptoms
Specify if: with onset during intoxication/with onset during withdrawal

300.00   Anxiety disorder NOS

Somatoform Disorders

300.81   Somatization disorder
300.82   Undifferentiated somatoform disorder
300.11   Conversion disorder
          Specify type: with motor symptom or deficit/with sensory symptom or deficit/with seizures or convulsions/with mixed presentation
307.xx   Pain disorder
     .80   Associated with psychological factors
     .89   Associated with both psychological factors and a general medical condition
          Specify if: acute/chronic
300.7   Hypochondriasis
          Specify if: with poor insight
300.7   Body dysmorphic disorder
300.82   Somatoform disorder NOS

Factitious Disorders

300.xx   Factitious disorder
     .16   With predominantly psychological signs and symptoms
     .19   With predominantly physical signs and symptoms
     .19   With combined psychological and physical signs and symptoms
300.19   Factitious disorder NOS

Dissociative Disorders

300.12   Dissociative amnesia
300.13   Dissociative fugue
300.14   Dissociative identity disorder
300.6   Depersonalization disorder
300.15   Dissociative disorder NOS

Sexual and Gender Identity Disorders

SEXUAL DYSFUNCTIONS
The following specifiers apply to all primary sexual dysfunctions:
    Lifelong type/acquired type
    Generalized type/situational type

Due to psychological factors/due to combined factors

Sexual Desire Disorders
302.71   Hypoactive sexual desire disorder
302.79   Sexual aversion disorder

Sexual Arousal Disorders
302.72   Female sexual arousal disorder
302.72   Male erectile disorder

Orgasmic Disorders
302.73   Female orgasmic disorder
302.74   Male orgasmic disorder
302.75   Premature ejaculation

Sexual Pain Disorders
302.76   Dyspareunia (not due to a general medical condition)
306.51   Vaginismus (not due to a general medical condition)

Sexual Dysfunction Due to a General Medical Condition
625.8   Female hypoactive sexual desire disorder due to . . . *[indicate the general/medical condition]*
608.89   Male hypoactive sexual desire disorder due to . . . *[indicate the general medical condition]*
607.84   Male erectile disorder due to . . . *[indicate the general medical condition]*
625.0   Female dyspareunia due to . . . *[indicate the general/ medical condition]*
608.89   Male dyspareunia due to . . . *[indicate the general medical condition]*
625.8   Other female sexual dysfunction due to . . . *[indicate the general medical condition]*
608.89   Other male sexual dysfunction due to . . . *[indicate the general medical condition]*
——.—   Substance-induced sexual dysfunction *(refer to Substance-Related Disorders for substance-specific codes)*
          Specify if: with impaired desire/with impaired arousal/with impaired orgasm/with sexual pain
          Specify if: with onset during intoxication
302.70   Sexual dysfunction NOS

PARAPHILIAS
302.4   Exhibitionism
302.81   Fetishism

302.89	Frotteurism
302.2	Pedophilia
	Specify if: sexually attracted to males/sexually attracted to females/sexually attracted to both
	Specify if: limited to incest
	Specify type: exclusive type/nonexclusive type
302.83	Sexual masochism
302.84	Sexual sadism
302.3	Transvestic fetishism
	Specify if: with gender dysphoria
302.82	Voyeurism
302.9	Paraphilia NOS

GENDER IDENTITY DISORDERS

302.xx	Gender identity disorder
.6	in children
.85	in adolescents or adults
	Specify if: sexually attracted to males/sexually attracted to females/sexually attracted to both/sexually attracted to neither
302.6	Gender identity disorder NOS
302.9	Sexual disorder NOS

Eating Disorders

307.1	Anorexia nervosa
	Specify type: restricting type; binge-eating/purging type
307.51	Bulimia nervosa
	Specify type: Purging type/nonpurging type
307.50	Eating disorder NOS

Sleep Disorders

PRIMARY SLEEP DISORDERS

Dyssomnias

307.42	Primary insomnia
307.44	Primary hypersomnia
	Specify if: recurrent
347	Narcolepsy
780.59	Breathing-related sleep disorder
307.45	Circadian rhythm sleep disorder
	Specify type: delayed sleep phase type/jet lag type/shift work type/unspecified type
307.47	Dyssomnia NOS

Parasomnias

307.47	Nightmare disorder
307.46	Sleep terror disorder
307.46	Sleepwalking disorder
307.47	Parasomnia NOS

SLEEP DISORDERS RELATED TO ANOTHER MENTAL DISORDER

307.42	Insomnia related to ... *[indicate the Axis I or Axis II disorder]*
307.44	Hypersomnia related to ... *[indicate the Axis I or Axis II disorder]*

OTHER SLEEP DISORDERS

780.xx	Sleep disorder due to ... *[indicate the general medical condition]*
.52	Insomnia type
.54	Hypersomnia type
.59	Parasomnia type
.59	Mixed type
——.—	Substance-induced sleep disorder *(refer to Substance-Related Disorders for substance-specific codes)*
	Specify type: insomnia type/hypersomnia type/parasomnia type/mixed type
	Specify if: with onset during intoxication/with onset during withdrawal

---

Impulse-Control Disorders Not Elsewhere Classified

312.34	Intermittent explosive disorder
312.32	Kleptomania
312.33	Pyromania
312.31	Pathological gambling
312.39	Trichotillomania
312.30	Impulse-control disorder NOS

Adjustment Disorders

309.xx	Adjustment disorder
.0	With depressed mood
.24	With anxiety
.28	With mixed anxiety and depressed mood
.3	With disturbance of conduct
.4	With mixed disturbance of emotions and conduct
.9	Unspecified
	Specify if: acute/chronic

Personality Disorders

Note: *These are coded-on Axis II.*

301.0	Paranoid personality disorder
301.20	Schizoid personality disorder
301.22	Schizotypal personality disorder
301.7	Antisocial personality disorder
301.83	Borderline personality disorder
301.50	Histrionic personality disorder
301.81	Narcissistic personality disorder
301.82	Avoidant personality disorder

301.6	Dependent personality disorder
301.4	Obsessive-compulsive personality disorder
301.9	Personality disorder NOS

Other Conditions That May Be a Focus of Clinical Attention

PSYCHOLOGICAL FACTORS AFFECTING MEDICAL CONDITION

316 ... *[specified psychological factor] affecting ... [indicate the general medical condition] Choose name based on nature of factors:*

Mental disorder affecting medical condition

Psychological symptoms affecting medical condition

Personality traits or coping style affecting medical condition

Maladaptive health behaviors affecting medical condition

Stress-related physiologic response affecting medical condition

Other or unspecified psychological factors affecting medical condition

MEDICATION-INDUCED MOVEMENT DISORDERS

332.1	Neuroleptic-induced parkinsonism
333.92	Neuroleptic-malignant syndrome
333.7	Neuroleptic-induced acute dystonia
333.99	Neuroleptic-induced acute akathisia
333.82	Neuroleptic-induced tardive dyskinesia
333.1	Medication-induced postural tremor
333.90	Medication-induced movement disorder NOS

OTHER MEDICATION-INDUCED DISORDER

995.2	Adverse effects of medication NOS

RELATIONAL PROBLEMS

V61.9	Relational problem related to a mental disorder or general medical condition
V61.20	Parent–child relational problem
V61.10	Partner relational problem
V61.8	Sibling relational problem
V62.81	Relational problem NOS

PROBLEMS RELATED TO ABUSE OR NEGLECT

V61.21	Physical abuse of child *(code 995.54 if focus of attention is on victim)*

V61.21	Sexual abuse of child *(code 995.53 if focus of attention is on victim)*
V61.21	Neglect of child *(code 995.52 if focus of attention is on victim)*
——.—	Physical abuse of adult
V61.12	(if by partner)
V62.83	(if by person other than partner) *(code 995.81 if focus of attention is on victim)*
——.—	Sexual abuse of adult
V61.12	(if by partner)
V62.83	(if by person other than partner) *(code 995.83 if focus of attention is on victim)*

ADDITIONAL CONDITIONS THAT MAY BE A FOCUS OF CLINICAL ATTENTION

V15.81	Noncompliance with treatment
V65.2	Malingering
V71.01	Adult antisocial behavior
V71.02	Child or adolescent antisocial behavior
V62.89	Borderline intellectual functioning **Note:** *This is coded on Axis II.*
780.9	Age-related cognitive decline
V62.82	Bereavement
V62.3	Academic problem
V62.2	Occupational problem
313.82	Identity problem
V62.89	Religious or spiritual problem
V62.4	Acculturation problem
V62.89	Phase-of-life problem

Additional Codes

300.9	Unspecified mental disorder (nonpsychotic)
V71.09	No diagnosis or condition on Axis I
799.9	Diagnosis or condition deferred on Axis II
V71.09	No diagnosis on Axis II
799.9	Diagnosis deferred on Axis II

Multiaxial System

Axis I	Clinical disorders Other conditions that may be a focus of clinical attention
Axis II	Personality disorders, Mental retardation
Axis III	General medical conditions
Axis IV	Psychosocial and environmental problems
Axis V	Global assessment of functioning

About the Authors

BENJAMIN JAMES SADOCK, M.D., is the Menas S. Gregory Professor of Psychiatry in the Department of Psychiatry at the New York University (NYU) School of Medicine. He is a graduate of Union College, received his M.D. degree from New York Medical College, and completed his internship at Albany Hospital. He completed his residency at Bellevue Psychiatric Hospital and then entered military service as a Captain in the United States Air force, where he served as Acting Chief of Neuropsychiatry at Sheppard Air Force Base in Texas. He has held faculty and teaching appointments at Southwestern Medical School and Parkland Hospital in Dallas and at New York Medical College, St. Luke's Hospital, the New York State Psychiatric Institute, and Metropolitan Hospital in New York City. Dr. Sadock joined the faculty of the NYU School of Medicine in 1980 and served in various positions: Director of Medical Student Education in Psychiatry, Co-Director of the Residency Training Program in Psychiatry, and Director of Graduate Medical Education. Currently, Dr. Sadock is Co-Director of Student Mental Health Services, Psychiatric Consultant to the Admissions Committee, and Co-Director of Continuing Education in Psychiatry at the NYU School of Medicine. He is on the staff of Bellevue Hospital and Tisch Hospital and is a Consulting Psychiatrist at Lenox Hill Hospital. Dr. Sadock is a Diplomate of the American Board of Psychiatry and Neurology and served as an Associate Examiner for the Board for more than a decade. He is a Distinguished Life Fellow of the American Psychiatric Association, a Fellow of the American College of Physicians, a Fellow of the New York Academy of Medicine, and a member of Alpha Omega Alpha Honor Society. He is active in numerous psychiatric organizations and was president and founder of the NYU-Bellevue Psychiatric Society. Dr. Sadock was a member of the National Committee in Continuing Education in Psychiatry of the American Psychiatric Association, served on the Ad Hoc Committee on Sex Therapy Clinics of the American Medical Association, was a Delegate to the Conference on Recertification of the American Board of Medical Specialists, and was a representative of the American Psychiatric Association Task Force on the National Board of Medical Examiners and the American Board of Psychiatry and Neurology. In 1985, he received the Academic Achievement Award from New York Medical College and was appointed Faculty Scholar at NYU School of Medicine in 2000. He is the author or editor of more than 100 publications (including 50 books), a reviewer for psychiatric journals, and lectures on a broad range of topics in general psychiatry. Dr. Sadock maintains a private practice for diagnostic consultations and psychiatric treatment. He has been married to Virginia Alcott Sadock, M.D., Professor of Psychiatry at NYU School of Medicine, since completing his residency. Dr. Sadock enjoys opera, golf, skiing, traveling, and is an enthusiastic fly fisherman.

VIRGINIA ALCOTT SADOCK, M.D., joined the faculty of the New York University (NYU) School of Medicine in 1980, where she is currently Professor of Psychiatry and Attending Psychiatrist at the Tisch Hospital and Bellevue

Hospital. She is Director of the Program in Human Sexuality at the NYU Langone Medical Center, one of the largest treatment and training programs of its kind in the United States. She is the author of more than 50 articles and chapters on sexual behavior and was the developmental editor of *The Sexual Experience*, one of the first major textbooks on human sexuality, published by Williams & Wilkins. She serves as a referee and book reviewer for several medical journals, including the *American Journal of Psychiatry* and the *Journal of the American Medical Association*. She has long been interested in the role of women in medicine and psychiatry and was a founder of the Committee on Women in Psychiatry of the New York County District Branch of the American Psychiatric Association. She is active in academic matters, served as an Assistant and Associate Examiner for the American Board of Psychiatry and Neurology for more than 20 years, and was also a member of the Test Committee in Psychiatry for both the American Board of Psychiatry and the Psychiatric Knowledge and Self-Assessment Program (PKSAP) of the American Psychiatric Association. She has chaired the Committee on Public Relations of the New York County District Branch of the American Psychiatric Association, has been a regional council member of the American Association of Sex Education Counselors and Therapists, a founding member of The Society of Sex Therapy and Research, and is President of the NYU Alumni Association of Sex Therapists. She has participated in the National Medical Television Network series *Women in Medicine* and the Emmy Award–winning PBS television documentary *Women and Depression* and currently hosts the radio program *Sexual Health and Well-being* (Sirius-XM) at NYU Langone Medical Center. She lectures extensively both in this country and abroad on sexual dysfunction, relational problems, and depression and anxiety disorders. She is a Distinguished Fellow of the American Psychiatric Association, a Fellow of the New York Academy of Medicine, and a Diplomate of the American Board of Psychiatry and Neurology. Dr. Sadock is a graduate of Bennington College, received her M.D. degree from New York Medical College, and trained in psychiatry at Metropolitan Hospital. She lives in Manhattan with her husband, Dr. Benjamin Sadock, where she maintains an active practice that includes individual psychotherapy, couples and marital therapy, sex therapy, psychiatric consultation, and pharmacotherapy. She and her husband have two children, James and Victoria, both emergency physicians, and two grandchildren, Emily and Celia. In her leisure time, Dr. Sadock enjoys theater, film, golf, reading fiction, and travel.